WORKBOOK IN PRACTICAL NEONATOLOGY

FIFTH EDITION

WORKBOOK IN PRACTICAL NEONATOLOGY

FIFTH EDITION

Richard A. Polin, MD

William T. Speck Professor of Pediatrics
College of Physicians and Surgeons
Columbia University
Director, Division of Neonatology
Morgan Stanley Children's Hospital of New York–Presbyterian
New York, New York

Mervin C. Yoder, MD

Distinguished Professor and Richard and Pauline Klingler Professor of Pediatrics
Assistant Dean for Entrepreneurial Research and Associate Director for
   Entrepreneurship for Indiana Clinical and Translational Sciences Institute
Indiana University School of Medicine
Associate Chair for Basic Research
Attending Neonatologist
Riley Hospital for Children
Indianapolis, Indiana

ELSEVIER
SAUNDERS

ELSEVIER
SAUNDERS

1600 John F. Kennedy Blvd.
Ste 1800
Philadelphia, PA 19103-2899

WORKBOOK IN PRACTICAL NEONATOLOGY   ISBN: 978-1-4557-7484-5

Notices

Knowledge and best practice in this field are constantly changing. As new research and experience broaden our understanding, changes in research methods, professional practices, or medical treatment may become necessary.

Practitioners and researchers must always rely on their own experience and knowledge in evaluating and using any information, methods, compounds, or experiments described herein. In using such information or methods they should be mindful of their own safety and the safety of others, including parties for whom they have a professional responsibility.

With respect to any drug or pharmaceutical products identified, readers are advised to check the most current information provided (i) on procedures featured or (ii) by the manufacturer of each product to be administered, to verify the recommended dose or formula, the method and duration of administration, and contraindications. It is the responsibility of practitioners, relying on their own experience and knowledge of their patients, to make diagnoses, to determine dosages and the best treatment for each individual patient, and to take all appropriate safety precautions.

To the fullest extent of the law, neither the Publisher nor the authors, contributors, or editors assume any liability for any injury and/or damage to persons or property as a matter of products liability, negligence or otherwise, or from any use or operation of any methods, products, instructions, or ideas contained in the material herein.

Library of Congress Cataloging-in-Publication Data

Workbook in practical neonatology / [edited by] Richard A. Polin, Mervin C. Yoder. -- Fifth edition.
     p. ; cm.
Includes bibliographical references.
ISBN 978-1-4557-7484-5 (alk. paper)
I. Polin, Richard A. (Richard Alan), 1945- editor. II. Yoder, Mervin C., editor.
[DNLM: 1. Infant, Newborn, Diseases--Programmed Instruction. WS 18.2]
RJ254
618.92'01--dc23

                                                                          2014014816

Senior Content Strategist: Kate Dimock
Content Development Specialist: Katy Meert
Publishing Services Manager: Jeff Patterson
Project Manager: Clay S. Broeker
Design Direction: Ellen Zanolle

Printed in China

Last digit is the print number: 9 8 7 6 5 4 3 2 1

CONTRIBUTORS

David H. Adamkin, MD
Professor of Pediatrics
Director of Division of Neonatology and
  Nutritional Research
Rounsavall Chair of Neonatal Medicine
Co-Director of Neonatal Fellowship
University of Louisville
Louisville, Kentucky
  Glucose Metabolism

Catalina Bazacliu, MD
Assistant Professor of Pediatrics
Georgia Regents University
Children's Hospital of Georgia
Augusta, Georgia
  Parenteral Nutrition

William E. Benitz, MD
Philip Sunshine Professor of Neonataoloy
Chief, Division of Neonatal and Developmental
  Medicine
Pediatrics, Stanford University School of
  Medicine
Stanford, California
Director of Nurseries and Chief of
  Neonatology
Lucile Packard Children's Hospital
Palo Alto, California
  Patent Ductus Arteriosus

Jatinder J.S. Bhatia, MD, FAAP
Professor of Pediatrics
Georgia Regents University
Children's Hospital of Georgia
Augusta, Georgia
  Parenteral Nutrition

Waldemar A. Carlo, MD
Edwin M. Dixon Professor of Pediatrics
University of Alabama at Birmingham
Physician, Department of Pediatrics
Children's of Alabama
Birmingham, Alabama
  Respiratory Distress Syndrome

Michael G. Caty, MD, MMM
Robert Pritzer Professor of Pediatric Surgery
  and Chief
Section of Pediatric Surgery
Yale University School of Medicine
Surgeon-in-Chief
Yale-New Haven Children's Hospital
New Haven, Connecticut
  Surgical Emergencies in the Newborn

Robert A. Cowles, MD
Associate Professor, Section of Pediatric
  Surgery
Yale School of Medicine
Attending, Department of Surgery
Yale-New Haven Children's Hospital
New Haven, Connecticut
  Surgical Emergencies in the Newborn

Alain Cuna, MD
Assistant Professor of Pediatrics
University of Missouri-Kansas City School
  of Medicine
Children's Mercy Hospitals and Clinics
Kansas City, Missouri
  Respiratory Distress Syndrome

Steven M. Donn, MD
Professor of Pediatrics
University Michigan Health System
Division of Neonatal-Perinatal Medicine,
  Pediatrics
C. S. Mott Children's Hospital
Ann Arbor, Michigan
  Principles of Mechanical Ventilation

Gabriel J. Escobar, MD
Regional Director for Hospital Operations
  Research, Kaiser Permanente Northern
  California
Research Scientist III, Kaiser Permanente
  Division of Research
Attending Physician, Department of Inpatient
  Pediatrics
Kaiser Permanente Walnut Creek Medical Center
Kaiser Permanente Antioch Medical Center
Walnut Creek, California
  Neonatal Sepsis

Cathy Hammerman, MD
Professor of Pediatrics
Hebrew University
Director, Newborn Nurseries
Shaare Zedek Medical Center
Jerusalem, Israel
Neonatal Hyperbilirubinemia

Elie G. Abu Jawdeh, MD
Assistant Professor of Pediatrics
Neonatal-Perinatal Medicine, Department
 of Pediatrics
Kentucky Children's Hospital
University of Kentucky
Lexington, Kentucky
Neonatal Apnea

Ben-Hur Johnson, MD
Assistant Professor of Pediatrics
University of Ottawa
Clinical Associate, Division of Neonatology
The Children's Hospital of Eastern Ontario
 and The Ottawa Hospital General Campus
Ottawa, Ontario, Canada
Bronchopulmonary Dysplasia

Michael Kaplan, MBChB
Professor of Pediatrics
Hebrew University
Director Emeritus, Department of Neonatology
Shaare Zedek Medical Center
Jerusalem, Israel
Neonatal Hyperbilirubinemia

Ganga Krishnamurthy, MBBS
Assistant Professor of Pediatrics
Columbia University Medical Center
Director, Neonatal Cardiac Care
Morgan Stanley Children's Hospital of New
 York-Presbyterian
New York, New York
Congenital Heart Disease in the Newborn Period

Satyan Lakshminrusimha, MD
Professor of Pediatrics
Chief, Division of Neonatology
Director, Center for Developmental Biology of
 the Lung
University at Buffalo
The Women and Children's Hospital of Buffalo
Buffalo, New York
*Persistent Pulmonary Hypertension of the
Newborn and Hypoxemic Respiratory Failure*

Tina A. Leone, MD
Assistant Professor of Pediatrics at CUMC
Pediatrics, Neonatology
Columbia University College of Physicians and
 Surgeons
Attending Neonatologist
Morgan Stanley Children's Hospital - New
 York Presbyterian
New York, New York
Neonatal Resuscitation

Stéphanie Levasseur, MD, FRCPC
Assistant Professor of Pediatrics
Director, Fetal Cardiology
Columbia University Medical Center
Morgan Stanley Children's Hospital of New
 York-Presbyterian
New York, New York
Congenital Heart Disease in the Newborn Period

Fangming Lin, MD, PhD
Associate Professor of Pediatrics
Columbia University College of Physicians and
 Surgeons
Morgan Stanley Children's Hospital
New York, New York
Renal Failure in Neonates

John M. Lorenz, MD
Professor of Pediatrics
Columbia University
Attending Neonatologist
Morgan Stanley Children's Hospital of New
 York-Presbyterian
New York, New York
*Fluid and Electrolyte Management in the
Newborn Intensive Care Unit*

Camilia R. Martin, MD, MS
Assistant Professor of Pediatrics
Harvard Medical School
Associate Director, NICU
Beth Israel Deaconess Medical Center
Boston, Massachusetts
Enteral Nutrition

Richard J. Martin, MD
Professor of Pediatrics, Reproductive Biology,
 and Physiology & Biophysics
Case Western Reserve University
Drusinsky/Fanaroff Professor
Division of Neonatology
Rainbow Babies and Children's Hospital
Cleveland, Ohio
Neonatal Apnea

Bobby Mathew, MBBS
Assistant Professor of Pediatrics
University of Buffalo
Attending Neonatologist, Associate Director
  Neonatal Perinatal Medicine Fellowship
  Program
The Women & Children's Hospital of Buffalo
Buffalo, New York
  Persistent Pulmonary Hypertension of the New-
  born and Hypoxemic Respiratory Failure

Josef Neu, MD
Professor of Pediatrics, Division of
  Neonatology
University of Florida College of Medicine
Gainesville, Florida
  Necrotizing Enterocolitis

Shahab Noori, MD
Associate Professor of Pediatrics
Keck School of Medicine of the Univer-
  sity of Southern California, Attending
  Neonatologist
Children's Hospital Los Angeles and the
  LAC+USC Medical Center
Los Angeles, California
  Neonatal Hypotension

Robin Kjerstin Ohls, MD
Professor of Pediatrics
University of New Mexico
Albuquerque, New Mexico
  Anemia

Eric B. Ortigoza, MD, MSCR
Neonatal-Perinatal Fellow
Department of Pediatrics, Division of
  Neonatology
University of Florida College of Medicine
Gainesville, Florida
  Necrotizing Enterocolitis

Jeffrey M. Perlman, MB, ChB
Professor of Pediatrics
Weill Cornell Medical College
Division Chief, Newborn Medicine
New York Presbyterian Hospital
Komansky Center for Children's Health
New York, New York
  Perinatal Asphyxia

Brenda B. Poindexter, MD, MS
Professor of Pediatrics
Section of Neonatal-Perinatal Medicine
Indiana University School of Medicine
Riley Hospital for Children at IU Health
Indianapolis, Indiana
  Enteral Nutrition

Karen M. Puopolo, MD, PhD
Associate Professor of Clinical Pediatrics
University of Pennsylvania Perelman School
  of Medicine
Chief, Section on Newborn Pediatrics
The Children's Hospital of Philadelphia
  Newborn Care at Pennsylvania Hospital
Philadelphia, Pennsylvania
  Neonatal Sepsis

Matthew A. Rainaldi, MD
Assistant Professor of Pediatrics
Division of Newborn Medicine
Weill Cornell Medical College, New York
  Presbyterian Hospital
Komansky Center for Children's Health
New York, New York
  Perinatal Asphyxia

Veniamin Ratner, MD
Assistant Professor of Pediatrics
Columbia University Medical Center
Neonatologist
Morgan Stanley Children's Hospital of New
  York-Presbyterian
New York, New York
  Congenital Heart Disease in the Newborn Period

Kimberly J. Reidy, MD
Assistant Research Professor of Pediatrics/
  Nephrology
Albert Einstein College of Medicine
Children's Hospital at Montefiore
Bronx, New York
  Renal Failure in Neonates

Ana Paula D. Ribeiro, MD
Neonatal-Perinatal Medicine Fellow
Department of Pediatrics, Rainbow Babies and
  Children's Hospital
Case Western Reserve University
Cleveland, Ohio
  Neonatal Apnea

S. David Rubenstein, MD
Professor of Pediatrics
Columbia University Medical Center
Director, Neonatal Intensive Care Unit
Morgan Stanley Children's Hospital of New
  York-Presbyterian
Director, Fellowship Training Program in
  Neonatal-Perinatal Medicine
New York Presbyterian Hospital, Columbia
  Campus
New York, New York
  Congenital Heart Disease in the Newborn Period

Istvan Seri, MD, PhD
Professor of Pediatrics
Keck School of Medicine of the University of
    Southern California
Director, Center for Fetal and Neonatal
    Medicine and Chief of Neonatal Medicine
Children's Hospital Los Angeles and the
    LAC+USC Medical Center
Los Angeles, California
    Neonatal Hypotension

Renée A. Shellhaas, MD, MS
Associate Professor
Pediatrics & Communicable Diseases (Division
    of Pediatric Neurology)
University of Michigan
Ann Arbor, Michigan
    Neonatal Seizures

Sunil K. Sinha, MD, PhD
Professor of Paediatrics and Neonatal Medicine
University of Durham
Stockton, United Kingdom
Consultant Paediatrician and Neonatologist
Directorate of Neonatology
The James Cook University Hospital
Middlesbrough, United Kingdom
    Principles of Mechanical Ventilation

Bernard Thébaud, MD, PhD
Professor of Pediatrics and Partnership
    Research Chair in Regenerative Medicine
University of Ottawa
Senior Scientist, Regenerative Medicine
    Program
Ottawa Hospital Research Institute
Neonatologist
Children's Hospital of Eastern Ontario
Ottawa, Ontario, Canada
    Bronchopulmonary Dysplasia

Andrew Whitelaw, MD, FRCPCH
Professor of Neonatal Medicine, School of
    Clinical Sciences
University of Bristol, Honorary Consultant
    Neonatologist, Neonatal Intensive Care Unit
Southmead Hospital
Bristol, United Kingdom
    Intraventricular Hemorrhage

Tai-Wei Wu, MD
Visiting Staff Physician
Division of Neonatal Medicine
Chang Gung Memorial Hospital
Chang Gung University
Linkou, Taiwan
    Neonatal Hypotension

Calvin J. Young, MD
Research Fellow, Department of Surgery
Yale School of Medicine
Resident, Department of Surgery
Yale-New Haven Hospital
New Haven, Connecticut
    Surgical Emergencies in the Newborn

PREFACE

This is the fifth edition of *Workbook in Practical Neonatology*. The original idea for the *Workbook* arose from an article that appeared in *Pediatrics in Review* more than 30 years ago on necrotizing enterocolitis. The interactive nature of that article was the inspiration of Dr. Frederick Burg (a prior editor), who wanted to create something that was fun and educational for the readership. The current edition of *Workbook in Practical Neonatology* continues that philosophy. Each chapter is centered on case histories in which the reader is asked to make management decisions. True-to-life clinical scenarios are chosen to involve the reader in the care of the babies described in each chapter. We still believe that providing active learning is a better way to promote reader comprehension than presenting concepts in a strictly didactic fashion.

For this edition, nearly every chapter has a new set of authors. We changed the authorship to get different perspectives on the management of critically ill infants. Much of the care we provide in the neonatal intensive care unit is more art than science. The *Workbook* authors were chosen for their expertise and their recognition as experts. We asked each of them to provide the latest evidence-based treatments; however, they also bring to the readership years of clinical experience caring for sick newborn infants. They were challenged to provide a comprehensive "state-of-the-art" review that used actual cases from their own nurseries. We hope that the reader of this book will take away as much about the style of teaching as about the book's content. The interactive, case-oriented format is as readily adaptable to bedside teaching as it is lecturing to large audiences. We also hope that this book will serve as an example that education (even about serious topics) can be delivered in an interesting fashion.

There are several individuals to whom we owe thanks. These include the phenomenal group of contributors who have provided us with well-written, informative, and absorbing chapters; Katy Meert and the staff at Elsevier; and Heidi Kleinbart for her technical, editorial, and organizational help. Most importantly, we would like to thank the great teachers of our past who taught us the importance of being effective and entertaining teachers.

SPECIAL DEDICATION

During the preparation of the fourth edition of the Workbook in Practical Neonatology, Dr. Frederic Burg passed away at the young age of 66. Fred had a distinguished academic career at the University of Pennsylvania and the University of Alabama. He was instrumental in the development of the first edition of the *Workbook* and served as a co-editor for three subsequent editions. Fred was a remarkable human being who genuinely cared about the health and welfare of children. He brought that caring and enthusiasm to every part of his professional life. The world has lost a wonderful pediatrician and an advocate for children—and we have lost a good friend. He will be remembered by all of us who worked with him.

Richard A. Polin
Mervin C. Yoder

CONTENTS

VIDEO CONTENTS

CHAPTER 1

NEONATAL RESUSCITATION

Tina A. Leone, MD

At the time of birth all infants undergo extensive physiologic changes in order to adapt to life outside of the uterus. Though most infants make this transition without a significant amount of assistance from caregivers, some infants do need assistance. The most commonly used interventions performed during the first several minutes of life help to facilitate the transition that is occurring naturally. However, more significant resuscitation is necessary when the infant does not initiate adequate spontaneous breathing or cannot maintain sufficient systemic perfusion. Though resuscitation practices are clearly important, measuring the actual impact of resuscitation on outcome is fairly difficult. Perhaps the best example of the importance of resuscitation interventions comes from recent experiences in limited-resource settings once resuscitation programs have been introduced. The introduction of neonatal resuscitation training to different limited-resource settings has decreased the stillbirth rate in those areas, suggesting that trained individuals are more likely to properly assess and respond to an infant who is not breathing and crying at birth (Goudar, 2013; Msemo, 2013).

The science of resuscitation is reviewed every 5 years by the International Liaison Committee on Resuscitation (ILCOR) leading to recommendations for evidence-based resuscitation interventions in each discipline (Perlman, 2010). Many national and international groups make recommendations based on the ILCOR review that are often similar to each other but not always identical. These recommendations are often used as the basis for training programs. In the United States the Neonatal Resuscitation Program (NRP), which was developed by the American Academy of Pediatrics and the American Heart Association, publishes a curriculum and resuscitation algorithm (Figure 1-1) that is used by most institutions as the basis for neonatal resuscitation training (Kattwinkel, 2011).

OVERVIEW OF NORMAL TRANSITIONAL PHYSIOLOGY

The unique aspects of neonatal resuscitation are based on the changing physiology of the fetal to neonatal transition, the most important characteristic of which is the change from placental to pulmonary gas exchange. The most frequent cause of physiologic instability after birth is inadequate breathing or ventilation. One striking difference between newborn resuscitation and other forms of resuscitation is the physiologic state of the lung as it transitions between fetal and newborn life. In fetal life the lungs are filled with fluid and the majority of the cardiac output bypasses the lungs in order to reach the placenta, where gas exchange takes place. Prior to birth at term gestation the amount of lung fluid begins to decrease. Further resorption of lung fluid takes place during labor and delivery, but most of the remaining lung fluid is cleared once the newborn infant takes the first breaths after birth. When an infant requires assisted ventilation the presence of fetal lung fluid must be anticipated in order to provide adequate ventilation. Understanding the normal process of fetal to neonatal transition allows the clinician to recognize deviations from normal and to facilitate resuscitation in a manner that will approximate the normal process as much as possible.

The basic principles of newborn resuscitation as currently practiced were based on studies of newborn animals that were asphyxiated by having their faces covered after birth (Dawes, 1968). The response of the animals was to have an initial period of apnea, which was called primary apnea, followed by a period of gasping breathing movements and finally, secondary apnea. Decreases in the heart rate followed by the blood pressure were noted with the occurrence of apnea. These changes also correlated with neonatal acidemia. In the human fetus, placental insufficiency or impaired fetal blood flow can be caused by a number of factors leading to fetal acidemia and perinatal depression.

BASIC TRANSITIONAL INTERVENTIONS FOR ALL NEWBORN INFANTS

There has been much debate in recent years over the appropriate timing of cord clamping. Immediate cord clamping became typical obstetric

Newborn Resuscitation

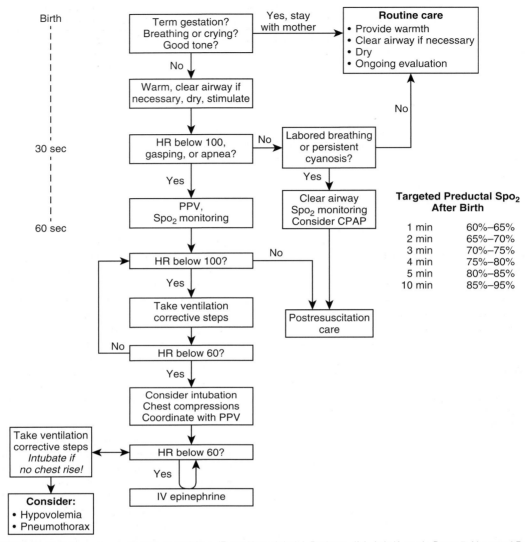

FIGURE 1-1 ■ **Newborn resuscitation algorithm.** (From Kattwinkel J, Perlman JM, Aziz K, et al.: Part 15: Neonatal Resuscitation 2010 American Heart Association guidelines for cardiopulmonary resuscitation and emergency cardiovascular care. *Circulation* 122:S909-919, 2010.)

practice as active management for prevention of postpartum hemorrhage. However, if the cord is clamped immediately, approximately 30% of the infant's blood volume remains in the placenta instead of approximately 10 ml/kg being transferred into the infant as the baby begins breathing and the uterus begins contracting. In preterm infants, delayed cord clamping for 30 to 60 seconds after birth has been shown to improve the cardiovascular transition and decrease the incidence of intraventricular hemorrhage. This practice is now recommended by the American College of Obstetrics and Gynecology (ACOG) for preterm infants. The recommendation was not made by

ACOG for term infants because there was not as significant a benefit in this population (Committee on Obstetric Practice, ACOG, 2012).

Before birth the temperature of the fetus is rigidly controlled approximately 0.5° C greater than the mother's temperature. After birth the newborn infant's temperature falls; a significant amount of heat is lost to the environment as cooler air moves around the infant (convection), fluid evaporates from the skin (evaporation), and the infant contacts cold items (conduction). Therefore, it is fairly common practice to place the infant after birth on the mother's chest or abdomen. The skin-to-skin contact with

TABLE 1-1	Risk Factors for Need for Resuscitation at Birth		
Maternal Factors	**Fetal Factors**		**Placental Factors**
Diabetes mellitus	Intrauterine growth restriction		Placenta previa
Preeclampsia	Known fetal anomalies		Placenta accreta
Chronic illness	Multiple gestation		Vasa previa
Poor prenatal care	Hydrops fetalis		Placental abruption
Substance Abuse	Oligohydramnios		
Uterine rupture	Polyhydramnios		
General anesthesia	Preterm birth		
Chorioamnionitis	Premature rupture of membranes		
	Fetal distress as indicated by fetal heart rate monitoring or tests of fetal well being		
	Breech presentation		
	Decreased fetal movement		

the mother helps to maintain the infant's body temperature. When the infant requires more interventions for stabilization, a radiant warmer is used to help maintain adequate body temperature. If the environment is not considered carefully the baby can become hypothermic after birth, leading to physiologic instability.

In the past it was routine to suction the mouth and nose of all infants after birth. However, this may not be necessary in all infants and suctioning can be associated with adverse effects including trauma and reflex bradycardia. Therefore, it is now recommended that suctioning be performed only in select cases when excessive fluid is noted to be present and obstructing the airway.

PREPARATION FOR RESUSCITATION

Individuals who care for newborn infants must anticipate problems with the transition from fetal to newborn life and respond to such problems quickly. Though most newborn infants will have no problem at the time of birth, it is essential that clinicians are able to provide assistance when needed. Identification of the infants most likely to need resuscitation is critical to providing adequate newborn resuscitation support. This allows the birth to occur in an area where help can be obtained quickly and equipment can be prepared ahead of time. Preparation may be the most important aspect of running a smooth resuscitation. Obtaining the history from the obstetrician is essential to determining the likelihood for needing resuscitation. It is best for the resuscitation team to discuss the intervention plans prior to the infant's birth. Tasks can be preassigned so that there is less chance for confusion during the actual resuscitation.

When considering which infants are likely to need resuscitation, it is helpful to consider the underlying causes that interfere with the normal transitional processes. Failure to initiate spontaneous breathing can result from perinatal depression associated with fetal acidemia or medications that cause respiratory depression. The infant can start breathing but have difficulty achieving adequate gas exchange owing to prematurity, perinatal illnesses, or a variety of congenital malformations. Table 1-1 lists the most important risk factors that predispose the infant to require neonatal resuscitation. Two of the factors that represent the greatest risk for resuscitation are preterm birth and delivery by emergency cesarean section (Aziz, 2008).

Immediately before an infant at high risk for needing resuscitation is born, it is important to assemble the appropriate personnel, discuss the plan for resuscitation, and ensure that all equipment is readily available and working. The suction and air flow to ventilation devices should be turned on and ready to use. The radiant warmer should be on and heat output increased to full power. A skin temperature servo-probe should be available to place on the infant if the infant will stay in that warmer for more than 10 minutes. As a safety precaution, radiant warmers are set to significantly decrease the heat output if left on full power for 15 minutes. Therefore, if the delivery is delayed the radiant warmer may need to be switched back to full power.

TEMPERATURE MANAGEMENT

Full-term infants who are expected to require resuscitation should be dried initially; wet towels should be discarded and the infant should be nursed under the radiant warmer using servo-control as discussed above. A hat should be placed on the infant's head to minimize heat loss from the large surface area of the scalp.

Temperature management of preterm infants is particularly important. Admission temperatures of extremely preterm infants are frequently in the hypothermic range and lower admission temperatures are associated with increased mortality. Covering the baby with plastic immediately after delivery has been shown consistently to increase admission temperatures in preterm infants (McCall, 2010; Vohra, 1999). This practice involves placing the body, excluding the head, in plastic wrap or a plastic bag without drying the baby (Figure 1-2). The plastic prevents evaporation and decreases heat loss from convective air movement around the baby. The head should be dried and can be covered with a hat. Other measures to increase body temperature of the preterm infant include maintaining the ambient temperature in the resuscitation room at least at 25° C and using a modern radiant warmer. A chemical heating pad or exothermic mattress that creates heat when activated can also be used to increase body temperature of extremely preterm infants. The infant's temperature should be monitored periodically during the first 30 minutes of life and hyperthermia should be avoided as well as hypothermia. Hyperthermia has been reported when multiple methods of increasing the infant's temperature are used together (McCarthy, 2013).

CASE STUDY 1

You are called urgently to a labor and delivery room for an infant who has recently been delivered and has not started crying. You and a neonatal intensive care unit (NICU) nurse rush in to assess the baby. When you arrive, the labor and delivery nurse has given stimulation and dried the infant. She has just started to put the facemask over the infant's mouth and nose to begin positive pressure ventilation (PPV). You take over the PPV and ask the NICU nurse for help.

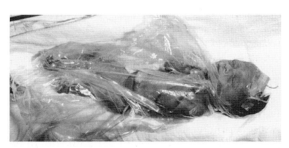

FIGURE 1-2 ■ Premature infant in polyethylene bag wrap. (From Vohra S, Frent G, Campbell V, et al.: Effect of polyethylene occlusive skin wrapping on heat loss in very low birth weight infants at delivery: a randomized trial. *J Pediatr* 134:547-551, 1999.)

EXERCISE 1

QUESTIONS

1. What is the first thing you ask the NICU nurse to do?

2. What else should you check as you make an initial scan of the resuscitation area?

3. What additional information would you want to obtain from the obstetric staff?

ANSWERS

1. In order to more completely assess the infant, you ask the NICU nurse to auscultate the heart rate. Determining the heart rate is the most important indicator of the infant's status at this time. Auscultation is the most reliable clinical method to determine heart rate but umbilical cord palpation can also be used. The nurse should communicate the heart rate to you by tapping out the rate. She should also count the rate for 6 seconds and multiply by 10, giving you the actual number.

2. Ensure that the radiant warmer has been turned on to full power. This may not have been done if the delivery was precipitous or expected to be completely uncomplicated. Check that the equipment you may need is readily available and the suction is turned on. Check the amount of oxygen being delivered with your ventilation device. You may need to ask the NICU or labor and delivery nurse to help you prepare other equipment as you are providing ventilation.

3. It would be helpful to confirm that this is a term infant, that the amniotic fluid was clear, and that the labor was otherwise uncomplicated. Specifically, you may ask if the fetal monitoring was reassuring, determine what medications were used during labor, and determine whether forceps or vacuum assistance was needed for delivery. Once the infant is stable, you can review the medical record in more detail to determine what other risk factors might be present for this infant such as the mother's group B *Streptococcus* status or presence of maternal diabetes.

CASE STUDY 1 (continued)

When you ask the obstetrician more about the labor and delivery you learn that this infant is 39 weeks' gestation and that the mother presented with rupture of membranes 10 hours prior to delivery and progressed to spontaneous labor. The amniotic fluid was clear and there was no fever during labor. The mother received an epidural for anesthesia. There was a reassuring fetal heart tracing and the delivery proceeded smoothly. There was a tight nuchal cord present that the obstetrician was able to reduce prior to delivery of the baby. Once you started giving PPV the baby began crying within 30 seconds and now appears vigorous. You are unsure of the cause of this baby's respiratory depression at birth, but are reassured that it was brief and the baby became vigorous so quickly. You observe the baby for a little longer and complete your review of the medical record.

ASSESSMENT AND MONITORING

After birth, careful assessment of the infant is important to ensure that the transition from fetal to neonatal life occurs smoothly. When the transition is progressing appropriately, the baby will begin crying and breathing spontaneously; the initial central blue color will become pink over several minutes. When the transition is not progressing normally, it is critical to assess the infant more closely. A more careful assessment begins with observation for spontaneous breathing and measurement of the heart rate. The infant should be placed on a radiant warmer with the head accessible to the end of the bed and the baby positioned in the neutral position for an optimally open airway (Figure 1-3). If the infant is not crying or breathing, a brief period of stimulation can be attempted to help the baby begin crying. However, other interventions should not be delayed for long if the infant does not begin crying and breathing quickly. Overly aggressive stimulation can in fact cause injury and should be avoided. If the infant was born through meconium stained amniotic fluid and is not vigorous, the current recommendations suggest that the infant be intubated for tracheal suctioning. A meconium aspirator can be connected to the end of the endotracheal tube following intubation so that suction can be directly applied to the tube. In the past all infants born through meconium stained amniotic fluid were intubated for tracheal suctioning. However, randomized controlled trials have shown that there is no benefit to this practice when infants are vigorous at birth (Wiswell, 2000). There have never been any controlled evaluations of this practice in nonvigorous infants and the data supporting that recommendation are not strong.

The heart rate will help determine the next steps necessary when resuscitation is required. An accurate heart rate can be obtained by auscultation, electrocardiogram (ECG), or pulse oximetry. However, in a complicated resuscitation it is preferable to use ECG and pulse oximetry monitoring. These monitoring devices allow for a continuous display of the heart rate providing the ability to respond to changes in an ongoing fashion. Furthermore, they free a member of the team to perform other tasks. The ECG provides the most rapid indication of heart rate, usually within approximately 30 to 45 seconds (Katheria, 2012). When placed quickly after birth, modern high-quality pulse oximeters can provide accurate signals by 1.5 minutes of life.

When these monitors are not available or not working it is necessary to determine the heart rate by clinical assessment. The most accurate method of clinical assessment is auscultation. A pulse can also be obtained by palpation of the umbilical cord, but is less reliable with a tendency to underestimate the true pulse rate. Palpation of the pulses at other sites is also quite unreliable and not recommended during resuscitation (Owen, 2004). When obtaining the heart rate by clinical assessment it is important for the individual making the assessment to indicate the rate to the other team members by tapping a finger. A heart rate that is below 100 beats per minute and not increasing is the most important indicator that an infant requires assistance. Because the vast majority of newborn infants have a low heart rate as a result of inadequate breathing, the initial intervention for a heart rate below 100 beats per minute is to provide assisted ventilation.

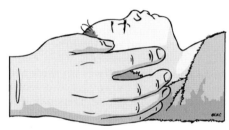

FIGURE 1-3 ■ Neutral newborn head positioning. (From Richmond S, Wyllie J: European Resuscitation Council guidelines for resuscitation 2010. *Resuscitation* 81:1389-1399, 2010.)

CASE STUDY 2

You are called to a cesarean section of an infant whose mother is past her due date at 41 weeks' gestation. Rupture of membranes occurred 2 hours prior to delivery and the amniotic fluid contained thick meconium. The fetal heart rate tracing had mild to moderate variable decelerations and labor had stopped progressing leading to the cesarean section. When you arrive in the operating room you prepare your equipment and await the delivery. Once the baby is delivered you hear a weak cry while the obstetrician is holding the baby, but when you place the baby on the radiant warmer you see that the baby is not crying or breathing.

The NICU nurse on your resuscitation team auscultates the heart rate and taps out a rate of approximately 80 beats per minute.

EXERCISE 2

QUESTION

1. What is your next step in the resuscitation of this infant?

ANSWER

1. This baby is not vigorous and the heart rate is low. Because there was thick meconium present in the amniotic fluid *and* the infant is depressed at birth, you should attempt to intubate the baby for tracheal suctioning. You should observe the suction catheter as you are withdrawing the endotracheal tube to see if there was meconium present in the trachea. Your NICU nurse should continue monitoring the heart rate throughout the procedure and if the bradycardia continues or the baby has not begun breathing after you have made one attempt to suction the trachea, you should begin providing PPV using a mask.

CASE STUDY 2 (continued)

Once you have intubated the baby and apply suction to the endotracheal tube you note that a small amount of meconium is suctioned from the trachea. The baby's heart rate is now 65 beats per minute and you decide to start giving mask PPV. After about 1 minute of PPV the heart rate increases to over 100 beats per minute. After 2 minutes of PPV the baby begins spontaneously breathing and crying.

EXERCISE 3

QUESTION

1. What else should you do to monitor this baby?

ANSWER

1. If not already done, you should place a pulse oximeter to ensure that the baby is achieving adequate postnatal oxygen saturations. The baby seems to have aspirated some meconium and could develop significant pulmonary disease that may require supplemental oxygen or more significant respiratory support. This baby is also at risk for developing persistent pulmonary hypertension of the newborn and would likely benefit from at least brief monitoring in the NICU to determine whether additional therapy will be necessary.

ASSISTING VENTILATION

Assisted ventilation is needed for 10% to 15% of newborns after birth (Aziz, 2005) and is most frequently provided with a facemask and bag or T-piece resuscitator. When beginning ventilation, it is important to ensure that the baby is positioned well with the airway open. The facemask should be placed gently on the face and held in place in a secure manner. Pushing down on the facemask may lead to reflex bradycardia. If the heart rate does drop suddenly when ventilation is started, release the mask and place it again more gently in an attempt to relieve any reflex bradycardia. The goal of assisting ventilation is to encourage the infant to begin spontaneous breathing. Before the infant initiates spontaneous breathing it may be necessary to provide higher airway pressures in order to deliver an adequate volume of gas to the lung. The normal process of spontaneous breathing after birth includes clearing the remaining lung fluid and maintaining air within the lung at the end of expiration, the functional residual capacity (FRC). When providing assisted ventilation it is difficult to know exactly how much air the infant needs to fill the lung. The volume of air that enters the lung when pressure is applied depends on the unobstructed continuity of the airway from the pressure device to the lung airspaces, the amount of leak in the system, the amount of pressure applied, and the compliance of the lungs.

Providing effective mask ventilation is one of the most important skills used in neonatal resuscitation. Assessing the effectiveness and making appropriate adjustments to ventilation requires some experience to master. When mask ventilation is provided and no signs of clinical improvement are apparent, the clinician must make adjustments to improve the ventilation. Initial adjustments to improve ventilation include ensuring that the mask is placed on the face correctly to minimize mask leak, repositioning the head and providing jaw thrust if necessary to ensure that the airway is open, and suctioning the airway if there is copious fluid present.

Obtaining the appropriate positioning for an open airway is probably the most important of these adjustments and can be difficult for inexperienced clinicians, especially when caring for very small babies. If the airway is positioned well and the infant is not improving, the ventilation pressure should be increased. Depending on the ventilation device in use the method of increasing pressure will vary. With a self-inflating bag or a flow-inflating bag the operator squeezes the bag harder to increase the pressure. This is often done without conscious effort if the infant is not improving and the operator is trying harder to give adequate ventilation. On the other hand, the operator must make a decision and turn a knob to increase pressure when a T-piece device is used. Although this is a limitation of the T-piece device, the benefit of this device is that the pressure delivered is much more consistent and closer to the desired target pressure (Bennett, 2005). In addition, T-piece devices are the only of the three types of ventilating devices that can reliably deliver positive end expiratory pressure (PEEP) and mask continuous positive airway pressure (CPAP), which are useful in establishing and maintaining FRC (Siew, 2009).

In addition to clinical improvement, the sign that the airway is open and the ventilating pressure is adequate is that chest rise occurs with each breath. However, the extent of chest rise is often difficult to estimate through observation and may be a sign of excessive pressure in small preterm infants. An alternate method of looking for an open airway and evidence of gas exchange is to use an end-tidal CO_2 detector in line with the mask and ventilating device. A simple colorimetric device provides a very rapid and reliable indication that gas exchange is occurring and often precedes other signs of clinical improvement (Finer, 2009). These devices should always be used to confirm endotracheal tube placement but may also be used with any ventilating device to confirm presence of an open airway and gas exchange. The color will not cycle as expected if there is not adequate cardiac output and pulmonary blood flow as occurs in a cardiac arrest.

If clinical improvement does not occur with optimal noninvasive ventilation, a more stable airway should be placed. To establish a more stable airway an endotracheal tube must be placed. Placement of an endotracheal tube is a skill that requires training and experience to develop proficiency. It is a procedure that can be associated with significant complications and may even destabilize the baby prior to allowing for improvement (O'Donnell, 2006). It should therefore only be performed if mask ventilation is not successful at achieving clinical stability or if prolonged ventilation is needed. When prolonged ventilation is needed (for example if the infant remains apneic), it is still preferable to place the endotracheal tube when the infant is well oxygenated with a good heart rate. Mask ventilation can frequently achieve effective ventilation prior to intubation even in the smallest infants. The one situation when mask ventilation should not be used as the first line of action to achieve clinical stability is in congenital diaphragmatic hernia. In this situation the intestines are displaced into the chest and will become distended with mask ventilation causing compression of the lungs and further clinical deterioration. Therefore endotracheal intubation is the necessary first step to avoid intestinal distention.

In some infants it may be difficult to place an endotracheal tube especially if the chin is small, the tongue is large, or there is a cleft palate or other airway anomaly. A laryngeal mask airway (LMA) can be used as an alternative airway if the endotracheal tube cannot be placed (see Figure 1-4). In cases of difficult airway management another alternative is to place a nasopharyngeal tube to deliver air closer to the larynx/trachea. PPV may be possible by this route even if it was not effective with a mask. An endotracheal tube can be used for the nasopharyngeal airway. Care should be used when placing this type of tube to ensure that it does not cause trauma. Though some units use nasopharyngeal tubes as the primary interface for assisted ventilation after birth, it has not been shown to be superior to mask ventilation and is a higher risk procedure (Kamlin, 2013; McCarthy, 2013b).

During assisted ventilation it is important to monitor the progress of the infant. Once clinical improvement is achieved, it is important to avoid excessive ventilation, which is not beneficial to the infant. It has been shown in animals that even a few excessively large assisted inflations can cause lung injury (Bjorklund, 1997). The methods available to monitor the size of the inflations include: looking for exaggerated chest rise, monitoring the inflation pressure, and monitoring the exhaled tidal volume. None of these methods is really ideal for ensuring that the inflations are not excessive. Observation for chest rise is quite subjective and using visible chest rise as the determinant of the inflating pressure has been associated with significant "over-ventilation" (Poulton, 2011). Although measuring the inflating pressure is simple, the correct inflating pressure is not known and the necessary pressure will vary for each infant, depending on the compliance of the lungs. Measuring the tidal volume and interpreting the measurements is technically more difficult, but often can be reliably determined once the infant is ventilated (Schilleman, 2013; Schmölzer, 2012).

Although preterm infants require resuscitation interventions more frequently than term infants, the reasons may be quite different. Although fetal acidosis leading to respiratory depression can occur in preterm infants as well as term infants, the most likely reasons that preterm infants require interventions immediately after

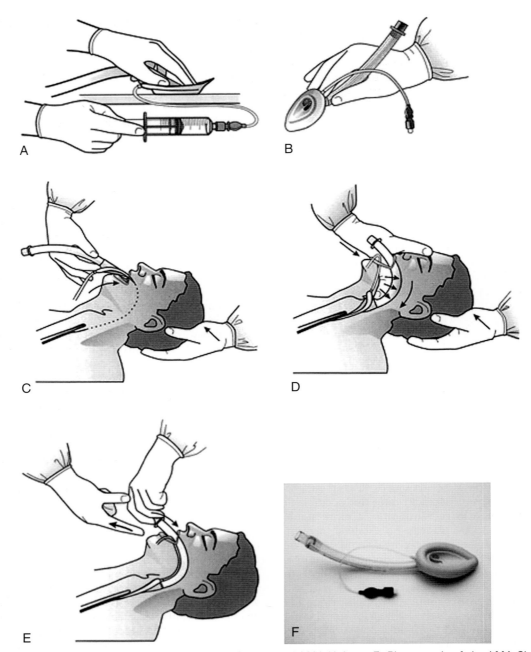

A

B

C

D

E

F

FIGURE 1-4 ■ **A–E**, Insertion technique for LMA-Classic and LMA-Unique. **F**, Photograph of the LMA-Classic. (From Pollack CV: The laryngeal mask airway: a comprehensive review for the emergency physician. *J Emerg Med* 20[1]:53-66, 2001.)

delivery relate to immaturity of the lung. The preterm infant's lungs may be surfactant deficient and the chest wall may be weak. These characteristics make it more difficult for the preterm infant to establish FRC without some degree of assistance. For some infants that assistance may be nasal CPAP alone, but others will need more support with PPV and supplemental oxygen. Even the smallest preterm infants can usually be

resuscitated with mask PPV initially and then intubated if necessary once stabilized.

CASE STUDY 3

You are called to attend a cesarean section for a preterm infant at 34 weeks' gestation who is being delivered owing to placenta accreta. The mother is receiving general anesthesia and has not had any signs of labor. After delivery you take the baby from the obstetrician and place the baby on a radiant warmer. You remove the wet towels, briefly dry the baby, and make your initial assessment. You note that the baby is apneic and you begin to stimulate the baby. Your assistant has started to auscultate the heart rate and notes that it is approximately 90 beats per minute.

EXERCISE 4

QUESTIONS

1. What factors place this infant at risk for needing resuscitation?

2. What is the most appropriate next step to care for this infant?

ANSWERS

1. The infant is at higher risk for requiring resuscitation because of the preterm gestational age and the mother has received general anesthesia.

2. Because the infant's heart rate is below 100 beats per minute, you should begin PPV. An additional team member should begin placing a monitor on the baby (ECG and pulse oximeter).

CASE STUDY 3 (continued)

When you begin PPV you note that the chest does not seem to be rising with each breath and the heart rate (now measured by ECG) is 82 beats per minute.

EXERCISE 5

QUESTION

1. What interventions should you make at this point?

ANSWER

1. Because the heart rate is not improving and you do not see chest rise, you need to readjust your PPV. You can begin by adjusting the mask position and ensure that the baby's head is in a neutral position with an open airway. If these maneuvers do not improve the infant's condition, begin to increase the ventilating pressure.

CASE STUDY 3 (continued)

Once you adjust the head position, you note improved chest rise and the heart rate on the ECG monitor is steadily increasing until it reaches 165 beats per minute. After approximately 1 more minute of assisted ventilation the infant begins taking some spontaneous breaths. By 5 minutes of life the infant is breathing consistently and you no longer need to give PPV.

EXERCISE 6

QUESTION

1. What interventions would you consider if the infant had not started spontaneously breathing?

ANSWER

1. If the infant has not begun spontaneously breathing after 5 to 10 minutes of PPV it is necessary to provide a more stable airway for continued support. The baby should be intubated at that point. Sometimes fentanyl is given with general anesthesia and could be suppressing the infant's spontaneous breathing. If it is known that the mother received an opiate prior to delivery, it is possible to give a trial dose of naloxone. Naloxone is given in a dose of 0.1 mg/kg intravenously (IV) or intramuscularly (IM) and is a competitive antagonist of the μ-opioid receptor blocking the action of opiates. Its duration of action is shorter than most opiates, so apnea may recur and the infant needs to be monitored carefully after naloxone use. Naloxone will not be effective if the cause of apnea is an anesthetic agent that is not an opiate. It is also very important to know that the mother is not chronically using any type of opiate, because if the infant has opiate dependence from chronic exposure, the naloxone dose can induce sudden withdrawal symptoms including seizures.

OXYGEN USE

Within the last 20 years there have been many studies aimed at determining whether supplemental oxygen is necessary and beneficial during resuscitation. These studies have shown that term infants respond to resuscitation better when room air (21% oxygen) is used as the initial ventilating gas with PPV. The infants ventilated with 21% oxygen started spontaneously breathing and crying slightly sooner (Saugstad, 1998). Furthermore, the metaanalysis of published randomized trials indicates there was also lower mortality among the infants resuscitated with room air as opposed to 100% oxygen (Rabi, 2007). There has been concern that oxygen itself can be toxic by generating free radicals, especially during reperfusion after prior ischemia, as is often the case when resuscitation is necessary. It is now the recommendation of the NRP as well as other international resuscitation guidelines, to start resuscitation with room air, 21% oxygen. However, if the heart rate is less than 60 beats per minute and chest compressions are indicated, 100% oxygen is recommended. After the infant has achieved an adequate heart rate, the oxygen can be titrated to maintain "normal" oxygen saturation values.

The understanding of normal oxygen saturation values has also changed over recent years. Fetal blood oxygen levels are lower than post-transitional newborn oxygen levels. Baseline fetal oxygen saturations are near 50% and may decrease even further throughout labor. After birth the oxygen saturation levels increase to values greater than 95% in healthy term newborns. The time that it takes to transition from fetal to newborn oxygen saturation levels has been determined in studies using pulse oximetry in infants making the transition from fetal to postnatal life without any assistance. The most recent study (Dawson, 2010), which has set the standard for normal newborn transitional oxygenation values, developed percentile curves of oxygen saturation values over the first 10 minutes of life from observations of well infants transitioning from fetal life without any assistance. The 25th, 50th, and 75th percentiles at each minute in the first 10 minutes of life are plotted in Figure 1-5. The consistent finding in all of these studies is that oxygen saturation values rise slowly and reach the 85% to 95% range over the first 10 to 15 minutes of life. There is, however, great variability among infants in the lowest levels of oxygen saturations and the speed with which the saturation levels increase. The recommended preductal SpO_2 reference range at each minute is displayed in the Newborn

Resuscitation Algorithm (Figure 1-1). As a rough guide, the minimum SpO_2 value begins with 60% at 1 minute and increases by 5% with each minute throughout the first 5 minutes of life.

Preterm infants have a slower increase in oxygen saturation values than term infants. In addition, preterm infants may be more vulnerable to oxidative stress owing to decreased antioxidant enzyme levels. On the other hand, preterm infants often need supplemental oxygen, most likely owing to immature lungs. Studies that have evaluated oxygen use in preterm infants have shown that most infants (<32 weeks' gestation) require some supplemental oxygen in order to achieve expected levels of oxygen saturation over the first 15 minutes of life (Dawson, 2009; Wang, 2008). In clinical practice it is common for otherwise well-appearing preterm infants to receive some supplemental oxygen. How much oxygen and when to provide it remains a question of some controversy. Some experts suggest starting with 21% oxygen and increasing it if the heart rate is low or saturation targets are not met. Others suggest starting with a higher percentage of oxygen (30% to 40% oxygen) and then adjusting the inspired oxygen concentration based on the heart rate and oxygen saturation levels. It is not clear which strategy is better, but it is possible that these strategies may vary in the total amount of oxygen used or in the need for other therapies during the resuscitation. Though currently unknown, it is possible that these differences may contribute to differences in clinical outcomes as well. Future studies are likely to address these questions. The recommendations from the NRP allow for either approach. It should be noted that

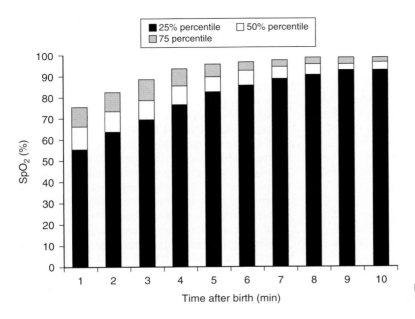

FIGURE 1-5 ■ **SpO_2 values at 1 to 10 minutes after birth.**

in order to provide an intermediate oxygen concentration between 21% and 100%, the resuscitation area must be equipped with compressed air and an oxygen blender. Therefore it is necessary for all hospitals that care for preterm newborn infants to have this equipment available in the area where babies will be delivered and managed after birth.

CASE STUDY 4

You have completed a prenatal consult for a 30-year old gravida 1, para 0 woman at 24 weeks' gestation with diamniotic dichorionic twins who has presented today with preterm labor. She has received one dose of betamethasone, and you have discovered that the estimated fetal weights of her twins are 550 grams and 580 grams. After you have reviewed the risks of morbidity and mortality and discussed what the family can expect if the babies are born at this gestational age, you go to write your note and the obstetric nurse calls you because the patient's labor has begun rapidly progressing and Baby A is about to deliver. You gather the other members of your resuscitation team and set up your resuscitation area.

EXERCISE 7

QUESTIONS

1. How should you organize the resuscitation teams for these infants?

2. What additional equipment and preparation do you need because these infants are 24 weeks' gestation?

ANSWERS

1. These infants are at high risk for needing resuscitation because of their extreme prematurity and they each need their own complete resuscitation team. You need to have a nurse and a respiratory therapist at the delivery to assist with *each* infant. You ask your colleague to help lead the resuscitation of one infant and you will lead the resuscitation of the other infant. For a high-risk resuscitation such as this it is best to have at least three individuals for each infant. It may even be beneficial to have additional individuals available to help if needed.

2. You will need to use plastic wrap for temperature management and should place the plastic wrap on the radiant warmers *before* the babies are born. Ensure that you have temperature probes available to use the radiant warmers in the servo-control mode. Prior to the infant being born, you should turn the radiant warmers up to

full power. Make sure, you have ECG leads with a heart monitor and pulse oximeter with probe.

CASE STUDY 4 (continued)

In this case, you have a T-piece resuscitator to provide PPV and you set your oxygen blender to 30%. You have suction turned on and you have a laryngoscope with a 00 blade available for each infant. You also have 2.5 French endotracheal tubes available in case you need to intubate these infants. You have colorimetric end-tidal CO_2 detectors available to determine if you have established a patent airway. Just as you complete your equipment preparation Baby A is delivered. You bring the baby to the radiant warmer, remove the blanket that you used to carry the infant and wrap the plastic around the baby's body. You note that the baby has made weak intermittent cries and has shallow breathing. Your NICU nurse places ECG leads and attaches them to the monitor. You quickly learn that the heart rate is 85 beats per minute. Meanwhile the respiratory therapist is placing the probe for the pulse oximeter on the right hand.

EXERCISE 8

QUESTION

1. What should be your next intervention for Baby A?

ANSWER

1. Because the heart rate is less than 100 beats per minute and the baby is making only weak respiratory efforts, begin PPV.

CASE STUDY 4 (continued)

You have the end-tidal CO_2 detector in between the facemask and T-piece resuscitator and you notice that there is no color change. You adjust the mask and head position ensuring that you have a neutral position and you provide slight jaw thrust. You continue to note that there is not adequate color change on the end-tidal CO_2 detector. You increase the pressure on the T-piece resuscitator by 10 cm H_2O and within two breaths you see color change on the end-tidal CO_2 detector. Within the next 10 seconds the heart rate has increased to 130 beats per minute. Baby A is now 4 minutes old and you note that the preductal SpO_2 is 80%, which is within the normal range so you keep the oxygen concentration at 30%. You transition the infant to nasal CPAP and continue close monitoring.

While you were managing Baby A, your colleague had received Baby B and is in the process of resuscitating Baby B. Because Baby A is now stable on CPAP, you check in with your colleague to see if he needs any help. Baby B is now 5 minutes old and is receiving mask PPV. Your colleague tells you that the baby had an initial heart rate of 65 beats per minute and no respiratory effort. Baby B did not respond initially to PPV until the pressure was increased. Currently the heart rate is 150 beats per minute and the SpO₂ is 35%; the infant is receiving 30% oxygen. Your colleague increases the oxygen concentration and follows the SpO₂. The SpO₂ increases to 85% once the infant is receiving 100% oxygen. The baby is currently not making continuous spontaneous breathing efforts.

EXERCISE 9

QUESTION

1. What should be your next step for Baby B?

ANSWER

1. You and your colleague decide that it is appropriate to intubate the baby at this point. Your colleague proceeds to perform the intubation and you assist. Once the tube is in place you note that the SpO₂ increases to 95% and you begin to decrease the oxygen concentration. You plan to give surfactant once you confirm that the tube is in good position.

CIRCULATORY SUPPORT

Reports of neonatal resuscitation interventions have documented that additional support beyond assisted ventilation is provided to approximately 1 to 3/1000 infants (Aziz, 2005; Perlman, 1995). Chest compressions are indicated if the heart rate is below 60 beats per minute and does not improve with adequate ventilation. The currently recommended technique for providing chest compressions is called the thumb technique. Using this technique the clinician encircles the infant's chest with her hands and compresses the sternum with both thumbs. The thumbs should be placed on the lower third of the sternum (below the nipple line and above the xiphoid) and the chest compressed one-third the anteroposterior diameter. The current recommendation is to provide chest compressions coordinated with ventilation in a 3:1 ratio. When truly needed, chest compressions are most effective when provided with the fewest possible interruptions. Therefore, once begun they should be continued for approximately 45 to 60 seconds before pausing to check the heart rate. It is helpful to have ECG leads and a pulse oximeter to monitor for increasing spontaneous heart rate during this time. It is important to remember though, that good chest compressions will cause a waveform to be displayed on the pulse oximeter. When providing chest compressions it is also necessary to increase the oxygen concentration to 100% if it has not been previously increased. Once chest compressions have been started, the team leader should anticipate the need for further interventions and begin preparing for intubation, umbilical venous catheter placement, and epinephrine administration. Because these tasks can take time to prepare, it is helpful to designate additional team members to begin the preparation as soon as it becomes apparent that they may be necessary.

An umbilical venous catheter should be placed when the heart rate remains below 60 beats per minute despite good ventilation and chest compressions. When used for resuscitation the umbilical venous catheter is placed in a shallow position, just past the body wall once good blood return is obtained. This positioning avoids infusion of medications into the liver, which can cause liver injury. An umbilical venous catheter is the preferred route for administration of epinephrine. If the infant remains bradycardic despite good ventilation and chest compressions, epinephrine should be administered as the next line of treatment. Epinephrine can also be given through the endotracheal tube but may not be as effective. The recommended dose of epinephrine when given IV is 0.01 to 0.03 mg/kg/dose but is increased to 0.05 to 0.1 mg/kg/dose when given by endotracheal tube. Repeat doses of epinephrine can be given every 3 minutes if the heart rate remains below 60 beats per minute.

If the infant has not responded to ventilation, chest compressions, and epinephrine the resuscitation team must consider administering volume. Though volume loss is not a frequent cause of perinatal depression, when it occurs it can be quite severe and the infant may not recover without receiving additional volume. Crystalloids can be given initially, but the resuscitation team must also consider the need for blood. Blood can be lifesaving in situations where the infant has had significant blood loss, but it must be given in a reasonable time to be effective. So as with all other aspects of resuscitation, the possibility of the need for volume must be considered ahead of time.

If the infant is not responding to resuscitation interventions it is also important to think of other complications that could be preventing improvement. A pneumothorax may have developed owing to excessive pressure administration during assisted ventilation. Check for equal breath sounds and consider using transillumination of the chest to evaluate for pneumothorax. Trans-illumination works well in preterm infants but may not be successful in term infants. If breath sounds are unequal without another obvious cause (displaced endotracheal tube or diagnosis of congenital diaphragmatic hernia) and the infant continues to deteriorate it may be necessary to attempt chest drainage prior to an x-ray. However, ideally a chest x-ray should always be obtained prior to "needling" the chest.

CASE STUDY 5

You receive a call from labor and delivery because a woman has just presented with profuse vaginal bleeding. She is at 30 weeks' gestation and on initial evaluation, the fetal heart rate was found to be 80 beats per minute. The obstetric team has started an emergency cesarean section. You and your resuscitation team go to the delivery room and prepare your equipment. The baby is handed to you and appears limp and pale and is not breathing. You place the infant on the radiant warmer and remove the wet blankets. The NICU nurse places the ECG leads and the respiratory therapist places a pulse oximeter on the right hand while you begin providing PPV. The initial heart rate is 56 beats per minute. You continue providing mask PPV making adjustments to the head positioning and ensuring that you have a good mask seal. The heart rate remains at approximately 55 beats per minute. You increase the amount of pressure that you are providing and you can see that you are now achieving good chest rise.

EXERCISE 10

QUESTION

1. The heart rate has not increased, what are your next steps?

ANSWER

1. Begin chest compressions and increase the inspired oxygen concentration to 100%

CASE STUDY 5 (continued)

You request that the NICU nurse begin chest compressions, which you coordinate in a 3:1 ratio of compression to breaths. Meanwhile you ask the respiratory therapist to increase the oxygen concentration to 100%. You also prepare for intubation, ensuring that you have all the necessary equipment. If you have additional help available you can ask another to person prepare and flush an umbilical venous catheter (UVC) for emergency placement. (If you had had adequate time to prepare the

UVC prior to delivery you would be able to save time and personnel with this step.) Meanwhile you perform the intubation. You are sure that the endotracheal tube has passed through the glottis and is in the trachea. You see good chest rise and hear equal breath sounds, but there is no color change on the end-tidal CO_2 detector. You suspect that this is caused by inadequate cardiac output and pulmonary blood flow. The infant is now 4 to 5 minutes old and the heart rate remains at 55 beats per minute.

EXERCISE 11

QUESTIONS

1. What is your next step?

2. If emergency blood will take too long to obtain, what other options do you have to support this infant?

ANSWERS

1. You place the emergency UVC and ask for a nurse to prepare one IV and one endotracheal tube (ET) dose of epinephrine. She has the ET dose of epinephrine prepared before you have the UVC in place so you give one dose in the endotracheal tube. Meanwhile you also request emergency blood. The circulating labor and delivery nurse has come to help and now goes to get the emergency blood.

2. You could administer IV normal saline to increase the circulating blood volume. In this infant there was a clear history of vaginal bleeding and the infant appears pale so you strongly suspect that the infant has lost a significant amount of blood. Therefore blood transfusion may be necessary in order to improve this infant's cardiac output and oxygen delivery. However, crystalloid infusion may help temporarily. In a true emergency if you cannot get O-negative emergency blood quickly enough, you could also use blood from the mother because it will have the same antibody profile as the baby's blood. The obstetrics team may be able to help draw blood from the mother so that you can administer it to the baby. Because the need for blood is so rare, this is an area that resuscitation teams should practice during simulation training.

CASE STUDY 5 (continued)

The infant is now 7 minutes old, you have given one dose of IV epinephrine after the one dose of ET epinephrine and the infant's heart rate is now 76 beats per minute. You have been able to obtain emergency O-negative blood and administer 10 mL/kg and the heart rate increases to 120 beats per minute.

EXERCISE 12

QUESTION

1. What are your next steps?

ANSWER

1. You should now continue mechanical ventilation and adjust the oxygen concentration as needed to maintain normal SpO$_2$ levels. You will obtain a blood sample for a blood gas and will check the hemoglobin/hematocrit. Because it is likely that the infant will need more than 10 mL/kg based on the clinical history and presentation, you plan to give an additional transfusion somewhat more slowly to correct the anemia.

SPECIAL CIRCUMSTANCES

There are certain conditions that require alternate or additional interventions compared with the standard resuscitation protocol. One such condition is congenital diaphragmatic hernia. In this condition the abdominal contents are displaced into the thorax. The lung on the side of the diaphragmatic hernia is hypoplastic and both lungs may have abnormal structural development. For resuscitation purposes, the best approach to management includes immediate intubation to avoid mask ventilation and distension of the intestines leading to further compression of lung tissue. Once the infant has been intubated a gastric suction tube should be placed to decompress any air that has accumulated in the gastrointestinal tract. Additionally, when providing PPV it is best to limit the peak pressures to approximately 20 cm H$_2$O and allow the baby to slowly increase oxygen saturations over time. Attempting to rapidly increase the oxygen saturation values using high ventilating pressure is likely to contribute to lung injury leading to increased difficulty with the resuscitation.

A second special circumstance of resuscitation involves infants with airway obstruction. Airway obstruction can occur owing to a variety of different problems such as micrognathia/Pierre Robin sequence, masses, etc. Prenatal diagnosis is extremely important in order to ensure adequate preparation. The most severe cases may be treated with an ex-utero intrapartum therapy (EXIT) procedure during which the mother is treated with general anesthesia and uterine relaxation while the infant is delivered and fetoplacental circulation is maintained until an airway can be secured. The airway may be secured by endotracheal intubation if possible, though it may be necessary to perform a tracheostomy. The EXIT procedure requires a large multidisciplinary team with a high level of coordination to be successful. It is a rarely needed but potentially lifesaving procedure.

A third circumstance requiring additional resuscitation interventions is that of fetal hydrops. The severity and presentation of fetal hydrops varies greatly and requires individualization of care depending on the presentation. Fetal hydrops is an accumulation of fluid in multiple body spaces including the pleural, peritoneal, pericardial, and interstitial spaces. The diagnosis prenatally is made by identifying fluid in at least two of these spaces. Prenatal management also includes a search for the underlying cause of the hydrops. It is helpful for the resuscitation team to know where the fluid is located and the extent of fluid that exists. Often fluid will need to be drained to allow for adequate ventilation. Fluid can be drained from the peritoneal cavity to improve breathing by decreasing upward pressure on the thorax from the abdomen. Pleural fluid may also require drainage in order to achieve adequate ventilation. It is likely that an umbilical venous line may be needed for intravascular volume replacement or epinephrine administration. It is best to have additional clinicians available to help perform these procedures in a coordinated fashion and to preassign roles for each clinician so that the tasks can be accomplished smoothly. The necessary equipment including umbilical catheters, catheters for peritoneal and pleural drainage, and chest tubes should be prepared ahead of time to minimize any delay in performing these procedures.

CASE STUDY 6

A 24-year-old woman at 36 weeks' gestation is transferred from a small local hospital because of a newly diagnosed hydrops fetalis that was discovered on ultrasound when the mother presented with decreased fetal movement. After an initial obstetric evaluation and a period of fetal monitoring a decision is made to proceed with delivery owing to nonreassuring fetal status. There are no noted fetal anomalies on ultrasound, the mother's blood type is O-positive, antibody screen negative, and there is no evidence of fetal anemia. The hydrops was diagnosed based on bilateral large pleural effusions, a moderate amount of ascites, and skin edema.

EXERCISE 13

QUESTIONS

1. As you are preparing for this delivery, what equipment do you prepare in addition to the standard equipment that you prepare for every delivery?

2. How will you assign tasks to your resuscitation team for this delivery?

ANSWERS

1. Because you may need to drain the pleural and peritoneal effusions, you should have at least three (plus additional spare) large-bore angiocatheters available to use for pleurocentesis and paracentesis. You will also need several large syringes, at least three stopcocks, and connector tubing. In addition you should have appropriately sized thoracostomy tubes with drainage equipment. You may choose initially to perform a pleurocentesis followed by more definitive thoracostomy tube placement (if necessary) once the baby is more stable. Alternatively, some individuals may choose to place a thoracostomy tube for the initial drainage. You must also be aware that a pneumothorax can develop as a complication of any of these procedures and you may need to perform another procedure to drain the pneumothorax. You should also have all of your intubation equipment (ensure that you have endotracheal tubes smaller than expected if needed because the appropriate size may be difficult to determine from the estimated fetal weight). Finally, it would be appropriate to have an umbilical venous catheter completely set up, flushed, and ready to use, as this infant may need resuscitation medications or intravascular fluid replacement.

2. For this resuscitation it would be best to have additional clinicians available to help perform drainage procedures if needed. You should assign an individual to monitor the heart rate and place a pulse oximeter and temperature probe. Another individual should be in charge of the airway. If you have two additional clinicians, one can be in charge of draining the left chest and the other can be in charge of draining the right chest. If you still have one more clinician, that individual can place a UVC and drain the ascites if necessary. Additional nurses can prepare syringes of epinephrine, flushes, and normal saline (for volume resuscitation if needed). You will need a team leader who may be the person in charge of the airway or preferably another individual without a specific task assignment. Although this may seem excessive at first glance, having plenty of people with preassigned tasks and a good understanding of how the decisions to proceed with each intervention will be made can make this very complicated resuscitation occur in a smooth and organized fashion. Because this is so complicated, it is best if this type of delivery can occur in the daytime when extra help is more readily available.

CASE STUDY 6 (continued)

Once the baby is delivered, she is handed to you and you note that she has an intermittent weak cry.

You bring her to the radiant warmer, dry her, and remove the wet blankets. The NICU nurse places the ECG leads and you learn that the heart rate is 90 beats per minute. He then places the pulse oximeter and temperature probe. You note that the baby is continuing to breathe and is crying weakly. You begin PPV using the T-piece resuscitator with facemask and end-tidal CO_2 detector. You note that there is color change on the end-tidal CO_2 detector but there is poor chest excursion with each breath. Your colleague auscultates the lungs and notes distant breath sounds bilaterally. On your initial survey of the infant you also note that the abdomen does not appear particularly distended. You determine that the infant is most likely having difficulty breathing because of the pleural effusions. One of your colleagues performs a pleurocentesis on the left and removes 60 mL of clear, straw-colored fluid. Another colleague performs pleurocentesis on the right and removes 30 mL of similar fluid. At this point the chest excursion is much greater and the heart rate is now 140 beats per minute.

The infant is now 5 minutes old and the SpO_2 is 25%. You increase the oxygen stepwise over the next several minutes but even when you have reached 100% oxygen the SpO_2 does not increase over 50%.

EXERCISE 14
QUESTION

1. What is your next step?

ANSWER

1. It would be appropriate to intubate the infant at this point. Though you were able to manage the infant initially with mask ventilation and the heart rate is now normal, you need more long-term ventilation because of the difficulty with oxygenation. Some clinicians may have chosen to intubate this infant prior to performing pleurocentesis, but your approach has kept the baby stable throughout the procedure and you can now intubate the baby while she has a normal heart rate.

CASE STUDY 6 (continued)

Once you intubate the infant, the SpO_2 increases to 80% and you move the baby back to the NICU for further evaluation and management.

POSTRESUSCITATION CARE

It is currently recommended that the resuscitation be stopped after 10 minutes of full resuscitation efforts if there has been no detectable heart rate. Infants who have required and responded to resuscitation after birth are at risk for ongoing clinical instability and must be evaluated closely. The need for significant resuscitation is often a sign of hypoxic-ischemic injury and the infant is at risk for encephalopathy. A careful assessment to determine whether the infant meets criteria for therapeutic hypothermia is always appropriate after a prolonged resuscitation. Each institution may have local guidelines for the use of therapeutic hypothermia, but if the institution does not provide this treatment, the clinicians must be ready to transfer the baby to another institution where the evaluation and treatment can be provided. The general criteria for use of therapeutic hypothermia include gestational age of greater than 35 weeks, history consistent with possible hypoxia-ischemia, a significant metabolic acidosis on cord or newborn blood gases, and physical examination consistent with encephalopathy. The therapy must be initiated as soon as possible, but within 6 hours from the hypoxic-ischemic event. Because the timing of the hypoxic-ischemic event is usually unknown, at least 6 hours from birth is used as the timeframe to initiate therapy.

Infants who have required significant resuscitation may subsequently have hemodynamic instability after the initial recovery of spontaneous circulation and breathing. Therefore, ongoing monitoring of systemic perfusion and blood pressure is important in the continued care of these infants. In the first day of life, infants make frequent physiologic adjustments as the circulatory pattern transitions from the fetal to the neonatal circulation. This transition can be impaired in infants requiring newborn resuscitation and persistent pulmonary hypertension can develop as a consequence. After resuscitation, glycogen stores can be depleted and the infant can develop hypoglycemia, requiring blood glucose monitoring and IV glucose infusion. Any infant who has received more than brief mask PPV should be observed more closely after resuscitation in an intensive care setting for a period of time depending on the significance of resuscitation and need for ongoing support.

APGAR SCORES

In 1953 Virginia Apgar published a report describing a scoring system to evaluate newborn infants 1 minute after birth. The score was intended to evaluate the effects of obstetric anesthesia on the condition of the newborn. Later the score was assigned at 5 minutes of life as well as at 1 minute. The Apgar score is composed of five parameters and each parameter is assigned a value of 0, 1, or 2 for a total of 10 possible points. The five parameters are heart rate, breathing, tone, color, and reflex irritability (responsiveness to stimuli). It is nearly universal that all infants throughout the world receive a 1-minute and a 5-minute Apgar score. If the score is less than 7 at 5 minutes it has become customary to assign repeat scores at 5-minute intervals through approximately 20 minutes or until the score is more than 7. Although there can be quite a bit of variability among scores assigned by different clinicians, most aspects of the score remain useful markers of an infant's ongoing condition.

CONCLUSION

Neonatal resuscitation is a critical skill for providers caring for newborn infants. Though most infants do not need extensive resuscitation interventions, careful assessment and basic interventions can be lifesaving. Assisted ventilation is the most important skill for providers to master and use appropriately. A well-prepared resuscitation team can perform interventions calmly and efficiently while minimizing adverse effects. Infants who have required more extensive resuscitation should be carefully evaluated for further necessary treatments.

SUGGESTED READINGS

Apgar V: A proposal for a new method of evaluation of the newborn infant, *Curr Res Anesth Analag* 32:260–267, 1953.

Aziz K, Chadwick M, Baker M, Andrews W: Ante- and intrapartum factors that predict increased need for neonatal resuscitation, *Resuscitation* 79:444–452, 2008.

Aziz K, Chadwick M, Downton G, et al.: The development and implementation of a multidisciplinary neonatal resuscitation team in a Canadian perinatal centre, *Resuscitation* 66:45–51, 2005.

Barber CA, Wyckoff MH: Use and efficacy of endotracheal versus intravenous epinephrine during neonatal cardiopulmonary resuscitation in the delivery room, *Pediatrics* 118:1028–1034, 2006.

Bennett SC, Finer NN, Rich W, Vaucher Y: A comparison of three neonatal resuscitation devices, *Resuscitation* 67:113–118, 2005.

Bjorklund LJ, Ingimarsson J, Curstedt T, et al.: Manual ventilation with a few large breaths at birth compromises the therapeutic effect of subsequent surfactant replacement in immature lambs, *Pediatr Res* 42:348–355, 1997.

Chalak LF, Barber CA, Hynan L, et al.: End-tidal CO_2 detection of an audible heart rate during neonatal cardiopulmonary resuscitation after asystole in asphyxiated piglets, *Pediatr Res* 69:401–405, 2011.

Committee on Obstetric Practice: American College of Obstetricians and Gynecologists. Committee Opinion No. 543: timing of umbilical cord clamping after birth, *Obstet Gynecol* 120:1522–1526, 2012.

Dawes GS: The natural history of asphyxia and resuscitation at birth. In: *Foetal and neonatal physiology: a comparative study of the changes at birth*, Chicago, IL, 1968, Yearbook Medical Publishers.

Dawson JA, Kamlin CO, Vento M, et al.: Defining the reference range for oxygen saturation for infants after birth, *Pediatrics* 125:1340–1347, 2010.

Dawson JA, Kamlin CO, Wong C, et al.: Oxygen saturation and heart rate during delivery room resuscitation of infants <30 weeks' gestation with air or 100% oxygen, *Arch Dis Child Fetal Neonatal Ed* 94:F87–91, 2009.

Finer NN, Rich W, Wang C, et al.: Airway obstruction during mask ventilation of very low birth weight infants during neonatal resuscitation, *Pediatrics* 123:865–869, 2009.

Goudar SS, Somannavar MS, Clark R, et al.: Stillbirth and newborn mortality in India after Helping Babies Breathe training, *Pediatrics* 131:e344, 2013.

Haddad B, Mercer BM, Livingston JC, et al.: Outcome after successful resuscitation of babies born with Apgar scores of 0 at both 1 and 5 minutes, *Am J Obstet Gynecol* 182:1210–1214, 2000.

Kamlin COF, Schilleman K, Dawson JA, et al.: Mask versus nasal tube for stabilization of preterm infants at birth: A randomized controlled trial, *Pediatrics* 132:e381–e388, 2013.

Katheria A, Rich W, Finer N: Electrocardiogram provides a continuous heart rate faster than oximetry during neonatal resuscitation, *Pediatrics* 130:e1777–1781, 2012.

Kattwinkel J, editor: *Textbook of neonatal resuscitation*, 6th ed, Elk Grove, IL, 2011, American Heart Association and American Academy of Pediatrics.

Kattwinkel J, Perlman JM, Aziz K, et al.: Part 15: Neonatal resuscitation: 2010 American Heart Association guidelines for cardiopulmonary resuscitation and emergency cardiovascular care, *Circulation* 122:S909–919, 2010.

McCall EM, Alderdice F, Halliday HL, Jenkins JG, Vohra S: Interventions to prevent hypothermia at birth in preterm and/or low birthweight infants, *Cochrane Database Syst Rev* (3), 2010. CD004210.

McCarthy LK, Molloy EJ, Twomey AR, et al.: A randomized trial of exothermic mattresses for preterm newborns in polyethylene bags, *Pediatrics* 132:e135–e141, 2013.

Msemo G, Massawe A, Mmbando D, et al.: Newborn mortality and fresh stillbirth rates in Tanzania after Helping Babies Breathe training, *Pediatrics* 131:e353–e360, 2013.

O'Donnell CPF, Kamlin COF, Davis PG, Morley CJ: Endotracheal intubation attempts during neonatal resuscitation: success rates, duration, and adverse effects, *Pediatrics* 117:e16–e21, 2006.

Owen CJ, Wyllie JP: Determination of heart rate in the baby at birth, *Resuscitation* 60:213–217, 2004.

Perlman J, Kattwinkel J, Wyllie J, et al.: Part 11: Neonatal resuscitation: 2010 International consensus on cardiopulmonary resuscitation and emergency cardiovascular care science with treatment recommendations, *Circulation* 122:S516–538, 2010.

Perlman JM, Risser R: Cardiopulmonary resuscitation in the delivery room: associated clinical events, *Arch Pediatr Adolesc Med* 149:20–25, 1995.

Poulton DA, Schmolzer GM, Morley CJ, et al.: Assessment of chest rise during mask ventilation of preterm infants in the delivery room, *Resuscitation* 82:175–179, 2011.

Rabi Y, Rabi D, Yee W: Room air resuscitation of the depressed newborn: a systematic review and meta-analysis, *Resuscitation* 72:353–363, 2007.

Richmond S, Wyllie J: European Resuscitation Council guidelines for resuscitation 2010. Section 7. Resuscitation of babies at birth, *Resuscitation* 81:1389–1399, 2010.

Saugstad OD, Rootwelt T, Aalen O: Resuscitation of asphyxiated newborn infants with room air or oxygen: an international controlled trial: the Resair 2 study, *Pediatrics* 102:e1, 1998.

Schilleman K, van der Pot CJM, Hooper SB, et al.: Evaluating manual inflations and breathing during mask ventilation in preterm infants at birth, *J Pediatr* 162:457–463, 2013.

Schmolzer GM, Morley CJ, Wong C, et al.: Respiratory function monitor guidance of mask ventilation in the delivery room: a feasibility study, *J Pediatr* 160:377–381, 2012. e2.

Siew ML, te Pas AB, Wallace MJ, et al.: Positive end-expiratory pressure enhances development of a functional residual capacity in preterm rabbits ventilated from birth, *J Appl Physiol* 106:1487–1493, 2009.

Trevisanuto D, Micaglio M, Ferrarese P, Zanardo V: The laryngeal mask airway: potential applications in neonates, *Arch Dis Child Fetal Neonatal Ed* 89:F485–F489, 2004.

Vohra S, Frent G, Campbell V, et al.: Effect of polyethylene occlusive skin wrapping on heat loss in very low birth weight infants at delivery: A randomized trial, *J Pediatr* 134:547–551, 1999.

Wang CL, Anderson C, Leone TA, et al.: Resuscitation of preterm neonates by using room air or 100% oxygen, *Pediatrics* 121:1083–1089, 2008.

Wiswell TE, Gannon CM, Jacob J, et al.: Delivery room management of the apparently vigorous meconium-stained neonate: results of a multicenter, international collaborative trial, *Pediatrics* 105:1–7, 2000.

Wood FE, Morley CJ, Dawson JA, et al.: Improved techniques reduce face mask leak during simulated neonatal resuscitation: study 2, *Arch Dis Child Fetal Neonatal Ed* 93:F230–F234, 2008.

CHAPTER 2

PERINATAL ASPHYXIA

Matthew A. Rainaldi, MD • Jeffrey M. Perlman, MB, ChB

The term asphyxia refers to a condition of impaired gas exchange in a subject, leading to progressive hypoxia, hypercarbia, and acidosis. During the perinatal period, this fetal state is most often a consequence of impaired placental blood flow, which in a subset of infants can progress to hypoxic-ischemic brain injury. However, one must be cautious in labeling a newborn infant with the diagnosis "asphyxia" as: (1) it lacks a specific biochemical definition; and (2) is often unjustly linked to poor neurologic outcome, resulting in costly litigation. Indeed, the presentation of neonatal encephalopathy at birth may be a result of asphyxia, but may be secondary to other etiologies, such as inborn errors of metabolism, genetic disorders, or intracranial hemorrhage. Before one can link an acute intrapartum hypoxic-ischemic event to a later case of cerebral palsy, the American Congress of Obstetricians and Gynecologists (ACOG) Task Force on Neonatal Encephalopathy and Cerebral Palsy define four essential criteria (ACOG, 2005): (1) evidence of a metabolic acidosis in fetal umbilical cord arterial blood obtained at delivery (pH <7 and base deficit ≥ 12 mmol/L); (2) early onset of severe or moderate neonatal encephalopathy in infants born at 34 weeks or more of gestation; (3) cerebral palsy of the spastic quadriplegic or dyskinetic type; and (4) exclusion of other identifiable etiologies such as trauma, coagulation disorders, infectious conditions, or genetic disorders.

In this chapter, we will follow the case of an asphyxiated term newborn from birth until hospital discharge, stopping for questions and discussion at key areas. The focus of this chapter will be on:

- Understanding the pathophysiology of interruption of placental blood flow on fetal well-being, including the fetal adaptive responses
- Interpreting clinical, laboratory, and electrographic data related to birth asphyxia
- Making management decisions regarding the care of a newborn infant following perinatal asphyxia
- Obtaining prognostic neurodevelopmental information throughout the case

CASE STUDY 1

A 36-year-old gravida 3, para 1011 African American woman at 40 weeks' gestation presents to the emergency department complaining of 30 minutes of back pain and contractions. Her prior obstetric history is significant for one elective abortion and one prior caesarean section for breech presentation. She has a history of leiomyomas requiring myomectomy. This pregnancy has been uneventful and her serologies were negative. Group B streptococcal testing was negative. In the emergency room, her physical examination is significant for vaginal bleeding and a firm uterus. She is transferred to the labor and delivery floor for further management. Fetal heart rate tracings upon hospital admission and 3 hours later are shown in Figure 2-1.

EXERCISE 1

QUESTIONS

1. What is your interpretation of the tracing in Figure 2-1, *A*? Choose the best answer.
   a. Reassuring fetal heart rate tracing
   b. Abnormal baseline fetal heart rate
   c. Excessive fetal heart rate variability
   d. Presence of fetal heart rate decelerations

2. What is your interpretation of the tracing in Figure 2-1, *B*? Choose best answer.
   a. Reassuring fetal heart rate tracing
   b. Abnormal baseline fetal heart rate
   c. Moderate fetal heart rate variability
   d. Presence of late fetal heart rate decelerations

3. The fetal heart rate pattern shown in Figure 2-1, *B* is most typically associated with:
   a. Maternal hypoxemia
   b. Uteroplacental insufficiency
   c. Cessation of oxytocin
   d. Head compression

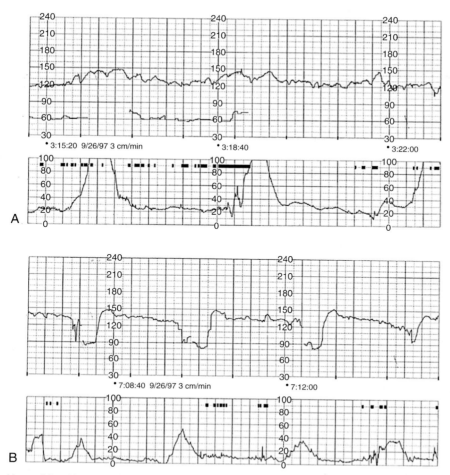

FIGURE 2-1 ■ Normal fetal heart rate tracing upon admission to the hospital **(A)**. Note the normal baseline rate, accelerations, moderate variability, lack of decelerations (*top panel*), as well as the periodic contractions (*bottom panel*). Three hours later, late decelerations **(B)** are seen. Note the periodic decreases in heart rate (*top panel*) beginning after a contraction starts (*bottom panel*), reaching a nadir after the peak of the contraction is reached, and the decreased heart rate variability compared to **(A)**. (Images courtesy of Dr. Amos Grunebaum.)

4. What is the likely cause of the decelerations and ultimately asphyxia in this case?
   a. Placental abruption
   b. Fetomaternal hemorrhage
   c. Nuchal cord
   d. Chorioamnionitis and funisitis

ANSWERS

1. **a.** The initial fetal heart rate tracing is reassuring (Figure 2-1, *A*). It has a normal baseline rate (110 to 160 beats/minute [bpm]) with accelerations, moderate variability, and absence of decelerations.

2. **d.** In contrast, the subsequent tracing (Figure 2-1, *B*) shows periodic decreases in the fetal heart rate that begin after a contraction starts and reach a nadir after the peak of the contraction is reached. These are categorized as late decelerations, an ominous finding. Note that they are followed by a lag in return to baseline of about 30 to 60 seconds.

3. **b.** Late decelerations are primarily associated with uteroplacental insufficiency; the associated bradycardia, if severe, can produce fetal hypotension. The occurrence of late decelerations is a worrisome finding, as it has been correlated with both fetal hypoxia and acidosis.

4. **a.** In addition to late decelerations, this woman has several signs and symptoms concerning for placental abruption including a history of leiomyomas, back pain, and vaginal bleeding. Although her symptoms are relatively acute, one must have a heightened suspicion for interruption of placental blood flow with potential compromise in fetal cerebral blood flow. This is a complex issue and appears to be related to the mechanism(s) resulting in interruption of placental blood flow. Thus studies in both monkeys and humans have suggested that duration of intermittent asphyxia of less than 1 hour is unlikely to lead to brain injury;

but severe "total" asphyxia (which may be occurring in this case) can cause brain injury much sooner (Low, Galbraith, Muir et al., 1984; Pasternak & Gorey, 1998; Volpe, 2008). The severity and duration of the uteroplacental insufficiency is often difficult to ascertain and may or may not become apparent as labor progresses.

CASE STUDY 1 (continued)

The fetal heart tracing worsens, with the late decelerations becoming more severe and the patient is taken to the operating room for an emergency caesarean section. Upon uterine incision, the obstetrician notes a large amount of blood loss and placental abruption. A newborn male emerges limp, pale, and apneic. He is placed on the radiant warmer for the pediatric team where profound bradycardia is noted. Initial resuscitation steps—including drying, stimulating, and gentle suctioning of the oropharynx—fail to increase his heart rate above 50 beats per minute.

EXERCISE 2

QUESTION

1. Fetal compensatory mechanisms in response to asphyxia aim to preserve blood flow to which of the following organs?
   a. Heart, brain, and adrenal glands
   b. Heart, brain, and lungs
   c. Heart and brain (only)
   d. Heart, brain, adrenal glands, and lungs

ANSWER

1. **a.** This newborn most likely suffered a decrease in placental blood flow as a result of the placental abruption. The pathophysiologic manifestation of this interruption of blood flow is termed asphyxia, a condition of impaired gas exchange leading to progressive hypoxia, hypercarbia, and acidosis. Crucial to understanding the pathophysiology of asphyxia and need for resuscitation in this newborn is the work of Dawes and colleagues (Dawes, Jacobson, Mott et al., 1963). Using rhesus monkeys, they initiated asphyxia by ligating the umbilical cord and covering the head with a small bag of warm saline and observed a characteristic series of changes. This was followed within 30 seconds by a brief period of rapid rhythmic respiratory effort culminating in apnea (primary) and a decrease in heart rate; this lasted for approximately 30 to 60 seconds (Figure 2-2). The animal then began to gasp after the onset of primary apnea, but spontaneous regular respiration could be induced via stimulation if done in a timely manner. Without interventions the gasping lasted for approximately 4 minutes, became weaker,

and a terminal "last gasp" occurred. This period is known as secondary apnea and unless resuscitation was initiated promptly, death ensued. Several additional relevant points include: (1) If the arterial pH was low (pH 7.00 to 7.10) as a result of uterine abruption, rhythmic respirations were often absent prior to primary apnea; and (2) If the pH was still lower (i.e., less than 6.80) often there was no gasping. In the presence of normal body temperature, pH at the time of delivery was the most important determinant of the time to the last gasp.

The disruption of placental blood flow initiates important adaptive mechanisms in the fetus including circulatory responses that redistribute cardiac output to protect more vital organs (e.g., brain, myocardium, and adrenal glands) (Figure 2-3). This preservation is at the expense of decreased blood flow to less vital organs such as the kidney, intestine, skin, and muscle. At baseline, oxygenated umbilical venous blood flow is preferentially directed through the ductus venosus, up the inferior vena cava and toward the foramen ovale through into the left atrium. The magnitude of shunting changes throughout gestation and is altered by hypoxemia. Additionally, peripheral vasoconstriction contributes to the preservation of central blood flow via catecholamine release triggered by arterial chemoreceptors.

With prolonged asphyxia, a critical threshold is reached, resulting in failure of the adaptive mechanisms and a decrease in cerebral perfusion and oxygen delivery. The infant described has presented with circulatory failure as a result of significant interruption of placental blood flow, but at this time it is not known whether the cerebral circulation has been compromised.

CASE STUDY 1 (continued)

Resuscitation is escalated and he is eventually stabilized following endotracheal intubation with positive pressure ventilation, chest compressions, and a dose of epinephrine via an umbilical venous catheter.

EXERCISE 3

QUESTION

1. Which of the following statements regarding oxygen supplementation in the delivery room is true?
   a. All healthy term newborns should appear pink by 5 minutes of life.
   b. Resuscitation should begin with 100% oxygen and titrated down if the infant is well saturated.
   c. A normal *in utero* oxygen saturation level is approximately 70%.
   d. Hyperoxia can be harmful and should be avoided.

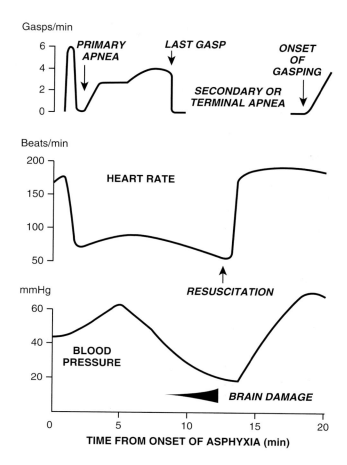

Pco$_2$	45	100	150	200	40
pH	7.3	7.0	6.8	6.75	7.1

FIGURE 2-2 ■ **Relationship between cardio-vascular parameters, respiratory effort, and acidosis in rhesus monkeys during asphyxia and resuscitation.** (From Dawes G et al.: The treatment of asphyxiated, mature foetal lambs and rhesus monkeys with intravenous glucose and sodium carbonate. *J Physiol* 16[1]:167-184, 1963.)

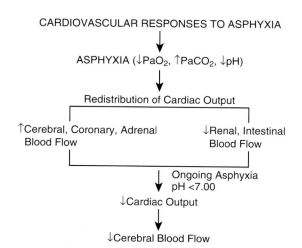

FIGURE 2-3 ■ **Circulatory responses to interruption of placental blood flow (asphyxia).** Note the redistribution of blood away from the lesser vital organs to preserve cerebral, myocardial, and adrenal blood flow.

ANSWER

1. **d.** Both insufficient and excessive oxygenation can be injurious to the neonate. Current Neonatal Resuscitation Program (NRP) guidelines recommend the use of pulse oximeters to measure preductal saturations when: (1) resuscitation is anticipated; (2) positive pressure ventilation is used for more than a few breaths; (3) cyanosis is persistent; or (4) supplementary oxygen is administered. It is preferable to begin resuscitation with room air, as 100% oxygen can have deleterious effects. Experimental data from animal models using 100% oxygen has demonstrated oxidative stress in multiple organs including the lungs and brain as compared to room air; and clinical data have shown increased mortality in neonates with the use of 100% oxygen versus room air. Increasing the oxygen concentration should be performed with

an air-oxygen blender and guided to maintain saturations in the interquartile range for healthy term newborns. As in this case, if the infant is bradycardic after 90 seconds of resuscitation with a lower concentration of oxygen, the concentration should be increased to 100% until the heart rate has increased to a normal range. It is important to recognize that healthy term newborns may take up to 10 minutes to increase from a normal *in utero* saturation of 60% to a normal postnatal saturation above 90%.

CASE STUDY 1 (continued)

Once stabilized, the oxygen concentration is weaned to room air. Apgar scores were 1, 2, 4, and 7 at 1, 5, 10, and 15 minutes respectively and he is transferred to the neonatal intensive care unit (NICU). Umbilical arterial cord gas shows: pH of 6.7, P_{CO_2} of 127 mmHg, P_{O_2} of 10 mmHg, and base deficit of 19 mEq/L. The placenta is sent for histopathologic evaluation.

EXERCISE 4

QUESTIONS

1. What is your interpretation of this umbilical arterial blood gas?
   a. Respiratory acidosis
   b. Metabolic acidosis
   c. Compensated metabolic acidosis
   d. Mixed respiratory and metabolic acidosis

2. Which statement regarding a low umbilical cord arterial pH is true?
   a. Umbilical venous cord pH is a more reliable indicator of fetal status.
   b. Infants with fetal acidemia are easily distinguished from those with a normal pH at birth.
   c. Acidemic infants who require significant resuscitation are at high risk for adverse neurologic outcome.
   d. Fetal pH is the best indicator of outcome.

ANSWERS

1. **d.** This blood gas indicates a mixed respiratory and metabolic acidosis in the fetus. Fetal acidemia (pH <7.20), or accumulation of acid occurs via three pathways: (1) excess carbon dioxide and in turn carbonic acid; (2) excess noncarbonic or metabolic acid (e.g., lactic, uric or keto acids); or (3) both carbonic and noncarbonic acids. Carbon dioxide quickly diffuses across the placenta and is excreted by the maternal lungs. Thus, alterations in fetal pH caused by carbon dioxide accumulation can occur and resolve quickly. In contrast, noncarbonic acids only slowly diffuse across the placenta into the maternal circulation. The primary noncarbonic acid, lactic acid, accumulates as a result of oxygen deprivation and anaerobic glycolysis and does so more slowly than carbonic acid. This results in a more sustained acidemia, the degree of which may relate to both the severity and duration of the hypoxic-ischemic insult.

   Because metabolic acids diffuse slowly into the maternal circulation for excretion by the maternal kidneys, some degree of acidemia may be seen in maternal prerenal or renal conditions such as diabetes, preeclampsia, or chronic hypertension. This may cause one to recover a more acidic pH in the umbilical artery not necessarily owing to fetal asphyxia.

2. **c.** Fetal acidemia is most helpful when it is interpreted in the context of the clinical situation. Even if cord blood acidemia is severe (pH <7.00) most infants will be triaged to a well-baby nursery and not have adverse outcomes. In a prospective study of 35 acidemic and 35 control newborns without fetal acidemia, there were no differences in terms of neurologic evaluation and outcome (King, Jackson, Josey et al., 1998). In contrast, acidemic infants who require significant resuscitation (e.g., CPR and epinephrine in the delivery room) are at a high risk for adverse neurologic outcome. This was demonstrated in a prospective study of 47 infants with severe fetal acidemia: the odds ratio of abnormal outcome (e.g., abnormal neurologic exam or seizures) was 234 (95% confidence limit: 12.9 to 4261) with persistent bradycardia requiring chest compressions (Perlman & Risser, 1993).

CASE STUDY 1 (continued)

In the NICU, his examination is significant for lethargy/stupor with pallor and poor central tone. The cranial nerve examination is pertinent for an absent suck and a weak gag. Reflexes are depressed but present. He slowly and weakly reacts during peripheral intravenous line placement. A peripheral blood culture is taken and antibiotics are started. As part of the evaluation for therapeutic hypothermia, an amplitude-integrated EEG (aEEG) is performed (Figure 2-4).

EXERCISE 5

QUESTIONS

1. What stage of encephalopathy is this clinical examination most consistent with?
   a. Stage 1
   b. Stage 2
   c. Stage 3

TABLE 2-1   **Relationship of Encephalopathy Stage to Outcome**

Sarnat Stage (Extent of Encephalopathy)	Outcome (Percent of Total Infants, Grouped by Encephalopathy Stage)		
	Deaths	Neurologic Sequelae	Normal
Stage I (Mild)	0%	0%	100%
Stage II (Moderate)	5%	24%	71%
Stage III (Severe)	80%	20%	0%
All	13%	14%	73%

Modified from Volpe JJ: Neurology of the newborn, 5th ed, Philadelphia, PA, 2008, Saunders/Elsevier. Data from Robertson C, Finer N: Term infants with hypoxic-ischemic encephalopathy: outcome at 3.5 years, Dev Med Child Neurol 27(4):473-484, 1985; and Thornberg E, et al.: Birth asphyxia: incidence, clinical course and outcome in a Swedish population, Acta Paediatr 84(8):927-932, 1995.

2. Which statement is false regarding encephalopathy staging?
   a. Severe encephalopathy is strongly correlated with adverse neurologic sequelae.
   b. Hypoxia-ischemia is one of several causes of neonatal encephalopathy.
   c. Infants with mild encephalopathy have similar outcomes to nonencephalopathic infants.
   d. None of the above are false.

3. What type of pattern does this aEEG show?
   a. Continuous with normal voltage
   b. Discontinuous with moderate voltage suppression
   c. Discontinuous with severe voltage suppression
   d. Isoelectric

4. Which of the following aEEG patterns is correlated with the best prognosis?
   a. Burst suppression
   b. Discontinuous low-voltage
   c. Continuous low-voltage
   d. Continuous normal-voltage

5. Would you treat this neonate with therapeutic hypothermia?

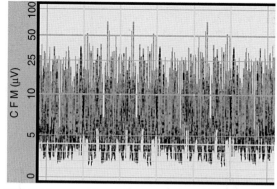

FIGURE 2-4 ■ **Amplitude-integrated EEG in a term infant with hypoxic-ischemic encephalopathy (see text).** Note the upper band is greater than 10 μV and the lower band is less than 5 μV, indicative of moderate suppression.

ANSWERS

1. **b.** Sarnat and Sarnat distinguished three clinical stages of neurologic dysfunction following perinatal hypoxia-ischemia (Sarnat & Sarnat, 1976). Stage 1 consists of hyperalertness, uninhibited Moro reflex, and predominance of sympathetic effects. In Stage 2, parasympathetic effects predominate and the infant is lethargic, hypotonic, and often has seizures. Infants in Stage 3 encephalopathy are stuporous, with little to no responsiveness. Only strong, noxious stimuli are reacted to, with withdrawal of an extremity or decerebrate posturing. Corneal and gag reflexes are absent.

   The lethargic/stuporous newborn in our case presents with a diminished level of consciousness, weak reflexes, and hypotonia and characterizes an infant in Stage 2 to early Stage 3 encephalopathy.

2. **d.** Clinical staging of encephalopathy is particularly valuable. A majority of the poor outcomes seen in infants with a history of hypoxic-ischemic encephalopathy is from those who presented with severe encephalopathy. As seen in data by Robertson and Thornberg, none of 115 infants with mild encephalopathy died or developed neurologic sequelae (Robertson & Finer, 1985; Thornberg, Thiringer, Odeback et al., 1995) (Table 2-1). Conversely, infants who progressed to severe encephalopathy had uniformly poor outcomes, e.g., either death or severe neurocognitive impairment in survivors.

3. **b.** aEEG delivers a continuous voltage recording of background cerebral activity that appears as a band and can be characterized by both band width and margins. This aEEG shows background activity with an upper margin above

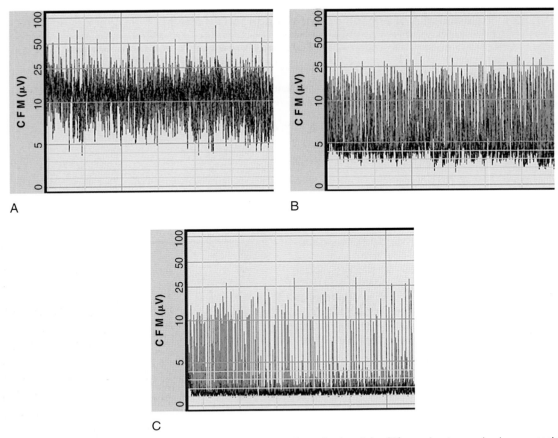

FIGURE 2-5 ■ Sample aEEG tracings demonstrating normal cerebral activity **(A)**, moderate cerebral suppression **(B)**, and severe cerebral suppression (burst suppression in this example) **(C)**.

10 μV and a lower margin below 5 μV. Using the classification system described by al Naqeeb, this is defined as a moderately suppressed aEEG. Normal activity consists of an upper margin above 10 μV and a lower margin above 5 μV (Figure 2-5). Severe suppression is classified as an upper margin below 10 μV and a lower margin below 5 μV, which is often accompanied by burst suppression (al Naqeeb, Edwards, Cowan et al., 1999).

4. **d.** Early use of aEEG has been shown to correlate with neurodevelopmental outcome. Unfavorable outcomes have been associated with flat, continuous low-voltage, and burst suppression tracings, with positive predictive values of 80% to 90% (Figure 2-5, *C*). Continuous normal-voltage tracings and rapid normalization of an abnormal aEEG is associated with favorable outcome. The best prognostic value, it appears, comes from the inclusion of both the aEEG and the neurologic examination, with a specificity of 94% and positive predictive value of 85% (Shalak, Laptook, Velaphi et al., 2003).

5. This infant is in at least Stage 2 (moderate) encephalopathy and has an abnormal, moderately suppressed aEEG. He meets criteria and should undergo therapeutic hypothermia (see criteria in Table 2-2).

HYPOTHERMIA AS A NEUROPROTECTIVE STRATEGY

Despite advances in neonatal care, the only effective neuroprotective therapy for treatment of hypoxic-ischemic encephalopathy is therapeutic hypothermia. Both total body cooling and selective head cooling have been shown to ameliorate brain injury following perinatal hypoxia-ischemia in the setting of an acute hypoxic-ischemic event, if implemented within the first 6 hours of life. A 2012 metaanalysis of seven randomized controlled trials examined data of more than 1200 newborns with moderate to severe hypoxic-ischemic encephalopathy (Tagin, Woolcott, Vincer et al., 2012). Hypothermia reduced the risk of death or severe disability in both moderate and severe

TABLE 2-2 Criteria for Treatment with Therapeutic Hypothermia (Candidates Must Meet All Three)

Criteria 1	Infant ≥36 weeks gestation age and at least one of the following: Apgar score ≤5 at 10 minutes Continued need for resuscitation including endotracheal or bag-mask ventilation at 10 minutes Acidosis defined as either umbilical cord arterial pH <7.00 or any arterial pH <7.00 within 60 minutes Base deficit ≥16 mmol/L in an umbilical cord sample or any blood sample obtained within 60 minutes of birth
Criteria 2	Evidence of moderate to severe encephalopathy on clinical exam (Sarnat stage 2 or 3)
Criteria 3	Amplitude-integrated EEG (aEEG) evidence of moderate to severe encephalopathy or seizures

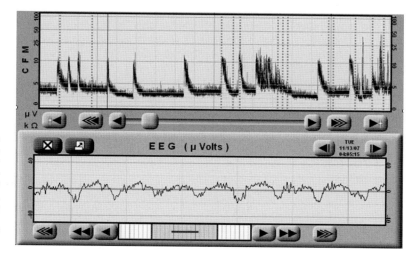

FIGURE 2-6 ■ Amplitude-integrated EEG in a term infant during hypothermia treatment for hypoxic-ischemic encephalopathy. Note the sharp and narrow increase in amplitude *(top panel)*. Note the repetitive activity on the single channel "raw EEG" consistent with seizures *(bottom panel)*.

encephalopathy (RR, 0.67; 0.56 to 0.81 and 0.83; 0.74 to 0.92, respectively).

CASE STUDY 1 (continued)

The infant meets criteria for cooling; selective head cooling is initiated at 4.5 hours of life. The aEEG is left in place to provide continuous monitoring of cortical activity. He is started on intravenous fluids at 60 cc/kg/day; his acidosis improves, but he develops hypoglycemia with a blood glucose level of 36 mg/dL. This is treated with a bolus of dextrose and a maintenance glucose infusion rate of 8 to 9 mg/kg/min.

EXERCISE 6

QUESTIONS

1. aEEG with single channel EEG tracing at 12 hours of life is shown in Figure 2-6. What aEEG pattern is depicted in this tracing?
   a. Seizure activity
   b. Burst suppression
   c. Isoelectric
   d. Continuous low-voltage

2. What is the appropriate next step in management of this neonate?
   a. Continue to observe because hypothermia will ameliorate seizure activity.
   b. Treat the seizures with phenobarbital.
   c. Remove the cooling apparatus to perform a full EEG.
   d. Both b and c

ANSWERS

1. **a.** This aEEG shows a baseline of severe suppression with a narrow-voltage bandwidth. Transient spikes of increased voltage interrupt this baseline activity. The raw EEG shows electrical activity in a rhythmic, repetitive fashion during one of these voltage spikes. This is characteristic of seizure activity, and in the absence of an observable clinical change is considered a subclinical seizure.

2. **b.** As seen in Figure 2-6, there has been relatively frequent seizure activity for several hours. Seizures of significant duration or frequency should be treated acutely and aggressively with antiepileptic therapy. Phenobarbital is the most

commonly used antiepileptic drug in neonates, although some prefer the use of phenytoin or benzodiazepines as a first-line.

CASE STUDY 1 (continued)

Phenobarbital (40 mg/kg) is given as a loading dose over 30 minutes and the seizures subside. The infant is also started on a continuous midazolam drip in part as a sedative and in part to control further seizures

His heart rate, which had previously been 120 to 130 bpm, decreases to 90 to 100 bpm. Mean arterial pressure correspondingly decreases from 45 to 50 mmHg to 35 to 40 mmHg. He makes only 5 mL of dark yellow urine in the first 12 hours of life. Serum electrolytes at this time show: sodium 131 mmol/L, potassium 4.9 mmol/L, chloride 102 mmol/L, bicarbonate 20 mmol/L, blood urea nitrogen 17 mg/dL, creatinine 1.2 mg/dL, calcium 8.6 mg/dL, magnesium 1.3 mEq/L, phosphate 4.3 mg/dL.

EXERCISE 7

QUESTIONS

1. What is the most likely cause of this newborn's bradycardia and hypotension?
   a. Severe myocardial ischemia and subsequent cardiac dysfunction
   b. Expected side effect of therapeutic hypothermia
   c. Adverse effect of antiepileptic therapies
   d. Both b and c

2. What is the most likely cause of electrolyte disturbances in this patient?
   a. Decreased renal perfusion as a result of redistribution of cardiac output prior to delivery
   b. Decreased renal perfusion to due postnatal hypotension
   c. Lack of appropriate electrolyte supplementation in the intravenous fluids
   d. Current electrolytes are entirely representative of the mother's electrolytes when sampled so soon after birth

3. What is the appropriate next step in the management of the oliguria in this patient?
   a. Volume resuscitation with crystalloid
   b. Diuretic therapy such as furosemide
   c. Decreasing fluid intake, i.e., "fluid restriction"
   d. Observation alone

4. What is the appropriate management of this patient's hyponatremia?
   a. Fluid restriction
   b. Addition of maintenance sodium while keeping the total fluid intake constant
   c. Addition of maintenance sodium while decreasing the total fluid intake
   d. Infusion of hypertonic saline

ANSWERS

1. **d.**
2. **a.**
3. **c.**
4. **a.**

Interruption of placental blood flow can lead to systemic organ injury, secondary to the redistribution of organ blood flow as discussed previously (Figure 2-7). Thus organ involvement is often seen in the kidneys, liver, gastrointestinal tract, and lungs.

Decreased renal blood flow can injure the tubular epithelium, leading to a spectrum of renal dysfunction. Mild injury may decrease renal concentrating ability, which may not be clinically apparent. Marked decreases in renal perfusion may cause acute tubular necrosis, as seen in this infant. Glomerular filtration rate is reduced, resulting in oliguria and azotemia. Accumulation of free water leads to hyponatremia. The syndrome of inappropriate antidiuretic hormone (SIADH) as a result of cerebral injury may also lead to oliguria and hyponatremia, complicating fluid management in these cases.

Other common electrolyte abnormalities to anticipate include both hypocalcemia and hypomagnesemia. The hypocalcemia is largely a reflection of depressed parathormone and elevated calcitonin concentration. Hypomagnesemia is seen with prolonged asphyxia and can disrupt the response to parathyroid hormone, worsening existing hypocalcemia.

Hypoglycemia in this infant is likely a manifestation of liver ischemia and a decrease in liver glycogen stores. It should be treated promptly as it can exacerbate ongoing brain injury. In a retrospective study of infants delivered in the presence of severe fetal acidemia (umbilical arterial cord pH <7.00) the presence of hypoglycemia was a strong predictor of abnormal outcome particularly in the presence of circulatory collapse.

Evidence of liver dysfunction includes elevated transaminase levels, which often persist for several days, and disrupted clotting factor production, which can lead to clinical bleeding. These can be associated with thrombocytopenia, transiently suppressed bone marrow hematopoietic activity, or disseminated intravascular coagulopathy in severe cases.

Although not clinically apparent in this infant, myocardial ischemia can affect contractility,

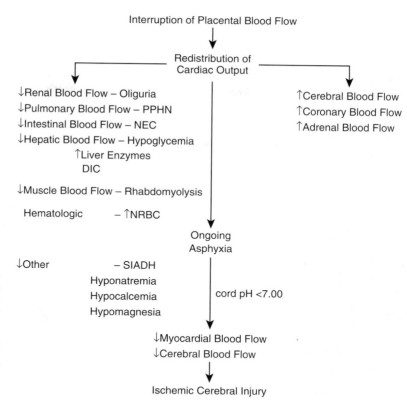

Interruption of Placental Blood Flow

Redistribution of Cardiac Output

↓Renal Blood Flow – Oliguria
↓Pulmonary Blood Flow – PPHN
↓Intestinal Blood Flow – NEC
↓Hepatic Blood Flow – Hypoglycemia
↑Liver Enzymes
DIC

↓Muscle Blood Flow – Rhabdomyolysis

Hematologic   – ↑NRBC

↑Cerebral Blood Flow
↑Coronary Blood Flow
↑Adrenal Blood Flow

Ongoing Asphyxia

↓Other   – SIADH
Hyponatremia
Hypocalcemia
Hypomagnesia

cord pH <7.00

↓Myocardial Blood Flow
↓Cerebral Blood Flow

Ischemic Cerebral Injury

FIGURE 2-7 ■ Systemic consequences of interruption of placental blood flow (asphyxia). *DIC,* Disseminated intravascular coagulation; *NEC,* necrotizing enterocolitis; *NRBC,* nucleated red blood cells; *PPHN,* persistent pulmonary hypertension of the newborn; *SIADH,* syndrome of inappropriate antidiuretic hormone release.

leading to reduced cardiac output, with hypotension and exacerbation of end-organ injury. Resulting pulmonary edema may impair gas exchange, worsening acidosis, and pulmonary vascular resistance may increase, leading to persistent pulmonary hypertension of the newborn (PPHN).

In addition to these consequences of hypoxia-ischemia, adverse effects related to therapeutic hypothermia must also be anticipated. As seen in this infant, bradycardia and mild hypotension are commonly encountered once the target rectal temperature of 34.5° C is reached. Rarely, treated infants may develop a coagulopathy, resulting in hemorrhage.

CASE STUDY 1 (continued)

To avoid worsening hyponatremia, the intravenous fluid rate is decreased to 50 cc/kg/day. A low-dose dopamine infusion (5 mcg/kg/min) is started to target both the hypotension and decreased kidney perfusion. Mean arterial pressures increase to 45 to 55 mmHg, and several hours later he begins to produce more urine. Blood sugar levels stabilize in a normal range (60 to 80 mg/dL) following the initial hypoglycemia. At 24 hours of life, urine output increases to 1.5 cc/kg/hr and a follow up serum electrolyte panel is significant for: sodium 134 mmol/L, potassium 4.9 mmol/L, bicarbonate 22 mmol/L, blood urea nitrogen 19 mg/dL, creatinine 1.4 mg/dL, calcium 9.0 mg/dL, and magnesium 1.5 mg/dL.

On Day 2, the urine output increases dramatically to 4.5 cc/kg/hr. Mean arterial pressures remain stable (50 to 55 mmHg) and the dopamine infusion is decreased to 2.5 mcg/kg/min. Serum electrolytes at 36 hours show: sodium 140 mmol/L, potassium 4.5 mmol/L, bicarbonate 23 mmol/L, blood urea nitrogen 11 mg/dL, creatinine 1.2 mg/dL, calcium 9.5 mg/dL, and magnesium 1.8 mg/dL. The intravenous fluid rate is increased to 70 cc/kg/day and maintenance sodium and potassium are added.

The cooling-associated hypotension in our case study infant was effectively managed with a dopamine infusion. This should be anticipated at the onset of therapeutic cooling and promptly addressed with the addition of a pressor.

Dopamine can improve renal perfusion through both the normalization of systemic blood pressure and direct vasodilatory effects on afferent and efferent renal arterioles. In this case study infant, fluid overload and worsening hyponatremia were avoided by decreasing the intravenous fluid rate while waiting for renal function to improve. Both normalization of blood pressure and direct renal effects of dopamine likely led to the relatively quick reestablishment of urine output. Fluid management was then transitioned back toward normal with the routine addition of sodium and potassium.

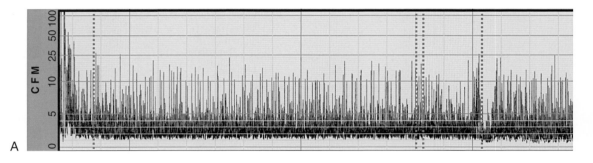

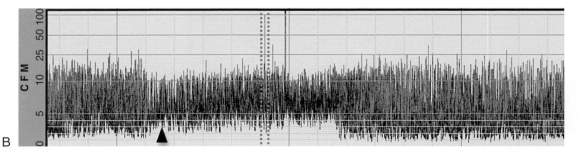

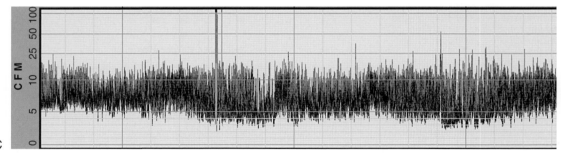

FIGURE 2-8 ■ aEEG tracings at 36 hours **(A)**, note the suppressed tracing; 60 hours **(B)**, note the upward shift of the integrated waveform (*arrowhead*) and a general widening of the wave form; and 96 hours **(C)**, note the appearance of cycling with an undulating pattern.

EXERCISE 8

QUESTIONS

1. The placental pathology is completed. Which statement regarding placental pathology is true?
   a. Placental pathology takes time to complete and is therefore of limited benefit in the management of ill neonates.
   b. Chorioamnionitis without maternal signs or symptoms is not a worrisome pathologic finding.
   c. Processes that lead to perinatal asphyxia are generally acute and readily known, obviating the need for placental pathology in these cases.
   d. Placental pathology can provide clues to the provider as to the etiology of the asphyxia as well as prognostic information that may be of benefit to the parents.

2. Representative aEEGs tracings at 36, 60, and 96 hours are shown (Figure 2-8, *A-C*). What is your interpretation of the aEEG findings?
   a. Gradual recovery of sleep-wake cycling
   b. Increase in voltage that could be related to seizure activity
   c. Widening of the bandwidth as the patient is returned to normothermia
   d. Emergence of cerebral activity as antiepileptics are metabolized

3. Which statement regarding sleep-wake cycling is incorrect?
   a. It is indicative of cerebral recovery.
   b. Timely recovery is associated with improved outcome.
   c. All infants will eventually recover sleep-wake cycling.
   d. It is present within the first several hours of birth in normal neonates.

ANSWERS

1. **d.** Placental histopathology is an often underutilized tool that can give important diagnostic and prognostic information to the pediatrician caring for a sick neonate. In addition to acute processes, such as placental abruption in this case, both subacute and chronic processes have the potential to compromise fetal blood flow and lead to hypoxia-ischemia. Importantly, clinically silent processes that would otherwise have gone undetected, such as histologic chorioamnionitis, can be recognized.

   Histologic chorioamnionitis refers to the subclinical inflammation, generally a result of infection by cervicovaginal organisms of the chorion and amnion, beginning with maternal tissue. In preterm infants, it is associated with white matter lesions such as periventricular leukomalacia. The fetal inflammatory response, funisitis, involves the umbilical cord and fetal vessels and is also associated with white matter lesions and cerebral palsy. Cytokine exposure to the developing brain is hypothesized to be the link between prenatal inflammation and central nervous system disease in infants and children. In addition to the deleterious effects of cytokines, severe necrotizing chorioamnionitis and funisitis may subacutely and acutely compromise placental blood flow by erosion of vessels.

   Placental abruption is often diagnosed clinically at the time of delivery, although pathology may reveal hemorrhage or thrombi. Other histopathologic diagnoses, such as fetal thrombotic vasculopathy, chronic villitis, and perivillous fibrin deposition, may shed light on a pathophysiologic process that led to perinatal asphyxia.

   In this case, the histopathology was consistent with placental abruption, without evidence of infection, vasculopathy, or other pathology.

2. **a.** These aEEG tracings represent the evolution of returning sleep-wake cycling. Normal sleep-wake cycles are seen as continuous, normal-voltage tracings, with periodic changes in bandwidth. This regular pattern is present in healthy term newborns and is disrupted by cerebral hypoxia-ischemia. At 36 hours, there is severe suppression of cerebral activity, as evidenced by a narrow bandwidth and low-voltage upper and lower margins (Figure 2-8, *A*). By 60 hours, sleep-wake cycling has started (Figure 2-8, *B*). And at 96 hours, cycling becomes more frequent and cerebral suppression is decreasing as the lower voltage margin increases (Figure 2-8, *C*).

3. **c.** The sleep-wake cycle is a marker of cerebral recovery, and both the pattern and chronology of the cycling have been correlated with the prognosis. Infants who go on to poor outcomes either do not recover sleep-wake cycling or have a higher percentage of suboptimal sleep-wake cycling during the encephalopathic period. The recovery to a normal aEEG background and timely return (within 120 hours) of normal sleep-wake cycling are predictors of normal outcome in those infants treated with hypothermia.

CASE STUDY 1 (continued)

Blood cultures remain negative at 48 hours and antibiotics are discontinued. The infant completes 72 hours of therapeutic hypothermia without other major events. His body temperature is slowly returned to normal physiologic range (i.e., 36.5° to 37° C) over 4 hours. Heart rate increases to 120 to 140 bpm and mean arterial pressures remain stable (45 to 55 mmHg). Dopamine is discontinued, and his urine output remains between 2 to 4 mL/kg/hr. Serum electrolytes further normalize by Day 4 with the creatinine decreased to 0.8 mg/dL. He is started on total parenteral nutrition. The midazolam drip is slowly weaned and discontinued. Over the next several days, his examination improves: tone increases and is normal by Day 6, posture is flexed, and his suck reflex becomes more vigorous. He is extubated from the ventilator to room air. Small volume feedings are introduced.

EXERCISE 9

QUESTION

1. Which statement regarding brain imaging is correct in this case?
   a. Imaging does not need to be performed in all cases of encephalopathy and can be reserved for those with prolonged recovery.
   b. Magnetic resonance imaging (MRI) is time consuming, costly, and provides little additional information over computed tomography or head ultrasound.
   c. MRI has the ability to capture the entire spectrum of neuropathologic changes seen with hypoxic-ischemic brain injury.
   d. MRI is most valuable within the first several hours after birth to provide prognostic information.

ANSWER

1. **c.** An MRI scan should be performed during the immediate neonatal period. MRI is the most accurate imaging modality in hypoxic-ischemic brain injury in the term newborn and has the ability to capture the entire spectrum of neuropathologic findings seen with this injury. Diffusion-weighted MRI (DWI), based on differences in the motion of water molecules, is more sensitive and shows injury earlier than conventional MRI.

CASE STUDY 1 (continued)

He has a brain MRI performed on Day 7 (Figure 2-9). Oral feeds are advanced and he is cleared for discharge home by Day 10.

USE OF MRI FOLLOWING HYPOXIC-ISCHEMIC BRAIN INJURY

Brain injury following hypoxia-ischemia is difficult to predict; neuropathologic features are inconsistent and vary depending on the type and duration of insult, gestational age, and whether the infant was treated with hypothermia.

The major patterns of neuropathologic injury seen in hypoxic-ischemic encephalopathy are: (1) selective neuronal necrosis; (2) parasagittal cerebral injury; (3) periventricular leukomalacia; and (4) focal ischemic brain necrosis.

Selective neuronal necrosis is often reflective of extensive death of neurons, is the most common type of injury seen in HIE, and can be further subdivided into three patterns (diffuse, cortical-deep nuclear, and deep nuclear-brain stem) (Table 2-3). Parasagittal cerebral injury refers to necrosis of the characteristic watershed region of the cortex and subcortical white matter with the parieto-occipital cortex particularly

vulnerable. Periventricular leukomalacia (PVL) is a spectrum of white matter necrosis and surrounding gliosis first described by Virchow in 1867 (Virchow, 1867). Although it is most commonly seen in premature infants, PVL accounts for a portion of the injury seen in term infants following hypoxia-ischemia. Focal ischemic necrosis (or arterial stroke) arises in specific vascular distributions of either one or multiple cerebral vessels. It can be seen concomitantly with the previously mentioned patterns of injury, as overlap between these lesions is frequently appreciated.

This DWI image (Figure 2-9) shows restricted diffusion isolated to the bilateral hippocampi. Involvement of the hippocampus is generally seen as part of a constellation of injury involving the basal ganglia and thalamus. This atypical lesion may be a reflection of hypothermia treatment, possibly representing neuroprotection of the basal ganglia and thalami. Perhaps this pattern of injury will be delineated further as more and more infants are treated with hypothermia.

MRI lesions associated with poor outcomes include basal ganglia and thalamic injury (often seen with changes in the central gyrus, see Figure 2-10), with loss of gray-white matter differentiation, and abnormal signal in the posterior limb of the internal capsule.

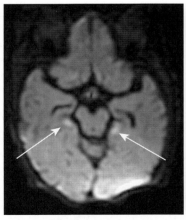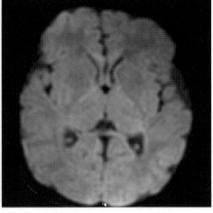

FIGURE 2-9 ■ **Diffusion-weighted MRI performed on Day 7** (see text). Note the hyperintensity in the bilateral hippocampi (*arrows*).

TABLE 2-3 Major Patterns of Selective Neuronal Injury and Relationship to Hypoxic-Ischemic Insult

Pattern	Usual Insult Severity	Usual Duration of Insult
Diffuse	Very severe	Very prolonged
Cerebral cortex-deep nuclear	Moderate to severe	Prolonged
Deep nuclear-brain stem	Severe	Abrupt

Modified from Volpe JJ: Neurology of the newborn, 5th ed, Philadelphia, PA, 2008, Saunders/Elsevier.

In this infant, the MRI was performed on Day 7, which is our standard practice. It is important to note that the timing of imaging may vary depending on institution protocol, stability of the infant to be transported out of the NICU, and availability of the MRI scanner. Evolution of brain injury must also be considered, as MRI-detected injury changes throughout the reperfusion period and as late as the second week of life. For example, diffusion and metabolic changes worsen on MRI until Day 4 or 5 and then begin to normalize, as highlighted by Barkovich and colleagues (Barkovich, Miller, Bartha et al., 2006).

EXERCISE 10

QUESTION

1. Which is an appropriate statement regarding counseling the family prior to discharge?
   a. Providing a specific prognosis during the neonatal period is difficult and often impossible to do.
   b. Close neurodevelopmental follow up is critical for recognizing and appropriately treating delays and/or deficits.
   c. The EEG, neurologic exam, and imaging findings each provide prognostic information that can guide counseling.
   d. All of the above

ANSWER

1. **d.** Determining prognosis in term infants following hypoxic-ischemic encephalopathy is very difficult, as most primary insults occur *in utero* and the extent of the injury is often unknown. This has become even more complex since the advent of therapeutic hypothermia.

Our approach is both optimistic and realistic. Although many factors are considered when counseling parents with regard to long-term prognosis, we focus on: (1) the EEG, e.g., a concerning sign is if the EEG remains abnormal (discontinuous or suppressed) as opposed to a positive sign of sleep-wake cycling; (2) the neurologic examination, e.g., an abnormal examination including the inability to suck/ swallow is concerning; and (3) neuroimaging, e.g., involvement of the basal ganglia portrays a high likelihood of abnormal neurodevelopment. Close neurodevelopmental follow up is crucial to recognizing delays and deficits and prompt referral for therapies is key to maximizing developmental progress.

CONCLUSION

Perinatal asphyxia as a result of interrupted placental blood flow can have significant immediate systemic and neurologic consequences. Anticipation and preparation in the delivery room is a key first step. Effective resuscitation is crucial to the recovery of spontaneous circulation and diligent care during the reperfusion period is critical to mitigating potential ongoing injury. Prompt use of therapeutic hypothermia for qualifying infants, or referral to a NICU capable of hypothermia, should be considered immediately once an infant is stabilized. Our practice employs selective head cooling and the use of continuous aEEG to treat seizures actively and aggressively. Whole-body cooling has shown an equally favorable effect. Similarly important is the correction and management of systemic abnormalities. Pertinent factors should be

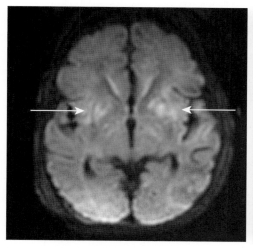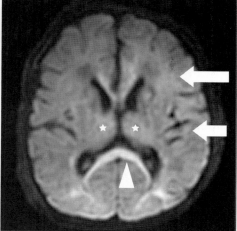

FIGURE 2-10 ■ Sample diffusion-weighted MRI images showing an example of diffuse injury to bilateral basal ganglia (*thin arrows*), thalami (*stars*), corpus callosum (*arrowhead*), and frontal and parietal lobes (*thick arrows*).

extracted from the history and physical examination, laboratory and radiologic data, and clinical course in providing parents with an appropriate long-term outlook.

SUGGESTED READINGS

American Congress of Obstetricians and Gynecologists: Committee Opinion, number 326. Inappropriate use of the terms fetal distress and birth asphyxia, *Obstet Gynecol* 106:1469–1470, 2005.

al Naqeeb N, Edwards AD, Cowan FM, et al.: Assessment of neonatal encephalopathy by amplitude-integrated electroencephalography, *Pediatrics* 103(6):1263–1271, 1999.

Barkovich A, Miller S, Bartha A, et al.: MR imaging, MR spectroscopy, and diffusion tensor imaging of sequential studies in neonates with encephalopathy, *Am J Neuroradiol* 27(3):533–547, 2006.

Barkovich AJ, Westmark K, Partridge C, et al.: Perinatal asphyxia: MR findings in the first 10 days, *Am J Neuroradiol* 16(3):427–438, 1995.

Cowan F, Pennock J, Hanrahan J, et al.: Early detection of cerebral infarction and hypoxic ischemic encephalopathy in neonates using diffusion-weighted magnetic resonance imaging, *Neuropediatrics* 25(4):172–175, 2008.

Dawes G, Jacobson H, Mott JC, et al.: The treatment of asphyxiated, mature foetal lambs and rhesus monkeys with intravenous glucose and sodium carbonate, *Journal Physiol* 169(1):167–184, 1963.

Kattwinkel J, Perlman JM, Aziz K, et al.: Neonatal resuscitation: 2010 American Heart Association Guidelines for Cardiopulmonary Resuscitation and Emergency Cardiovascular Care, *Pediatrics* 126(5):e1400–e1413, 2010.

King TA, Jackson GL, Josey AS, et al.: The effect of profound umbilical artery acidemia in term neonates admitted to a newborn nursery, *Pediatrics* 132(4):624–629, 1998.

Krägeloh–Mann I, Helber A, Mader I, et al.: Bilateral lesions of thalamus and basal ganglia: origin and outcome, *Dev Med Child Neurol* 44(7):477–484, 2002.

Low JA, Galbraith R, Muir D, et al.: Factors associated with motor and cognitive deficits in children after intrapartum fetal hypoxia, *Am J Obstet Gynecol* 148(5):533, 1984.

Martin RJ, Fanaroff AA, Walsh MC: *Fanaroff and Martin's neonatal-perinatal medicine: diseases of the fetus and infant,* 9th ed., Philadelphia, PA, 2011, Mosby/Elsevier.

Martín-Ancel A, García-Alix A, Cabañas FGF, et al.: Multiple organ involvement in perinatal asphyxia, *J Pediatr* 127(5):786–793, 1995.

Pasternak JF, Gorey MT: The syndrome of acute near-total intrauterine asphyxia in the term infant, *Pediatr neurol* 18(5):391–398, 1998.

Perlman J, Tack E, Martin T, et al.: Acute systemic organ injury in term infants after asphyxia, *Am J Dis Child* 143(5):617, 1989.

Perlman JM, Risser R: Severe fetal acidemia: Neonatal neurologic features and short-term outcome, *Pediatr Neurol* 9(4):277–282, 1993.

Polin RA, Fox WW, Abman SH: *Fetal and neonatal physiology,* 4th ed., Philadelphia, PA, 2011, Elsevier/Saunders.

Robertson C, Finer N: Term infants with hypoxic–ischemic encephalopathy: outcome at 3.5 years, *Dev Med Child Neurol* 27(4):473–484, 1985.

Rutherford MA, Pennock JM, Counsell SJ, et al.: Abnormal magnetic resonance signal in the internal capsule predicts poor neurodevelopmental outcome in infants with hypoxic-ischemic encephalopathy, *Pediatrics* 102(2):323–328, 1998.

Salhab WA, Wyckoff MH, Laptook AR, et al.: Initial hypoglycemia and neonatal brain injury in term infants with severe fetal acidemia, *Pediatrics* 114(2):361–366, 2004.

Sarnat HB, Sarnat MS: Neonatal encephalopathy following fetal distress: a clinical and electroencephalographic study, *Arch Neurol* 33(10):696, 1976.

Shalak LF, Laptook AR, Velaphi SC, et al.: Amplitude-integrated electroencephalography coupled with an early neurologic examination enhances prediction of term infants at risk for persistent encephalopathy, *Pediatrics* 111(2):351–357, 2003.

Tagin MA, Woolcott CG, Vincer MJ, et al.: Hypothermia for neonatal hypoxic ischemic encephalopathy: an updated systematic review and meta-analysis, *Arch Pediatrics Adolesc Med* 166(6):558–566, 2012.

Takenouchi T, Rubens EO, Yap VL, et al.: Delayed onset of sleep-wake cycling with favorable outcome in hypothermic-treated neonates with encephalopathy, *J Pediatr* 159(2):232–237, 2011.

Tan A, Schulze A, O'Donnell CP, et al.: Air versus oxygen for resuscitation of infants at birth, *Cochrane Database Syst Rev* 2004 (3):CD002273. doi: 10.1002/14651858. CD002273.pub3.

Thoresen M, Hellström-Westas L, Liu X, et al.: Effect of hypothermia on amplitude-integrated electroencephalogram in infants with asphyxia, *Pediatrics* 126(1):e131–e139, 2010.

Thornberg E, Thiringer K, Odeback A, et al.: Birth asphyxia: incidence, clinical course and outcome in a Swedish population, *Acta Paediatr.* 84(8):927–932, 1995.

Thorp JA, Rushing RS: Umbilical cord blood gas analysis, *Obstet Gynecol Clinics North Am* 26(4):695–709, 1999.

Verma UL, Archbald F, Tejani NA, et al.: Cerebral function monitor in the neonate, I: normal patterns, *Dev Medicine Child Neurol* 26(2):154–161, 1984.

Virchow R: Congenitale Encephalitis und Myelitis, *Archiv für pathologische Anatomie und Physiologie und für klinische Medicin* 38(1):129–138, 1867.

Volpe JJ: *Neurology of the newborn,* 5th ed., Philadelphia, PA, 2008, Saunders/Elsevier.

Wyka KA, Mathews PJ, Rutkowski JA: *Foundations of respiratory care,* Clifton Park, NY, 2011, Delmar, Cengage Learning.

CHAPTER 3

FLUID AND ELECTROLYTE MANAGEMENT IN THE NEWBORN INTENSIVE CARE UNIT

John M. Lorenz, MD

Fluid and electrolyte management is an important and challenging part of the initial care of any very premature or critically ill newborn. The transition from fetal to neonatal life is associated with major changes in fluid and electrolyte homeostasis and total body balance. Before birth the fetus has a constant and ready supply of water and electrolytes; homeostasis is largely a function of maternal and placental mechanisms. After birth, newborns must rapidly assume responsibility for their own fluid and electrolyte homeostasis in an environment in which water and electrolyte availability and losses are much more variable and less subject to feedback control than *in utero*. Moreover, significant contraction of the extracellular fluid (ECF) space occurs with the transition from fetal to neonatal life. In very premature newborns, this transition is also associated with a change in internal potassium (K) balance: K shifts from the intracellular fluid (ICF) space to the ECF space. The goal of fluid and electrolyte therapy in the immediate postnatal period is not to maintain fluid and electrolyte balance, but to allow the appropriate changes in balance to occur without detrimental perturbations in fluid and electrolyte status.

BODY WATER AND SODIUM

A weight loss of about 5% to 12% is almost invariable during the first week of life in preterm infants (Bauer, 1989; Lorenz, 1982; Shaffer, 1987). Although inadequate caloric intake may contribute to this weight loss, multiple studies have found that it results in large part from contraction of the ECF space after birth (Bauer, 1989; Bauer, 1991; Hartnoll, 2000; Heimler, 1993; Shaffer, 1986; Shaffer & Meade, 1989) (Figure 3-1). The following data suggest that contraction of the ECF space is physiologic:

- It occurs in spite of large variation in water and sodium (Na) intake (Lorenz, 1982; Shaffer & Meade, 1989).
- It occurs even if caloric/protein intake mitigates postnatal weight loss (Heimler, 1993).
- When postnatal weight loss is regained, ECW volume per kg body weight remains stable at the new lower level (Singhi, 1995).
- Attenuation of this decrease may be associated with increased morbidity (Bell & Acarregui, 2008; Costarino, 1992; Hartnoll, 2000).

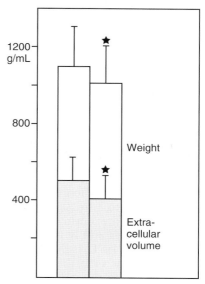

FIGURE 3-1 ■ **Postnatal changes in body weight, extracellular fluid volume, and sodium balance in very premature infants.** (From Bauer K, Versmold H: Postnatal weight loss in preterm neonates less than 1,500 grams is due to isotonic dehydration of the extracellular volume, *Acta Paediatr Scand Suppl* 360:37-42, 1989.)

TABLE 3-1   **Postnatal Renal, Fluid, and Electrolyte Adaptation in Very Premature Newborns**

Phase	Prediuretic	Diuretic/Natriuretic	Homeostatic
Age	~ Birth-2 days	~ 1-5 days	After ~ 2-5 days
Urine output	Low	Abrupt ↑↑	↓ then α intake
Sodium excretion	Minimal	Abrupt ↑↑	↓ then α intake
Potassium excretion	Minimal	Abrupt ↑↑	↓ then α intake
Water balance	< intake-IWL	Markedly negative	~ α sodium balance
Sodium balance	~ negative	Markedly negative	Stable, then positive w/growth
Potassium balance	~ negative	Markedly negative	Stable, then positive w/growth
ECF volume (mL)	Stable or ~ ↓	Abrupt ↓↓	1. α sodium balance 2. ↑ w/ growth
Creatinine clearance	Low	Abrupt ↑↑	± ↓, then gradual ↑ with maturation
FENa	Variable	↑	Gradual ↓
FEK	Variable	No change	No change
Urine osmolality	Moderately hyposmotic	Moderately hyposmotic	Moderately hyposmotic
Common problems	Water intoxication with lower IWL than anticipated		Water and sodium retention with PDA, CLD
	Hypernatremia with higher IWL than anticipated	Hypernatremia	Water and sodium depletion with or without hyponatremia
	Hyperkalemia		Hypokalemia
		Hyperglycemia	

DIURESIS AND NATRIURESIS

Negative total body water (TBW) and total body sodium (TBNa) balances are associated with contraction of ECF space. In most infants, the excretion of water and Na that occurs as a result of contraction of the ECF space in the first few days of life is not gradual. In fact, a characteristic pattern of fluid and electrolyte adaptation, which is largely independent of fluid and electrolyte intake, is observed in the first week of life in the majority of very low birth weight newborns (Bidiwala, 1988; Costarino, 1985; Lorenz, 1982; Lorenz, 1995). Usually, three phases can be distinguished. Table 3-1 summarizes the changes in fluid and electrolyte balance, ECF volume, and renal function associated with each phase. Table 3-2 summaries recommended water, Na, and K intakes in the first week of life.

During the first 12 to 48 hours of life, the urine flow rate is low (0.5 to 3 mL/kg/hour), regardless of intake. Therefore, during this prediuretic phase, excretion of Na and K is also quite low; insensible water loss (IWL) is the major route of water loss. At the same time, the low glomerular filtration rate (GFR) in the immediate perinatal period limits the infant's ability to excrete water and electrolyte loads.

As the diuretic/natriuretic phase begins, an abrupt increase in urinary water and Na occurs independent of water and Na intake, and heralds contraction of the ECF space. Early in the diuretic/natriuretic phase, serum Na concentration ($[Na^+]$) often rises because water balance is more negative than sodium balance. The majority of body weight loss occurs during this phase. A fall in serum K concentration ($[K^+]$) can be anticipated as increased delivery of water and Na to the distal nephron stimulates K secretion and kaliuresis. As the ECF space stabilizes at an appropriate volume, urinary water and electrolyte excretion decrease and begin to vary appropriately with intake.

This negative TBW and TBNa balance and reduction of ECF volume during this postnatal diuresis/natriuresis in the immediate newborn period may represent excretion of fetal pulmonary fluid, which is absorbed from the alveolar space and interstitium of the lung prior to delivery and in the immediate postnatal period.

POTASSIUM

The serum $[K^+]$ rises in the first 24 to 72 hours after birth in very premature infants, even in the absence of exogenous K intake or renal failure (Lorenz, 1997; Sato, 1995). This increase results from the shift of K from the ICF space to the ECF space; urine outputs are usually normal in affected infants (i.e., nonoliguric hyperkalemia). The magnitude of this shift correlates roughly

TABLE 3-2 **Guidelines for Initiating and Adjusting Fluid and Electrolyte Therapy in Appropriate for Gestational Age Infants Nursed Naked in an Incubator with 50% Ambient Humidity and Ambient Air Temperature in the Neutral Thermal Range**

	Day of Life 1	Adjustment During Prediuretic Phase	Adjustment During Diuretic/Natriuretic Phase	Adjustment During Homeostatic Phase
Water	23-24 wk: 150 mL/kg/d 25-27 wk: 120 mL/kg/d 28-30 wk: 100 mL/kg/d 31-36 wk: 80 mL/kg/d >36 wk: 60 mL/kg/d	**Increase if:** Wt loss >2 %/day or serum [Na$^+$] increases **Decrease if:** Wt increases or serum [Na$^+$] increases	**Increase** 10-30 mL/kg/d if: wt loss >5 %/day or serum [Na] >150 mL/kg/d with no sodium intake **Decrease** 10-30 mL/kg/d if: wt loss <1%/day	Increase volume to optimize caloric intake without fluid retention
Na	None	None	**Begin** 1-2 mmol/kg/d if: serum [Na$^+$] <135 mmol/L with wt loss or serum [Na$^+$] <130 mmol/L with no change or gain in wt	Approximate sodium loss ± growth allowance—sodium requirement will be inversely proportional to gestational age
K	None	None	**Begin** 1-2 mmol/L/d if: serum [K$^+$] is <5 mmol/L and serum [K$^+$] is not ↑ing and urine output is >1 mL/kg/hr	≥2-3 mmol/kg/d to maintain serum [K$^+$] normal
Glucose	4-8 mg/kg/min; adjust to maintain normal serum glucose concentration	Change in fluid requirement may require change in dextrose concentration	↑ fluid requirement may require ↓ dextrose concentration	↑ as tolerated to maximize caloric intake

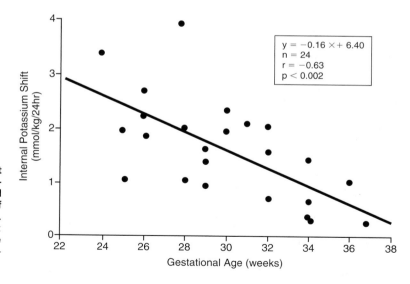

FIGURE 3-2 ■ **Magnitude of the shift in potassium from the intracellular fluid to the extracellular fluid space during the first 24 hours of life as a function of gestational age.** (From Sato K, Kondo T, Iwao H, et al.: Internal potassium shift in premature infants: cause of nonoliguric hyperkalemia, *J Pediatr* 126:109-113, 1995.)

with the degree of prematurity and has been associated with decreased levels of Na/K ATPase. Clinically significant nonoliguric hyperkalemia rarely occurs after 30 to 32 weeks of gestation (Sato, 1995) (Figure 3-2). However, it affected 25% to 50% of infants weighing less than 1000 grams at birth or born before 28 weeks' gestation (Fukada, 1989; Gruskay, 1988; Lorenz, 1997; Shaffer, 1992; Stephano, 1993) prior to the more prevalent use of antenatal steroids

(ANS). ANS are associated with decreased risk of nonoliguric hyperkalemia (Omar, 1992) and are likely the major factor responsible for the decreased prevalence of nonoliguric hyperkalemia in NICUs today.

GLUCOSE

With the clamping of the umbilical cord at birth, the supply of glucose and other nutrients from the mother ceases and neonatal glucose production begins. As a result, serum glucose concentration ([GLU]) falls sharply over the first 45 to 90 minutes of life (Heck, 1987; Metzger, 2010; Srinivasan, 1984). In response to this fall in serum glucose concentration, there are abrupt increases in the levels of epinephrine, norepinephrine, and glucagon with a concomitant fall in insulin. Although the effect of these counterregulatory hormones on glucose metabolism is not as robust as in the adult, these responses mobilize glucose from glycogen stores and promote gluconeogenesis. Glucose utilization averages 4 to 8 mg/kg/minute in term and preterm newborns (Bier, 1977; Sunehag, 1993). Endogenous glucose production may be inadequate to maintain a normal serum [GLU] in infants with prematurity, perinatal stress, or intrauterine growth restriction. In this case exogenous administration of glucose at a rate that matches the rate of glucose utilization is necessary to conserve glycogen stores and prevent hypoglycemia (Tryala, 1994).

Premature infants are also at increased risk for hyperglycemia with exogenous glucose infusions because of a decreased hepatic responsiveness to insulin and a greater metabolic clearance rate for insulin (Farrag, 1997). As will be obvious later in this chapter, neonatal hyperglycemia is associated with increased morbidity and mortality.

CASE STUDY 1

Ms. M presents at 23 weeks' gestation in normal spontaneous preterm labor with intact membranes. She is tocolyzed with MgSO₄ and receives a course of betamethasone. Contractions subside, but recur after 4 days. When she develops a low-grade fever tocolysis is discontinued, and a 550-gram male infant is delivered at 24 weeks' gestation. The baby is stabilized on synchronous intermittent mechanical ventilation (SIMV) support and nursed in an incubator with 50% relative humidity. Abdominal skin temperature is servo-controlled to a temperature of 36.5° C. An umbilical venous catheter (UVC) and an umbilical arterial catheter (UAC) are placed.

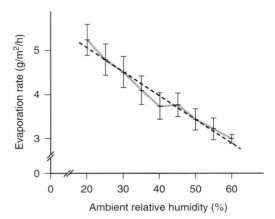

FIGURE 3-3 ■ **Transepidermal water loss (IWL from the skin) as a function of ambient humidity.** Mean ± SE; dashed line = regression line (R = −0.986). (From Hammarlund K, Nilsson GE, Oberg PA, et al.: Transepidermal water loss in newborn infants. Relation to ambient humidity and site of measurement and estimation of total transepidermal water loss, *Acta Paediatr Scand* 66:553-562, 1977.)

EXERCISE 1

QUESTIONS

1. At what rate should intravenous fluid be started?

2. What should be infused though the UAC?

3. How much sodium and potassium should be administered?

4. What should the concentration of dextrose be in the umbilical venous line infusate?

ANSWERS

1. As discussed, during the prediuretic period, the total water infusion rate (UVC + UAC) should approximate estimated IWL. IWL varies with environmental humidity (Figure 3-3), gestational and postnatal age (Figure 3-4), and exposure to ANS. IWL decreases with increasing ambient humidity (Hammarlund, 1977), increasing gestational and postnatal age (see Figure 3-3) (Hammarlund, 1983), and ANS exposure (Dimitriou, 2005; Omar, 1999). The accuracy of IWL estimation is critical because this will be by far the major route of water loss at this gestational and postnatal age and is not subject to feedback control. However, estimation of IWL is imprecise for several reasons. First, IWL is highly variable among individual neonates even when all variables affecting it are equal. Second, values for transepidermal water loss (cutaneous IWL, excluding respiratory IWL) are likely to overestimate IWL because they are calculated on the assumption

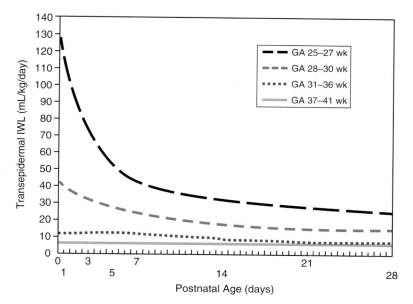

FIGURE 3-4 ■ **Transepidermal water loss as a function of gestational and postnatal age.** (From Lorenz JM: Maintenance fluid requirements. In Polin RA, Spitzer A, editors: *Fetal and neonatal secrets,* 2nd ed, Philadelphia, PA, Hanley & Belfus, Inc, 2007, pp 154-190. Drawn from data from Hammarlund K, Sedin G, Strömberg B: Transepidermal water loss in newborn infants VIII. Relation to gestational age and post-natal age in appropriate and small for gestational age infants, *Acta Paediatr Scand* 72:721-728, 1983.)

that the baby's entire body surface area is exposed to the gaseous environment (which is not the case when the baby is lying on a mattress), and most of the data are from an era in which the use of ANS (which decrease IWL) was much less prevalent than today. Third, there are no measurements of IWL in newborns delivered at 23 weeks' gestation and the data from infants 24 to 25 weeks' gestation is extremely sparse (Agren, 1998). Based on the data of Agren and colleagues, mean (95% CI) IWL for the newborn in this case study would be 164 (range 74 to 254) mL/kg/day during the first day of life if the mother received ANS. Because only about two-thirds of the baby's surface area is exposed to the gaseous environment (the Hooven correction), IWL would range from 50 to 170 mL/kg/day. To err on the side of caution, total water intake should be 120 to 150 mL/kg/dL (because of the risk of hypernatremia if IWL is underestimated in combination with the amount of Na administered via the UAC [see below]).

2. An incredible array of UAC infusates are used in different NICUs with astonishingly little data. In a survey of 13 NICUs, 0.25 normal saline, 0.5 normal saline, and D_5W were most commonly used; use of normal saline was the least common (Fletcher, 1994). Saline solutions offer the advantage of facilitating accurate determination of serum [GLU] and serum [Na+], but can deliver significant exogenous sodium at a time when excretion of a Na load is limited by low GFR. A lower Na concentration in the infusate will decrease the Na intake, but increase the

risk of obtaining a spuriously low serum [Na+] owing to dilution of the sample with the infusate. Moreover, the more hypotonic the saline solution, the greater the risk of hemolysis of red blood cells in the solution drawn to clear the line and during subsequent flushing of the line (Jackson, 2000). Dextrose solutions (D_5W is isotonic) have the advantage of avoiding Na intake, but have a greater risk of obtaining spuriously low serum [Na+] and spuriously high serum [GLU] (Brown, 1975). There are no data regarding the minimal infusion rate necessary to maintain UAC patency (with or without heparin), but 1 mL/hr is commonly used. In this case, 0.5 normal saline is infused at 1 mL/hr in order facilitate accurate determination of serum [GLU] and serum [Na+] on samples obtained from the UAC (Brown, 1975), minimize hemolysis (Jackson, 2000), and limit sodium intake. This will provide 44 mL/kg/d of water and 3.4 mmol/kg/d of Na (1 mL/hr × 77 mmol/L × 1 L/1000 mL × 24 mL/hr/day × 1/0.55 kg).

3. None. Urinary Na losses are low during the prediuretic period (1 to 3 mmol/kg/day) (Bidiwala, 1988; Lorenz, 1993) because the GFR is low. Furthermore, Na losses from the gastrointestinal (GI) tract are minimal. Therefore, Na intake via the UAC is already in excess of estimated losses. Moreover, if IWL is underestimated, any exogenous Na intake will exacerbate hypernatremia. Urinary K secretory capacity and excretion will also be low and there is still a possibility of nonoliguric hyperkalemia, even with ANS exposure. Therefore, no K intake should be administered until it is certain that the serum [K] is *not rising* and renal function is known to be normal.

4. The concentration of dextrose depends on the rate of dextrose to be provided and the volume infused; 75 to 105 mL/kg/day of 5% dextrose water (D_5W) will provide 2.2 to 3.1 mg/kg/minute; 75 to 105 mL of 10% dextrose water ($D_{10}W$) will provide 4.5 to 6.3 mg/kg/minute. The latter is in the range of endogenous glucose production, so $D_{10}W$ should be infused though the UVC.

CASE STUDY 1 (continued)

Total fluid intake is held constant at 140 mL/day of water, which provides 5.8 mg/kg/minute of glucose. Over the first 36 hours of life, the urine out averaged 2.1 mL/kg/hr, but it has been increasing over the last 8 hours. The serum [Na+] is 139 mmol/L at 8 hours, 137 mmol/L at 20 hours and 140 mmol/L at 32 hours of life. The serum glucose concentration ([GLU]) has ranged from 6.7 to 7.8 mmol/L (120 to 140 mg/dL). Over the next 12 hours, the urine output increases to 3.5 mL/kg/hr and the serum [Na+] rises to 148 mmol/L. The body weight is 525 grams. Fluid intake is increased to 170 mL/kg/day because of the rising serum [Na+] and 9% loss of body weight in the first 2 days of life. Over the next several hours, the serum glucose concentration increases to 8.9 to 10 mmol/L (160 to 180 mg/dL). The urine output is now 4 mL/kg/hr.

EXERCISE 2

QUESTIONS

1. Is the baby hyperglycemic?

2. Why has the infant developed an elevated serum [GLU]?

3. What are the risks of hyperglycemia?

4. What should be done to decrease the serum [GLU]?

ANSWERS

1. There is no consensus regarding a definition for hyperglycemia in the newborn. Serum [GLU] >8.3 and >10 mmol/L (>150 and >180 mg/dL) have both been used. "Normal" serum glucose concentration is <6.6 mmol/L (<120 mg/dL).

2. When the infusion rate through the UVC was increased and the dextrose concentration in the infusate was held constant, the glucose administration rate increased to 7.5 mg/kg/minute and was not tolerated.

3. Regardless of the exact threshold, hyperglycemia is associated with increased risk of severe intracranial hemorrhage, late-onset bacterial infection, necrotizing enterocolitis, and retinopathy of

prematurity in preterm infants (Bottino, 2011). There are no data, however, to confirm that lowering serum [GLU] below these thresholds prevents these morbidities or mortality.

A serum [GLU] >8.3 mmol/L (>150 mg/dL) is associated with glucosuria in moderately preterm newborns; more immature infants exhibit glucosuria at lower serum glucose values (Stonestreet, 1980). Glucosuria can be associated with increased urinary Na losses, although these are generally not clinically significant.

4. It is not clear that there is any benefit in treating hyperglycemia except perhaps in the unusual circumstance in which osmotic diuresis causes dehydration. If treatment is required, it is best to treat hyperglycemia by decreasing the dextrose infusion rate whenever possible. Alternatively, if intravenous lipids are being given, the rate of infusion can be reduced or even temporarily discontinued if the hyperglycemia persists. Another alternative is to initiate an insulin drip. However, insulin pharmacokinetics have not been well delineated in extremely low birth weight infants and hypoglycemia is more common with insulin therapy (Beardsall, 2008). Moreover, insulin is absorbed by intravenous tubing, which decreases its bioavailability. Impregnating the tubing with 5 IU/L of insulin for 20 minutes reduces absorption, but 100% bioavailability is not achieved until 8 hours even with this strategy (Fuloria, 1998).

CASE STUDY 2

Baby girl A is an 840-gram, 25-weeks' gestation infant delivered by emergent cesarean section because of severe maternal preeclampsia. One dose of betamethasone was given shortly before delivery. She is placed in an incubator with 50% relative humidity and started on 10% dextrose in water at 120 mL/kg/day. At 12 hours of age, the serum [Na+] is 146 mmol/L. The only sodium intake has been via the UAC (as 0.5 normal saline) at 1 mL/hour. Urine output has averaged 1.1 mL/kg/hour.

EXERCISE 3

QUESTIONS

1. Why is the baby hypernatremic?

2. What are the risks of hypernatremia?

3. What do you anticipate will happen in the next 12 to 24 hours if no changes are made in water or Na intake?

4. Given this expectation, what changes, if any, should be made in water and/or Na intake?

5. When should serum [Na+] be rechecked?

ANSWERS

1. Serum [Na+] is determined by TBW volume and TBNa content. Serum [Na+] may be high because either TBW is abnormally low or TBNa is abnormally high, or both. However, during the first day of life changes in serum [Na+] are largely the result of changes in water balance because Na losses in the prediuretic period are low. Sodium intake is only 1.1 mmol/day via the UAC. Therefore, it is unlikely that TBNa balance is positive enough to be responsible for the increase in serum [Na+]. In this case, hypernatremia is a result of IWL in excess of that anticipated. This conclusion would be supported by a decrease in body weight, although this information is not available.

2. Compared to the rate of water diffusion, even small ions, like Na, diffuse slowly across the blood–brain barrier into the interstitial fluid (ISF) space of the central nervous system. Thus, when the serum (and thereby osmolality) rises rapidly, osmotic equilibrium between serum and central nervous system ISF initially must be maintained by the movement of water from the brain. This causes the central nervous system ISF space pressure to fall, causing capillaries in the brain to dilate and possibly rupture. High-pitched cry, irritability, seizures, impaired consciousness, intracranial hemorrhage, cerebral infarction, long-term neurodevelopmental disability, or death may result. The risk of intracranial hemorrhage depends on the degree and rapidity of the increase in serum [Na+], but does not generally occur with serum [Na+] <150 mmol/L.

3. IWL will continue to be high; therefore, it is likely that serum [Na+] will continue to increase. Furthermore, diuresis/natriuresis can be expected to begin over the next 12 to 24 hours. Although water and Na balance are both expected to be negative during the diuretic/natriuretic period, serum [Na+] may rise—even if water intake is sufficient for IWL—because change water balance may be more negative than change Na balance during this period.

4. Water intake should be increased; however, how much of an increase can only be roughly estimated. Note, however, that the percent change in TBW will be greater than the percent change in serum [Na+] because the increase in ECF [Na+] is blunted by the movement of water from the ICF to the ECF space. This must occur to maintain osmolality equilibrium across cell membranes. In this case, if we assume the baby's serum [Na+] concentration at birth was approximately 140 mmol/L (which would be the case if maternal serum [Na+] was normal), serum [Na+] increased 4%. Therefore, an increase in water intake a little more than this will be necessary to stabilize serum [Na+] and a substantially greater increase in water intake will be needed to decrease serum [Na+]. An increase in water intake of 8% to 10% (or an increase of ~10 mL/kg/day to 130 mL/kg/day) is a rough estimation. With the onset of diuresis/natriuresis, a further increase might be necessary.

5. With all the variables involved, the appropriateness of any estimated change in water intake is subject to error. Therefore, serum [Na+] should be rechecked in 6 to 8 hours to be sure that serum [Na+] is *gradually* changing in the right direction. Once the water and sodium distribution across the blood–brain barrier have both reached equilibrium, too rapid a decrease in serum [Na+] will result in water movement into the brain faster than Na can move out, resulting in cerebral edema.

CASE STUDY 3

Baby girl N was born at 39 weeks' gestation after an unremarkable pregnancy. Apgar scores were 9 and 9. She is rooming in with her mother and breastfeeding. The morning after delivery, mother reports that the baby—now 28 hours of age—was fussy overnight, but is now quieter. The nurse notes bilious emesis on the crib sheet. When she takes the baby from the mother and removes the blanket, she finds more bilious emesis. The baby is listless with acrocyanosis and abdominal distension. The diaper is dry. A NICU fellow is called and immediately transports the baby to the intensive care nursery. On admission, the heart rate is 165 bpm, respiratory rate 68/minute, temperature 98.6° F, mean blood pressure 32 mmHg, and oxygen saturation 95%. The weight is unchanged from delivery. The baby is listless but responsive. The hands and feet are cool, the capillary refill time is 4 seconds, and the pulses are diminished. The abdomen is distended and firm. A peripheral IV is started.

EXERCISE 4

QUESTIONS

1. What is the likely pathophysiology responsible for the poor perfusion and hypotension?

2. What is your differential diagnosis?

3. What is the first thing to do for this baby?

ANSWERS

1. The hypotension in this case is likely caused by a relative decrease in the blood volume, secondary to sepsis-induced vasodilatation or a decrease in ECF volume owing to an intraabdominal process.

A normal hematocrit does not exclude the possibility of an intraabdominal hemorrhage, because there are usually no changes in the hematocrit with acute blood loss until the blood volume is replaced with either crystalloid or plasma. A decrease in ECF volume can result from accumulation of fluid in the intestinal lumen with bowel obstruction or movement of ECF water and sodium into injured cells. The latter occurs with impaired function of the Na^+K^+-ATPase pump in the cell membrane secondary to hypoxia or ischemia. With impaired function of the Na^+K^+-ATPase pump, there is net movement of solute (and secondarily water) into the cell. "Loss" of Na and water into the bowel lumen or the ICF space is referred to as *third space losses*. The stable body weight does not exclude either blood loss or loss of ECF into ICF space, because there is no loss from the body. Vasodilatation owing to sepsis might be independent of the intraabdominal process (in which case the abdominal distention could be caused by an ileus) or associated intraabdominal pathology.

2. The short list of differential diagnoses is intestinal obstruction, necrotizing enterocolitis, or sepsis. Bilious emesis is most consistent with proximal intestinal distension. The systemic signs suggest that the proximal bowel obstruction is associated with intestinal perforation or ischemic bowel. The combination of bilious emesis and systemic signs of illness are most consistent with midgut volvulus, which requires an urgent laparotomy.

3. The baby's compromised hemodynamic status requires *immediate* volume resuscitation. At this time distinguishing among the possible etiologies of the hypotension is unimportant for deciding what blood product or solution should be used. Therefore, regardless of whether the problem is hypovolemia (decreased blood or plasma volume or vasodilatation owing to shock) or a decreased extracellular volume, the emergent treatment is the same: volume expansion with normal saline. Although 5% albumin might be considered for hypovolemia, studies have not shown it to be superior to normal saline for treatment of hypotension (Oca, 2003; So, 1997). The volume of saline must be titrated to therapeutic response because body weight is of no help in estimating the endogenous loss.

CASE STUDY 3 (continued)

Blood pressure and perfusion improve after three (10 mL/kg) boluses of normal saline (total 30 mL/kg). Bilious fluid is suctioned from the stomach after placement of the nasogastric tube. Abdominal films demonstrate complete obstruction of the proximal intestine without free air. The baby is taken directly to the operating room for an exploratory laparotomy for suspected midgut volvulus. In the operating room, malrotation with midgut volvulus is confirmed, necrotic bowel is resected, and the baby returns to the NICU with an ileostomy and mucous fistula.

EXERCISE 5
QUESTION

1. Is this a true or false statement? "Because the necrotic bowel has been resected, third space loss is no longer concerning."

ANSWER

1. **False**. Handling of viable bowel during the exploratory laparotomy may result in transient cellular dysfunction that can lead to third space losses.

CASE STUDY 4

Baby boy O-B is a 668-gram, 26-weeks' gestation, first of twins, who was delivered by cesarean section after spontaneous onset of preterm labor and breech presentation. His mother received no ANS. Apgar scores are 1 at 1 min and 4 at 5 min and positive pressure ventilation and intubation are needed in the delivery room. An umbilical arterial blood gas shows a pH of 6.87 and a base excess of –27 mmol/L. He is started on mechanical ventilation and placed under a radiant warmer. A UAC is placed and $D_{10}W$ (with no Na added) is started via a peripheral IV for a total fluid intake of 110 mL/kg/d. The mean arterial blood pressure is 28 mmHg and the baby is warm and well perfused. By 8 hours of age the baby has largely cleared the metabolic acidosis and is stable on low IMV support after a dose of surfactant. The weight is 643 grams. There has been 0.6 mL/kg/hr of urine output since birth. Serum [Na^+] is 132 mmol/L, serum [K^+] 6.5 mmol/L, serum [Creat] is 88 μmol/L (1.0 mg/dL), serum [GLU] 8.8 mmol/L (9159 mg/dL), and base excess –12 mmol/L. He is in normal sinus rhythm with a heart rate of 135 beats per minute.

EXERCISE 6
QUESTIONS

1. Is the baby's renal function normal?

2. Does this baby have nonoliguric hyperkalemia?

3. Would you treat the hyperkalemia?

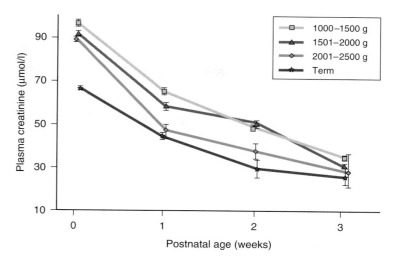

FIGURE 3-5 ■ **Change in plasma [Creat] in the first 3 weeks of life in healthy full-term infants and premature infants with uncomplicated postnatal courses (88 μmol/L creatinine = 1 mg/dL).** (From Bueva A, Guignard JP: Renal function in pre-term neonates, *Pediatr Res* 36:572-577, 1994.)

ANSWERS

1. It is too soon after birth to evaluate the baby's renal function. Initially, the newborn's serum [Creat] is a function of mother's serum [Creat] (Guignard & Drukker, 1999). A single serum [Creat], therefore, indicates nothing about the baby's GFR at this age. Renal function is best reflected by the *change* in serum [Creat] over time. This urine flow rate is not necessarily abnormal in the immediate newborn period (Bidiwala & Lorenz, 1995).

2. Nonoliguric hyperkalemia occurs by definition in spite of normal renal function. It is too early to assess this infant's renal function; therefore, it is impossible to differentiate nonoliguric hyperkalemia from renal failure. However, because the serum [K+] has increased from birth with no K intake, then it is likely caused by a shift of K from the ICF to ECF space.

3. There is no consensus about the criteria for treating hyperkalemia in the newborn. Considerations included the rate of rise in serum [K+], the degree of hyperkalemia, and the presence of electrocardiographic changes or arrhythmias consistent with hyperkalemia. Cardiac arrhythmias are unusual with serum [K+] <7 to 8 mmol/L. In this case, the serum [K+] is very likely to continue to increase and measures should be taken to lower the serum [K+].

CASE STUDY 4 (continued)

No therapy for hyperkalemia in initiated. By 16 hours of age, the infant's weight is 630 grams. He remains on 100 mL/kg/day and receives no K. There has been 0.4 mL/kg/hr of urine output in the last 8 hours. Serum [Na+] is 141 mmol/L, serum [K+] 7.8 mmol/L, serum [GLU] 13.5 mmol/L (175 mg/dL), *serum [Creat] is 115 μmol/L (1.3 mg/dL), and base excess is −10 mmol/L. Serum ionized calcium concentration ([Ca++]) is low normal. He remains in a normal sinus rhythm with a heart rate of 120 beats per minute. Mean blood pressure is stable at 28 mmHg.*

EXERCISE 7

QUESTIONS

1. Is the baby in acute renal failure?

2. Does this baby have nonoliguric hyperkalemia?

3. Would you treat the hyperkalemia?

4. What changes would you make in fluid and electrolyte intake?

ANSWERS

1. Although urine output is still not abnormal for an infant of this age, an increase in serum creatinine concentration [Creat] of 26 μmol/L (0.3 mg/dL) over 8 hours is abnormal and probably indicative of renal failure. The rate of change in serum [Creat] after birth depends largely on the GFR. Because GFR increases with gestational age, the rate of change in serum [Creat] after birth varies with gestational age (Figure 3-5) (Bueva & Guignard, 1994). In extremely preterm infants, serum creatinine may rise 9 to 26 μmol/L (0.1 to 0.3 mg/dL) over the first few days of life, then return to the original base line and decrease slowly (Figure 3-6) (Choker & Gouyon, 2004; Miall, 1999).

2. This infant requires immediate treatment for hyperkalemia. Furthermore, additional increases in serum [K+] are likely. The slightly lower heart rate could be caused by hyperkalemia.

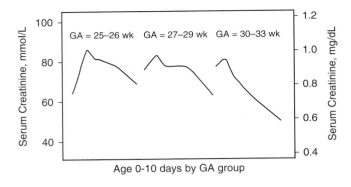

FIGURE 3-6 ■ **Change in plasma [Creat] in preterm infants without risk factors for acute renal failure over the 10 days of life as a function of gestational age.** (From Bateman BA, Thomas W, Paraviccini E, Lorenz JM: Unpublished data, 2013.)

3. Treatment strategies should first include preventing hyperkalemia and antagonizing its cardiac toxicity. These include: (1) withholding K from the intravenous fluids given to extremely preterm infants after birth until the serum [K+] is normal and not rising and renal function is judged to be normal; and (2) preventing/treating hypocalcemia aggressively. Hypocalcemia potentiates the cardiotoxic effects of hyperkalemia. Slow intravenous pushes of 0.5 to 1.0 mEq/kg elemental calcium (1 to 2 mL/kg of 10% calcium gluconate solution) can be given to treat life-threatening arrhythmias, although the effect is short lived. The second strategy is to stimulate the cellular uptake of K by maximizing glucose administration (with or without exogenous insulin), and/or by using inhaled albuterol (Hu, 1999; Malone, 1991; Singh, 2002). Albuterol inhalation therapy has been shown to be effective, but there are limited safety data. Insulin therapy is also effective, but is subject to the difficulties in regulating serum [GLU] as discussed above. In extreme circumstances, total body K can be decreased by removing K with peritoneal dialysis. Ion exchanges resins, which increase colonic secretion of K, are not recommended because of lack of efficacy compared to insulin therapy (Hu, 1999; Malone, 1991) and risk of serious intestinal complications (Bennet, 1996; Grammatikopoulos, 2003; Ohlsson & Hosking, 1987).

4. The total fluid intake should be increased. In spite of the low urine output and the possibility of acute renal failure, the baby's weight loss and increase in serum [Na+] from 132 to 141 mmol/L suggests that water balance is negative. It is important to remember that the serum glucose concentration will likely rise with any increase in the UVC infusion rate (if the same concentration of dextrose is infused through the UVC). However, the serum [GLU] is only mildly elevated at present and a slightly higher serum [GLU] may be advantageous to stimulate endogenous insulin secretion and promote movement of K into cells. However, serum [GLU] should be followed closely. A decrease in the glucose administration rate or initiation of an insulin drip will be necessary if serum [GLU] continues to increase.

CASE STUDY 4 (continued)

The heart rate increases after the intravenous infusion of calcium gluconate. The clinicians start albuterol inhalation treatments every 2 hours and the serum [K] falls to 6.8 mmol/L by 24 hours. Fluid intake is increased to 130 mL/kg/day. The new body weight is 645 grams. Over the last 8 hours, urine output has averaged 0.5 mL/kg/hr. Serum [Na+] is 135 mmol/L, serum [Creat] is 150 μmol/L (1.7 mg/dL), serum [GLU] is 9 mmol/L (162 mg/dL), and base excess is −5 mmol/L. The hematocrit is stable at 45%, the mean arterial blood pressure is normal, and the baby is well perfused. He remains in a normal sinus rhythm, but is now tachycardic with a heart rate of 175 beats per minute. Mean blood pressure is stable.

EXERCISE 8

QUESTIONS

1. Is the baby in acute renal failure?

2. What is the significance of the tachycardia?

3. Should the albuterol inhalation treatment be discontinued?

ANSWERS

1. This infant is definitely in acute renal failure. An increase in serum [Creat] of 62 μmol/L (0.7 mg/dL) over 16 hours is clearly abnormal and indicative of a very low GFR. Note that anuria/oliguria is not a necessary criteria for acute renal failure in the newborn (Karlowicz & Adelman, 1995). The cause of the acute renal failure must be considered now to determine if it is reversible or not; this will determine management. Oligoanuria may be prerenal, intrinsic (owing to

renal parenchymal maldevelopment or injury), or postrenal in origin. Prerenal failure (e.g., owing to decrease in renal blood flow as the result of dehydration, hypovolemia, decreased effective blood volume, decreased cardiac output) is most common in the newborn intensive care unit and very often difficult to exclude; importantly, though, *prerenal failure may progress to intrinsic renal failure if the cause is not promptly treated.* If prerenal failure is suspected, a 10 to 20 mL/kg intravenous bolus of normal saline should be given over 30 minutes), unless ECF volume expansion is strongly contraindicated by a concomitant condition. If there is no response, a second bolus of normal saline may be given. If there is no correction of the oliguria or anuria, intrinsic renal failure is likely and low-dose dopamine (0.5 to 2 μg/kg/minute) might be considered. Although there is some evidence that this improves urine output in newborns with normotensive oliguria (Lynch, 2003), a beneficial effect on GFR has not been demonstrated convincingly (Prins, 2001).

2. The tachycardia could be caused by the albuterol inhalation treatments, but hypovolemia or excessive contraction of the ECF space are diagnostic possibilities. If the baby has prerenal failure, volume expansion will likely improve renal function and prevent progression to intrinsic renal failure. In this case, however, prerenal failure is unlikely—the baby has largely cleared the metabolic acidosis at birth, there is no identifiable internal hemorrhage, and body weight is down only 3%.

3. Albuterol should be continued. If acute renal failure persists, serum [K+] will increase if albuterol is discontinued. However, heart rate and blood pressure should continue to be monitored closely.

CASE STUDY 4 (continued)

The baby is given 10 mL/kg of normal saline without a decrease in the heart rate. Tachycardia persists despite a second 10 mL/kg bolus. A cranial ultrasound shows bilateral germinal matrix hemorrhages. Albuterol inhalation treatments are discontinued. The heart rate gradually decreases to 150 bpm. At 32 hours of age, the serum [GLU] increases to 10 mmol/L (180 mg/dL) and the serum [K+] increases to 8.3 mmol/L. The body weight is 665 grams. Urine output over the previous 8 hours was 0.6 mL/kg/hr. Serum [Na+] is 130 mmol/L and serum [Creat] is 204 μmol/L (2.3 mg/dL). Serum ionized [Ca++] is mildly elevated after the administration of calcium gluconate intravenously for a decline in heart rate to 110 beats per minute.

EXERCISE 9

QUESTIONS

1. What is the etiology of the acute renal failure?

2. How should the hyperkalemia be treated?

ANSWERS

1. The baby has intrinsic renal failure, probably owing to perinatal asphyxia.

2. An insulin drip should be started. Another albuterol treatment could be considered while the infusion is ordered, prepared, and the tubing impregnated with insulin.

CASE STUDY 4 (continued)

An insulin drip is initiated at 0.05 IU/kg/hr. The baby remains oliguric, but the body weight is stable. The serum [GLU] decreases to 6.7 to 7.8 mmol/L (120 to 140 mg/dL). It remains stable after changing fluid intake to 100 mL/kg/day of D$_{12.5}$W. The serum [K+] is 8.8 mmol/L at 36 hours, 7.9 mmol/L at 42 hours, and 6.7 mmol/L at 48 hours. The infant weighs 665 grams. Urine output averages 0.5 mL/kg/hr. The serum [Na+] is 130 mmol/L and serum [Creat] 212 μmol/L (2.4 mg/dL). At 60 hours of age, the body weight is 580 grams. Urine output has steadily increased and is now averaging 4.3 mL/kg/hr. Repeat serum chemistries demonstrate that the serum [Na+] is 128 mmol/L, serum [K+] 6 mmol/L, serum [Creat] 221 μmol/L (2.5 mg/dL), and serum [GLU] 4.4 mmol/L (80 mg/dL). The insulin drip is discontinued. Urine osmolality is 308 on a "spot" urine. Urine [Na+] is 112 mmol/L and urine [Creat] is 85 μmol/L (4.7 mg/dL). Fraction excretion of Na (FENa) is 47%.

EXERCISE 10

QUESTIONS

1. Why has the urine output increased?
   a. Urine output is improving because the GFR is improving with resolution of acute renal failure.
   b. The physiologic diuresis/natriuresis has begun.
   c. The baby is in the polyuric phase of acute renal failure.
   d. Water and sodium retained over the first 2.5 days of life are being excreted appropriately.

2. Why has serum [Na+] fallen further in spite of a markedly negative fluid balance as judged by a 7% decrease in body weight and urine output in excess of water intake over the previous 12 hours?

3. What, if any, changes should be made in fluid and electrolyte intake?

4. How frequently should body weight and serum electrolytes be checked?

ANSWERS

1. **c.** The baby is in the polyuric phase of acute renal failure.

    The isotonic urine is consistent with and the very high FENa is diagnostic of renal tubular injury, i.e., acute tubular necrosis. Serum [Creat] has not decreased; therefore, the GFR has probably not changed. The polyuria in the face of low GFR is the result of decreased reabsorption of the water and Na load. In this case, the FENa indicates that approximately half of the filtered Na load is reabsorbed. Physiologic diuresis/natriuresis (and excretion of water and sodium) may be difficult to distinguish from ATN after oliguric acute renal failure; the FENa is elevated in both of these circumstances, but usually not to this degree with the physiologic diuresis/natriuresis (Bidiwal, 1988; Lorenz, 1997). It is important, however, to differentiate these conditions. Physiologic diuresis/natriuresis and excretion of retained water and sodium are self-limited and the water and sodium loss is appropriate and should not be replaced. With ATN there is no feedback control of water and sodium excretion and it will persist until the renal tubules recover; if water and sodium losses are not replaced during this period, dehydration (abnormal decrease in ECF volume) will result.

2. Serum [Na+] fell in spite of a 7% decrease in body weight with the onset of the polyuric phase of ATN; Na (as well as water balance) is negative. If the spot urine is representative of that voided in the previous 12 hours, the urinary Na losses were 5.8 mmol/kg, whereas Na intake via the UAC was only 1.4 mmol/kg.

3. The baby has already lost 13% of body weight, indicating that contraction of the ECF space has occurred; further contraction caused by urinary water and Na losses that are not under homeostatic control may be deleterious. In this case, maintenance water and electrolytes should be provided (along with parenteral nutrition) or perhaps increased a little given the degree of weight loss. Given estimated changes in water balance associated with the varying fluid intake during the period of oliguria, a reasonable starting point would be 100 mL/kg/day of fluid intake with 2 to 3 mmol/kg/day Na. K should be added when it is confirmed that serum [K+] continues to fall. *In addition to this, urinary water and Na losses should be replaced.*

4. Obligatory urinary water and Na losses will continue for an unknown period of time and may vary considerably over time. Given the magnitude of these losses, urine output and serum and urine electrolytes and creatinine should be assessed every 6 hours. Urinary water and Na loss in the previous 6 hours should be replaced over the ensuing 6 hours. It would also be helpful to follow body weight every 6 to 12 hours depending on how this is tolerated by the baby.

CLINICAL SUMMARY

Careful attention to fluid and electrolyte balance in newborns requiring an intensive care period is a critical part of their management. It is important to monitor the ability of the critically ill newborn to assume fluid and electrolyte homeostasis as the transition from fetal to neonatal life occurs. Pathologic conditions for which low urine output is a hallmark can be particularly difficult to diagnose in the immediate newborn period when urine output is normally low. In every newborn, but especially those born prematurely, the ability to assume control of fluid and electrolyte homeostasis is seriously limited by increased insensible losses of water through the skin and respiratory tract. Water loss by this route is not under homeostatic control. Moreover, in the first day or two of life the ability of the newborn to excrete excessive water and Na intake is limited by a low GFR. Thus, a reasonably accurate estimation of IWL (taking into account gestational age, the environment in which the infant is cared for, and whether antenatal steroids were given) is particularly important in the immediate newborn period. In extremely premature infants, a shift of K from the ICF to the ECF space should be anticipated during the first several days of postnatal life and may result in life-threatening hyperkalemia. It is also important to provide dextrose at a rate that meets requirements, so that limited glucose stores can be preserved and hypoglycemia and hyperglycemia can be avoided. Although glucose requirements are similar across gestational ages, fluid requirements are quite variable. Therefore, the glucose concentration ordered will depend upon the amount of fluid administered, so that the targeted dextrose administration rate can be achieved.

After the first 1 or 2 days of life, self-limited diuresis and natriuresis occur that are largely independent of water and Na intake and result in a physiologically appropriate postnatal contraction of the ECF space. This contraction of the ECF space should be allowed to occur at a rate that avoids hypernatremia. Failure to allow this physiologic contraction of the ECF space may be associated with patent ductus arteriosus, necrotizing enterocolitis, and bronchopulmonary dysplasia. During this period urinary K secretion is high, usually requiring the initiation of K supplementation if hypokalemia is to be avoided. It is important to distinguish physiologic diuresis/natriuresis from the polyuric phase of acute renal failure, because the latter is not self-limited and will result in dehydration and hypokalemia if the attendant water, Na, and K losses are not appropriately replaced.

Finally, with the cessation of diuresis/natriuresis, water and electrolyte excretion begin to vary appropriately with intake, although the premature infant is at risk for hyponatremia secondary to excessive urinary sodium loss as the result of renal immaturity. Fluid intake is now maximized to optimize caloric intake while avoiding fluid retention. Principles of fluid and electrolyte maintenance and management of perturbations in fluid and electrolyte homeostasis during this phase are the same as in older children.

It must be emphasized that appropriate fluid and electrolyte management during the first week of life requires *anticipation* of fluid and electrolyte losses that are likely to occur and the changes in water and electrolyte balance that are appropriate. Consideration of these factors then allows the water, Na, and K requirements to be *estimated*. These requirements are quite variable among infants. Therefore, intakes must be individualized and evaluation of fluid and electrolyte balance that results from these estimated intakes must be periodically reevaluated so that fluid and electrolyte intake can be appropriately adjusted. Parameters useful in evaluating fluid and electrolyte balance include change in body weight, intakes and outputs, and serum and urine electrolyte and creatinine concentrations.

SUGGESTED READINGS

Agren J, Sjors G, Sedin G: Transepidermal water loss in infants born at 24 and 25 weeks of gestation, *Acta Paediatr* 87:1185–1190, 1998.

Bauer K, Bovermann G: Roithmaier, Götz M, Prölss A, Versmold HT. Body composition, nutrition, and fluid balance during the first two weeks of life in preterm infants weighing less than 1500 grams, *J Pediatr* 18:615–620, 1991.

Bauer K, Versmold H: Postnatal weight loss in preterm neonates less than 1500 g is due to isotonic dehydration of the extracellular volume, *Acta Paediatr Scand Suppl* 360:37–42, 1989.

Beardsall K, Dunger D: Insulin therapy in preterm newborns, *Early Hum Devel* 84:839–842, 2008.

Bell EF, Acarregui MJ: Restricted versus liberal water intake for preventing morbidity and mortality in preterm infants, *Cochrane Database Syst Rev* (1): CD000503, 2008.

Bennet LN, Myers TF, Lambert GH: Cecal perforation associated with sodium polystyrene sulfonate-sorbitol enemas in a 650 gram infant with hyperkalemia, *Am J Perinatol* 13:167–170, 1996.

Bidiwala KS, Lorenz JM, Kleinman LI: Renal function correlates of postnatal diuresis in preterm infants, *Pediatrics* 82:50–58, 1988.

Bier DM, Leake RD, Haymond MW, et al.: Measurement of true glucose production rates in infancy and childhood with 6,6-dideuteroglucose, *Diabetes* 26:1016–1023, 1977.

Bottino M, Cowett RM, Sinclair JC: Interventions for treatment of neonatal hyperglycemia in very low birth weight infants, *Cochrane Database Syst Rev* (10): CD007453, 2011.

Brown DR, Fenton LJ, Tsang RC: Blood sampling through umbilical catheters, *Pediatrics* 55:257–260, 1975.

Bueva A, Guignard JP: Renal function in pre-term neonates, *Pediatr Res* 36:572–577, 1994.

Choker G, Gouyton JB: Diagnosis of acute renal failure in very preterm infants, *Biol Neonate* 86:212–216, 2004.

Costarino AT, Baumgart S, Norman ME, et al.: Renal adaptation to extrauterine life in patients with respiratory distress syndrome, *Am J Dis Child* 139:1060–1063, 1985.

Costarino AT, Gruskay JA, Corcoran L, et al.: Sodium restriction versus daily maintenance replacement in very low birth weight premature neonates: a randomized, blind therapeutic trial, *J Pediatr* 120:99–106, 1992.

Dimitriou G, Kavvadia V, Marcou M, Greenough A: Antenatal steroids and fluid balance in very low birthweight infants, *Arch Dis Child Fetal Neonatal Ed* 90:F509–F513, 2005.

Farrag HM, Nawrath LM, Healey JE, et al.: Persistent glucose production and greater peripheral sensitivity to insulin in the neonate vs. the adult, *Am J Physiol* 273:E86–E93, 1997.

Fletcher MA, Brown DR, Landers S, Seguin J: Umbilical arterial catheter use: report of an audit conducted by the Study Group for Complications of Perinatal Care. Umbilical arterial catheter use: report of an audit conducted by the Study Group for Complications of Perinatal Care, *Am J Perinatol* 11:94–99, 1994.

Fukada Y, Kojima T, Ono A, et al.: Factors causing hyperkalemia in premature infants, *Am J Perinatol* 6:76, 1989.

Fuloria M, Friedberg MA, DuRant RH, Aschner JL: Effect of flow rate and insulin priming on the recovery of insulin from microbore infusion tubing, *Pediatrics* 102:1401–1406, 1998.

Grammatikopoulos T, Greenough A, Pallidis C, et al.: Benefits and risks of calcium resonium therapy in hyperkalaemic preterm infants, *Acta Paediatr* 92:118–127, 2003.

Gruskay J, Costarino AT, Polin RA, Baumgart S: Nonoliguric hyperkalemia in the premature infant weighing less than 1000 grams, *J Pediatr* 113:381–386, 1988.

Guignard J-P, Drukker A: Why do newborn infants have a high plasma creatinine? *Pediatrics* 103:e49, 1999.

Hammarlund K, Nilsson GE, Oberg PA, et al.: Transepidermal water loss in newborn infants. Relation to ambient humidity and site of measurement and estimation of total transepidermal water loss, *Acta Paediatr Scand* 66:553–562, 1977.

Hammarlund K, Sedin G, Stromberg B: Transepidermal water loss in newborn infants VIII. Relation to gestational age and post-natal age in appropriate and small for gestational age infants, *Acta Paediatr Scand* 72:721–728, 1983.

Hartnoll G, Bétrémieux P, Modi N: Randomized controlled trial of postnatal sodium supplementation on oxygen dependency and body weight in 25-30 week gestational age infants, *Arch Dis Child Fetal Neonatal Ed* 82:F19–F23, 2000.

Heck LJ, Erenberg A: Serum glucose values during the first 48 hours of life, *J Pediatr* 110:119–122, 1987.

Heimler R, Doumas BT, Jendrzejcak BM, Nemeth PB, Hoffman RG, Nelin LD: Relationship between nutrition, weight change, and fluid compartments in preterm infants during the first week of life, *J Pediatr* 122:110–114, 1993.

Hu PS, Su BH, Peng CT, et al.: Glucose and insulin infusion versus kayexalate for early treatment of non-oliguric hyperkalemia in very-low-birth-weight infants, *Acta Paediatr Taiwan* 40:314–318, 1999.

Jackson JK, Derleth DP: Effects of various arterial infusions solutions on red blood cells in the newborn, *Arch Dis Child Fetal Neonatal Ed* 83:F130–F134, 2000.

Karlowicz MG, Adelman RD: Nonoliguric and oliguric acute renal failure in asphyxiated term neonates, *Pediatr Nephrol* 9:718–722, 1995.

Lorenz JM, Kleinman LI, Ahmed G, et al.: Phases of fluid and electrolyte homeostasis in the extremely low birth weight infant, *Pediatrics* 96:484–489, 1995.

Lorenz JM, Kleinman LI, Kotagal UR, et al.: Water balance in very low-birth-weight infants: relationship to water and sodium intake and effect on outcome, *J Pediatr* 101:423–432, 1982.

Lorenz JM, Kleinman LI, Markarian K: Potassium metabolism in extremely low birth weight infants in the first week of life, *J Pediatr* 131:81–86, 1997.

Lynch SK, Lemley KV, Polak MJ: The effect of dopamine on glomerular filtration rate in normotensive, oliguric premature neonates, *Pediatric Nephrology* 18:649–652, 2003.

Malone TA: Glucose and insulin versus cation-exchange resin for the treatment of hyperkalemia in very low birth weight infants, *J Pediatr* 118:121–123, 1991.

Metzger BE, Persson B, Lowe LP, et al.: Hyperglycemia and adverse pregnancy outcomes study: neonatal glycemia, *Pediatrics* 126:e1545–e1552, 2010.

Miall LS, Henderson MJ, Turner AJ, et al.: Plasma creatinine rises dramatically in the first 48 hours of life in preterm infants, *Pediatrics* 104:e76, 1999.

Oca MJ, Nelson M, Donn SM: Randomized trial of normal saline versus 5% albumin for the treatment of neonatal hypotension, *J Perinatol* 23:473–476, 2003.

Ohlsson A, Hosking M: Complications following oral administration of exchange resins in extremely low-birth-weight infants, *Eur J Pediatr* 146:571–574, 1987.

Omar SA, DeCristofaro JD, Agarwal BI, LaGamma EF: Effects of prenatal steroids on water and sodium homeostasis in extremely low birth weight neonates, *Pediatrics* 104:482–488, 1999.

Omar SA, DeCristofaro JD, Agarwal BI, LaGamma EF: Effect of prenatal steroids on potassium balance in extremely low birth weight neonates, *Pediatrics* 106:561–567, 2000.

Prins I, Plotz FB, Uiterwaal CS, van Vught HJ: Low-dose dopamine in neonatal and pediatric intensive care: a systematic review, *Inten Care Med* 27:206–210, 2001.

Sato K, Kondo T, Iwao H, et al.: Internal potassium shift in premature infants: cause of nonoliguric hyperkalemia, *J Pediatr* 126:109–113, 1995.

Shaffer SG, Bradt SK, Hall RT: Postnatal changes in total body water and extracellular volume in preterm infants with respiratory distress syndrome, *J Pediatr* 109:509–514, 1986.

Shaffer SG, Kilbride HW, Hayes LK, et al.: Hyperkalemia in very low birth weight infants, *J Pediatr* 121:275–279, 1992.

Shaffer SG, Meade VM: Sodium balance and extracellular volume regulation in very low birth weight infants, *J Pediatr* 115:285–290, 1989.

Shaffer SG, Quimiro CL, Anderson JV, et al.: Postnatal weight changes in low birth weight infants, *Pediatr* 79:702–705, 1987.

Singh DS, Sadiq HF, Noguchi A, et al.: Efficacy of albuterol inhalation in treatment of hyperkalemia in premature infants, *J Pediatr* 14:16–20, 2002.

Singhi S, Sood V, Bhakoo ON, Gnanuly NK, Kaur A: Composition of postnatal weight loss and subsequent weight gain in preterm infants, *Indian J Med Res* 101:157–162, 1995.

So KW, Fok TF, Ng PC, Wong WW, Cheung KL: Randomised controlled trial of colloid or crystalloid in hypotensive preterm infants, *Arch Dis Child Fetal Neonatal Ed* 76:F43–F46, 1997.

Srinivasan G, Pildes RS, Cattamanchi G, et al.: Plasma glucose values in normal neonates: a new look, *J Pediatr* 105:114–119, 1984.

Stefano JL, Norman ME: Nitrogen balance in extremely low birth weight infants with nonoliguric hyperkalemia, *J Pediatr* 623:632–635, 1993.

Stonestreet BS, Rubin L, Pollak A, Cowett M, Oh W: Renal functions of low birth weight infants with hyperglycemia and glucosuria produced by glucose infusions, *Pediatrics* 66:561–564, 1980.

Sunehag A, Ewald U, Larsson A, et al.: Glucose production rate in extremely immature neonates (<28 weeks) studied with use of deuterated glucose, *Pediatr Res* 33:97–100, 1993.

Tyrala EE, Chen X, Boden G: Glucose metabolism in the infant weighing less than 1100 grams, *J Pediatr* 125:283–287, 1994.

CHAPTER 4

GLUCOSE METABOLISM

David H. Adamkin, MD

CASE STUDY 1

A 30-year-old primigravida after an uncomplicated pregnancy is admitted in labor at 38 weeks' gestation. The perinatal screening tests are negative including a negative screen for group B Streptococcus (GBS) at 36 weeks of gestation. Membranes rupture occurred 2 hours prior to vaginal delivery. Apgar scores were 8 and 9 at 1 and 5 minutes, respectively. The male infant weighs 3200 grams. The mother has planned to exclusively breastfeed the baby and she begins in the delivery room with what is described as a "successful" first feed. Shortly thereafter, mother and baby are transferred to a postpartum room.

Prior to the baby being breastfed at 8 hours of age, the nurse on a routine assessment thinks the baby has slight tremors and she performs a point-of-care glucose level and it is 36 mg/dL. Apparently the infant looks well enough to breastfeed because the nurse advises the mother to feed again. The nurse also advises that after this feeding the mother should supplement the infant with one ounce of a term formula. She tells the mother that she will check the glucose again 1 hour after the formula feed to make sure the baby is no longer hypoglycemic. The mother is very disappointed that she will have to abandon her plan to exclusively breastfeed and wonders if it is absolutely necessary to give the formula.

The nurse calls you at home and discusses the findings and what is going on and that the mother is disappointed about having to give formula supplement to her baby.
  - *Is the nurse offering correct advice to this mother?*
  - *Do you have orders for screening and management of glucose levels for the well baby?*

You have your smart phone with you and you pull up the "Glucose App, Sugar Wheel" (Figure 4-1) based on the algorithm from the Clinical Report—Postnatal Glucose Homeostasis in Late-Preterm and Term Infants published in Pediatrics in March 2011 from the American Academy of Pediatrics (AAP) Committee on Fetus and Newborn.

EXERCISE 1

QUESTIONS

1. Should this term, appropriate for gestational age breastfeeding infant been screened at all?

2. Is this infant symptomatic? Because the glucose value was <40 mg/dL, should the infant have received intravenous glucose?

3. Should a plasma glucose concentration have been sent to the lab?

4. Should the infant simply have been left to continue breastfeeding?

5. Do infants that are exclusively breastfed tend to have lower plasma glucose concentrations than those fed infant formulas?

ANSWERS

1. Yes, if the tremors were really symptoms.

2. The tremors may not have been related to hypoglycemia because the level is not particularly low.

3. Always send confirmatory value to lab for plasma glucose if you are concerned about symptoms.

4. Yes, if the symptoms are really not symptoms or related to the plasma glucose level, which is not low.

5. Breastfed infants probably do have lower plasma glucose levels than formula fed.

CASE STUDY 1 (continued)

This case demonstrates a few of the issues that we will consider in the chapter. Cornblath and Reisner established (nearly 50 years ago) that neonatal hypoglycemia was a significant cause of neonatal mortality and morbidity, yet the definition and management of neonatal hypoglycemia have remained unclear. We will examine the controversies and discuss what constitutes clinically significant

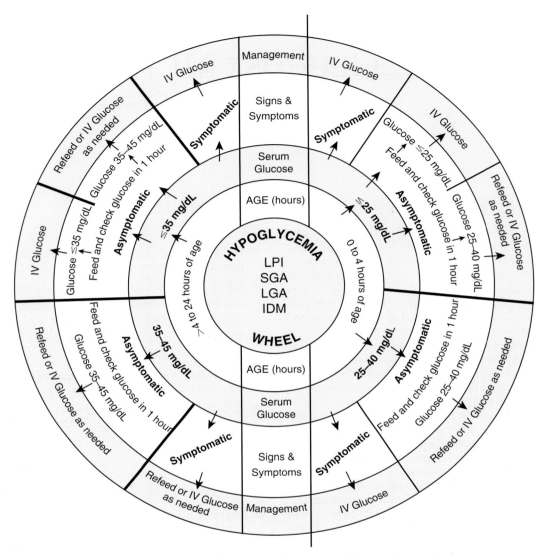

FIGURE 4-1 ■ **Sugar Wheel nomogram for postnatal glucose homeostasis.**

hypoglycemia, who should be screened and when, laboratory methods, and the relationship between "low" plasma glucose concentrations and long-term neurologic outcomes.

INTRODUCTION

After birth, the normal newborn infant's plasma glucose concentration falls below levels that were prevalent in fetal life. This is part of the normal transition to an extrauterine existence and through a series of triggers, the infant activates endocrine and metabolic events associated with successful adaptation. When this adaptation fails, perhaps secondary to immaturity or illness, there is a limitation of substrate supply, which may disturb cerebral function and potentially

result in neurologic sequelae. A low plasma glucose may be indicative of this process but is not per se diagnostic. What is meant by "low"? How low is "too low?" At what glucose level does hypoglycemia lead to irreversible changes in brain structure or function?

More than a decade ago, Cornblath and colleagues summarized the contemporary state of knowledge relating to neonatal hypoglycemia by stating the following: "Unfortunately, untoward long-term outcomes in infants with one or two low blood glucose levels have become grounds for litigation and for alleged malpractice, even though the causative relationship between the two is tenuous at best. . . . The definition of clinically significant hypoglycemia remains one of the most confused and contentious issues in contemporary neonatology."

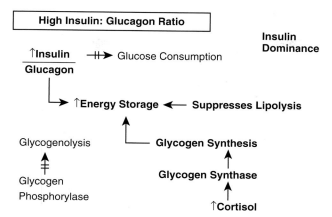

FIGURE 4-2 ■ **Fetal maintenance of anabolic state promoting energy storage.**

Four years ago a workshop report from the Eunice Kennedy Shriver National Institute of Child Health and Human Development was published in the *Journal of Pediatrics*, after a group of experts from around the world was assembled in Washington, D.C. to focus on gaps in knowledge and suggest research needs for understanding and treating neonatal hypoglycemia. Conclusions from the workshop included: "There is no evidence-based study to identify any specific plasma glucose concentration (or range of glucose values) to define pathologic hypoglycemia." "Monitoring for and prevention and treatment of neonatal hypoglycemia remain largely empirical." Finally the report concludes, "at present data are insufficient to produce definitive guidelines." At the same time as this conference was taking place, the Committee on Fetus and Newborn for the American Academy of Pediatrics was working on a clinical report to provide guidance and an algorithm for the screening and subsequent management of neonatal hypoglycemia.

GLUCOSE HOMEOSTASIS

Maintenance of glucose homeostasis via initiation of glucose production is one of the critical transitional physiologic events that must take place as the fetus adapts to extrauterine life. It is not uncommon that the transition may be difficult and result in an alteration in glucose homeostasis and an infant with a low plasma glucose level.

The fetus depends on maternal supply and the placental transfer of glucose, amino acids, free fatty acids, ketones, and glycerol for its energy supply. The normal lower limit of fetal glucose concentration is approximately 54 mg/dL (3 mmol/L) over most of gestation. Fetal glucose production does not take place under normal conditions.

The ratio of insulin to glucagon in the fetal circulation plays a critical role in regulating the balance between glucose consumption versus energy stored. The high fetal ratio results in activation of glycogen synthesis and suppression of glycogenolysis through the regulation of hepatic enzymes used for these pathways (Figure 4-2). Therefore, in the fetus glycogen synthesis is enhanced and glycogenolysis is minimized. There is a rapid increase in hepatic glycogen during the last 30% of fetal life. This marked increase is associated with an increase in both circulating insulin and cortisol. The high insulin/glucagon ratio also suppresses lipolysis, which allows for energy to be stored as subcutaneous fat. This subcutaneous and hepatic reservoir establishes a ready substrate supply for the fetus to transition metabolically and establish postnatal glucose homeostasis (Figure 4-2).

The dependence of the fetus on maternal glucose necessitates significant changes in regulation of glucose metabolism at birth following the abrupt cessation of umbilical glucose delivery. A number of physiologic changes allow the newborn to maintain glucose homeostasis (Figure 4-3). Catecholamine concentrations increase immediately after delivery and this stimulates glucagon secretion. Therefore, there is a decrease in the insulin/glucagon ratio. This ratio is important because it drives events in utero and in transition that explain fetal preparedness for transition and the postnatal adaptation and glucose homeostasis.

When glycogen synthase is inactivated and glycogen phosphorylase is activated, this leads to

Glucose Homeostasis in Newborn

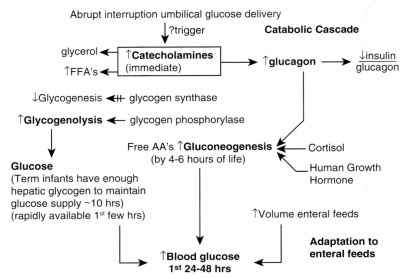

FIGURE 4-3 ■ **Adaptations around delivery and over the first 24 hours of life to establish postnatal glucose homeostasis.**

stimulation of glycogenolysis and inhibition of glycogen synthesis, which is the exact opposite of the in utero fetal milieu. The release of glucose from glycogen provides the rapidly available source of glucose for the neonate the first few hours after delivery. The estimates are that for the term infant the hepatic glycogen supplies enough glucose for the first 10 hours. It is very important that other mechanisms come into play to maintain glucose homeostasis (Figure 4-3).

The next important pathway for postnatal glucose homeostasis is gluconeogenesis. The high insulin/glucagon ratio after delivery induces enzymes required for gluconeogenesis. Free fatty acids are released secondary to surging catecholamines that lead to the availability of glycerol and amino acids from the circulation. By 4 to 6 hours of life, the term infant is capable of significant gluconeogenesis.

Until an exogenous supply of glucose is provided, either enterally or intravenously, hepatic glucose production is the most significant source of glucose to meet the needs of the infant. To maintain normal levels of hepatic glucose production, the infant must have the following:

- Adequate stores of glycogen and gluconeogenic precursors (fatty acids, glycerol, amino acids, and lactate)
- Concentrations of hepatic enzymes necessary for glycogenesis and gluconeogenesis
- Normally functioning endocrine system (counterregulatory hormones, human growth hormone [HGH], and cortisol)

If any of these systems are not in place, then there is a disruption of glucose homeostasis, which increases the chances that there will be neonatal hypoglycemia.

It has long been thought that preterm infants during the first 3 days of life had lower glucose values than term infants and they tolerated these lower levels better. This misconception came from the observation of lower plasma glucose levels in preterm infants when these infants were commonly starved the first few days of life. These low values are no longer observed in preterm infants because of early intravenous therapy and/or enteral feedings. In fact, the preterm infant has a significantly greater fall in glucose within the first few hours after birth than in term infants, suggesting that they are less able to adapt to the cessation of intrauterine nutrition. Gluconeogenic ability is limited in preterm infants, possibly owing to immaturity of the enzymatic pathways.

CASE STUDY 2

A term appropriate for gestational age (AGA) male infant was born after an uneventful pregnancy to a 30-year-old gravida 2 woman. The mother had no evidence of hyperglycemia and no chronic diseases. Apgar scores were 5, 7, and 8 at 1, 5, and 10 minutes, respectively. The baby received blow-by oxygen in the delivery room because of cyanosis. At approximately 1 hour of age, a bedside glucose determination was obtained; the value was 27 mg/ dL. The infant then received his first feeding of formula after a plasma glucose level was sent to the lab. The plasma glucose concentration run by the lab was 35 mg/dL and the repeat bedside glucose 1 hour after the feeding was 36 mg/dL.

EXERCISE 2

QUESTIONS

1. Should this baby have received the initial screening bedside glucose at 1 hour of age?

2. What is the significance of 27 mg/dL at 1 hour of age prior to feeding?

3. Why does the plasma glucose concentration of 35 mg/dL (from the laboratory) differ from the bedside screen, which was 27 mg/dL?

4. The repeat bedside glucose is 36 mg/dL at 2 hours of age after a feeding of formula. Is that level still actionable?

ANSWERS

1. Cyanosis at delivery is very unlikely due to these levels of plasma glucose. It was the reason the infant was screened.

2. The bedside screen of 27 mg/dL is typical of the nadir during metabolic transition (the actual plasma value was 35 mg/dL).

3. Bedside screening values are not as accurate as plasma levels, particularly at low levels of glucose.

4. The repeat level of 35 mg/dL is still actionable. However, this infant probably should not have been screened and was asymptomatic and well.

DEFINITION OF HYPOGLYCEMIA

A consistent definition of hypoglycemia does not exist in the literature or in clinical practice. When the first neonates were recognized as having significant hypoglycemia in the mid-1950s, the infants had striking clinical manifestations, often seizures, and their blood sugar values were consistently below 20 to 25 mg/dL (1.1 to 1.4 mmol/L). The abnormal signs cleared quickly after increasing the blood glucose concentration to (>40 mg/dL, 2.2 mmol/L). Now 60 years later, after hypoglycemia was first described and "40" mg/dL became a "classic" standard for defining hypoglycemia, our understanding of the metabolic disturbances and genetic defects underlying aberrations in postnatal glucose homeostasis has increased dramatically. However, this growth of knowledge, if anything, has led us further from what we need to know about

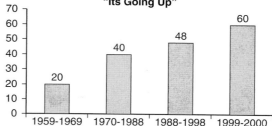

FIGURE 4-4 ■ **Plasma glucose concentrations considered representing hypoglycemia over the last 40 years.**

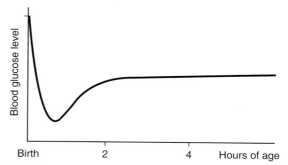

FIGURE 4-5 ■ **Blood glucose concentration transition from fetus to neonatal over the first hours of life.** (From Srinivasan G, Pildes RS, Cattaman G: Plasma glucose values in normal neonates: a new look, *J Pediatr* 109[1]:114-117, 1986.)

blood glucose concentrations in the newborn: "How low is too low?"

In a review of current textbooks, there is no consensus for the definition of hypoglycemia; values range from 18 mg/dL (1 mmol/L) to 70 to 100 mg/dL (3.8 to 5.5 mmol/L). It is interesting to note that the definition of neonatal hypoglycemia has gone up decade by decade over the last forty years (Figure 4-4); however, the higher blood glucose values that have been proposed are without scientific justification. The easiest diagnosis may be the situation in which the symptoms associated with a low blood sugar resolve when the blood sugar concentration is increased. Apart from this clinical situation, the diagnosis of hypoglycemia is much more complex.

The blood glucose concentrations during the immediate postnatal period are important to understand to determine what may or may not constitute a low blood sugar concentration. At birth, the blood glucose concentration in the umbilical venous blood is 70% to 90% of that in the maternal venous blood. Blood glucose concentration falls rapidly after birth, reaching a nadir by 1 hour of age or so and then rises to stabilize by 3 hours of age despite the absence of any nutritional support (Figure 4-5). During this period, plasma insulin levels are falling as glucagon levels surge. This surge of glucagon combined with low insulin levels is the key hormonal adaptation in the newborn infant that leads to mobilization of glycogen. Plasma glucose concentrations are lowest at 1 to 2 hours of age and may reach a nadir as low as approximately 30 mg/dL (1.8 mmol/L), or even lower (Figure 4-6), after which time the infant's normal physiologic responses increase the glucose concentrations to values greater than 45 mg/dL (2.5 mmol/L), which are maintained over the first days of life (Figure 4-6).

Several approaches have been taken to determine normal reference ranges for blood glucose concentrations in normal newborns. The first was to sample umbilical venous blood at various times during gestation and establish reference ranges for blood glucose concentrations for the normal fetus and then apply these glucose concentrations to the newborn. This method demonstrated a range of 54 to 90 mg/dL with a mean concentration of 70 mg/dL. Another approach was to measure the glucose values in full-term, appropriately grown newborn infants without any prenatal or neonatal complications over the first few hours. These values are shown in Figures 4-5 and 4-6.

In using these approaches one can arrive at a statistical definition of hypoglycemia in the normal term after 12 hours of life of 36 to 45 mg/dL. However, the literature does not provide a consensus for a threshold blood or plasma glucose concentration that specifically defines hypoglycemia or when and how much treatment should be provided. Attempts have also been made to identify the threshold blood glucose concentration in which there is substantial likelihood of functional impairment, particularly the brain. These methods can be categorized into five approaches: epidemiologic, clinical, metabolic-endocrine, neurophysiologic, and neurodevelopmental.

The epidemiologic approach simply defines blood concentrations in a cohort of healthy infants, and then uses an empirically derived cut-off such as <2 standard deviations below the mean. Any single value is unlikely to represent a threshold of abnormality, because the data represents a continuum from normal. Most important is that a statistical abnormality does not imply a biologic impairment. This method shows the vast majority have blood glucose concentrations >40 mg/dL.

The clinical approach is based on the importance of glucose levels when signs of hypoglycemia appear. However, jitteriness is just as likely

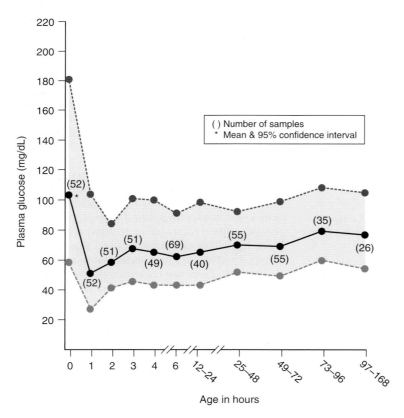

FIGURE 4-6 ■ **Plasma glucose concentrations in full-term, appropriately grown newborns without any prenatal or neonatal complications.** (From Srinivasan G, Pildes RS, Cattaman G: Plasma glucose values in normal neonates: a new look, *J Pediatr* 109[1]:115, 1986)

among normoglycemic infants and those with a variety of other conditions. Also, equally low blood glucose levels are found in infants with no signs ("asymptomatic hypoglycemia"). This is often seen in the first few hours after birth when fuels other than glucose are providing neural energy and the brain is protected despite the "low plasma glucose screen." Therefore, the presence or absence of signs and symptoms cannot be used to discriminate between normal and abnormal blood glucose values.

The metabolic-endocrine approach is not practical and needs more data. The premise is that the concentration of glucose at which metabolic counterregulation occurs can be used to define a "safe" lower limit for blood glucose concentration. Premature infants are unable to mount a mature counterregulatory response to low blood glucose levels compared to term infants, thus making them more vulnerable during periods of insufficient fuel.

Similarly, the neurophysiologic approach has attempted to measure neurophysiologic changes in relation to various blood glucose concentrations. Studies use somatosensory evoked potentials. The studies have had small numbers and some studies have failed to show effects of hypoglycemia on evoked responses. Changes in cerebral blood flow with very low blood glucose concentrations have been studied in preterm infants. However, the practicality of this technology and application remain unclear.

The neurodevelopmental approach has taken on the most significance for many investigators to define significant hypoglycemia and also is pivotal in the Canadian Pediatric Statement and algorithm on screening and management of hypoglycemia. An important and very influential article from the United Kingdom published in 1988 by Lucas and colleagues opened with "there has been considerable debate over what should be chosen as a safe lower limit for blood glucose concentration in the neonatal period." The article provided data on 661 infants who weighed <1850 g at birth, and from the data the authors concluded that "moderate hypoglycemia may have serious neurodevelopmental consequences, and reappraisal of current management is urgently required." They used statistical strategies to analyze for a threshold value that reliably predicted an adverse outcome. They suggested that a glucose concentration <47 mg/dL (<2.5 mmol/L) offered the greatest predictive power. They found that the number of days that these infants experienced moderate hypoglycemia was strongly related to reduced scores for mental and motor development at 18 months corrected age, even after adjustment for a wide range of factors

known to influence development. However, the monitoring of blood glucose was not standardized; sicker infants had more frequent blood glucose determinations. The fact that hypoglycemia was not a primary focus of this prospective controlled feeding study is apparent from the observation that some infants were permitted to have plasma glucose values <20 mg/dL (<1.1 mmol/L) for as long as 3 to 7 days without intervention. In addition, the glucose value reported and used in their analyses for prognosis was the first one obtained each day and the number of days <47 mg/dL were usually not consecutive.

The adjustment for confounding variables and the large sample size were positive aspects of this study. Therefore for high-risk infants with birthweight <1850 g, a first glucose value of <47 mg/dL on 5 or more days correlated positively with abnormal neurologic and developmental outcomes at 18 months of age. However, by 7.5 to 8 years of age, only deficiencies in arithmetic and motor test scores were present. This suggested the findings at 18 months were not permanent. Thus, doubt was cast on the importance of a threshold value <47 mg/dL as a marker for neuroglycopenia or, alternatively, it suggests that early adversity may be attenuated by later environmental factors.

A second retrospective study gained importance in trying to define a "threshold" level for increased risk of brain injury. The study included small for gestational age preterm infants <32 weeks' gestation, the majority of whom had symmetric growth restriction including head circumference. They reported 73% of these infants had hypoglycemia (i.e., <47 mg/dL), and that recurrent episodes of hypoglycemia strongly correlated with physical growth deficits and persistent neurodevelopmental delays. In this study, the initial bedside screen was not confirmed with a laboratory plasma glucose in many of the infants.

A prospective controlled clinical trial with a strict protocol for measuring frequent blood glucose levels at specific times and with explicit indications is necessary. The approach that links statistically based hypoglycemia with outcome measures like abnormal neuromotor and intellectual performance at 18 months of age or older cannot be validated without this prospective study.

Recently another group in the United Kingdom, Tin and colleagues, completed a prospective study that evaluated neurodevelopmental outcomes at 2 and 15 years later for preterm infants who had a low blood glucose level during the first 10 days of life. This study was designed to test the hypothesis that recurrent low blood glucose levels <47 mg/dL, even in the absence of any suggestive clinical signs, can harm a preterm infant's long-term development.

All children born <32 weeks in the north of England in 1990 to 1991 had laboratory blood glucose levels measured daily for the first 10 days of life. Forty-seven of the 566 who survived to 2 years had a blood glucose level <47 mg/dL for more than 3 days. All were matched with hypoglycemia-free controls matched for appropriate variables. No differences in developmental progress or physical disability were detected at 2 years of age.

The families were seen again when the children were 15 years old, and 38 (81%) of the original cohort and matched controls were nearly identical for full scale IQ. Even children who had a level <47 mg/dL for >4 days and another group <36 mg/dL on 3 different days did not alter these results. Tin concluded "they found no evidence that recurrent low blood glucose levels (<47 mg/dL) in the first 10 days of life pose a hazard to preterm infants."

Tin's study doesn't imply that low blood glucose concentrations cannot be damaging in the preterm infant even in the absence of overt recognizable signs. However, the data suggest that the danger threshold must be lower than many had come to think it was.

A recent analysis of all 18 reported eligible studies through 2005 on neonatal hypoglycemia and subsequent neurodevelopmental outcomes concluded that the overall methodologic quality was poor in 16 and high in two studies. None of the studies provided a valid estimate of the effect of neonatal hypoglycemia on neurodevelopmental outcomes. They developed a proposal for a well-designed prospective study, which the second UK study by Tin and colleagues represents.

Rozance and Hay, reviewing features associated with adverse outcomes in infants with hypoglycemia, conclude that attributing long-term neurologic impairment to neonatal hypoglycemia is difficult and controversial. They also suggest there are no definitive studies that have been able to address this issue. Conditions to consider when entertaining this possibility are listed in Box 4-1.

CASE STUDY 3

A term male infant is born to a 21-year-old primigravida who had no prenatal care. Because of failure to progress, a cesarean section was performed. Apgar scores were 6 and 7 at 1 and 5 minutes, respectively. The infant weighed 4550 grams and the length and head circumference both plotted out at the 50th percentile on the fetal growth curve. At 6 hours of age, the infant appears lethargic, feeding poorly at the breast, and jittery. A bedside glucose determination was performed and the reading was 10 mg/dL. A plasma glucose was sent to the laboratory.

EXERCISE 3

QUESTIONS

1. When should this infant with macrosomia and no prenatal care be screened for neonatal hypoglycemia?

2. Do you consider this infant asymptomatic with a low blood glucose concentration, or a symptomatic infant with a low blood glucose concentration?

BOX 4-1	**Conditions That Should Be Present Before Considering That Long-Term Neurologic Impairment Might Be Related to Neonatal Hypoglycemia**

1. Blood or plasma glucose concentrations below 1 mmol/L (18 mg/dL). Such values definitely are abnormal, although if transient there is no study in the literature confirming that they lead to permanent neurologic injury.
2. Persistence of such severely low glucose concentrations for prolonged periods (hours, >2 to 3 hours, rather than minutes, although there is no study in human neonates that defines this period)
3. Early mild-to-moderate clinical signs (primarily those of increased adrenalin [epinephrine] activity), such as alternating central nervous system (CNS) signs of jitteriness/tremulousness vs. stupor/lethargy or even brief convulsion, that diminish or disappear

with effective treatment that promptly restores the glucose concentration to the statistically normal range (>45 mg/dL)
4. More serious clinical signs that are prolonged (many hours or longer), including coma, seizures, respiratory depression and/or apnea with cyanosis, hypotonia or limpness, high-pitched cry, hypothermia, and poor feeding after initially feeding well; these are more refractory to short-term treatment
5. Concurrence of associated conditions, particularly persistent excessive insulin secretion and hyperinsulinemia with repeated episodes of acute, severe hypoglycemia with seizures and/or coma (although subclinical, often severe, hypoglycemic episodes occur in these conditions and might be just as injurious)

From Rozance P, Hay W: Hypoglycemia in newborn infants: features associated with adverse outcomes, Biol Neonate 90:84, 2006.

3. Would you immediately feed this infant or would you be providing intravenous glucose by mini-bolus and/or glucose infusion?

ANSWERS

1. This infant with macrosomia should have been screened 30 minutes after the first feeding, which should have taken place by 1 hour of age.

2. This infant has signs that can be consistent with hypoglycemia.

3. The infant that is symptomatic with hypoglycemia and demonstrates a low bedside glucose and/or plasma screen should be treated immediately.

OPERATIONAL THRESHOLDS

Hypoglycemia represents an imbalance between glucose supply and utilization and may result from many different regulatory mechanisms (Box 4-2). In 2000, Cornblath proposed an operational definition for neonatal hypoglycemia. An operational threshold is an indication for action but it not diagnostic of a disease. One uses available clinical and experimental data for these infants using conservative estimates for designating the lower level of normoglycemia. The belief is that the neonate can safely tolerate these levels at specific ages and under established conditions.

Cornblath first suggested an operational level for plasma glucose of 30 to 36 mg/dL during the first 24 hours or less for the healthy full-term or late preterm (34 to 37 weeks' gestation) formula-fed infant. If the glucose concentration fell below that operational level after a feeding or recurred, he suggested increasing the plasma glucose levels above 45 mg/dL. This absolutely does not imply that the lower plasma glucose concentrations alone produce mental or developmental abnormalities. He also suggested that the operational threshold might be increased to 45 to 50 mg/dL (2.5 to 2.8 mmol/L) or higher in a sick, low birth weight, or premature infant suspected of having increased glucose requirements as a result of sepsis, hypoxia, or other major systemic illness.

Finally, he recommended that beyond 24 hours of age, this operational threshold may be increased to 40 to 50 mg/dL. Values below the operational threshold level are an indication to raise the plasma glucose levels and do not imply neuroglycopenia or neurologic injury. Infants at all ages and gestations with repetitive, reliable plasma glucose values less than 20 to 25 mg/dL should be given parenteral glucose and be monitored at regular intervals to ensure that these low values do not persist or recur.

When the low plasma glucose levels are prolonged or recurrent, they may result in acute systemic effects and neurologic sequelae. Cornblath stresses that it is not possible to define a plasma glucose level that requires intervention in every

---

BOX 4-2 Pathogenesis of Hypoglycemia in Neonates

EXCESS UTILIZATION

Hyperinsulinism: IDM, erythroblastosis, LGA, SGA, or islet cell or other endocrine pathology

Increased calorie expenditure for thermoregulation in LBW and SGA infants

Increased calorie expenditure owing to excess muscle activity: increased work of breathing in respiratory distress, drug withdrawal, CNS irritability

Circulatory or respiratory diseases that shift energy metabolism from aerobic to anaerobic pathways: hypoxemia, hypotension, hypoventilation, septic shock

Relative excess of glucose-dependent tissues: high brain-to-liver ratio in SGA infants

Inborn errors of metabolism resulting in inadequate glucose-sparing substrates: free fatty acids, ketones, glycerol, amino acids, lactate

Acute brain injury causing increased brain glucose utilization: seizures, intoxication, meningitis, encephalitis, or hypermetabolism following acute brain injury (hypoxia-ischemia, trauma, hemorrhage)

INADEQUATE PRODUCTION OR SUBSTRATE DELIVERY

Inadequate or delayed feedings or parenteral delivery of calories

Aberrant hormonal regulation of glucose or lipid metabolism: hypothalamic, pituitary, and peripheral endocrine disorders

Transient developmental immaturity of critical metabolic pathways reducing endogenous production of glucose and/or other substrates

Deficient metabolic reserves of precursors or glucose-sparing substrates

Deficient brain glucose transporters: posthypoxia-ischemia, inherited glucose transporter defects

Suppression of gluconeogenesis, glycogenolysis, and hepatic glucose release by inappropriately high circulating insulin levels in conditions associated with hyperinsulinism.

IDM, Infant of diabetic mother; *LBW*, low birth weight; *LGA*, large for gestational age; *SGA*, small for gestational age.
From Cornblath M, Ichord R. Hypoglycemia in the neonate, Semin Perinatol 24(2):138, 2000.

newborn infant because there is uncertainty over the level and duration of hypoglycemia that causes damage, and little is known of the vulnerability of the brain at various gestational ages for such injury. He emphasized significant hypoglycemia is not and can never be defined by a single number that can be applied universally to every individual patient. Rather, it is characterized by a value(s) that is unique to each individual and varies with both their state of physiologic maturity and the influence of pathology. It can be defined as the concentration of glucose in the blood or plasma at which the individual demonstrates a unique response to the abnormal milieu caused by the inadequate delivery of glucose to a target organ (for example, the brain).

Treatment should be guided by clinical assessment and not by glucose concentration alone. The infant displaying neurologic signs requires more urgent elevation of plasma glucose concentration than the asymptomatic one, regardless of the individual plasma glucose concentration.

The National Institutes of Health conference on Knowledge Gaps and Research Needs for Neonatal Hypoglycemia concluded the following concerning operational thresholds: "The so called operational thresholds are useful guidelines to take appropriate actions. However, the recommendations are not based on evidence of significant morbidity if no actions are taken. Similarly, there is no evidence that outcomes improve if actions are taken at the operational threshold value. All published definitions providing singular values or ranges have been arbitrary and developed for analytical and grouping purposes."

PHYSIOLOGIC RESPONSES TO HYPOGLYCEMIA AND BRAIN INJURY

There is no definitive study of glucose insufficiency in human infants in relation to hypoglycemia and acute neuronal injury. Glucose concentration is only an indicator of glucose insufficiency; the other factors to consider when determining glucose insufficiency include cerebral blood flow, cerebral glucose utilization rate, and cerebral uptake and metabolism of alternative fuels, as well as the duration of the hypoglycemia and the presence of associated clinical complications. Plasma or blood glucose concentration, however, may be the only practical laboratory measure available to assess glucose insufficiency and response to treatment. A thorough physical exam assessing for signs and symptoms of hypoglycemia and particularly neurologic abnormalities may help distinguish those infants with low blood glucose concentrations who are adequately compensating. Figure 4-7 shows the many factors (neuronal fuel economy) that must be considered in evaluating the infant with a low blood glucose concentration.

Some studies have shown increased cerebral blood flow in the hypoglycemic infant compared to normal, healthy euglycemic infants; after treatment the cerebral blood flow returned to normal in 30 minutes, as did epinephrine levels, which had risen as well with hypoglycemia. However, studies have not shown a change in cerebral rate of glucose utilization in relation to the change in cerebral blood flow.

Another important neuroprotective response to hypoglycemia is the capacity to accommodate changes in the rate of cerebral glucose metabolism by substituting alternate energy substrates. The best characterized alternative fuel for the brain during hypoglycemia is lactate. Observations from animal data indicate that lactate entry into and metabolism by the tricarboxylic acid cycle may help compensate for decreased glucose metabolism. Lactate is the product of an astrocyte-neuronal lactate shuttle, which can supply the neurons with lactate for energy during periods of glucose deprivation. Brain glycogen is stored in the astrocyte, which makes this shuttle another important source of neuroprotection.

It appears that the human brain has the capacity to metabolize ketone bodies. Therefore the ability of the neonatal brain to utilize ketone bodies is almost certainly another form of neuroprotection during hypoglycemia. In healthy, term infants, plasma ketone bodies increased to a maximum concentration on days 2 and 3. Additionally, the ketone bodies increased further

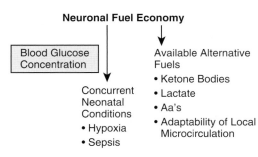

Neuronal Fuel Economy

Blood Glucose Concentration

Concurrent Neonatal Conditions
- Hypoxia
- Sepsis

Available Alternative Fuels
- Ketone Bodies
- Lactate
- Aa's
- Adaptability of Local Microcirculation

Given complexity of defining adequacy of neuronal fuel adequacy–concept of rigid threshold for blood glucose is challenged

Clinical exam is more important than glucose level

FIGURE 4-7 ■ **Factors that play a role in energy available for the central nervous system including blood glucose concentrations.**

when the glucose concentration in the blood was low. However, preterm infants did not show similar patterns of ketone response and appear to have a lower capacity to mobilize ketones as an alternative fuel. It is also clear that formula feeding as a clinical intervention for hypoglycemia has a suppressive effect on early ketogenesis.

There are considerable differences in regional susceptibility in the brain to hypoglycemia that contribute to the pattern and distribution of injury; however, the reported changes have not been consistent. Some animal and human neonatal imaging studies have indicated vulnerability to hypoglycemia in the occipital region, striatum, cingulate cortex, and hippocampus. However, recent clinical and imaging studies have indicated more diverse cerebral injury in infants with significant clinical symptoms of hypoglycemia. A study including 35 term infants with symptomatic hypoglycemia (86% of infants with a blood glucose <35 mg/dL and seizures) extended the spectrum of magnetic resonance imaging (MRI) abnormalities to the white matter, deep nuclear gray matter, and cortical infarction. Therefore an MRI should be a routine investigation for the newborn infant with symptomatic hypoglycemia to define the nature of any cerebral injury.

It must be emphasized, however, that studies like these relate to infants who sustained severe and prolonged hypoglycemia with encephalopathy. There is currently no imaging evidence that mild hypoglycemia of any duration causes brain injury or that asymptomatic hypoglycemia of any duration causes brain injury.

CASE STUDY 4

A 37-year-old gravida 4 para 4 woman delivers a 3400 g male infant with Apgar scores of 9 and 9 at 1 and 5 minutes, respectively, after an uncomplicated pregnancy and labor. The mother has breastfed all of her other children successfully and breastfeeds this infant at 45 minutes of age in the delivery room. A bedside glucose is obtained right after the feeding and it is 27 mg/dL.

EXERCISE 4

QUESTIONS

1. Should this infant have been screened for hypoglycemia?

2. Should the screen occur immediately follow the feeding?

3. Do breastfeeding babies have higher ketone levels and lower blood glucose levels than formula-fed infants?

ANSWERS

1. This infant does not meet any of the risk categories for screening and management of postnatal glucose homeostasis.

2. Glucose screens during the first 4 hours of life are taken 30 minutes after feedings. Thereafter, screens precede feedings for optimal management.

3. Breastfeeding infants are believed to have higher ketone levels, the principal alternate metabolic fuel for the brain, thus sparing glucose.

BREASTFEEDING

In most term infants who are formula fed, the plasma glucose concentration exceeds 40 mg/dL by 6 to 12 hours of postnatal age. Infants who are exclusively breastfed tend to have lower blood glucose concentrations that those fed formula. One study noted that nearly 50% of breastfed infants had blood glucose levels remaining below 36 mg/dL during the first 24 hours after delivery. Other studies show a very wide range of glucose concentrations during the first 72 hours with lower limits at 23 mg/dL in healthy breastfed infants (Table 4-1). Furthermore, breastfed infants tend to have higher ketone concentrations, the principal

TABLE 4-1 **Plasma Glucose Concentrations (mmol/L) in Term, Appropriate Size for Gestation, Breastfed Infants at Four Different Ages**

Age (hr)	Mean	Median	Interquartile Range	Range
3	54 (19)	50.4	25.2-149.4	41.4-59.4
6	53.1 (13.5)	50.4	28.8-97.2	43.5-59.4
24	52.02 (14.2)	52.2	23.4-136.8	46.8-59.4
72	54 (14.2)	50.4	25.2-127.8	46.8-59.4

Repeated analysis of variance, $p = 0.9$

From Wight N: Hypoglycemia in breastfed neonates, Breastfeed Med 1(4):253, 2006.

alternate metabolic fuel for the brain. There-fore, studies indicate that breastfed term infants have lower blood glucose concentra-tions and higher levels of ketone bodies than formula-fed infants. Data extended out to 1 week of age showed that breastfed infants still had significantly lower mean blood glucose levels (range 27 to 95 mg/dL) with mean of 58 mg/dL versus formula-fed of the same age at (range 45 to 111 mg/dL) and mean of 72 mg/dL. A unique observation is that the breastfed infants losing the most weight postnatally had the highest ketone body concentrations. This suggests alternate fuel neuroprotection as a normal adaptive response to a transiently low nutrient intake with modest breastfeeding vol-umes as they increase the first week of life. For the breastfed infant, the only correlation with glucose concentration was the interval between feeds. This emphasizes the need for lactation support, monitoring, and frequent on-demand nursing.

Wight promotes early and exclusive breast-feeding as meeting the nutritional needs of the healthy, term infant and that these infants do not develop symptomatic hypoglycemia simply as a result of underfeeding. She advises against routine supplementation of these healthy infants with water, glucose water, or formula because these may interfere with the establishment of normal breastfeeding.

Healthy term infants should initiate breast-feeding within 30 to 60 minutes of life and con-tinue on demand, recognizing that crying is a very late sign of hunger. Frequent feedings are best 10 to 12 times per 24 hours, which also helps prevent hyperbilirubinemia in the first few days after birth.

If a breastfed term infant meets criteria for glucose screening it should not preclude early initiation of breastfeeding. The infant can be monitored and further clinical decisions should be based on subsequent glucose moni-toring and clinical exam. If such an infant does develop hypoglycemia, it is important to reas-sure the mother that there is nothing wrong with her breast milk and that supplementation or whatever treatment is necessary is usually temporary and the intent is not to jeopardize breastfeeding her infant. In some cases, the mother may want to express or pump milk that is then fed to her infant. It is important to maintain her milk supply until the baby is back to latching and suckling well. Trying to keep the baby on the breast or returning to the breast as soon as is safely possible is impor-tant to maintain breastfeeding for mother and baby.

POSTNATAL GLUCOSE HOMEOSTASIS IN LATE-PRETERM AND TERM INFANTS

The clinical report from the Committee on the Fetus and Newborn provides a practical guide for the screening and subsequent management of neonatal hypoglycemia in at-risk late pre-term (34 to 36 6/7 weeks' gestational age) and term infants. The report does not identify any specific value or range of plasma glucose con-centrations that potentially could result in brain injury. Instead, it is a pragmatic approach to a controversial issue for which evidence is lack-ing but guidance is needed. Recommendations include: which infants to screen, when to screen them, laboratory data, clinical signs, and finally management.

WHICH INFANTS TO SCREEN

Healthy full-term infants born after an entirely normal pregnancy and delivery and who have no clinical signs do not require screening. Routine measurement of blood glucose concentration should only be undertaken in infants who have clinical manifestations or who are known to be at risk of compromised metabolic adaptation. The AAP clinical report was not inclusive of all pre-mature infants and focused only on the late pre-term infant. This was based on the assumption that the vast majority of more premature infants would be cared for in intermediate care or in the neonatal intensive care unit, where routine screening is already in place.

Because plasma glucose homeostasis requires gluconeogenesis and ketogenesis to maintain normal rates of fuel use, neonatal hypoglycemia most commonly occurs in infants with impaired gluconeogenesis and/or ketogenesis, which may occur with excessive insulin production, altered counterregulatory hormone production, an inadequate substrate supply, or a disorder of fatty acid oxidation. Neonatal hypoglycemia commonly occurs in infants who are small for gestational age, infants born to mothers who have diabetes, and late preterm infants. Included as well are large for gestational age infants because it is difficult to exclude maternal diabe-tes or maternal hyperglycemia (prediabetes) with standard-glucose tolerance tests.

A large number of additional maternal and fetal conditions may also place infants at risk of neonatal hypoglycemia (Box 4-2). For the AAP clinical report, it was assumed that clinical signs would be common with these conditions and it

Screening and Management of Postnatal Glucose Homeostasis in Late Preterm and Term SGA, IDM/LGA Infants

[(LPT) Infants 34-36$_{6/7}$ weeks and SGA (screen 0-24 hrs): IDM and LGA ≥34 weeks (screen 0-12 hrs)]

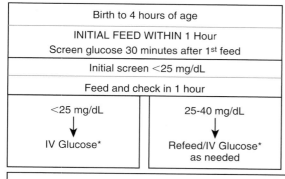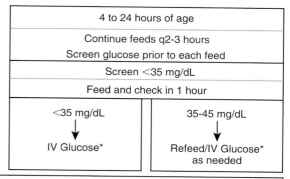

Symptomatic and <40 mg/dL ⟶ IV Glucose

ASYMPTOMATIC

Birth to 4 hours of age	4 to 24 hours of age
INITIAL FEED WITHIN 1 Hour Screen glucose 30 minutes after 1st feed	Continue feeds q2-3 hours Screen glucose prior to each feed
Initial screen <25 mg/dL	Screen <35 mg/dL
Feed and check in 1 hour	Feed and check in 1 hour

<25 mg/dL	25-40 mg/dL	<35 mg/dL	35-45 mg/dL
↓	↓	↓	↓
IV Glucose*	Refeed/IV Glucose* as needed	IV Glucose*	Refeed/IV Glucose* as needed

Target Glucose screen ≥45 mg/dL prior to routine feeds

*Glucose dose = 200 mg/kg (dextrose 10% at 2 mL/kg) and/or IV infusion at 5 to 8 mg/kg/min (80-100 mL/kg/d) to achieve plasma glucose 40-50 mg/dL.

Symptoms of hypoglycemia include: Irritability, tremors, jitteriness, exaggerated Moro reflex, high-pitched cry, seizures, lethargy, floppiness, cyanosis, apnea, poor feeding.

Pediatrics March 2011, COFN, AAP, Adamkin

FIGURE 4-8 ■ **Screening and management of postnatal glucose homeostasis from the AAP Committee on Fetus and Newborn.** (From Adamkin DH: Postnatal glucose homeostasis in late-preterm and term infants, *Pediatrics* 127[2]:576, 2011)

is likely that patients with such conditions would be monitored and that plasma glucose analyses were being performed. Therefore for practicality, "at risk" in the management approach outlined in Figure 4-8 includes only infants who are small for gestational age, infants who are large for gestational age, infants who were born to mothers with diabetes, and late preterm infants.

WHEN TO SCREEN

Plasma glucose should be measured as soon as possible (minutes, not hours) in any infant who manifests clinical signs (Box 4-3, Figure 4-8) compatible with low blood glucose concentration (i.e., the symptomatic infant). Neonatal glucose concentrations decrease after birth to as low as 30 mg/dL or less during the first 1 to 2 hours after birth, and then increase to higher more stable concentrations, generally above 45 mg/dL by 12 hours after birth. Values <40 to 45 mg/dL occur in as many as 5% to 15% of normal newborn infants. Data on the optimal timing and intervals for glucose screening are limited. It seems inappropriate to make early blood glucose measurements on any baby during this immediate fall because the normal cannot be distinguished from

BOX 4-3	Signs and Symptoms of Hypoglycemia in Newborn Infants

General findings
   Abnormal cry
   Poor feeding
   Hypothermia
   Diaphoresis
Neurologic signs
   Tremors and jitteriness
   Hypotonia
   Irritability
   Lethargy
   Seizures
Cardiorespiratory disturbances
   Cyanosis
   Pallor
   Tachypnea
   Apnea
   Cardiac arrest

From Rozance P, Hay W: Hypoglycemia in newborn infants: features associated with adverse outcomes, Biol Neonate 90:81, 2006.

the abnormal. Fortunately, even in the absence of any enteral nutrition intake, the blood glucose rises by 3 hours of age. Even in the "at-risk" infant for hypoglycemia, blood glucose measurement is best avoided during the first 2 hours after birth. There is the real danger that measurements made at this time are self-fulfilling prophecies. No studies have demonstrated harm from a few hours of asymptomatic hypoglycemia during this normal postnatal period of establishing "physiologic homeostasis."

Blood glucose concentrations show a cyclic response to an enteral feed, reaching a peak by about an hour after the feed, and the nadir just before the next feed is due. Because the purpose of blood glucose monitoring is to identify the lowest blood glucose level, it makes most sense to measure a value immediately before the next feeding.

The AAP guideline recommends the frequency and duration of screening for at-risk groups based on risk factors specific to the individual infant. After 24 hours, repeated screening before feeds should be continued if plasma glucose concentrations remain lower than 45 mg/dL.

LABORATORY MEASUREMENTS OF GLUCOSE

Accurate and rapid measurement of blood glucose concentration is the cornerstone of the management of glycemic status in the neonate. Ideally it would be rapid, accurate, inexpensive, and require a small volume of blood. Unfortunately none of the available devices or methods has met all the required attributes for detection of low blood glucose in the neonatal population. When neonatal hypoglycemia is suspected, the plasma or blood glucose must be determined immediately by using one of the laboratory enzymatic methods (glucose oxidase, hexokinase, or dehydrogenase method). Plasma glucose tends to be 10% to 18% higher than whole-blood values because of the higher water content of plasma.

Although a laboratory determination is the most accurate method of measuring the glucose concentration, the results are not available quickly enough for rapid diagnosis of a low blood glucose level, which thereby delays potential interventions and treatments. Bedside reagent test-strip glucose analyzers can be used if the test is performed carefully and the clinician is aware of the limited accuracy of these devices. This bedside or point-of-care testing is done to obtain an estimate of the glucose concentration quickly and conveniently. Although the results of these tests are used for clinical decisions, there are several pitfalls. At present, there is no point-of-care method that is sufficiently reliable and accurate in the low range of blood glucose to allow it to be used as the sole method to screen for hypoglycemia. Test-strip results may vary as much as 10 to 20 mg/dL versus the actual plasma glucose concentration. Unfortunately, this variation is greatest at the low blood glucose concentrations.

Because of limitation with "rapid" bedside methods, the blood or plasma glucose concentration must be confirmed by laboratory testing ordered "stat." A long delay in processing the specimen can result in a falsely low concentration because erythrocytes in the sample metabolize the glucose in the plasma. This problem can be avoided by transporting the blood in tubes that contain a glycolytic inhibitor such as fluoride.

Treatment of the suspected neonatal hypoglycemia should not be postponed while waiting for laboratory confirmation. However, there is no evidence that such treatment will mitigate neurologic sequelae.

CLINICAL SIGNS OF HYPOGLYCEMIA

The clinical signs of neonatal hypoglycemia are not specific and include a wide range of local or generalized manifestations that are common in sick neonates (Box 4-3). The signs and systems of isolated hypoglycemia can be viewed as systemic manifestations of glucopenia (e.g., episodes of cyanosis, apnea, irritability, poor sucking or feeding,) and/or hypothermia accompanied by manifestations of central nervous system glucose deficiency (neuroglycopenia; e.g., changes in level of consciousness, tremors, irritability, lethargy, seizures, exaggerated Moro reflex, coma). The manifestations of neuroglycopenia include the full spectrum of acute encephalopathy. Coma and seizures may occur with prolonged neonatal hypoglycemia (plasma or blood glucose concentrations lower than 10 mg/dL range) and repetitive hypoglycemia.

Because avoidance and treatment of cerebral energy deficiency is the principal concern, greatest attention should be paid to neurologic signs. The clinical manifestations should subside within minutes to hours in response to adequate treatment with intravenous glucose if hypoglycemia alone is responsible. Cornblath and colleagues have suggested that the Whipple triad be fulfilled: (1) a low blood glucose concentration, (2) signs consistent with neonatal hypoglycemia, and (3) resolution of signs and symptoms after restoring blood glucose concentrations to normal values.

MANAGEMENT

The plasma glucose concentration at which intervention is indicated needs to be tailored to the clinical situation and the particular characteristics of the infant. The AAP clinical report on postnatal glucose homeostasis applies to the first 24 hours after birth. It considers symptoms, mode of feeding, risk factors, and hours of age in a pragmatic approach for these infants. Immediate intravenous glucose treatment might be instituted for an infant with clinical signs and a plasma glucose <40 mg/dL, whereas an at-risk but asymptomatic term formula-fed infant with the same value may only require an increased frequency of feeding and would receive intravenous glucose only if the glucose values decreased to <25 mg/dL (birth to 4 hours of age) or 35 mg/dL (4 to 24 hours of age) (Figure 4-8). Follow-up glucose concentrations and clinical evaluation must be obtained to ensure that postnatal glucose homeostasis is achieved and maintained.

All strategies for the management of neonatal hypoglycemia should be based on the infant's glucose concentration, its trend over time, response to enteral feedings, and clinical signs and symptoms. Because severe, prolonged, symptomatic hypoglycemia may result in neuronal injury, prompt intervention is necessary for infants who manifest clinical signs and symptoms. A reasonable (although arbitrary) cutoff for treating symptomatic infants is 40 mg/dL. This value is higher than the physiologic nadir and higher than concentrations usually associated with clinical signs (Figure 4-8). If the decision is to treat, a plasma sample must be sent to the laboratory just before giving the intravenous minibolus of glucose (200 mg/k of glucose per kg, 2 mL/kg dextrose 10% in water, D10W, intravenously) and/or starting a continuous infusion of glucose (D10W at 80 to 100 mL/k/d). A reasonable goal is to maintain plasma glucose concentration in symptomatic infants between 40 and 50 mg/dL (Figure 4-8).

This algorithm (Figure 4-8) is based on the following observations from Cornblath and Ichord: (1) Almost all infants with proven symptomatic neonatal hypoglycemia during the first hours of life have plasma glucose concentrations lower than 20 to 25 mg/dL; (2) persistent or recurrent neonatal hypoglycemia syndromes present with equally low plasma glucose concentrations; and (3) little or no evidence exists to indicate that asymptomatic neonatal hypoglycemia at any concentration of plasma glucose in the first days of life results in any adverse sequelae in growth or development.

Figure 4-8 is divided into two time periods (birth to 4 hours and 4 to 24 hours) and accounts for the changing values of glucose that occur over the first 24 hours after birth. The recommended values for intervention are intended to provide a margin of safety over concentrations of glucose associated with clinical signs. The intervention recommendations also provide a range of values over which the clinician can decide to refeed or provide intravenous glucose. The target plasma glucose is >45 mg/dL before each feeding. At-risk infants should be fed by 1 hour of age and screened 30 minutes after the feeding. The initial feeding recommendation is consistent with that of the World Health Organization. For infants who are able to tolerate enteral feeds, increasing feeding volume should be the first strategy for actionable thresholds. Milk contains nearly twice the amount of energy as an equivalent volume of 10% dextrose, and breast milk in particular promotes ketogenesis. Gavage feeding may be considered in infants who are not nippling well. Glucose screening should continue for 12 hours of age for infants born to mothers with diabetes and those who are large for gestational age and maintain plasma glucose >40 mg/dL. Late-preterm and infants who are small for gestational age require glucose monitoring for at least 24 hours after birth, because they are more vulnerable to low glucose concentrations, especially if regular feedings or intravenous fluids are not yet established (Figure 4-8).

If inadequate postnatal glucose homeostasis is documented, the clinician must be certain that the infant can maintain normal plasma glucose concentrations on a routine diet for a reasonably extended period (through at least three feed–fast periods) before discharge.

It is recommended that the at-risk asymptomatic infants who have glucose concentrations <25 mg/dL (birth to 4 hours of age) or <35 mg/dL (4 to 24 hours of age) be refed and that the glucose value be rechecked 1 hour after refeeding. Subsequent concentrations, <25 mg/dL, or lower than 35 mg/dL, respectively, after attempts to refeed, necessitate treatment with intravenous glucose (Figure 4-8). Persistent hypoglycemia can be treated with a minibolus (200 mg/k, 2 mL/k D10W) and/or intravenous infusion of D10W at 5 to 8 mL/k per minute, 80 to 100 mL/k/d; the goal is to achieve a plasma glucose concentration >40 to 50 mg/dL (higher concentrations will only stimulate further insulin secretion). Plasma glucose concentration should be checked 30 minutes after the minibolus or glucose infusion, then every 1 to 2 hours until stable and in the normal range. If a subsequent value falls in the treatment range, the bolus can be repeated and the infusion rate increased by 10% to 15%. In some cases, it may require as much as 12 to 15 mg/k/min of intravenous glucose to maintain normoglycemia. In such cases, it may be necessary to place an umbilical venous catheter or peripheral central venous catheter to allow administration of intravenous solution with dextrose concentration greater than 12.5%. If it is not possible to maintain blood glucose concentration of >45 mg/dL after 24 hours of using this rate of glucose infusion, consideration should be given to the possibility of hyperinsulinemia, which is the most common cause of severe persistent hypoglycemia in the newborn period.

CASE STUDY 5

A 32-year-old gravida 2 is delivered by cesarean section because of failure to progress. Fetal macrosomia was suspected during the pregnancy. Apgars were 6, 7, and 8 at 1, 5, and 10 minutes respectively. The infant's birthweight was 4.6 kg. The infant was breastfed in the delivery room and was screened with a bedside glucose determination 30 minutes after the feeding and the result was 15 mg/dL. A plasma glucose concentration performed at the same time by the laboratory was 18 mg/dL. The infant remained asymptomatic and was breastfed again. One hour later the next bedside screen was 20 mg/dL and the laboratory value was 23 mg/dL.

EXERCISE 5

QUESTIONS

1. What would you do next?

2. What diagnosis are you most concerned about?

ANSWERS

1. The infant should receive intravenous glucose because the level has remained <25 mg/dL despite two feedings.

2. Macrosomia suggests hyperinsulinism.

CASE STUDY 5 (continued)

A minibolus is given and this is followed by an infusion of 5 mg/k/min after the second bedside glucose value of 20 mg/dL. The infant is rescreened with bedside glucose measurements and plasma glucose levels; and despite advancing glucose infusion rate to 16 mg/kg/min, the plasma glucose levels never exceed 40 mg/dL and at 24 hours of age the infant has a seizure. The mother reveals that her previous child had a similar course to this one.

WHEN ARE FURTHER INVESTIGATIONS REQUIRED?

Infants with persistent hypoglycemia or those with inadequate responses to treatment need further evaluation. Recurrent or persistent

TABLE 4-2 Causes of Recurrent or Persistent Hypoglycemia

Hormone Deficiencies	
Multiple endocrine deficiency or congenital hypopituitarism	Anterior pituitary "aplasia"
	Congenital optic nerve hypoplasia
Primary endocrine deficiency	Isolated growth hormone deficiency
	Adrenogenital syndrome
	Adrenal hemorrhage
Hormone excess with hyperinsulinism	Beckwith-Wiedemann syndrome
	Hereditary defects of pancreatic islet cells
Hereditary deficits in carbohydrate metabolism	Glycogen storage disease
	Fructose intolerance
	Galactosemia
	Glycogen synthase deficiency
	Fructose, 1-6 diphosphatase deficiency
Hereditary deficits in amino acid metabolism	Maple syrup urine disease
	Propiionic acidemia
	Methylmalonic acidemia
	Tyrosinosis
	3-OH-3 methyl glutaryl COA lyse deficiency
Hereditary defects in fatty acid metabolism	Acyl CoA dehydrogenase—medium, long chain Deficiency
	Mitochondrial β-oxidation and degradation defects

From Cornblath M, Ichord R: Hypoglycemia in the neonate, Semin Perinatol 24:145, 2000.

hypoglycemia (Table 4-2) is defined as conditions that: (1) require infusions of large amounts of glucose (>12 to 16 mg/k/min) to maintain normoglycemia or (2) persist or recur beyond the first 7 to 14 days of life. These infants require specific diagnostic determinations as well as a rapid trial of therapeutic-diagnostic agents to determine cause and therapy. Table 4-2 shows a brief list of these syndromes. Hyperinsulinism, hypopituitarism, and fatty acid oxidation disorders are probably the most common of these rather uncommon causes of neonatal hypoglycemia.

An underlying metabolic or hormonal etiology should be suspected when the hypoglycemia is of unusual severity or occurs in an otherwise low-risk infant. Some clues to a possible underlying metabolic-hormonal disorder include:

- Symptomatic hypoglycemia in a healthy, well grown term infant
- Hypoglycemia with seizures or abnormalities of consciousness
- Persistent or recurrent hypoglycemia

- Hypoglycemia in association with other abnormalities (midline defects, micropenis, exophthalmos, labile thermoregulation)
- Hypoglycemia requiring >10 mg/kg/min of glucose
- Family history of sudden infant deaths or developmental delay

CONCLUSION

Current evidence does not support a specific concentration of glucose that can discriminate euglycemia from hypoglycemia or can predict the acute or chronic irreversible neurologic damage that will result. Once observed, a significantly low concentration of glucose in the plasma of an at-risk asymptomatic infant should be confirmed and treated to restore glucose values to a normal physiologic range. Recognizing infants at risk of disturbances in postnatal glucose homeostasis and providing a margin of safety by early measures to prevent (feeding) and treat (feeding and intravenous glucose infusion) are the goals of management.

SUGGESTED READINGS

Adamkin DH: Committee on Fetus and Newborn. Clinical report—postnatal glucose homeostasis in late-preterm and term infants, *Pediatrics* 127:575, 2011.

Adamkin DH: Update on neonatal hypoglycemia, *Arch Perinat Med* 11(3):13–15, 2005.

Boluyt N, van Kempen A, Offringa M: Neurodevelopment after neonatal hypoglycemia: a systematic review and design of an optimal future study, *Pediatrics* 117:2231–2243, 2006.

Burns C, Rutherford M, Boardman J, Cowan F: Patterns of cerebral injury and neurodevelopmental outcomes after symptomatic hypoglycemia, *Pediatrics* 122(1):65–74, 2008.

Cornblath M, Ichord R: Hypoglycemia in the neonate, *Semin Perinatol* 24(2):136–149, 2000.

Cornblath M, Hawdon JM, Williams AF, et al.: Controversies regarding definition of neonatal hypoglycemia: suggested operational thresholds, *Pediatrics* 105(5):1141–1145, 2000.

Deshpande S, Ward Platt M: The investigation and management of neonatal hypoglycemia, *Semin Fetal Neonatal Med* 10(4):351–361, 2005.

Hay W, Raju TNK, Higgins RD, Kalhan SC, Devaskar SU: Knowledge gaps and research needs for understanding and treating neonatal hypoglycemia: workshop report from Eunice Kennedy Shriver National Institute of Child Health and Human Development, *J Pediatr* 155(5):612–617, 2009.

Inder T: Commentary: How low can I go? The impact of hypoglycemia on the immature brain, *Pediatrics* 122(2):440–441, 2008.

Lucas A, Morley R, Cole TJ: Adverse neurodevelopmental outcome of moderate neonatal hypoglycemia, *Br Med J* 297:1304–1308, 1988.

McGowan JE: Neonatal hypoglycemia, *Pediatrics in Review* 20(7):6–15, 1999.

Platt MW, Deshpande S: Metabolic adaptation at birth, *Semin Fetal Neonatal Med* 10(4):341–350, 2005.

Rozance PJ, Hay WW: Hypoglycemia in newborn infants: features associated with adverse outcomes, *Biol Neonate* 90:74–86, 2006.

Srinivasan G, Pildes RS, Cattamanchi G: Plasma glucose values in normal neonates: a new look, *J Pediatr* 109:114–117, 1986.

Tin W, Brunskill G, Kelly T, Fritz S: 15 year follow-up of recurrent "hypoglycemia" in preterm infants, *Pediatrics* 130(6):1497–1503, 2012.

Wight NE: Hypoglycemia in breastfed neonates, *Breastfeed Med* 1(4):253–262, 2006.

Williams AF: Neonatal hypoglycemia: clinical and legal aspects, *Semin Fetal Neonatal Med* 10(4):363–368, 2005.

CHAPTER 5

NEONATAL HYPERBILIRUBINEMIA

Michael Kaplan, MBChB • Cathy Hammerman, MD

Neonatal jaundice is the most common physiologic variant encountered in the newborn. About 60% of healthy, term neonates, and even a greater percentage of breastfed infants, display some degree of visible jaundice during the first week of life. Usually the body's regulatory mechanisms succeed in keeping the serum total bilirubin (STB) level within physiologic—and therefore nontoxic—concentrations. Indeed, STB concentrations within this range may even have beneficial, antioxidant properties.

On occasion STB levels may increase and hyperbilirubinemia may develop. Not all degrees of hyperbilirubinemia are necessarily dangerous, but because of the potential for the STB to continue to rise, phototherapy may be indicated, limiting further rise of STB and preventing the potential for bilirubin neurotoxicity. Rarely the STB may increase to extreme levels at which bilirubin neurotoxicity may occur. In these cases, bilirubin, especially the unbound fraction, may enter the basal ganglia of the brain, causing bilirubin encephalopathy and an increased likelihood of choreoathetoid cerebral palsy (kernicterus).

It is not our intention in this chapter to provide yet another all-inclusive treatise on neonatal hyperbilirubinemia. Rather, following some background information regarding neonatal hyperbilirubinemia, the reader will be presented with some actual clinical cases drawn from the authors' experience. The reader is encouraged to put himself in the "driver's seat" and actually manage the patients, making clinical decisions from the options provided. The cases will provide the opportunity for in-depth discussions of the issues at hand and focus on practical issues with which the practitioner may come in contact on a daily basis.

THE SERUM TOTAL BILIRUBIN: WHAT DOES IT REPRESENT?

CASE STUDY 1

A 36-weeks' gestation, otherwise healthy infant aged 48 hours was being discussed on rounds in the regular newborn nursery. The STB was 15.0 mg/dL. The professor asked the residents what this value actually meant.

EXERCISE 1

QUESTION

1. The following possibilities were suggested. Which answer do you think is correct?
   a. One resident plotted the result on the hour-specific bilirubin nomogram. Because the value was greater than the 95th percentile, this resident concluded that increased hemolysis was present.
   b. The second resident related to the late prematurity of this infant. The bilirubin-conjugating system is clearly immature, he claimed, resulting in the increased STB.
   c. The third resident claimed that the pathogenesis of the high STB value was multifactorial and that both increased bilirubin production and hemolysis contributed to its development.

ANSWER

1. c. The third resident correctly argued that several physiologic or pathophysiologic processes contributed to the STB. His claim that no single process is responsible for an STB value at any point in time—but that the STB value represents a combination of processes acting in tandem—must be taken into account. The first resident's

answer (a) was incorrect in that, although increased hemolysis may have been present, he did not take bilirubin elimination into account. Similarly, the second resident (b) correctly identified late prematurity and a diminished conjugation ability of the infant as risk factors, but neglected to take the potential for increased hemolysis into account.

The STB: A Delicate Balance of Forces

Equilibrium Between Bilirubin Production and Elimination

The STB at any point in time, in any newborn, represents a combination of forces both affecting heme catabolism and therefore bilirubin production, on the one hand, and bilirubin elimination—primarily by the process of bilirubin conjugation, but also excretion—on the other. As long as these processes remain in equilibrium the STB may rise to physiologic levels, but should not pose a threat to an otherwise healthy, term newborn.

Lack of Aforesaid Equilibrium

Should this delicate balance become compromised, and bilirubin production exceeds bilirubin elimination, the equilibrium will fail and hyperbilirubinemia may result. Severe hemolysis *per se* or immature bilirubin conjugation in and of itself may not necessarily result in hyperbilirubinemia. For example, an infant with blood type "A," born to a woman with blood type "O" who has a positive direct antiglobulin test (DAT-Coombs) can be expected to be a strong bilirubin producer, but may not necessarily develop hyperbilirubinemia should the bilirubin conjugation and elimination processes be well functioning. On the other hand, moderate hemolysis coupled with immaturity of uridine diphosphate (UDP)-glucuronosyltransferase 1A1 (UGT1A1) (the bilirubin-conjugating enzyme)—as might occur in a late-preterm infant—may result in lack of equilibrium between the aforementioned processes with resultant hyperbilirubinemia.

This concept has been likened to a sink of water. Provided the drainage is functional, an influx of water may not result in the water level increasing. Partial blockage of the drain may lead to a high water level even with a partly opened tap. The concept has been demonstrated mathematically by using a "production-conjugation index." The blood carboxyhemoglobin concentration (corrected for inspired CO), an accurate index of heme catabolism, and the serum total conjugated bilirubin (a reflection of intrahepatocytic conjugated bilirubin) have been used as components of this index. A rising index suggests an increasing lack of equilibrium between production and excretion.

It should be obvious that when evaluating a hyperbilirubinemic infant, both etiologic factors contributing to increased bilirubin production as well as diminished bilirubin conjugation should be taken into consideration. Given the unreliability of hematologic indices to reflect hemolysis in the newborn as well as the current unavailability of a clinical tool such as end tidal CO evaluation with which to assess the presence of ongoing hemolysis, it may be difficult to distinguish disorders associated with increased production or increased excretion. These processes may include exaggerated heme catabolism (hemolysis), immaturity of UGT1A1, and reabsorption of bilirubin from the bowel to reenter the bloodstream. Immaturity in the enzyme UGT1A1 may be compounded by presence of the $(TA)_n$ polymorphism in the promoter of the *UGT1A1* gene, resulting in diminished gene expression with decreased enzyme activity (Gilbert syndrome). Factors affecting lack of equilibrium between the processes contributing to the STB are summarized in Box 5-1.

Is the STB Predictive of Bilirubin Neurotoxicity?

Although the STB is used as a tool for the management of neonatal hyperbilirubinemia, this test is actually a poor predictor of bilirubin-related neurologic outcome. Although it is unlikely that an otherwise healthy, term infant with no obvious hemolytic condition will develop bilirubin neurotoxicity at STB levels <25 mg/dL,

BOX 5-1	Factors Affecting Lack of Equilibrium Between the Processes Contributing to the Serum Total Bilirubin at Any Specific Point in Time

1. Increased hemolysis
2. Immaturity of the bilirubin-conjugating enzyme, UDP-glucuronosyltransferase 1A1 (UGT1A1)
3. (TA)n promoter polymorphism of the encoding gene *UGT1A1* with resultant diminished gene expression and enzyme activity (associated with Gilbert syndrome in adults)
4. Enterohepatic circulation

there is actually no specific cut off point at which an STB level will, or will not, be predictive of neurotoxicity. Certainly, not all newborns with extreme hyperbilirubinemia go on to develop choreoathetoid cerebral palsy. For example, in one study of 140 newborns with total serum bilirubin (TSB) values >25 mg/dL who were treated with phototherapy or exchange transfusion, overall, 5-year outcomes were not significantly different from those of randomly selected controls. In a reanalysis of data from the Collaborative Perinatal Project, there was no relationship, overall, between maximum STB levels and subsequent intelligence quotient (IQ) scores. However, in both these studies presence of a positive DAT resulted in a poorer prognosis. (See the section on Increased Hemolysis). Similarly, of 249 newborns admitted to a children's hospital in Cairo, Egypt, all of whom had STB values ≥25 mg/dL, there was little correlation between admission STB and acute bilirubin encephalopathy. However, in babies with hemolytic risk factors including Rh incompatibility, ABO incompatibility, and sepsis, the threshold STB for identifying babies with bilirubin encephalopathy was lower relative to those without these factors.

Predictive Value of Serum Unbound Bilirubin

If the STB is not a good predictor of bilirubin neurotoxicity, then what is? Several studies have suggested that the unbound bilirubin fraction may be a more accurate predictor of bilirubin toxicity than STB, both in term and preterm infants. Use of the unbound fraction as an indication for institution of phototherapy or for performing exchange transfusion would take much of the guesswork out of the decision-making process and permit better identification of the infant at risk for brain damage. Currently, however, unbound bilirubin determinations are unavailable for routine clinical use and STB remains the cardinal laboratory indication used for clinical decision-making in hyperbilirubinemic newborns.

DEFINITIONS

Jaundice and Hyperbilirubinemia

The terms jaundice and hyperbilirubinemia are sometimes, incorrectly, used interchangeably.

Jaundice refers to a yellow coloring of the sclera, skin, and mucous membranes, due to infiltration from the serum of the yellow pigment bilirubin. *Hyperbilirubinemia*, on the other hand, relates to a measurement of serum or transcutaneous bilirubin, the result of which is greater than an accepted norm.

The Hour-Specific Bilirubin Nomogram

In infants ≥35 weeks gestation, a useful definition of hyperbilirubinemia is an STB value greater than the 95th percentile for age in hours on the hour-specific bilirubin nomogram (Figure 5-1). Use of the nomogram adjusts for the dynamic changes in STB during the first postnatal week and obviates the concept whereby a single STB value is regarded as representative of hyperbilirubinemia. Thus an infant with an STB value of 10.0 mg/dL at 12 hours will be regarded as hyperbilirubinemic, whereas the same concentration 48 hours later will have little significance.

Variations on This Definition

Because phototherapy may be indicated in newborns with lower gestational ages or with risk factors for hyperbilirubinemia, at levels of STB below the 95th percentile, adherence to the 2004 American Academy of Pediatrics (AAP) guidelines would prevent many newborns from actually meeting the above criteria for hyperbilirubinemia. Variations on this definition, to accommodate intervention with phototherapy, include an STB value within 1 mg/dL of the indications for phototherapy or an STB value exceeding the 75th percentile on the bilirubin nomogram.

Bilirubin Encephalopathy and Kernicterus

The terms bilirubin encephalopathy and kernicterus are often used interchangeably, although the AAP recommends differentiating these two conditions (AAP, 2004).

Acute bilirubin encephalopathy relates to the acute manifestations of bilirubin neurotoxicity seen during or immediately following an episode of extreme hyperbilirubinemia. Permanent features of choreoathetoid cerebral palsy may ensue, but reversal, when appropriately treated, has been reported.

Kernicterus, on the other hand, refers to cases manifesting chronic and permanent sequelae attributable to bilirubin neurotoxicity, the result of bilirubin deposition in the target nuclei of the brain.

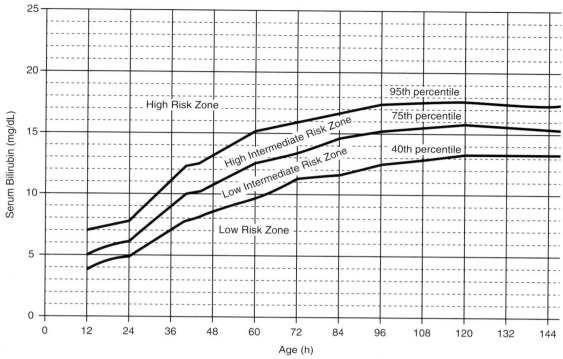

FIGURE 5-1 ■ Nomogram for designation of risk in 2840 well newborns at ≥36 weeks' gestational age with birth weight of ≥2000 g or ≥35 weeks' gestational age and birth weight of ≥2500 g based on the hour-specific serum bilirubin values. (Reproduced with permission from Bhutani VK, Johnson L, Sivieri EM: Predictive ability of a predischarge hour-specific serum bilirubin for subsequent significant hyperbilirubinemia in healthy term and near-term newborns, *Pediatrics* 103:6-14, 1999.)

PHYSIOLOGY OF BILIRUBIN PRODUCTION AND METABOLISM

An understanding of the basic concepts of bilirubin physiology is necessary for perceptive management of the hyperbilirubinemic newborn. Because detailed reviews of this subject are available in standard texts, only an outline will be provided here as a basis for comprehension of the subsequent portions of the chapter. Variations in bilirubin physiology peculiar to the newborn, contributing to the development of hyperbilirubinemia, are interspersed among the descriptions of basic bilirubin physiology

A. Bilirubin Formation

Most heme is produced by the destruction of red blood cells (RBC) in the reticuloendothelial system. This substance is further catabolized to biliverdin by the enzyme heme oxygenase 1 and thence to bilirubin. This bilirubin component is termed unconjugated or indirect bilirubin. In newborn infants, the RBC mass is larger, the turnover of the RBC is more rapid, and this cell lifespan is shorter than in adults. There is thus a relatively large heme load, which contributes to the bilirubin pool.

B. Bilirubin Binding to Serum Albumin; Unbound Bilirubin

To facilitate transportation to the liver, indirect bilirubin is bound to serum albumin. This step is very important in our current understanding of the pathophysiology of bilirubin neurotoxicity. As long as the bilirubin molecule is bound to albumin it is not expected to cross the blood–brain barrier and bilirubin neurotoxicity should not occur. Should the albumin binding sites become saturated and the bilirubin be unable to bind unbound—or free—bilirubin will result. This "free" bilirubin fraction can enter brain cells and cause neurotoxic damage. Potential causes of unbound bilirubin formation, raising the risk for neurotoxicity, should always be kept in mind when evaluating an infant for hyperbilirubinemia. Some causes of unbound bilirubin formation are listed in Box 5-2.

C. Bilirubin Uptake

Uptake Genes

Uptake of bilirubin into the liver is controlled by the solute carrier organic anion transporter protein 1B1, *SLCO1B1*, also known as *OATP2*.

BOX 5-2	**Some Causes of Unbound Bilirubin Formation**

Hypoalbuminemia
Excessive hemolysis even in the presence of
    normal serum albumin concentrations
Metabolic acidosis
Hypothermia
Sepsis
Drugs such as sulfa-containing antimicrobials
Prematurity (possible)

Varying expression of this sinusoidal transporter gene, the result of polymorphisms, may affect bilirubin kinetics and metabolism. For example, the *SLCO1B1*1b* variant is associated with neonatal hyperbilirubinemia in Taiwanese newborns, especially when coupled with *UGT1A1* variants. Similarly coexpression of *SLCO1B1*1b* with glucose-6-phosphate dehydrogenase (G-6-PD) A- was associated with hyperbilirubinemia in a U.S.-based study.

D. Bilirubin Conjugation and Elimination

The Importance of UDP-Glucuronosyltransferase 1A1 (UGT1A1)

Following uptake into the hepatocyte, indirect bilirubin is conjugated with glucuronic acid to form water-soluble mono- and diglucuronides. These complexes are known as conjugated or direct bilirubin. The enzyme controlling the conjugation process is UGT1A1. Immaturity of UGT is an important contributor to hyperbilirubinemia in both term and preterm infants. In term infants activity of UGT is only about 1% that of adults and is even less in preterm infants. Developmental immaturity with slowing of the conjugation process is actually the bottleneck of the neonatal bilirubin elimination process and the reason why the majority of newborns exhibit some degree of visible jaundice during the postnatal period.

E. Excretion of Bilirubin into the Bowel and the Enterohepatic Circulation

Direct bilirubin is secreted into the bile and then to the bowel from which it is excreted in the stool. The presence of the enzyme beta-glucuronidase in the colon deconjugates bilirubin-glucuronides and allows the reabsorption of bilirubin into the bloodstream, thereby adding to the bilirubin pool. A delay in enteral feeding may diminish intestinal motility. The resultant increased bowel stasis with decreased elimination will allow for even greater reabsorption of bilirubin.

Genetic Control of Bilirubin Conjugation

There is increasing appreciation that the modulation of serum bilirubin levels and the development of hyperbilirubinemia may be under genetic control. A detailed account of all the genes contributing to bilirubin metabolism is beyond the scope of this text. Because of the practical nature of the enzyme UGT1A1, its genetic control is discussed in some detail.

The enzyme UGT1A1 is encoded by the gene *UGT1A1*, mapped to chromosome 2q37. This gene contains both a noncoding promoter region and a coding region. Polymorphisms of the promoter region, such as the $(TA)_n$ polymorphism, result in diminished expression of a normally formed enzyme and are associated with Gilbert syndrome. On the other hand, coding area mutations, as seen in Crigler-Najjar syndrome, result in an abnormally structured enzyme that has little or no conjugating ability. Coexpression of genes, presence of several mutations or polymorphisms, and interactions with environmental factors may potentiate the genetic contribution to the pathophysiology of neonatal hyperbilirubinemia. A paradigm of this concept may be found in the pathophysiology of neonatal hyperbilirubinemia in G-6-PD–deficient neonates, in which interaction between environmental factors triggering hemolysis, the G-6-PD deficiency in and of itself, and $(TA)_n$ promoter polymorphisms of *UGT1A1* (*UGT1A1*28*) may potentiate severe hyperbilirubinemia.

INCREASED HEMOLYSIS: A RISK FACTOR FOR BILIRUBIN NEUROTOXICITY

ABO Isoimmunization

CASE STUDY 2

Baby AB was born at term gestation to a blood group O, Rh-negative mother. The nurses thought that the baby's skin had a yellow tinge on admission to the nursery. The physician believed this was only very mild jaundice and chose to ignore it. An astute nurse, however, took an STB at age 12 hours, the result of which was 9.2 mg/dL. "Not very high" responded the physician. By the next day (28 hours) the STB value was 15 mg/dL.

EXERCISE 2

QUESTION

1. What should you do?
   a. Observe the baby and repeat the STB in another 24 hours.
   b. Place the infant under "intense" phototherapy and repeat the STB in 4 to 6 hours.
   c. Begin phototherapy and proceed to exchange transfusion.

ANSWER

1. **b.** However, this baby had not been correctly managed from the outset. A baby born to a blood group O mother may be at risk for neonatal hyperbilirubinemia if the infant's blood type is A or B. The second risk factor for severe hyperbilirubinemia was the presence of jaundice shortly after birth, with an STB concentration significantly above the 95th percentile. Answers "a" and "c" are incorrect. There is no need at this point to proceed to exchange transfusion as the rise in STB in many cases of ABO isoimmunization may be modulated by intense phototherapy and intravenous immune globulin (IVIG) administration.

CASE STUDY 2 (continued)

One hour after commencing phototherapy, the following laboratory results were reported: infant's blood group B, Rh positive, DAT strongly positive, Hb 12.0 mg/dL, Hct 36%, reticulocyte count 6%. The anemia in association with an elevated reticulocyte count suggests that hemolysis is occurring.

EXERCISE 3

QUESTION

1. After 6 hours of intensive phototherapy a repeat STB value is 18.3 mg/dL. What should be done now?
   a. Continue phototherapy and repeat the STB in 12 hours.
   b. Exchange transfusion.
   c. Administer IVIG, 1 gm/kg.

ANSWER

1. c.

Intravenous Immune Globulin (IVIG) in Immune Hemolytic Anemia

Answer "a" is incorrect because waiting 12 hours might allow the bilirubin to rise to a dangerous level. Answer "b" might be considered a valid option. However, in the authors' experience, administration of IVIG has virtually eliminated the need for exchange transfusion in infants with ABO incompatibility.

In an infant with ABO incompatibility, administration of IVIG is very effective in preventing a further increase in STB and decreasing the need for exchange transfusion. In other isoimmunizations such as Rh, anti-c or anti-e, IVIG therapy may be less effective but may be instrumental in gaining time to allow for stabilization of the baby before performing an exchange transfusion. As suggested by carboxyhemoglobin (COHb) studies, IVIG is assumed to diminish the rate of hemolysis (CO is a sensitive index of heme catabolism). IVIG therapy is recommended in the therapeutic armamentarium of the AAP guideline (2004) for the management of immune-mediated hemolysis.

In fact, this baby did respond to an infusion of IVIG. The rise in STB was curtailed and exchange transfusion avoided. In the authors' experience, an aggressive approach to ABO-incompatible infants—including: (1) a high rate of awareness of babies born to blood group O mothers, (2) identification of early jaundice either by visual inspection or transcutaneous bilirubin (TcB) examination, (3) intense phototherapy according to AAP recommendations, and (4) IVIG administration should the STB continue to rise despite phototherapy—has circumvented the need for exchange transfusion in ABO-incompatible newborns.

Increased Risk for Bilirubin Neurotoxicity Associated with Hemolysis

It is generally believed that neonates with hemolytic disease are at a higher risk for bilirubin-induced neurotoxicity than those whose hyperbilirubinemia is not caused by a hemolytic process. Whereas an STB concentration of 20 to 24 mg/dL may be associated with bilirubin encephalopathy and kernicterus in a neonate with Rh isoimmunization, in the absence of a hemolytic condition a healthy, term infant will rarely be endangered by STB concentrations in this range. The mechanism by which hemolysis increases the risk of bilirubin neurotoxicity has not been elucidated. Because the unbound bilirubin fraction is thought to be that which crosses the blood–brain barrier, it seems logical that babies with hemolytic conditions should have higher unbound bilirubin fractions than their nonhemolyzing counterparts. However, to date, this has not been demonstrated. A high rate of bilirubin production over a short period of time, typical of increased hemolysis, may offset the effect of bilirubin distribution into the tissues, a process that may be effective in moderating the rise in STB.

Several studies support the concept of increased severity of bilirubin neurotoxicity in the face of hemolysis. In a study performed in Turkey, a positive DAT—used as a presumed marker of hemolysis in infants with Rh isoimmunization or ABO incompatibility—was associated with lower IQ scores and a higher incidence of neurologic abnormalities than in controls who were not DAT positive. A similar observation was made in Norway in the 1960s; DAT-positive males who had STB levels >15 mg/dL for longer than 5 days had IQ scores lower than that observed in the general population. In the Jaundice and Infant Feeding Study, IQ values in the subgroup of DAT-positive infants with TSB >25 mg/dL were significantly lower than hyperbilirubinemic infants who were DAT negative. Finally, in a reanalysis of the data from the Collaborative Perinatal Project, the presence of a positive DAT in infants with a TSB of ≥25 mg/dL was associated with decreased IQ scores.

Recent case series of infants with kernicterus from the United States, Canada, the United Kingdom and Ireland, and Denmark indicate that hemolysis (with or without isoimmunization) plays a major role in the etiology of hyperbilirubinemia. Hemolytic conditions including ABO incompatibility—with or without a positive DAT—and G-6-PD deficiency topped the list of conditions in which a specific etiology for the hyperbilirubinemia was determined. Although Rh isoimmunization is rarely encountered in Western countries, the condition is still rampant in developing countries.

AAP Recommendations Regarding Babies with Hemolysis

In its 2004 guidelines, the AAP placed special emphasis on identifying neonates with hemolytic conditions. Infants with early jaundice (<24 hours postdelivery) or those who have rapidly increasing bilirubin values (that "jump percentiles" on the hour-specific bilirubin nomogram) should be suspected of having ongoing hemolysis. Similarly, blood group incompatibility with a positive DAT and other known hemolytic disease including G-6-PD deficiency are regarded as major risk factors for the development of severe hyperbilirubinemia. Although the complete blood count may be helpful in detecting hemolysis in cases of isoimmunization, there may be overlap in values between babies with and without hemolysis. G-6-PD deficiency is especially notorious in demonstrating normal values in the presence of extremely high STB values, which can only be attributed to hemolysis.

In cases of overt hemolysis including isoimmune hemolytic disease and G-6-PD deficiency, the Subcommittee on Hyperbilirubinemia of the AAP recommends a more aggressive approach to management of hyperbilirubinemia including initiation of phototherapy or performing exchange transfusions at lower levels of STB than in neonates without obvious hemolytic etiologies. A list of some commonly occurring etiologies of hemolysis can be seen in Box 5-3. For a comprehensive listing the reader is referred to standard textbooks.

G-6-PD Deficiency: an Important Cause of Kernicterus

CASE STUDY 3

Baby GP, male, was born at term in the United States to parents who were recent immigrants from Greece. The parents reported that a previous

BOX 5-3	Some Important or Commonly Occurring Causes of Increased Hemolysis

IMMUNE CONDITIONS

ABO immunization
Rh (D) isoimmunization (in the main eliminated in Westernized countries, still common in developing countries)
Some rarer immune conditions
    Anti-c, anti-C
    Anti-e, anti-E
    Anti-Kell
    Anti-Duffy
    Anti-Kidd

NON–IMMUNE CONDITIONS

Red cell enzyme deficiencies
    G-6-PD deficiency
    Pyruvate kinase deficiency
    Other rare RBC enzyme deficiencies
Red cell membrane defects
    Hereditary spherocytosis
    Elliptocytosis
    Ovalocytosis
    Stomatocytosis
    Pyknocytosis
Hemoglobinopathies
    Unstable hemoglobinopathies
General conditions
    Sepsis
    Extravasated blood (cephalhematoma, ecchymosis, adrenal hemorrhage, subdural hemorrhage)

child in their family had been treated with phototherapy. At the time of discharge at 48 hours, the STB was 11.0 mg/dL (the 75th percentile on the bilirubin nomogram). The infant was breastfeeding, apparently successfully.

EXERCISE 4

QUESTION

1. What should you advise the parents?
   a. See a pediatrician within 2 to 3 days in accordance with AAP guidelines (2004).
   b. Assess the baby as being relatively risk free for hyperbilirubinemia. See a pediatrician by age 2 weeks.
   c. This infant is at high risk for significant neonatal hyperbilirubinemia. He should be seen by a pediatrician or medical professional within 48 hours (or sooner should the infant become yellow).

ANSWER

1. None of these answers is correct. This infant was at high risk for severe hyperbilirubinemia based on the history of a sibling requiring phototherapy and the family's Mediterranean-basin origin. The discharging pediatrician did not recognize those risk factors. Furthermore, the STB was already in the intermediate high-risk zone. Based on these risk factors in a male, breastfeeding baby (additional risk factors), this infant should have had a repeat STB within 24 hours. The parents should have been instructed how to recognize jaundice and what to do should their infant become jaundiced.

   At age 5 days the baby became lethargic and refused to nurse. They called the pediatrician's office, but were told that the first available appointment was at 2:00 PM the following day. Following onset of seizures the parents took the baby to the emergency room. The triage nurse exclaimed: "This baby looks like a pumpkin!" While waiting to be seen by a doctor the baby became apneic and required intubation and ventilation. Phenobarbital was administered. One and one half hours later the STB was reported as 35 mg/dL. The baby was admitted to the pediatric ward, an IV placed, antibiotics administered, and phototherapy commenced. Blood was ordered for an exchange but because of a technical problem delivery of the blood was delayed for 3 hours.

Acute Bilirubin Encephalopathy: to Exchange or Not to Exchange?

While waiting for the blood for the exchange transfusion, there was a discussion among the doctors attending to this case regarding the efficacy of performing an exchange transfusion in a baby who already had signs of bilirubin encephalopathy.

- One physician argued that kernicterus is associated with irreversible neurologic injury. Therefore why perform a potentially dangerous procedure in a baby who is already damaged?
- Another physician stated that the early signs of kernicterus can be reversed when the STB is promptly lowered by exchange transfusion and intense phototherapy. Some of these infants develop normally.

The second physician is correct. There have been reports of reversal of the bilirubin neurotoxicity process with prompt lowering of the STB by exchange transfusion, even in cases already manifesting signs of bilirubin encephalopathy. The AAP guideline (2004) recommends immediate performance of exchange transfusion should an infant manifest signs of acute bilirubin encephalopathy (see the following). The initiation of intensive phototherapy while waiting for the blood for the exchange transfusion is the correct response.

In the current case, exchange transfusion via the umbilical vein was commenced 7 hours after arrival at the emergency room. A G-6-PD assay on blood that had been sampled prior to the exchange transfusion was very low, indicative of G-6-PD deficiency. On interrogation it became apparent that a neighbor had prepared a meal for the parents that included fava beans, a Mediterranean ethnic dish. The infant was probably exposed to the bean metabolites via breast milk. The child is currently 7 years old and has severe choreoathetotic cerebral palsy.

Severe Hyperbilirubinemia Associated with G-6-PD Deficiency: Unpredictable and Unpreventable

The AAP regards kernicterus as a condition that should generally be preventable. G-6-PD deficiency, however, may be one important reason why this goal may be unreachable. G-6-PD–deficient newborns sometimes have acute episodes of severe jaundice in which STB rises in an exponential fashion. These episodes are by and large unpreventable and unpredictable and occur even when all preventive measures are undertaken. However, much can be done to facilitate treatment in the early stages of the hyperbilirubinemia, prior to the onset of signs of bilirubin encephalopathy, or at a point when bilirubin encephalopathy may, with appropriate treatment, still be reversible.

BOX 5-4	Population Subgroups at Risk for G-6-PD Deficiency in the United States

African American
Italian
Greek
Middle East through India, Asia, and China
Sephardic Jews, especially of Middle Eastern origin
Central and Western Africa
Brazil

What went wrong? This baby was inadequately managed and evaluated by the pediatricians, both in the hospital and in the community setting. Many pediatricians in North America regard G-6-PD deficiency as a condition prevalent in the Middle East or Mediterranean basin, with little relevance to their own practices. As a result, most states do not screen for that disorder. Although the indigenous distribution of G-6-PD deficiency characteristically includes central and west Africa, Mediterranean countries, the Middle East, and parts of Asia, G-6-PD–deficient individuals are widely distributed because of ease of travel and immigration patterns. Furthermore, about 12% of African American males are G-6-PD deficient. Therefore, it is not surprising that G-6-PD deficiency comprised more than 20% of the 125 cases reported in the U.S.-based Kernicterus Registry (Johnson and Bhutani), making it overrepresented relative to estimated U.S. G-6-PD frequency. A list of population subgroups in the United States at risk for G-6-PD deficiency appears in Box 5-4.

Will G-6-PD Screening Help?

The parents of this baby should have been warned of the high-risk nature of their ethnic background with regard to the potential for G-6-PD deficiency. Had the baby been born in Greece, G-6-PD deficiency would have been screened for as part of a national screening program. In the United States, except for Washington, D.C. and Pennsylvania, there is no obligation to screen otherwise healthy babies for this condition. Discussions, however, have commenced regarding feasibility and whether it is economically worthwhile to establish such a program in the United States. Screening will not prevent the acute hemolytic attacks, but knowledge that their infant is G-6-PD deficient, in combination with parental education, should heighten parental and medical caretaker awareness, facilitate earlier referral to medical centers, and result in earlier institution of effective therapy. Because

so many infants are discharged as healthy but readmitted with bilirubin encephalopathy at or around 5 days of age, it will be important to perform screening for G-6-PD deficiency, obtain the results, and instruct the parents prior to discharge from the birth hospital. Recent studies have shown that this goal is feasible.

Although the trigger of hemolysis in G-6-PD–deficient babies can frequently not be identified, the parents of this baby should have been warned of the dangers of eating fava beans, using clothes that had been stored in naphthalene-containing mothballs, or of using any drugs or medications without consulting a doctor beforehand. The office pediatrician should have given instructions to his staff that an infant whose parents complain of jaundice should be seen immediately and not be given an appointment for the following day. Similarly, the emergency room triage nurse who recognized the extreme jaundice in this baby should have recognized the emergent nature of the situation and called a physician immediately. An STB should have been taken immediately and intensive phototherapy should have been started even prior to the results becoming available. Attention to these details may have prevented permanent bilirubin neurotoxicity.

Moderate G-6-PD Deficiency Associated Hyperbilirubinemia: a Potentially High-Risk Setup

Some G-6-PD–deficient infants develop a more moderate form of hyperbilirubinemia. We do not know the natural history of this form because most infants are treated with phototherapy with good response, although a few do require exchange transfusion. The pathophysiology of the jaundice is attributed to a moderate degree of increased heme catabolism, as demonstrated by COHbc studies, in combination with diminished bilirubin conjugation, the result of presence of a promoter polymorphism of UGT1A1, associated with Gilbert syndrome. These infants are at risk for severe hyperbilirubinemia because the imbalance between bilirubin production and conjugation may be exacerbated should the infant come into contact with a hemolytic trigger, or if prematurity further diminishes the bilirubin conjugation ability.

CLINICAL EFFECTS OF SEVERE NEONATAL HYPERBILIRUBINEMIA

Kernicterus: a Never Event?

Kernicterus has been regarded as a preventable condition. However, despite formulation of comprehensive guidelines, in the United States, Canada, and other countries (including the United Kingdom, South Africa, Israel, Netherlands, Norway), kernicterus continues to occur in westernized countries that have well-organized healthcare systems. Although the incidence of kernicterus relative to the number of deliveries in any developed country is low, the results of bilirubin neurotoxicity are permanent and long lasting, with major implications for the affected infants, their families, and society. The incidence of extreme hyperbilirubinemia and kernicterus in industrialized countries varies. Kernicterus is estimated to occur in Denmark at the rate of 1/64,000 (1994-1998) or 1/79,000 (1994-2003); the United Kingdom and Ireland 1/150,000; Canada 1/43,000; and California 0.44/100,000.

Bilirubin toxicity—manifest as acute bilirubin encephalopathy (or kernicterus), or the less devastating bilirubin auditory neuropathy and bilirubin-induced neurologic dysfunction (BIND)—has not been encountered by the majority of readers. On the other hand, pediatricians and neonatologists spend much of the time devoted to newborns in predicting, monitoring, and treating hyperbilirubinemia to prevent the STB from reaching a neurotoxic level. Although a comprehensive account of bilirubin neurologic disease is beyond the scope of this chapter, we will in the ensuing paragraphs briefly describe the clinical picture of newborns who have been exposed to and affected by high levels of STB.

Acute Bilirubin Encephalopathy

The early clinical features giving rise to the suspicion of acute bilirubin encephalopathy include severe lethargy and poor feeding in a baby who has previously been feeding well. Granted, these signs are nonspecific, but in the presence of severe jaundice, encephalopathy should be suspected and therapy instituted without delay. Spasm of the extensor muscles results in opisthotonus and back arching. Muscle tone may subsequently fluctuate between hypo- and hypertonia and a high-pitched cry frequently develops. Impairment of upward gaze results in the "setting sun sign," and fever, seizures, apnea, and death may follow.

Associated with acute bilirubin encephalopathy may be a "kernicteric facies" (Figure 5-2). This includes a combination of facial features: (1) the setting sun sign (paresis of upward gaze); (2) eyelid retraction; and (3) facial dystonia. In combination, these signs make the infant seem stunned, scared, or anxious. A fourth sign, dysconjugate or wandering eyes, may also occur. Recognition of this peculiar facial pattern should

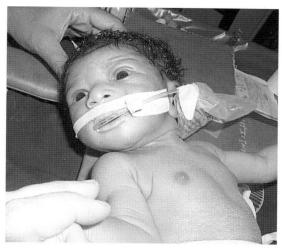

FIGURE 5-2 ■ Kernicteric facies in a baby with acute bilirubin encephalopathy. Note the setting sun sign (paresis of upward gaze), eyelid retraction, and facial dystonia, making the infant seem stunned, scared, or anxious. (Photograph courtesy Tina Slusher, MD, from that physician's personal collection, taken in Nigeria with mother's permission.)

help identify a baby who is developing bilirubin encephalopathy.

Chronic Athetoid Cerebral Palsy: Kernicterus

The clinical picture of kernicterus is a result of deposition of bilirubin in the basal ganglia neural tissue. The condition comprises a tetrad including:

- Abnormal muscle control, movements and muscle tone typical of choreoathetoid cerebral palsy
- Auditory processing disturbance, with or without hearing loss
- Oculomotor impairments resulting in paralysis of upward gaze
- Enamel dysplasia of the teeth

The description of 25 cases of kernicterus in California portrays the dismal picture of these chronically affected children. Seventy-two percent were male. At a mean (SD) age of 7.8 (3.9) years, 60% did not walk at all, while only 16% were able to walk independently. Only 52% could self-feed while a feeding tube was in place in 12%. Severe or profound mental retardation or severe disablement was found in 36%. There was no evidence of mental retardation in 32%. Epilepsy was found in 20%. Severe, profound, or untestable visual or hearing impairment was documented in 25% and 56% of cases, respectively, while only 36% had normal hearing. Motor spasticity was seen in

32%, ataxia and dyskinesis in 12% each, and hypotonia in 8%.

SUBTLE BILIRUBIN ENCEPHALOPATHY AND AUDITORY NEUROPATHY

Bilirubin-Induced Neurologic Dysfunction (BIND)

Bilirubin encephalopathy may not always manifest as the classic, chronic picture of kernicterus. In some, BIND may result in subtle bilirubin encephalopathy. These children have less severe injury than those with classic kernicterus, but nevertheless attributable to bilirubin neurotoxicity. The spectrum of neurologic manifestations in BIND includes subtle disturbances of hearing; disorders of auditory processing known as auditory neuropathy/dyssynchrony; visual motor paralysis; and disorders of speech, language, and cognition. Hearing loss or auditory neuropathy may be isolated or in combination with additional manifestations of kernicterus. Cognitive disturbances may also be evident.

Auditory Neuropathy/Dyssynchrony

Auditory neuropathy associated with hyperbilirubinemia is not simply a sensorineural hearing loss, but rather is the result of dysfunction at the level of the auditory brainstem or nerve. Thus the cochlear hair cells remain intact, but the central auditory nerve tissue or auditory brain center are affected. Functionally, auditory neuropathy or dyssynchrony is characterized by absent or abnormal brainstem auditory evoked potentials, but with normal inner ear function. In these cases, hearing screening utilizing automated auditory brainstem responses (testing neural tissue) will identify the condition. However, evoked otoacoustic emission studies, reflecting cochlear hair cell inner ear function, may be normal. If the latter technology is used exclusively, the auditory neuropathy may remain undiagnosed. Affected patients may be able to hear, as documented on audiogram, and able to respond to sounds appropriately, but their ability to decode speech and language and interpret the sounds they are hearing may be hindered. Awareness of bilirubin auditory neuropathy is of practical importance because cochlear implantation has been used successfully in children with this condition. The mechanism by which hearing is improved is not clear, because the implant is actually proximal to the neural lesion.

Late Prematurity

CASE STUDY 4

A 36-weeks' gestation, male breastfed infant was to be discharged at 48 hours. The predischarge STB was 11.0 mg/dL. Both mother's and infant's blood groups were O, Rh positive. The parents are Caucasian.

EXERCISE 5
QUESTION

1. Which of the following physicians is correct in his/her assessment?
   a. The first pediatrician was not concerned because the STB was "not very high" in his evaluation. He claimed that this was a case of nonhemolytic jaundice.
   b. His partner, in contrast, insisted that this baby has risk factors for neonatal hyperbilirubinemia and requires very close observation.

ANSWER

1. **b.**

Every STB Value Should Be Plotted on the Bilirubin Nomogram

The pediatrician did not plot the STB value on the nomogram. Had he done so he would have seen that the value was on the 75th percentile (the beginning of the intermediate high-risk range). Because of bilirubin dynamics during the first week of life, it is essential to plot each and every STB value on the nomogram. A value of 11.0 mg/dL at 24 hours will be >95th percentile in the high-risk zone; at 48 hours it will fall on the 75th percentile (at the beginning of the intermediate high-risk zone); and at 72 hours on the 40th percentile, bordering on the low-risk zone. Each percentile has different risk values for the potential to develop hyperbilirubinemia.

Regardless of the actual STB value, the higher the hour-specific percentile value the greater the risk for subsequent hyperbilirubinemia. Furthermore, should more than one STB determination be available, the STB trajectory can be evaluated. A trajectory running parallel to the graph may be reassuring, whereas a trajectory that is "jumping percentiles" may be indicative of hemolysis and predictive of subsequent hyperbilirubinemia. Although the low-risk zones on the nomogram (<75th percentile) have traditionally been regarded as minimal or moderate risk for subsequent hyperbilirubine-mia, this may not be entirely true. Recent studies of newborns readmitted for hyperbilirubinemia determined a false negative predischarge bilirubin screen in many instances. For example, in a study from Israel, of 143 readmitted infants, 4.2% had predischarge STB values in ≤40th percentile (low-risk zone) range, while 28% were in the intermediate low-risk zone (41st to 75th percentile) predischarge. These and other results support the AAP recommendation that every newborn should be seen by a health authority within a few days of discharge, in order to detect those with increasing jaundice that may not be recognized by the parents.

In this case, the pediatrician did not take some risk factors into consideration. The conjugating ability of ≤37-weeks' gestation newborns is very different from those born more at term gestation. Studies have demonstrated that a combination of predischarge STB in conjunction with gestational age has an excellent predictive accuracy for subsequent hyperbilirubinemia (see later). Breastfeeding and male sex further add to the complexities of this case and compound the risk for hyperbilirubinemia.

Physician "b" was correct. Although it is not mandatory to observe this infant in hospital, he should have been seen by a healthcare professional within 1 or 2 days of discharge. Whether the jaundice in this infant was "nonhemolytic" or not will be discussed in the following.

Jaundice Associated with Prematurity

Jaundice in premature infants is more common and severe than in full-term neonates. STB concentrations peak around the 5th day of life. The major reason for the frequency of jaundice in premature infants is developmental immaturity of the UGT1A1 bilirubin-conjugating enzyme. In premature infants, bilirubin toxicity may occur at lower concentrations of bilirubin than in term infants and any visible jaundice in a preterm infant should be closely monitored.

Jaundice Associated with Late-Preterm Infants

Late-preterm gestation (newborns born between 34⁴⁄₇ and 36⁶⁄₇ completed weeks) is another important risk factor for the development of severe neonatal hyperbilirubinemia. Immature bilirubin conjugative capacity is implied in the potential severity of jaundice in these infants. Coexpression of late prematurity with additional icterogenic factors such as G-6-PD deficiency

may enhance the jaundice. Management of late preterm infants as if they were term infants, with lack of appropriate follow up, may be a major contributor to the bilirubin-related morbidity in these cases.

"Nonhemolytic Jaundice": Is There Such an Entity?

In the absence of known or obvious etiologies for neonatal hyperbilirubinemia, some pediatricians have used the term "nonhemolytic jaundice." Although there may be some cases of true nonhemolytic jaundice, such as delayed breast-feeding jaundice or Crigler-Najjar syndrome, categorization of hyperbilirubinemic newborns as "nonhemolytic" may lessen the degree of concern regarding the potential for bilirubin neurotoxicity. The presence of a hemolytic condition does not categorically imply that the jaundice or hyperbilirubinemia is necessarily due to this condition. Conversely, absence of an identifiable etiology does not necessarily imply that increased hemolysis is not participant to the pathophysiology of the jaundice. Studies utilizing the endogenous production of CO, an accurate index of heme catabolism, have demonstrated that many jaundiced babies do, in fact, have a hemolytic component to their jaundice, even in the absence of a defined hemolytic condition.

In a multicenter, multinational study utilizing end tidal CO concentration, the mean ETCOc value for 1370 infants who completed the study was 1.48 ± 0.49 ppm. The 120 newborns who developed any TSB concentration >95th percentile on the hour-specific nomogram had significantly higher ETCOc values than those who did not (1.81 ± 0.59 ppm vs. 1.45 ± 0.47 ppm, $p <0.0001$). However, high bilirubin production was not a prerequisite for the development of hyperbilirubinemia; some babies with low bilirubin production did, nevertheless, develop hyperbilirubinemia, while others with high production rates did not. These findings confirm that both bilirubin production and its elimination contribute to the STB at any point in time. Additional studies utilizing both ETCOc and blood carboxyhemoglobin (COHbc) levels have demonstrated greater endogenous production of CO—reflective of increased heme catabolism—in many newborns, even in the absence of a specific diagnosis associated with increased hemolysis. It appears, therefore, that many hyperbilirubinemic babies do have some degree of increased heme catabolism with the potential of bilirubin neurotoxicity. Absence of an obvious etiology associated with increased hemolysis for hyperbilirubinemia should not result in us labeling newborns as "nonhemolytic." This practice may result in a sense of complacency and lack of recognition of babies with increased potential for bilirubin neurotoxicity. Even in cases in which hemolysis is not a major contributor to severe neonatal jaundice, such as Crigler-Najjar syndrome, kernicterus may occur (see subsequent section).

DIMINISHED BILIRUBIN CONJUGATION AND NEONATAL HYPERBILIRUBINEMIA

Diminished bilirubin conjugation may result in hyperbilirubinemia independently, or in conjunction with increased bilirubin production. Some important causes of hyperbilirubinemia owing to diminished conjugation may be found in Box 5-5.

Gilbert Syndrome

Gilbert syndrome is a benign disorder that produces mild unconjugated bilirubinemia in about 6% of adults. Both defective hepatic uptake of bilirubin and decreased hepatic UGT activity have been demonstrated. In individuals with Gilbert syndrome, the UGT1A1-conjugating enzyme is normally structured, but not fully functional because of diminished gene expression. This is because the noncoding, rather than coding, area of the gene is affected. The genetic basis of the reduced gene expression lies in the presence of additional TA repeats [$(TA)_7$ or occasionally $(TA)_8$ instead of the wild type $(TA)_6$] in the TATAA box in the promoter region of the *UGT1A1* gene. In and of itself, the $(TA)_7$ promoter polymorphism has not been associated with hyperbilirubinemia, but when in combination with additional factors, it may. A dose-dependent genetic interaction between

---

BOX 5-5	Some Important Causes of Hyperbilirubinemia Due to Diminished Bilirubin Conjugation

Prematurity
Late prematurity
Hypothyroidism
Pyloric stenosis
Gilbert syndrome
Crigler-Najjar syndromes types 1 and 2

G-6-PD deficiency and $(TA)_7$ promoter polymorphism increased the incidence of a STB >15 mg/dL dramatically when these two factors were in combination. In Asian populations, interaction between G-6-PD deficiency and coding area UGT1A1 mutations similarly exacerbate hyperbilirubinemia, while a similar interaction between $(TA)_7$ promoter polymorphism and hereditary spherocytosis has been documented.

Breastfeeding and Breast Milk Jaundice

CASE STUDY 5

A male, term infant was born to parents who were second cousins. The infant was breastfed. The STB was 20.0 mg/dL on day 3 of life. Phototherapy was instrumental in decreasing the STB value and the baby was discharged, only to be readmitted 3 days later with an STB value of 23.0 mg/dL.

EXERCISE 6

QUESTION

1. What is the most likely diagnosis?

ANSWER

1. At this point, the leading diagnosis is *breastfeeding jaundice*. Breastfeeding jaundice occurs in the first weeks of life. Lack of proper technique, engorgement, cracked nipples, small amounts of milk and fatigue may impair effective breastfeeding on the part of the mother. Neonatal factors such as an ineffective suck may be common in late-preterm infants. The result may be ineffective breastfeeding, underhydration, delayed meconium passage, and intestinal stasis leading to an increased enterohepatic circulation and increased bilirubin load.

   Breast milk jaundice, on the other hand, occurs after the first 3 to 5 days of life. Mutations of the *UGT1A1* gene, including a $(TA)_7$ promoter polymorphism, or G71R mutation can contribute to the development of hyperbilirubinemia in breastfed infants. More severely affected neonates may achieve peak levels as high as 20 to 30 mg/dL with no obvious evidence of hemolysis or illness. Interruption of nursing and substitution with formula feeding for 1 to 3 days usually causes a prompt decline of the TB concentration. However, it is not generally recommended unless TB concentrations reach levels that might be of danger to the infant. On resumption of nursing, the TB does not usually increase. Most infants with breast milk jaundice can be observed without other interventions. However, one must determine that other pathology is not existent. Therefore, fractionation of bilirubin, thyroid testing and urine cultures are indicated.

CASE STUDY 5 (continued)

In the baby presented earlier, the sequence of readmission and phototherapy repeated itself several more times. Laboratory investigations revealed a normal complete blood count (CBC), a direct bilirubin value of 0.3 mg/dL, normal thyroid function tests, and no evidence of sepsis. Both maternal and newborn blood groups were A Rh positive and the DAT was negative.

EXERCISE 7

QUESTION

1. What if anything, should be done next?
   a. This is clearly a nonhemolytic situation and no further testing or interventions are necessary.
   b. Indirect hyperbilirubinemia in a breastfed infant indicates breastfeeding jaundice. Breastfeeding should be discontinued.
   c. Pay attention to the family history: the parents are second cousins. Consider evaluation for Crigler-Najjar syndrome. Treat the baby with phototherapy to prevent the STB concentrations from rising to potentially neurotoxic levels.

ANSWER

1. **c.**

Crigler-Najjar Syndrome

Although breastfeeding jaundice should definitely be taken into consideration, it does not usually result in in a sequence of readmissions for hyperbilirubinemia. Response "b" was the correct response early on in this baby's management, but the repeated readmissions should have made the breastfeeding jaundice an unlikely possibility. The *UGT1A1* gene was sequenced in the baby and both parents. A coding area mutation associated with Crigler-Najjar syndrome was found, homozygous in the baby and heterozygous in both parents.

Crigler-Najjar syndrome type I is a rare autosomal recessive disease characterized by an almost complete absence of hepatic UGT activity. In this situation, the coding area of the *UGT1A1* gene is mutated, resulting in a structurally abnormal enzyme with little or no bilirubin-conjugating

ability. Severe unconjugated hyperbilirubinemia may develop and kernicterus may occur should the STB not be vigorously controlled with phototherapy. The diagnosis can now be obtained by sequencing the *UGT1A1* gene. Liver transplant offers the only definitive treatment for the disease; however, in a multicenter report, 7 of 21 (33%) of transplanted children had already developed some form of brain damage by the time of their transplantation.

Crigler-Najjar Syndrome Type II

Crigler-Najjar syndrome type II is more common than type I disease and is typically benign. The occurrence of kernicterus is rare. Unconjugated hyperbilirubinemia occurs in the first days of life, and may be exacerbated by fasting, illness, and anesthesia. Phenobarbital may be used as a simple clinical tool to differentiate between type II and type I diseases. Jaundiced neonates with type II disease respond to oral administration of phenobarbital with a sharp decline in TSB, while individuals with type I disease do not respond in this way. Beyond the neonatal period, there should be no long-term risk of kernicterus.

Hypothyroidism

About 10% of congenitally hypothyroid neonates may develop prolonged jaundice owing to diminished UGT activity, and testing for thyroid function should be performed in these cases. With modern methods of routine metabolic screening the diagnosis of hypothyroidism should be available in the first week of life. The mechanism of this association may be impairment of hepatic uptake and reduced hepatic ligandin concentrations. Absence of thyroid hormone may delay hepatic bilirubin enzyme and transport development.

EFFECT OF RACE AND ETHNIC BACKGROUND ON NEONATAL HYPERBILIRUBINEMIA

CASE STUDY 6

A term, male infant was born to African American parents. There was no blood group incompatibility. The infant was breastfed and apparently healthy. At 50 hours of life, a predischarge STB result was 10.0 mg/dL. When plotted on the hour-specific nomogram, it fell between the 40th and 75th percentiles.

EXERCISE 8

QUESTION

1. Which of the following statements is correct?
    a. This is a term infant with an STB value in the intermediate low-risk range. He can be safely sent home; there are no special concerns.
    b. This infant is of African American heritage and at very low risk for neonatal hyperbilirubinemia.
    c. This infant is at potentially high risk and should be followed according to AAP guidelines with the same vigilance as a Caucasian infant.

ANSWER

1. **c.** Within the African American population, there is a subset at risk for extreme hyperbilirubinemia and kernicterus. Additional risk factors in this case include male sex and breastfeeding. Until recently, black heritage has been regarded as protective against hyperbilirubinemia. Indeed, the AAP (2004) statement on hyperbilirubinemia lists black ethnicity among conditions *decreasing* the risk of hyperbilirubinemia. However, black race does seem to contribute to the development of kernicterus. Black ethnicity comprises 25% of the U.S.-based Kernicterus Registry and increased the incidence of bilirubin encephalopathy significantly in the United Kingdom and Ireland survey. Both figures are out of proportion to the number of black individuals in the background populations studied. Some of these cases may be caused by concurrent G-6-PD deficiency and others owing to disadvantaged social status. Kernicterus is rampant in Western and Central Africa. In a recent study from California, Wickremasinghi and colleagues confirmed a lower incidence of moderate hyperbilirubinemia (STB ≥20 mg/dL) in black infants, an equal incidence of STB ≥25 mg/dL in black and Caucasian infants, and an increased incidence of hazardous hyperbilirubinemia (STB ≥30 mg/dL) in black neonates compared with white infants. Low-risk categorization of black newborns may therefore no longer be appropriate, and answers "a" and "b" are incorrect.

Additional Racial Aspects of Hyperbilirubinemia

Another population group at risk for neonatal hyperbilirubinemia includes Asians. Some of these may result from a high incidence of the G71R mutation of UGT1A1, associated with Gilbert syndrome, in Asian populations. Native Americans are also at high risk for neonatal hyperbilirubinemia.

PREDISCHARGE EVALUATION FOR PREDICTION OF HYPERBILIRUBINEMIA

In normal, healthy term babies, there is a natural progression of STB levels during the first days of life to a peak between the 3rd and 5th postnatal day. Current practice in many countries is to discharge babies around 48 hours (or earlier). This means that the peak STB will be reached when the infant is already at home, thereby placing much of the onus for recognition of hyperbilirubinemia on the parents and community services. It is therefore essential to assess each and every infant for the risk of developing subsequent hyperbilirubinemia, and to ensure adequate follow up to detect developing hyperbilirubinemia.

Universal Predischarge Screening

In their clarification to the 2004 AAP guideline, Maisels and colleagues recommend universal predischarge bilirubin screening, using either STB or TcB readings, to assess the risk of subsequent severe hyperbilirubinemia. These authors suggest a structured approach incorporating not only the bilirubin reading reflected as a percentile value, but also gestational age and the presence or absence of risk factors. The underlying concept to this approach is that the higher the predischarge bilirubin percentile, the lower the gestational age and the higher the number of risk factors, the greater will be the chance of developing subsequent hyperbilirubinemia. These recommendations are not evidence-based but representative of expert opinion. The risk factors that are most predictive of significant hyperbilirubinemia include:

- Lower gestational age
- Exclusive breastfeeding, the latter especially if the nursing is not going well and there is excessive weight loss
- Jaundice appearing in the first 24 hours
- Bilirubin trajectory crossing percentiles on the nomogram
- Hemolytic conditions
    - Isoimmune hemolytic disease of the newborn
    - G-6-PD deficiency
- Previous sibling with jaundice
- Cephalhematoma or ecchymosis
- East Asian race

A Practical Approach to Follow Up for Hyperbilirubinemia

In order to ease the screening process and facilitate formulation of a follow up plan, Maisels and colleagues provide an algorithm for the predischarge screen. Those neonates who do not meet the AAP criteria for phototherapy are followed up according to a suggested protocol based on predischarge STB or TcB risk zone, gestational age 35 to 37 weeks or ≥38 weeks, and the presence of risk factors.

False Negative Predischarge Bilirubin Screening

Recent studies have shown that some infants readmitted for hyperbilirubinemia had a predischarge bilirubin screen in the low-risk zones on the nomogram indicating a false negative screen. A predischarge screen in the low-risk zones should not, therefore, result in complacency, and the results of these studies confirm the AAP (2004) recommendations that each and every newborn should be evaluated for developing jaundice within 2 to 3 days of discharge.

TRANSCUTANEOUS BILIRUBINOMETRY

Transcutaneous bilirubinometry (TcB) is a relatively new technology for the noninvasive, instantaneous point-of-care estimation of the STB. To date, this technique has been used primarily in the hospital setting, but has been successful in the outpatient setting as well. Visual inspection, which was for decades the mainstay for deciding which infant needs a bilirubin test performed, is notoriously inaccurate. TcB takes the guesswork out of bilirubinometry. TcB should be regarded as a screening tool and not as a substitute for actual STB measurement. The technique involves a flash of light entering the skin and subcutaneous tissues and measurement of the degree of yellowness. After correcting for skin color and hemoglobin, an estimated STB level is reported.

TcB tends to underestimate the actual STB. As a result, in their clarification to the 2004 AAP guidelines, Maisels and colleagues suggest measuring STB if: (1) the TcB is 70% of the STB value recommended for phototherapy, (2) the TcB is >75th percentile on the bilirubin nomogram or >95th percentile on a TcB nomogram, and (3) a postdischarge TcB value is >13 mg/dL.

TREATMENT OF NEONATAL HYPERBILIRUBINEMIA

Newborns ≥35 Weeks' Gestation

The mainstays of treatment for neonatal hyperbilirubinemia include phototherapy and exchange transfusion. The indications, technologies, and equipment required have been comprehensively described in the 2004 AAP hyperbilirubinemia guidelines with clarifications in the 2009 statement of Maisels and colleagues, and a 2011 technical report on phototherapy by Bhutani and colleagues from the Committee on the Fetus and Newborn. These statements relate to infants ≥35 weeks' gestational age and are still applicable. The indications take into account not only the actual STB value, but also the time and percentile of this value, gestational age, and the presence of risk factors. The higher the STB percentile, the lower the gestational age and the greater the number of risk factors, the sooner treatment should be initiated. The 2004 AAP guidelines emphasize that in considering the indications for phototherapy and exchange transfusion the direct-reacting (or conjugated) bilirubin level should not be subtracted from the total. However, the statement continues, in unusual circumstances in which the direct bilirubin is >50% of the total bilirubin, and because there are no good data to provide guidance for therapy, consultation with an expert in the field is recommended.

With regard to phototherapy, the 2009 clarification emphasizes the need to take risk factors for bilirubin neurotoxicity into account when making the decision to initiate phototherapy or perform exchange transfusion. Neurotoxicity risk factors may increase the risk of neurologic damage in infants with severe hyperbilirubinemia. Neurotoxicity risk factors listed in the statement include:

- Isoimmune hemolytic disease
- G-6-PD deficiency
- Asphyxia
- Sepsis
- Acidosis
- Albumin ≤3.0 mg/dL

The statement also provides algorithms with providing recommendations for management, phototherapy, and follow up taking into account not only bilirubin measurements, but gestation and risk factors for subsequent hyperbilirubinemia.

TABLE 5-1   Guidelines for Phototherapy and Exchange Transfusion in Premature Infants*

	Phototherapy	Exchange Transfusion
GESTATIONAL AGE (WK)	INITIATE PHOTOTHERAPY TOTAL BILIRUBIN (mg/dL)	TOTAL SERUM BILIRUBIN (mg/dL)
<27⁶⁄₇	5-6	11-14
28⁶⁄₇-29⁶⁄₇	6-8	12-14
30⁶⁄₇-31⁶⁄₇	8-10	13-16
32⁶⁄₇-33⁶⁄₇	10-12	15-18
34⁶⁄₇-34⁶⁄₇	12-14	17-19

Summary of Maisels and colleagues' (2012) comments to their table:
1. The levels of STB at which phototherapy or exchange transfusion is recommended are not based on good evidence.
2. The wide ranges and overlapping of values between gestational age groups reflects a degree of uncertainty in the formulation of these guidelines.
3. Use the lower values in any given range for babies at high risk for bilirubin neurotoxicity, including lower gestational age, sepsis, clinical instability, serum albumin level <2.5 gm/dL, and rapidly rising STB levels suggestive of hemolysis.
4. Indications for exchange transfusion apply to infants in whom STB levels continue to rise to exchange transfusion levels despite intense phototherapy.
5. Exchange transfusion is indicated in a baby who shows signs of acute bilirubin encephalopathy.
6. Use the total bilirubin value for decision-making. Do not subtract the direct or conjugated bilirubin value from the total value.
7. Use the postmenstrual (adjusted) age for phototherapy indications.
8. Prophylactic phototherapy is an option in premature infants ≤26 weeks' gestation.
9. In infants <1000 gm birth weight, because of possible increased mortality associated with phototherapy in this group, start with lower levels of irradiance and increase this should the STB levels continue to rise.

*These guidelines were formulated by four United States–based neonatologists who were involved in the preparation of the 2004 AAP guidelines, the 2009 clarification, or both.
From Maisels MJ, Watchko JF, Bhutani VK, Stevenson DK. An approach to the management of hyperbilirubinemia in the preterm infant less than 35 weeks of gestation. J Perinatol 32:660-664, 2012.

Cardinal points of the 2011 Committee on Fetus and Newborn technical report include that the effectiveness of phototherapy light is enhanced by:

- Emission of light in the blue-green range that overlaps the in vivo plasma bilirubin absorption spectrum (460 to 490 nm)
- Irradiance of at least 30 $\mu W.cm^{-2}.nm^{-1}$ (confirmed with an appropriate irradiance meter calibrated over the appropriate wavelength range)
- Illumination of maximal body surface
- Demonstration of a decrease in total bilirubin concentrations during the first 4 to 6 hours of exposure

Additional points in the technical report include measurements of serial bilirubin based on the rate of decrease. Phototherapy should be introduced urgently in cases of excessive hyperbilirubinemia and procedures should be conducted while the infant receives phototherapy. Phototherapy may be interrupted briefly for feeding, parental bonding, or nursing care once a decrease in serum bilirubin has been detected. Possible rebound should be taken into consideration following discontinuation of phototherapy.

Premature Infants <35 Weeks' Gestation

Management of hyperbilirubinemia in the premature infant <35 weeks has been unclear, with a wide range of STB values suggested for various gestational ages and birth weights. Recently, a suggested protocol—albeit non–evidence-based—has been proposed, which will hopefully standardize the treatment delivered to these infants (Maisels and colleagues, 2012) (Table 5-1). Other protocols including guidelines for premature infants include the U.K.-based NICE guidelines, and Norwegian, Dutch, and South African guidelines.

SPECIAL INVESTIGATIONS IN KERNICTERUS

Magnetic Resonance Imaging (MRI) Findings in Kernicterus

The MRI pattern seen in infants affected with kernicterus is typified by the appearance of hyperintensity (frequently bilateral) of the globus pallidus, subthalamic nucleus, and other brainstem nuclei. It is not known, however, whether these MRI changes are apparent in all cases of kernicterus and what their relationship is to long-term prognosis. For example, in a recent Canadian study, MRI findings consistent with kernicterus were initially present in three infants who were subsequently clinically and developmentally normal. On the other hand, the same authors report two infants with a normal MRI early on, but who subsequently had abnormal developmental outcomes on follow up.

Brainstem Auditory Evoked Response (BAER)

Because auditory neural tissue is sensitive to the effects of bilirubin toxicity, the BAER offers an early and sensitive measure of bilirubin-induced central nervous system dysfunction. Early signs include increased latency and decreased amplitude of waves III and V, progressing to absence of these waveforms, and finally to complete absence of all activity. Automated brainstem response (ABR) can be used at the bedside as a rapid test of auditory function in a neonate with severe hyperbilirubinemia. Absence of automated ABR—or change from "pass" prior to the hyperbilirubinemia to "refer" following its appearance—may be indicative of bilirubin neurotoxicity.

SUGGESTED READINGS

American Academy of Pediatrics Subcommittee on Hyperbilirubinemia: Management of hyperbilirubinemia in the newborn infant 35 or more weeks of gestation, *Pediatrics* 114:297–316, 2004.

Bhutani VK, Johnson L, Sivieri EM: Predictive ability of a predischarge hour-specific serum bilirubin for subsequent significant hyperbilirubinemia in healthy term and near-term newborns, *Pediatrics* 103:6–14, 1999.

Bhutani VK, Stark AR, Lazzeroni LC, et al.: the Initial Clinical Testing Evaluation and Risk Assessment for Universal Screening for Hyperbilirubinemia Study Group. Predischarge screening for severe neonatal hyperbilirubinemia identifies infants who need phototherapy, *J Pediatr* 162:477–482, 2013.

Bhutani VK, The Committee on Fetus and Newborn: Technical report: phototherapy to prevent severe neonatal hyperbilirubinemia in the newborn infant 35 or more weeks gestation, *Pediatrics* 128:e1046–e1052, 2011.

Bromiker R, Bin-Nun A, Schimmel MS, Hammerman C, Kaplan M: Neonatal hyperbilirubinemia in the low-intermediate-risk category on the bilirubin nomogram, *Pediatrics* 130(3):e470–e475, 2012.

Brooks JC, Fisher-Owens SA, Wu YW, Strauss DJ, Newman TB: Evidence suggests there was not a "resurgence" of kernicterus in the 1990s, *Pediatrics* 127:672–679, 2011.

Ebbesen F, Bjerre JV, Vandborg PK: Relation between serum bilirubin levels ≥450 μmol/L and bilirubin encephalopathy; a Danish population-based study, *Acta Paediatr* 101:384–389, 2012.

Gamaleldin R, Iskander I, Seoud I, et al.: Risk factors for neurotoxicity in newborns with severe neonatal hyperbilirubinemia, *Pediatrics* 128(4):e925–e931, 2011.

Hansen TW: The role of phototherapy in the crash-cart approach to extreme neonatal jaundice, *Semin Perinatol* 35:171–174, 2011.

Harris MC, Bernbaum JC, Polin JR, Zimmerman R, Polin RA: Developmental follow-up of breastfed term and near-term infants with marked hyperbilirubinemia, *Pediatrics* 107:1075–1080, 2001.

Johnson L, Bhutani VK, Karp K, Sivieri EM, Shapiro SM: Clinical report from the pilot USA Kernicterus Registry (1992 to 2004), *J Perinatol* 29(Suppl 1):S25–S45, 2009.

Kaplan M, Bromiker R, Hammerman C: Severe neonatal hyperbilirubinemia and kernicterus: are these still problems in the third millennium? *Neonatology* 100:354–362, 2011.

Kaplan M, Hammerman C: Glucose-6-phosphate dehydrogenase deficiency and severe neonatal hyperbilirubinemia: a complexity of interactions between genes and environment, *Semin Fetal Neonatal Med* 15:148–156, 2010.

Kaplan M, Hammerman C, Maisels MJ: Bilirubin genetics for the nongeneticist: hereditary defects of neonatal bilirubin conjugation, *Pediatrics* 111:886–893, 2003.

Kaplan M, Herschel M, Hammerman C, Hoyer JD, Stevenson DK: Hyperbilirubinemia among African American, glucose-6-phosphate dehydrogenase-deficient neonates, *Pediatrics* 114(2):e213–e219, 2004.

Kaplan M, Muraca M, Hammerman C, et al.: Imbalance between production and conjugation of bilirubin: a fundamental concept in the mechanism of neonatal jaundice, *Pediatrics* 110(4), 2002. e47.

Kaplan M, Renbaum P, Levy-Lahad E, Hammerman C, Lahad A, Beutler E: Gilbert syndrome and glucose-6-phosphate dehydrogenase deficiency: a dose-dependent genetic interaction crucial to neonatal hyperbilirubinemia, *Proc Natl Acad Sci U S A* 94:12128–12132, 1997.

Keren R, Luan X, Friedman S, Saddlemire S, Cnaan A, Bhutani VK: A comparison of alternative risk-assessment strategies for predicting significant neonatal hyperbilirubinemia in term and near-term infants, *Pediatrics* 121(1), 2008. e1.

Kuzniewicz MW, Escobar GJ, Newman TB: Impact of universal bilirubin screening on severe hyperbilirubinemia and phototherapy use, *Pediatrics* 124:1031–1039, 2009.

Lin Z, Fontaine J, Watchko JF: Coexpression of gene polymorphisms involved in bilirubin production and metabolism, *Pediatrics* 122:e156–e162, 2008.

Maisels MJ: Neonatal hyperbilirubinemia and kernicterus —not gone but sometimes forgotten, *Early Hum Dev* 85:727–732, 2009.

Maisels MJ, Bhutani VK, Bogen D, Newman TB, Stark AR, Watchko JF: Hyperbilirubinemia in the newborn infant > or = 35 weeks' gestation: an update with clarifications, *Pediatrics* 124:1193–1198, 2009.

Maisels MJ, Watchko JF, Bhutani VK, Stevenson DK: An approach to the management of hyperbilirubinemia in the preterm infant less than 35 weeks of gestation, *J Perinatol* 32:660–664, 2012.

Manning D, Todd P, Maxwell M, Jane Platt M: Prospective surveillance study of severe hyperbilirubinaemia in the newborn in the UK and Ireland, *Arch Dis Child Fetal Neonatal Ed* 92:F342–F346, 2007.

Newman TB, Liljestrand P, Jeremy RJ, et al.: Jaundice and Infant Feeding Study Team. Outcomes among newborns with total serum bilirubin levels of 25 mg per deciliter or more, *N Engl J Med* 354:1889–1900, 2006.

Nkhoma ET, Poole C, Vannappagari V, Hall SA, Beutler E: The global prevalence of glucose-6-phosphate dehydrogenase deficiency: a systematic review and meta-analysis, *Blood Cells Mol Dis* 42:267–278, 2009.

Oh W, Stevenson DK, Tyson JE, et al.: Influence of clinical status on the association between plasma total and unbound bilirubin and death or adverse neurodevelopmental outcomes in extremely low birth weight infants, *Acta Paediatr* 99:673–678, 2010.

Sgro M, Campbell DM, Kandasamy S, Shah V: Incidence of chronic bilirubin encephalopathy in Canada, 2007-2008, *Pediatrics* 130(4):e886–e890, 2012.

Shapiro SM: Bilirubin toxicity in the developing nervous system, *Pediatr Neurol* 29:410–421, 2003.

Stevenson DK, Fanaroff AA, Maisels MJ, et al.: Prediction of hyperbilirubinemia in near-term and term infants, *Pediatrics* 108:31–39, 2001.

Strauss KA, Robinson DL, Vreman HJ, Puffenberger EG, Hart G, Morton DH: Management of hyperbilirubinemia and prevention of kernicterus in 20 patients with Crigler-Najjar disease, *Eur J Pediatr* 165:306–319, 2006.

Watchko JF, Kaplan M, Stark AR, Stevenson DK, Bhutani VK: Should we screen newborns for glucose-6-phosphate dehydrogenase deficiency in the United States? *J Perinatol* 33:499–504, 2013.

Watchko JF, Lin Z, Clark RH, Kelleher AS, Walker MW, Spitzer AR: Complex multifactorial nature of significant hyperbilirubinemia in neonates, *Pediatrics* 124(5):e868–e877, 2009.

Wennberg RP, Ahlfors CE, Bhutani VK, Johnson LH, Shapiro SM: Toward understanding kernicterus: a challenge to improve the management of jaundiced newborns, *Pediatrics* 117:474–485, 2006.

Wickremasinghe AC, Kuzniewicz MW, Newman TB: Black race is not protective against hazardous bilirubin levels, *J Pediatr* 162:1068–1069, 2013.

Zipursky A, Paul VK: The global burden of Rh disease, *Arch Dis Child Fetal Neonatal Ed* 96:F84–F85, 2011.

CHAPTER 6

PARENTERAL NUTRITION

Catalina Bazacliu, MD • Jatinder J.S. Bhatia, MD, FAAP

INDICATIONS

Parenteral nutrition (PN) is used to provide fluid, energy, and nutrients to patients who cannot tolerate—or have contraindications to—enteral nutrition (Table 6-1). It can be classified as "total" when all the energy/nutrition is administered parenterally, or "partial" or "supplemental" when used along with enteral nutrition.

One of the most common indications for PN is prematurity. The majority of somatic growth and nitrogen and mineral accretion takes place during the third trimester. The ideal postnatal nutrition for premature infants is one that results in a postnatal growth similar to that of the fetus *in utero*. Achieving this rate of growth postbirth is difficult and challenging. Most of the "growth restriction" develops in premature infants after birth for several reasons, including: diseases that may preclude enteral nutrition, delay in starting appropriate PN, intolerance to enteral feeds, and inappropriate feedings or feeding strategies. There is growing evidence that inadequate nutrition early in life delays the time to regain birth weight and subsequently leads to extrauterine growth restriction. The latter is difficult to overcome and poorer growth during the neonatal period is associated with long-term adverse neurocognitive effects. The components of the PN are protein, carbohydrates, lipids, minerals, vitamins, and trace elements.

CASE STUDY 1

A 1.1 kg infant is born following a 28-week gestation. Parenteral nutrition with 10% dextrose and amino acids is started on day 1 of life and intravenous fat is added on day 2. The infant is nursed in an isolette with 70% humidity.

EXERCISE 1

QUESTIONS

1. How many calories are needed to achieve a growth rate of 15 to 20 g/kg/day in this infant on PN?
   a. 90 to 100 kcal/kg/day
   b. 60 to 80 kcal/kg/day
   c. 110 to 130 kcal/kg/day
   d. 140 to 160 kcal/kg/day

2. Which of the following statements about carbohydrate intake is true?
   a. Carbohydrates should provide 50% to 60% of total caloric intake.
   b. Excess carbohydrate intake increases CO_2 production.
   c. Glucose intolerance and hyperglycemia does not occur at glucose infusion rates <10 mg/kg/min.
   d. The glucose utilization rate is 2 to 4 mg/kg/min.

3. Which of the following statements about protein requirements in this newborn infant is correct?
   a. Preterm infants should receive 2.0 to 2.5 g/kg/day of protein when receiving PN.
   b. Protein intakes of 4.0 to 4.5 g/kg/day are recommended for preterm infants with slow weight gain.
   c. The protein requirements of preterm infants are greater than that of term infants.

TABLE 6-1	Indications for Parenteral Nutrition
Medical	Prematurity
	Ileus
	Hypoxic-ischemic encephalopathy/cooling
	Feeding intolerance
	Short gut syndrome
	Failure to thrive secondary to cardiac/renal/pulmonary diseases
Surgical	Hirschsprung disease
	Intestinal atresias
	Surgical necrotizing enterocolitis (NEC)/bowel perforation
	Gastrointestinal malformations (e.g., gastroschisis, omphalocele, imperforate anus, esophageal atresia/tracheoesophageal fistula)
	Diaphragmatic hernia

d. Protein intakes >3.5 g/kg/day may result in high uric acid and creatinine levels.

4. Which of the following statements about lipid emulsions is true?
   a. None of the commercially available lipid emulsions provides linolenic acid.
   b. To meet essential fatty acid requirements, at least 3.0 g/kg/day of 20% emulsions should be given.
   c. 10% emulsions are cleared more quickly than 20% emulsions.
   d. Lipid emulsions should be given over 6 to 12 hours.
   e. Lipid emulsions should provide 40% to 50% of total energy intake.

5. Which of the following statements about mineral requirements is true?
   a. In infants weighing <1000 grams, no sodium should be provided in the first few days of life unless the serum sodium concentration is <130 mEq/L.
   b. All infants should receive potassium beginning on day 1 of life.
   c. Calcium contained in PN is sufficient to prevent osteopenia.
   d. Raising the pH of the PN solution increases the solubility of calcium and phosphorous and allows more to be delivered.
   e. Infants with PN-induced cholestasis should receive supplemental manganese and copper.

ANSWERS

1. **a.** The energy provided should meet the basal metabolic rate plus the energy cost of growth and losses (gastrointestinal, urinary, skin, others). The estimated energy needs of a premature infant to achieve growth at a rate of 15 to 20 g/kg/day is estimated to be 110 to 130 kcal/kg/day enterally. When all nutrition is administered parenterally, 90 to 100 kcal/kg/day might meet the growth needs because there is no energy spent for digestion and absorption, and fecal losses are minimal. Energy losses are minimized by the use of a controlled thermoneutral environment and fluid losses are ameliorated by the use of humidification. Because of intolerance to rapid advancement of parenteral or enteral nutrition (see later), energy intakes are advanced slowly with the goal of achieving full intake by the end of the second week of life.

2. **b.** Glucose in the form of dextrose is the main source of carbohydrates in PN and should provide 35% to 50% of calories. Other carbohydrate sources such as fructose, galactose, sorbitol, glycerol, and ethanol have been used in the past. One gram of glucose provides 3.4 kcal.

The glucose utilization rate of a preterm infant is 5 to 8 mg/kg/min. The glucose infusion rate (GIR) can be increased up to 12 mg/kg/min (if tolerated) to optimize the energy intake. This is usually achieved by increasing the dextrose concentration slowly, thereby advancing the GIR by 1 to 2 mg/kg/min daily (to avoid hyperglycemia). Increasing GIR above 13 mg/kg/min is not considered beneficial because it increases the CO_2 production, induces lipogenesis, and may contribute to the development of a fatty liver. Early provision of carbohydrate is protein sparing and with the addition of protein, infants can achieve positive nitrogen balance within the first 3 days of life.

Glucose intolerance can occur in premature infants even at GIR of 6 mg/kg/min or lower. This is attributed to elevated endogenous glucose production in very low birth weight (VLBW) infants compared to term infants—especially when glucose is infused without amino acids, and to lower peripheral glucose utilization. In addition, end-organ insulin resistance, decreased glucose transporters, and absence of enteral nutrition have been implicated in the pathogenesis of hyperglycemia. Several strategies have been proposed to manage hyperglycemia (Table 6-2). Infants of extremely low birth weight (ELBW) are very susceptible to hyperglycemia, further aggravating the overall nutritional status of these fragile infants.

3. **c.** Pediatric amino acid solutions had been formulated to meet the requirements of infants and children and provide a plasma amino acid profile similar to that of term 30-day-old breast-fed infants. These solutions contain essential amino acids and conditionally essential amino acids such as tyrosine, cysteine, and taurine. The delivery of amino acids along with adequate energy results in positive nitrogen balance and a decrease in loss of body weight, thereby reducing time to return to birth weight. It is estimated that, in the absence of exogenous intake, endogenous protein losses are 0.5 to 1.0 g/kg/day for infants receiving only dextrose in the infusion. Based on accretion rates in the fetus, protein requirements are estimated to be 2.5 to 3.5 g/kg/day for preterm infants and 1.9 to 2.5 g/kg/day for term infants. Infants receiving PN have protein requirements at the higher end of that range. Protein should provide 8% to 10% of total calories, and should not exceed

TABLE 6-2   Management of Glucose Intolerance

Strategy	Advantages	Limitations
Decrease GIR	Easy	Solution tonicity Minimum GIR necessary for brain metabolism is 4 mg/kg/min
Administration of exogenous insulin	Controls hyperglycemia Low risk for hypoglycemia Improves energy intake and growth	Metabolic acidosis due to: • Increased lactic acid • Increased lipogenesis with fat deposition in liver and increased CO_2 production Risk of hypoglycemia
Administration of amino acids	Increases endogenous insulin secretion Prevents proteolysis	None at recommended doses

12%. One gram of protein provides 4 kcal. Early introduction of amino acids in PN is safe, results in a positive nitrogen balance, and improves glucose tolerance. More recent studies reveal that higher amino acid intake of 3 g/kg/day administered in the first few days of life is safe and decreases the incidence of extra uterine growth restriction. The current recommendations for preterm infants are to start amino acids at minimum 2.5 g/kg/day in the first day of life and advance to 3.5 g/kg/day by day 3. Intakes of amino acids higher than 3.5 g/kg/day early in life may increase the risk of metabolic acidosis, hyperammonemia, and adversely affect cognitive scores and anthropometric measurements at 18 months of age (but not at 24 months). A lower incidence of chronic lung disease has been reported in infants receiving higher intakes (4 g/kg/day) than in those receiving 3 g/kg/day. It should be underscored that nitrogen retention increases with increasing energy intake, and therefore appropriate protein-to-energy ratios of 3.8 to 2.6 grams protein per 100 kcal must be maintained to avoid inadequate protein intake in the face of excessive energy intake.

Glutamine, the most abundant amino acid in plasma and human milk, is not included in PN solutions owing to decreased solubility. However, supplementation of glutamine in preterm infants did not improve mortality, rates of sepsis, or length of stay. Therefore glutamine supplementation is not currently recommended.

Cysteine may be considered an essential amino acid in preterm infants, especially in infants less than 33 to 34 weeks' gestation. Cysteine is important for protein accretion, and is added as cysteine hydrochloride 40 mg/g amino acid (not to exceed 100 mg/kg/day).

The ideal PN solution for premature infants is unknown. Currently, three formulations are available in the United States and data to date do not allow firm conclusions of superiority of one over the other (Table 6-3). Tyrosine is not present in these solutions, but may be added as N-acetyl tyrosine.

Carnitine is another essential amino acid not included in available solutions. It is important in mitochondrial transport of long chain fatty acids and plasma levels decline without dietary supplementation. It is an accepted additive for long-term PN, despite lack of evidence of altered fatty acid metabolism.

4. **e.** Fat emulsions are a source of essential fatty acids (linoleic and linolenic acid) and energy (2 kcal/mL of 20% emulsion). Lipids should provide 40% to 50% of the daily energy intake. Lipid emulsions, derived mainly from soybean and safflower oil, contain neutral triglycerides, glycerol, and phospholipids for emulsification. Olive oil–based emulsions containing medium chain fatty acids, alpha-tocopherol, and decreased amounts of n-6 polyunsaturated fatty acids are available in Europe. Fish oil–based lipid emulsions can provide very long chain omega-3 fatty acids and are available in United States under compassionate-use protocol only. Omega-3 fatty acids or very long chain polyunsaturated fatty acids (VLPUFA) have beneficial effects on the developing brain and retina and may be considered conditionally essential in preterm infants. Studies have demonstrated that the use of these emulsions reverses hepatic dysfunction in infants and children with parenteral-nutrition–associated cholestatic liver disease, but the quantity of fish oil emulsion required has not been determined.

Commercial lipid emulsions are available in 10%, 20%, and 30% concentrations. For infants, the 20% concentration is preferred because of the lower phospholipid content and more rapid clearance than 10% emulsions. It is recommended to start intravenous lipids the

TABLE 6-3   Composition of 10% Amino Acid Solutions Available Commercially in the United States

		TrophAmine (mg/100 mL)	Premasol (mg/100 mL)	Aminosyn-PF (mg/100 mL)
Essential amino acids	Isoleucine	820	820	760
	Leucine	1400	1400	1200
	Lysine	820	820	677
	Methionine	340	340	180
	Phenylalanine	480	480	427
	Threonine	420	420	512
	Tryptophan	200	200	180
	Valine	780	780	673
Conditionally essential amino acids	Cysteine	<16	<16	-
	Taurine	25	25	70
	Tyrosine	284	240	44
Nonessential amino acids	Alanine	540	540	698
	Arginine	1200	1200	1227
	Aspartic acid	320	320	527
	Glutamic acid	500	500	820
	Glycine	360	360	385
	Histidine	480	480	312
	Proline	680	680	812
	Serine	380	380	495
Total nitrogen (g/L)		15.5	15.5	15.2

day following birth at a dose of 0.5 to 1 g/kg/day and to increase the amount by 0.5 to 1 g/kg/day, depending on tolerance, up to 3 to 4 g/kg/day. Preterm infants have decreased tolerance to intravenous lipids owing to decreased lipoprotein lipase activity, the enzyme responsible for lipid clearance. Furthermore, tolerance to increasing doses of lipid may also vary with the disease status. A recent study demonstrated that administering 3 g/kg/day of lipid on day 1 of life is well tolerated even in VLBW infants. However, most preterm and small for gestational age infants do not tolerate excessive amounts of lipids; lipid infusion rates are generally maintained <0.25 g/kg/h to enhance clearance and to decrease the incidence of hypertriglyceridemia. Higher rates of lipid administration in small preterm infants (over 4 to 6 hours) have been associated with impaired oxygenation. It is generally recommended to infuse lipids without interruption over 24 hours to avoid variable triglyceride concentrations. Most clinicians monitor triglycerides and maintain them less than 200 mg/dL although there are no studies to demonstrate adverse effects of higher levels. However, a theoretical concern with hypertriglyceridemia is the concomitant increase in free fatty acids that may displace bilirubin from albumin. A lipid emulsion dose as low as 0.5 to 1 g/kg/day is sufficient to prevent essential fatty acid

TABLE 6-4   Mineral Requirements for Parenteral Nutrition

Component	Amount/kg/day
Sodium (mEq)	2-5
Potassium (mEq)	2-4
Calcium (mg)	50-100
Magnesium (mg)	3-6
Chloride (mEq)	2-3
Phosphorus (mg)	40-60
Zinc (μg)	200-400
Copper (μg)	20
Iron (μg)	100-200

Modified from Mundy C, Bhatia J: Feeding the premature infant. In Berdanier CD, Dwyer J, Heber D, editors: Handbook of nutrition and food, 3rd ed, Boca Raton, FL, 2013, CRC Press, pp 279-289.

deficiency that can become manifest as early as 3 to 5 days after birth.

5. **a.** Guidelines for mineral intakes are summarized in Table 6-4.

Sodium is not needed during the first few days of life. All infants are born with an expanded extracellular fluid space and increased total body sodium content. The postnatal diuresis is responsible for removing fluid and ridding the body of excess sodium. A delayed diuresis or provision of maintenance sodium in the first few days of life has been associated with an increased risk of bronchopulmonary dysplasia. Furthermore, most ill preterm infants receive significant amounts of sodium in arterial line solutions and drugs such as sodium ampicillin, calcium gluconate, and heparin. In the first few days of life, sodium should be added to the PN solution only when fluid intake has first been restricted and if the serum sodium decreases below 130 mEq/dL. Excess fluid intake is probably the most common cause of hyponatremia in the neonatal intensive care unit (NICU). After the first few days of life, 2 to 5 mEq/kg/day of sodium is usually sufficient, but requirements can increase in infants with renal losses. Potassium should be added in PN after renal function is established. It should be used with caution in ELBW infants who are at increased risk for nonoliguric hyperkalemia for the first 5 days of life. The balance between chloride and acetate is based on acid–base status of the infant. Acetate is commonly added to PN fluids in infants with a metabolic acidosis secondary to bicarbonate wasting in the urine. Cysteine hydrochloride added to PN fluids is a minor source of chloride. However, the addition of cysteine decreases the pH of the solution allowing delivery of increased amounts of calcium and phosphorus because of enhanced solubility.

Calcium and phosphorus supplementation in PN accounts for 60% to 70% of the intrauterine mineral requirements, higher amounts being limited by solubility in solution. Preterm infants are relatively osteopenic at birth because calcium is transferred mainly during the third trimester. It is recommended that calcium supplementation be started as soon as possible after birth especially in the smaller premature infants; a calcium/phosphorus ratio of 1.7:1 by weight is considered ideal. The intake of elemental calcium generally ranges from 50 to 75 mg/kg/day and phosphorus 0.5 to 1 mMol/kg/day. Hypercalcemia secondary to hypophosphatemia and hyperphosphatemia resulting in hypocalcemia should be avoided. Although the intake of calcium and phosphorus can be increased by separate delivery of calcium and phosphorus on alternate days, this is not recommended because of the resultant hypercalciuria and hypercalcemia on days phosphorus is not provided, and hyperphosphaturia and hyperphosphatemia when calcium is omitted.

Iron supplementation in PN is still controversial. Preterm infants have low iron stores and they are at increased risk of developing iron deficiency anemia in early infancy. Because of concerns regarding iron overload, production of reactive oxygen species, and altered immune function, the timing of iron supplementation remains controversial. However, with restrictive transfusion criteria,

TABLE 6-5 Trace Elements for Parenteral Nutrition*

Nutrient	Amount/kg/day <14 Days	Amount/kg/day >14 Days
Manganese (µg)	0-0.75	1.0
Chromium (µg)	0-0.05	0.2
Selenium (µg)	0-1.3	2.0
Iodine (µg)	0-1.0	1.0
Molybdenum (µg)	0	0.25

Modified from Mundy C, Bhatia J. Feeding the premature infant. In Berdanier CD, Dwyer J, Heber D, editors: Handbook of nutrition and food, 3rd ed, Boca Raton, FL, 2013, CRC Press, pp 279-289.
*Commercially available Trace Pack contains copper as well.

TABLE 6-6 Vitamin Components for Parenteral Nutrition

Component	Amount/5 mL
C (mg)	80
A (mg)	0.7 (= 2300 USP units)
D (µg)	10 (= 400 USP units)
B1 (mg)	1.2
B2 (mg)	1.4
B6 (mg)	1
Niacinamide (mg)	17
Dexpanthenol (mg)	5
E (mg)	7
Folic acid (µg)	140
B12 (µg)	1
Biotin (µg)	20
K (µg)	200

From Manufacturer's instructions, M.V.I. Pediatric, Hospira, Inc., Lake Forest, IL.

some experts recommend enteral iron supplementation as early as 2 weeks of life at 1 to 2 mg/kg/day.

Trace elements such as zinc, copper, manganese, iodine, chromium, and selenium can be added (Table 6-5).

Vitamins for PN are provided as MVI-Pediatric (Table 6-6). The recommended dose is 1 mL/kg/day and it should not exceed 2 mL/kg/day.

Heparin 0.5 to 1 unit/mL should be added to PN solutions administered through a central catheter to maintain the patency of the catheter. Care should be taken to avoid using greater than 100 units/kg/day of heparin in very small infants.

Ranitidine is no longer recommended as an additive. Recent studies show that it increases the risk of central line–associated bloodstream infections, necrotizing enterocolitis, and death in preterm infants.

TABLE 6-7	Routes of Parenteral Nutrition Administration	
	Peripheral	Central
Advantages	Preferred for short term	Better caloric intake
	Easy vascular access	Deliver solutions with higher osmolarity
Disadvantages	Osmolarity <1200 mOsm/L	Difficult to obtain
	Dextrose <12.5%	Risk of significant complications related to central catheters
	Lower calcium concentrations	
	Lower caloric intake and increased risk of inadequate growth	
	IV burns from infiltrates	Require heparin

TABLE 6-8	Complications of Parenteral Nutrition		
Metabolic	Short term	Hypoglycemia	
		Hyperglycemia	
		Metabolic acidosis	
		Electrolyte imbalance	
		Hyperlipidemia	
	Long term	PN-associated liver disease (PNALD)	
		Metabolic bone disease	
		Postnatal growth restriction	
Related to administration route	Infectious	Sepsis (staphylococcus spp., Candida, Malassezia furfur)	
		Liver abscess	
	Mechanical	Infiltration	
		Extravasation	
		Thrombosis	
		Pericardial effusion	
		Pleural effusion	
		Arrhythmias	

Delivery route. Parenteral nutrition can be delivered peripherally or centrally through a PICC (percutaneous inserted central catheter), UVC (umbilical venous catheter), or a centrally placed (Broviac) catheter. If it is anticipated that PN is needed for longer than 2 weeks, a centrally placed line (PICC or Broviac) should be used. The advantages and disadvantages of central and peripheral administration are summarized in Table 6-7.

Complications. Complications associated with PN use can be classified as metabolic (generally short-term complications), hepatotoxic (long-term complication), mechanical, or infectious (short- and long-term) (Table 6-8). Most of the metabolic complications can be prevented using a stepwise advancement in the constituents and careful monitoring. Infectious complications can be prevented by aseptic line insertion and careful maintenance, including: sterile change of infusion solutions, minimizing access to the line for administering other medications or blood products, and removing the catheters when enteral feeds are progressing well and have reached 80 to 100 mL/kg/day.

Hepatic dysfunction, including PN-associated liver disease (PNALD), is of multifactorial etiology and can manifest after only 2 weeks of initiation of PN. The risk factors are the duration of PN, the delay in initiation of enteral feeding, and the degree of prematurity. The earliest biochemical derangement is an increase in serum bile acids. This is followed by a rise in direct bilirubin, alkaline phosphatase, and gamma-glutamyl transferase; transaminases

increase last. At the cellular level, it manifests as cholestasis that can advance to portal fibrosis and cirrhosis. Multiple strategies have been proposed for prevention and treatment of PNALD, including decreasing the amino acid intake, limiting the amount of lipid infused, use of fish oil–based lipid emulsions, "cycling" of PN (not generally recommended in premature infants), use of ursodeoxycholic acid to treat cholestasis, and the early introduction and continuation of enteral feeds.

Monitoring the infant and adjusting the PN to his or her needs is of paramount importance to prevent complications and achieve the desired growth and development. Suggested guidelines for monitoring infants on TPN are presented in Table 6-9.

TIPS FOR STARTING AND ADVANCING PN

- Choose a dextrose concentration that allows a GIR of at least 4 mg/kg/min for term infants and 6 mg/kg/min for premature infants. Be careful to adjust the dextrose concentration as the total parenteral nutrition volume increases to prevent an inadvertent increase in the GIR.
- Begin administering amino acids on the first day of life.
- Add calcium to PN on day 1 of life, especially in premature infants and infants of diabetic mothers.

TABLE 6-9 Monitoring of Infants on PN

	Initial	Later
Glucose	Daily until stable	PRN
Electrolytes (Na, K, Cl, CO₂), BUN, creatinine	Daily until stable	Weekly/biweekly
Triglycerides	After every lipid change	Weekly/biweekly
Ca, Phosphorus	Daily until stable	Weekly/biweekly
Magnesium	Initial	Weekly/biweekly
Bilirubin	Initial	Weekly/biweekly
Transaminase (ALT, AST)	Initial	Weekly/biweekly
Gamma GT	Initial	Weekly/biweekly
CBC with reticulocytes	Initial	Weekly/biweekly
Weigh	Daily	Daily
Length	Weekly	Weekly
Head circumference	Weekly	Weekly

Modified from Mundy C, Bhatia J. Feeding the premature infant. In Berdanier CD, Dwyer J, Heber D, editors: Handbook of nutrition and food, 3rd ed, Boca Raton, FL, 2013, CRC Press, pp 279-289.

- In preterm infants with respiratory distress, add sodium once the postnatal diuresis is well established and serum sodium is <130 mEq/L (usually by day 3).
- Start intravenous fat emulsions on the first or second day of life.
- Monitor serum glucose levels.
- Obtain electrolytes at 12 to 24 hours of life, especially in the VLBW infant.
- Advance GIR by 1 to 2 mg/kg/min daily if tolerated (maintain a serum glucose lower than 130 mg/dL). Remember, when fluid intake is increased the glucose delivery rate is also increased for the same dextrose concentration.
- In preterm infants advance the amino acid intake to 3 to 3.5 g/kg/day (this should be achieved by day 2 to 3 of life).
- Advance lipids by 1 g/kg/day as long as triglycerides are less than 175 to 200 mg/dL to maximum of 3.5 g/kg/day.
- Check electrolytes daily until stable, and then weekly.
- Add potassium after renal function is normal; however, be very cautious in adding potassium to ELBW infants who are at risk for nonoliguric hyperkalemia.
- Check magnesium level before adding it in PN, especially in infants born to mothers receiving magnesium sulfate before delivery. Start magnesium when the serum level is <2 mMol/dL.

EXERCISE 2

QUESTION

1. In which of the following cases should PN be initiated?
   a. Term infant with gastroschisis
   b. One-month-old former 26-week preemie with abdominal distension and portal venous air on abdominal x-ray
   c. Three-month-old former 26-week premature infant with chronic lung disease and failure to thrive
   d. 35-weeks' gestational age (GA) preterm infant in septic shock secondary to group B *Streptococcus* (GBS) sepsis
   e. All of the above
   f. None of the above

ANSWER

1. **e.** See Table 6-1.

CASE STUDY 2

A baby girl was born by cesarean section at 25 weeks' gestation to a 25-year-old primigravida woman. Apgar scores were 5 and 7 at 1 and 5 minutes of life. She required positive pressure ventilation, intubation, and surfactant administration in the delivery room. Her birth weight was 720 grams. She was admitted to the NICU, placed on mechanical ventilation, and umbilical arterial and venous catheters were inserted.

EXERCISE 3

QUESTIONS

1. Of the following, the most appropriate IV solution for this newborn is:
   a. 10% dextrose and calcium (20 mg/kg/day) at a fluid rate of 100 mL/kg/day
   b. 5% dextrose, amino acid solution (1.5 g/kg/day), and calcium (20 mg/kg/day) at a fluid rate of 100 mL/kg/day
   c. 10% dextrose, amino acid solution (2.5 g/kg/day), and calcium (20 mg/kg/day) at a fluid rate of 100 mL/kg/day
   d. 10% dextrose, amino acid solution (1.5 g/kg/day), and calcium (20 mg/kg/day) at a fluid rate of 100 mL/kg/day
   e. Donor breast milk at 3 mL/h (100 mL/kg/day)

2. What are the advantages of using a central line for parenteral administration?

a. Central lines have a lower rate of infectious complications than the peripheral intravenous catheters.
b. Central lines can deliver dextrose concentrations >12.5%, but peripheral intravenous lines cannot.
c. Lipid emulsions can only be administered through a central catheter.
d. Central lines require lower doses of heparin than peripheral intravenous lines.
e. Central lines may be left in place until discharge from the hospital and used as needed.

ANSWERS

1. **c.** Solution "c" provides a GIR of 5.2 mg/kg/min, the recommended amount of amino acids (2.5 g/kg/day) and calcium (20 mg/kg/day). Calcium can be administered IV every 6 hours as a bolus or as a continuous infusion of calcium gluconate. Choice "a" is incorrect because no protein is given. Choice "b" provides inadequate amount of protein and glucose. Choice "d" provides adequate amount of glucose, but insufficient amount of protein. Choice "e" is incorrect because premature infants cannot tolerate large amounts of enteral feed this early in life.

   GIR can be calculated as (% dextrose × total fluids in mL/kg/day)/144

   Example: What is the GIR provided by a 5% dextrose solution administered at a rate of 3 mL/h to a 720-gram infant?

   The infant receives TF of (3 mL/h × 24 hours)/0.72 kg = 100 mL/kg/day.

   5 (% dextrose) × 100/144 = 3.47 mg/kg/min.

2. **b.** See Table 6-7.

CASE STUDY 2 (continued)

At 27 hours of life, the GIR is increased from 5.2 to 6 mg/kg/min, amino acids are maintained at 2.5 g/kg/day, and lipids are provided at 1 g/kg/day. Six hours after the new solution is begun, the serum glucose concentration is 250 mg/dL.

EXERCISE 4
QUESTION

1. Which of the following strategies may be helpful in reestablishing euglycemia?
   a. Decrease the dextrose concentration from 10% to 3%.
   b. Increase the dose of amino acids to 3 g/kg/day.
   c. Decrease the dose of intravenous lipid.

d. Administer insulin and check serum glucose in 30 minutes.
e. Decrease total fluids from 100 mL/kg/day to 50 mL/kg/day and check the glucose level in 6 hours.

ANSWER

1. **d.** Administration of lipid can result in elevated glucose concentrations but there is no evidence that lipid restriction treats hyperglycemia. Decreasing the dextrose concentration to 3% (choice "a") decreases the GIR to less than 4 mg/kg/min and may result in hemolysis because the solution is hypotonic. Increasing the amount of amino acids infused (choice "b") might decrease the serum glucose concentration by increasing endogenous insulin secretion, but this infant is already receiving 2.5 g/kg/day of amino acids and it is unlikely that increasing the amount of amino acids will decrease serum levels of glucose. Insulin can be used (choice "d") but is difficult to titrate and increases the risk of hypoglycemia.

CASE STUDY 2 (continued)

The following laboratory values are obtained on day 2: Na 145 mEq/L, K 4.8 meq/L, Cl 118 mEq/L, HCO$_3$ 18 mg/dL, BUN 40 mg/dL, creatinine 0.81 mg/dL, glucose 127 mg/dL, Ca 8.0 mg/dL, Mg 1.8 mg/dL, PO$_4$ mg/dL 4.1, triglycerides (TG) 130 mg/dL, total bilirubin 7 mg/dL with direct bilirubin 0.5 mg/dL. The infant's urine output is 0.8 mL/kg/h. She is receiving 100 mL/kg/day of a 10% dextrose solution, 3 g/kg/day of amino acids, 1 g/kg/day of lipids, and calcium (20 mg/kg/day).

EXERCISE 5
QUESTIONS

1. What changes should be made in her TPN?
   a. Increase total fluid intake to 125 mL/kg/day, increase the dextrose concentration to 12.5 %, decrease the intake of amino acids to 2.0 g/kg/day, and increase the dose of lipids to 2.0 g/kg/day. Add potassium phosphate.
   b. Leave the PN solution unchanged.
   c. Increase total fluid intake to 125 mL/kg/day, leave the concentration of dextrose unchanged (10%), increase the amino acid intake to 3.5 g/kg/day, and leave the dose of lipids unchanged (1.0 g/kg/day). Add potassium phosphate.
   d. Decrease total fluid intake to 80 mL/kg/day, increase the dose of amino acids to 3.5 g/kg/day, leave the concentration of dextrose unchanged (10%) and increase lipid dose to 2.0 g/kg/day. Add potassium phosphate.

e. Increase total fluids to 125 mL/kg/day, increase the concentration of dextrose to 12.5%, increase the dose of amino acids to 3.5 g/kg/day, and increase the dose of lipids to 2.0 g/kg/day.

2. What lab tests should be ordered for the next day?
   a. Serum chemistries (Na, K, Cl, CO_2, BUN, glucose, Mg, Ca, PO_4) and triglyceride levels
   b. Serum chemistries (Na, K, Cl, CO_2, BUN, glucose, Mg, Ca, PO_4) and liver function studies (transaminases and alkaline phosphatase)
   c. Serum ammonia and lipid profile

3. Which of the following is the most correct statement regarding mineral requirements in PN for this infant?
   a. Sodium, iron, and calcium should be added as soon as PN is initiated.
   b. Sodium should be routinely added if the serum Na is <130 mEq/dL. Potassium should be added when renal function is adequate.
   c. Maintenance sodium should be added once the diuresis is well established. Potassium should be withheld until renal function is adequate and nonoliguric hyperkalemia is unlikely.
   d. Copper should be added whenever hepatic dysfunction is suspected.

ANSWERS

1. **e.** The infant is mildly dehydrated as evidenced by a rising serum sodium concentration (secondary to a free water diuresis) and decreased urine output. Therefore, total fluids should be increased. Amino acids should be increased to 3.5 g/kg/day to meet protein requirements for a preterm infant. An increase in BUN to 40 mg/dL may be a sign of mild dehydration (or increased protein utilization). However, it is a normal value and the protein intake should be advanced (not decreased). Increasing the amount of amino acids will permit the addition of more calcium and phosphorus in the parenteral solution because the pH will be lowered and the solubility of calcium increased. The infant is euglycemic. Therefore the dose of intravenous lipids should be increased by 0.5 to 1 g/kg/day, to increase the caloric intake.

2. **a.** This infant needs monitoring of routine serum chemistries and triglyceride levels. Triglyceride levels should be determined whenever the dose of intravenous lipid is increased. Liver function tests should only be checked if the direct bilirubin is elevated. In infants needing PN for more than 1 week, liver function tests should be obtained biweekly.

3. **c.** There is a physiologic contraction of the extracellular fluid space that occurs secondary to a postnatal diuresis in every newborn infant. Sodium should not be added to the intravenous solution until the diuresis is well established. If the serum sodium concentration decreases to a concentration <130 mEq/L, fluid restriction should be tried first before supplemental sodium is given. However, when the serum sodium concentration is <125 mEq/L additional sodium should be given. Potassium should be withheld until renal function is established and nonoliguric hyperkalemia is unlikely. Calcium should be started on day 1 of life. The optimal timing for iron supplementation is controversial. Most experts would recommend supplementation only if PN continues for more than 2 weeks. Copper can be hepatotoxic and is not recommended in infants with liver dysfunction.

CASE STUDY 2 (continued)

On day 4 the infant receives a solution containing 12.5% dextrose (at a rate of 100 mL/kg/day), 3.5 g/kg/day amino acid, and 20% lipids (0.5 mL/h) continuously over 24 hours. The infant's weight is 0.72 kg.

EXERCISE 6

QUESTION

1. What amount of energy does she receive from the non–protein calories in PN?
   a. 78 kcal/kg/day
   b. 80 kcal/kg/day
   c. 92 kcal/kg/day
   d. 100 kcal/kg/day
   e. 125 kcal/kg/day

ANSWER

1 **c.**
   - *Lipid emulsion: The emulsion concentration is 20%, which means there are 20 grams of fat in 100 mL of emulsion. The caloric density of 20% intravenous fat emulsion is 2 kcal/mL. The fat calories delivered can be easily calculated as the amount of intravenous lipid received (mL) multiplied by the caloric density of 2 kcal/mL (12 mL/day × 2 kcal/mL = 24 kcal/day). The "fat calories"/kg = 24/0.72 (infant's weight) = 33 kcal/kg/day.*
   - *There are 12.5 grams of glucose in 100 mL of 12.5% dextrose solution. If the infant is receiving 100 mL/day, he is receiving 12.5 grams glucose/day. Since one gram of glucose provides 3.4 kcal, then 12.5 g/day × 3.4 kcal/g = 42.5 kcal/day or 59 kcal/kg/day).*

- Total energy intake from non–protein calories (kcal/kg/day) is: 33 + 59 = 92 kcal/kg/day.

CASE STUDY 2 (continued)

On day 6 the same baby becomes lethargic, hypotensive, and requires increased ventilator support. She has an increased white blood count and a left shift. Because of suspicion of sepsis, a blood culture has been drawn and antibiotics given.

EXERCISE 7

QUESTIONS

1. What changes should be made in her total PN?
   a. Increase the amount of lipids to provide more energy.
   b. Change the PN to a peripherally suitable solution because the central line should be removed.
   c. Adjust the dextrose concentration according to serum levels and monitor triglyceride levels.
   d. Increase the amount of heparin to improve lipid tolerance.
   e. Decrease the amount of intravenous lipid infused because lipids can decrease the ability to clear the infection.

2. Assuming that at 2 weeks of life this infant is still receiving TPN, what is her targeted growth?
   a. 10 to 15 g/day
   b. 15 to 20 g/day
   c. 30 to 35 g/day
   d. An infant on TPN is unlikely to gain weight

ANSWERS

1. **c.** The infants can become either hypo- or hyperglycemic in response to sepsis. It is reasonable to monitor blood glucose whenever an acute illness presents. They can also become lipid intolerant. Triglyceride level should be checked and lipids adjusted accordingly. Although intravenous lipid is a risk factor for central line–associated bloodstream infections, it does not decrease the ability of the infant to clear the infection. Heparin should not be used to increase lipid tolerance because it does not increase lipid utilization. Central catheters have to be removed in a limited number of cases (e.g., *Candida spp.* or *S. aureus* sepsis). The most frequent catheter-related infections, caused by coagulase negative staphylococcus, do not usually require removal or replacement of the catheter, but the antibiotic treatment should

be administered through that central catheter. Total fluids and electrolytes should be managed according to the infant's hydration status.

2. **b.** Ideally, postnatal growth should mimic *in utero* fetus growth. At 27 weeks the expected weight gain is 15 to 20 g/day.

CASE STUDY 3

A term infant is born vaginally to a 17-year-old mother with no prenatal care. The Apgar scores are 8 and 9 at 1 and 5 minutes. Immediately after delivery he is noticed to have a gastroschisis. The infant is transferred to the NICU for further care. The birth weight is 3 kg. Gestational age by physical assessment is 39 weeks. While awaiting surgery evaluation a peripheral IV is placed.

EXERCISE 8

QUESTION

1. Which of the following would be the most appropriate fluid solution for this infant?
   a. 5% dextrose with 2.0 g/kg/day amino acids at a rate of 8.5 mL/h
   b. 10% dextrose at a rate of 10 mL/h
   c. 5% dextrose with 0.25 g/kg/day amino acids at a rate of 20 mL/h
   d. 10% dextrose and 0.25% NS at a rate of 12.5 mL/h
   e. 10% dextrose with 2 g/kg/day amino acids at a rate of 12.5 mL/h

ANSWER

1. **e.** This is a term infant with higher insensible losses (secondary to the gastroschisis) and a clear contraindication to enteral feedings. Healthy term infants generally receive 60 to 80 mL/kg/day during the first 24 hours of life; however, this infant should receive at least 25% more to compensate for the higher insensible water losses. The protein requirements for term infants are lower than preterm infants, so 2 to 2.5 g/kg/day is sufficient. Higher amounts may be needed for wound healing postsurgery. Sodium-containing fluids should be avoided in the first day of life, but the serum sodium concentration should be monitored closely. Choice "a" is incorrect because the total fluid intake (68 mL/kg/day) and the GIR (2.4 mg/kg/min) are both inadequate. Choice "b" is incorrect because no protein is given. Choice "c" is incorrect because the fluid intake is too high (160 mL/kg/day) and protein intake inadequate. Choice "d" is incorrect because sodium should

not be given in the first 24 hours of life and no protein is given.

CASE STUDY 3 (continued)

The infant is electively intubated and sedated. A silo is placed, through which the bowel looks well perfused. By the size of the defect you estimate that it might take more than a week before the defect can be closed.

EXERCISE 9

QUESTION

1. With regard to venous access in this infant, which of the following would be appropriate?
   a. There is no need for vascular access; the baby can be fed breast milk by gavage.
   b. Place a UVC.
   c. Insert a new peripheral intravenous line for lipid emulsions.
   d. No central line is necessary because the infant will be able to feed immediately after defect closure.
   e. Place a PICC because you anticipate that he will need total PN for more than 2 weeks.

ANSWER

1. **e.** A central indwelling catheter placement is indicated in this infant, who will likely require PN for more than 2 weeks. Umbilical line placement should be avoided in infants with abdominal wall defects. Lipids and other components in PN can be given through the same line.

CASE STUDY 3 (continued)

The abdominal wall was closed on day 8 of life. Over the next 2 weeks infant failed multiple attempts to feed enterally. A contrast study was consistent with bowel obstruction. An exploratory laparotomy done 2 weeks later revealed multiple areas of atresia in the proximal ileum. Approximately 50 cm of small bowel were resected and an ostomy was created.

EXERCISE 10

QUESTION

1. What complications related to provision of nutrition do you anticipate in this case?
   a. Parenteral nutrition associated cholestasis and hepatocellular injury
   b. Metabolic bone disease and anemia
   c. Central line–associated bloodstream infections
   d. Short bowel syndrome and "dumping"
   e. All of the above

ANSWER

1. **e.** This infant is at risk for sepsis, PNALD, thrombosis, dumping, short bowel syndrome, anemia, failure to thrive, and metabolic bone disease (more common in preterm infants).

CASE STUDY 3 (continued)

Low-volume enteral feeds were started and stopped due to a high ostomy output. He is now 9 weeks old and weighs 3300 grams. The following laboratory data were obtained: total bilirubin 12 mg/dL with direct bilirubin 10.3 mg/dL, alkaline phosphatase 720 I U/L, gamma glutamyl transferase 250, AST 90 IU/L, ALT 75 IU/L, triglyceride 130 mg/mL, albumin 2.1 g/dL, and sodium 126 mEq/L.

EXERCISE 11

QUESTION

1. What should be done to decrease the liver injury?
   a. Write a compassionate-use protocol request for fish oil–based lipid emulsion, as this infant developed PNALD.
   b. Administer probiotics to decrease the dumping and allow enteral feeds to restart.
   c. Start ursodeoxycholic acid and sodium chloride supplements via gavage, to decrease cholestasis and replenish sodium. Request a surgery consult for bowel reanastomosis.
   d. Start phototherapy to decrease bilirubin.

ANSWER

1. **d.** This infant developed PNALD. The most helpful action in preventing the progression of disease would be to restart enteral feeds. Bowel reanastomosis could potentially resolve the dumping and allow him to tolerate enteral feedings. Intravenous lipids should be decreased as there is a strong association with lipid emulsions and continued hepatocellular injury. He is not a candidate for compassionate use of fish oil emulsion because other options have not been tried and the treatment is still investigational. Ursodeoxycholic acid is given enterally so it cannot be used in this infant. Direct hyperbilirubinemia is a contraindication for phototherapy.

SUGGESTED READINGS

Adamkin AH: *Nutritional Strategies for the Very Low Birth Weight Infant*, New York, 2009, Cambridge University Press, pp 1-77.
Bartley JH, Nagy S, Frank M, Bhatia J: Inadvertent sodium load in the first 5 days of life in extremely low-birth-weight infants, *J Perinatol* 25:593, 2004.

Collins Jr JW, Hope M, Brown K: A controlled trial of insulin infusion on parenteral nutrition in extremely low birth weight infants with glucose intolerance, *J Pediatr* 118:921, 1991.

Dinerstein A, Neito RM, Solana CL, et al: Early and aggressive nutritional strategies (parenteral and enteral) decreases postnatal growth failure in very low birth weight infants, *J Perinatol* 26:436–442, 2006.

Georgieff MK: Iron. In Thureen PJ, Hay WW, editors: *Neonatal nutrition and metabolism*, Cambridge, UK, 2006, Cambridge University Press.

Gura K, Duggan CP, Collier SB, et al: Reversal of parenteral nutrition-associated liver disease in two infants with short bowel syndrome using parenteral fish oil: implications for future management, *Pediatrics* 118: e197-e201, 2006.

Ibrahim HM, Jeroudi MA, Baier RJ, et al: Aggressive early total parental nutrition in low-birth-weight infants, *J Perinatol* 24:482–486, 2004.

Mitton SG, Garlick PJ: Changes in protein turnover after the introduction of parenteral nutrition in premature infants: comparison of breast milk and egg protein-based amino acid solutions, *Pediatr Res* 32:447–454, 1992.

Mundy C, Bhatia J: Feeding the premature infant. In Berdanier CD, Dwyer J, Heber D, editors: *Handbook of nutrition and food*, 3rd ed, Boca Raton, FL, 2013, CRC Press, pp 279–289.

Parenteral nutrition. In Klienman RE, editor: *Pediatric nutrition handbook*, 6th ed, American Academy of Pediatrics, 2009, pp 519–540.

Poindexter B, Denne S: Nutrition and metabolism in the high-risk neonate. In Martin RJ, Fanaroff AA, Walsh MC, editors: *Fanaroff and Martin's neonatal-perinatal medicine: diseases of the detus and infant*, St. Louis, MO, 2011, Mosby, pp 643-651.

Poindexter BB, Erenkrantz RA, Stoll BJ, et al: National Institute of Child Health and Human Development Neonatal Research Network. Parenteral glutamine supplementation does not reduce the risk of mortality or late-onset sepsis in extremely low birth weight infants, *Pediatrics* 113:1209–1215, 2004.

Rollins MD, Scaife ER, Jackson WD, et al: Elimination of soybean lipid emulsion in parenteral nutrition and supplementation with enteral fish oil improve cholestasis in infants with short bowel syndrome, *Nutr Clin Pract* 25:199–204, 2010.

Sengupta A, Lehmann C, Diener-West M, et al: Catheter duration and risk of CLABSI in neonates with PICCs, *Pediatrics* 125:648–653, 2010.

Soden JS, Lovell MA, Brown K, et al: Failure of resolution of portal fibrosis during omega-3 fatty acid lipid emulsion therapy in two patients with irreversible intestinal failure, *J Pediatr* 156:327–331, 2010.

te Braake FW, van den Akker CH, Wattimena DJ, et al: Amino acid administration to premature infants directly after birth, *J Pediatr* 147:457–461, 2005.

Terrin G, Passariello A, De Curtis M, et al: Ranitidine is associated with infections, necrotizing enterocolitis and fatal outcome in newborns, *Pediatrics* 129(1):e40–e45, 2012.

The American Society of Parenteral and Enteral Nutrition, Carney LN, Nepa A, Cohen SS, et al: Parenteral and enteral nutrition support: determining the best way to feed. In Corkins MR, Balint J, Bobo E, Yaworki JA, editors: *Pediatric nutrition support core curriculum*, The American Society of Parenteral and Enteral Nutrition, 2010, pp 433-447.

CHAPTER 7

ENTERAL NUTRITION

Brenda B. Poindexter, MD, MS • Camilia R. Martin, MD, MS

Evidence is increasingly accumulating that nutritional inadequacies in the early neonatal period can have both short- and long-term consequences. Nonetheless, provision of adequate nutritional support to the high-risk premature infant remains a significant clinical challenge. Among extremely premature infants, postnatal growth failure remains a nearly universal complication of neonatal intensive care. This chapter contains exercises designed to help those who care for premature infants to review enteral nutrient requirements, identify strategies to optimize provision of nutrition, and describe the importance of adequate postnatal growth. In addition, areas where further research is needed to determine optimal nutritional support to improve outcomes in this population are emphasized.

NUTRIENT REQUIREMENTS

Recommendations for nutrient requirements for the premature infant are largely based on the goal of duplicating rates of fetal nutrient accretion and growth to optimize long-term outcomes. Based on the available evidence, recommendations for enteral nutrient supply for premature infants were made by an expert panel convened by the Committee on Nutrition of the European Society of Pediatric Gastroenterology, Hepatology, and Nutrition (ESPGHAN) (Agostoni et al, 2010). A summary of these recommendations is shown in Table 7-1. During the early phase of nutritional support of very low birth weight (VLBW) and extremely low birth weight (ELBW) infants, it is important to recognize that a combination of both parenteral and enteral nutrition is needed to meet requirements to avoid nutrients deficits, which contribute to postnatal growth failure.

Meeting these recommendations can be particularly challenging in the extremely premature infant owing to high incidence of feeding intolerance and the fear of necrotizing enterocolitis (NEC) if feeds are advanced too quickly. In addition, human milk must be fortified in order to meet these nutrient requirements to support optimal growth and outcomes.

INITIATION AND ADVANCEMENT OF ENTERAL NUTRITION

Initiation of Minimal Enteral Nutrition

CASE STUDY 1

HR is a 2-day-old, 27-week gestation female whose birth weight was 635 grams. She was delivered by cesarean section because of worsening maternal preeclampsia. She initially was intubated and received a total of three doses of exogenous surfactant for respiratory distress syndrome and has subsequently weaned to low ventilatory support and <30% oxygen. Indomethacin is being given for intraventricular hemorrhage (IVH) prophylaxis. Upon admission to the neonatal intensive care unit (NICU), intravenous amino acids were immediately initiated to provide 3 g/kg/day; total parenteral nutrition with 10% dextrose (15 g/kg/day carbohydrate), 3.5 g/kg/day amino acids, and 3 g/kg/day lipids is now infusing at 150 mL/kg/day (providing a total of 92 kcal/kg/day). Umbilical arterial and venous lines remain in place. Mom is expressing breast milk every 3 hours. On rounds, her bedside nurse inquires as to when the baby will start to receive enteral feedings.

TABLE 7-1	Nutrient Requirements for Enterally Fed Premature Infants	
	Per kg/day	**Per 100 kcal**
Fluid, mL	135-200	
Energy, kcal	110-135	
Protein, g		
<1000 g body weight	4.0-4.5	3.6-4.1
1000-1800 g body weight	3.5-4.0	3.2-3.6
Lipid, g	4.8-6.6	4.4-6.0

EXERCISE 1

QUESTION

1. Which of these statements reflects an evidence-based decision related to the initiation of enteral feedings in this infant?
   a. Parenteral nutrition (PN) is supplying the infant with all necessary nutrients; enteral feeding should be delayed until the infant is no longer at risk of developing NEC.
   b. Feedings cannot be initiated until both umbilical lines are removed.
   c. Feedings can be initiated using half-strength human milk or premature formula at 40 to 60 mL/kg/day.
   d. Trophic or minimal enteral feedings (10 to 20 mL/kg/day) with full-strength human milk should be initiated today.

ANSWER

1. **d.** Although the infant is receiving a reasonable intake from PN, it is important that consideration is given to begin enteral feedings as early as possible. There are known benefits of minimal enteral feedings in premature neonates, and conversely, potential detriment to postnatal intestinal adaptation with a prolonged absence of any enteral feedings.

Delayed Initiation of Enteral Nutrition

In a piglet model of neonatal nutrition, a delay in enteral feedings resulted in a decrease in intestinal cell proliferation, a decrease in superior mesenteric artery blood flow, and an increase in apoptosis. Although, studies specifically evaluating the effects of delayed feedings (>4 days) compared to feedings initiated within 48 hours are few, none have shown significant morbidity when feedings are delayed. However, evidence does demonstrate that with delayed feedings, the number of days to achieve full enteral feedings is greater. Additionally, for every week delay in initiating the first feeding, the risk of late-onset sepsis progressively increased.

The presence of umbilical lines, including an umbilical arterial catheter, is not a reason to withhold enteral nutrition. Current evidence has not supported the theoretical concern of the umbilical catheter reducing intestinal blood flow or increasing medical complications during trophic feedings. In addition, the common practice of withholding enteral feedings during treatment for a patent ductus arteriosus has been called into question recently. A randomized clinical trial demonstrated that continuation of trophic feedings at 15 mL/kg/day during treatment with indomethacin (versus no enteral feedings) resulted in fewer days to achieve full enteral feedings (defined as 120 mL/kg/day) with no increase in complications, including NEC or spontaneous intestinal perforation (Clyman et al, 2013).

Minimal Enteral Nutrition

Minimal enteral feedings, also known as trophic feedings, are typically defined as low-volume feedings that do not provide sufficient calories to support somatic growth but rather help to promote maturation of the structure and function of the premature intestinal tract. Several clinical studies have demonstrated reductions in the number of days to achieve full enteral feeding, total number of days that enteral feeds are withheld, and days of hospital stay. If available, full-strength expressed mother's milk should be given. There is no evidence to suggest that use of diluted formula is an effective strategy to decrease the risk of NEC.

Advancement of Enteral Nutrition and Necrotizing Enterocolitis

Even under the best of circumstances, it takes a substantial amount of time to achieve full enteral feedings in premature neonates. Among ELBW infants cared for at participating centers of the Eunice Kennedy Shriver National Institute of Child Health and Human Development (NICHD) Neonatal Research Network, the mean age at which full enteral feedings (defined as ≥110 kcal/kg/day) were achieved was as long as 35 days. Neither early versus late initiation of enteral feedings nor slow versus fast enteral advancement reduces the risk of NEC as summarized in recent systematic reviews. Several studies have shown a decrease in the incidence of NEC with the implementation of standardized feeding protocols. Regardless of the approach, PN should be maintained until enteral nutrition is supplying a minimum of 100 mL/kg/day.

Intrauterine Growth Restriction (IUGR)

According to the 2013 Fenton Growth Curve, HR's birth weight is at the 9th percentile and is thus considered growth restricted. IUGR infants have an increased risk of NEC. As a result, it is common practice to delay initiation of enteral nutrition, theoretically to reduce the compromise to an already perceived compromised gut. However, this strategy is not evidence-based and has been challenged recently in a study that showed that a delay in the initiation of enteral feedings (>48 hours) in growth restricted infants with abnormal umbilical artery Doppler waveforms did not lead to a lower risk of NEC. In contrast, feedings initiated within 48 hours reduced the time to full enteral feedings (with a concomitant reduction in the days requiring PN) and reduced the incidence of cholestasis (Leaf et al, 2012).

ENTERAL FEEDING REGIMENS

Benefits of Human Milk

CASE STUDY 2

The attending obstetrician requests a prenatal consult for Mrs. B, a 26-year-old primigravida, who has presented at 24 weeks' estimated gestational age with premature labor with rupture of membranes, and imminent delivery. After discussing the morbidity and mortality risks associated with extreme prematurity, you encourage the mother to consider expressing human milk for her infant.

EXERCISE 2

QUESTION

1. Which of the following statements should be included in your discussion regarding provision of human milk to premature infants?
   a. Mother's own milk supports the preterm infant's developing immune system.
   b. Premature infants who receive their mother's own milk have a lower incidence of sepsis and NEC.
   c. Premature infants who receive mother's own milk demonstrate improved developmental outcomes compared with formula-fed premature infants.

ANSWER

1. All of the above statements are true. Given these and other important benefits, the use of mother's own milk should be encouraged for all premature infants. The use of mother's own milk as the primary diet for preterm infants was affirmed in a recent policy statement from the American Academy of Pediatrics (AAP) and European Society of Paediatric Gastroenterology, Hepatology and Nutrition (ESP-GHAN) (AAP Section on Breastfeeding, 2012; Agostoni et al, 2009).

   Several studies have demonstrated the immunologic benefits of human milk for premature infants, including higher concentrations of secretory IgA, lysozyme, lactoferrin, and interferon in preterm human milk. Provision of mother's own milk may also enhance colonization of the infant's intestinal tract with beneficial commensal

organisms. The incidence of infection and NEC are decreased in preterm infants who receive mother's own milk. In addition, observational studies in ELBW infants have shown an association between exposure to mother's own milk and improved neurodevelopmental outcomes at 18 to 22 months' corrected age (CA). In one study, maternal milk was also found to decrease the need for rehospitalization between NICU discharge and 30 months' CA (Vohr et al, 2006 and 2007).

It is important to recognize that many mothers who deliver prematurely will choose to express milk for their infant once they are properly informed of the numerous benefits. For many mothers with a critically ill infant, expressing breast milk provides a means to make a contribution to their child's welfare, where they otherwise have very little control. All caregivers providing care to ELBW and VLBW infants should be knowledgeable with respect to the many benefits of mother's own milk and must be committed to ensuring that all mothers in their care are equipped to express their breast milk. Many units have successfully implemented quality improvement initiatives to increase human milk feedings in preterm infants.

Composition of Premature Human Milk

CASE STUDY 3

Two hours after completing your prenatal consult, EB is born weighing 710 g. After being informed of the advantages of human milk and being instructed in use of an electric breast pump, the mother has begun pumping every 3 hours. Colostrum is immediately provided to the infant via orogastric tube.

EXERCISE 3

QUESTION

1. After 2 weeks of established lactation, which of the following statements regarding the composition of this mother's milk are true?
   a. The protein content is lower now than it will be after 4 weeks of lactation.
   b. Milk expressed at 2 weeks is sufficient to meet all nutrient requirements.
   c. Expressed milk has higher content of calcium and phosphorus than preterm formula.

ANSWER

1. None of the above statements is true. A thorough understanding the nutrient content of

human milk is needed in order to make informed decisions about provision of optimal nutritional support to premature infants. The composition of milk expressed by women who deliver prematurely is different from that of women who deliver at term. In the first 2 weeks of lactation, the protein content of preterm human milk is typically 1.4 to 1.6 g/dL. Over time, the protein content steadily declines to that of term milk (average 1.0 g/dL). Despite the higher content of protein and some minerals, preterm human milk alone does not meet all nutrient requirements of extremely premature infants.

Banked Donor Human Milk

CASE STUDY 4

After observing your conversation with the mother, the neonatal nurse practitioner in the NICU asks your opinion regarding the use of banked donor human milk if the mother is unable to provide enough milk for her infant.

EXERCISE 4

QUESTION

1. Which of the following statements are true based on currently available evidence?
   a. Donor milk is pasteurized to minimize risk of infection.
   b. Pasteurization preserves all immunologic benefits of human milk.
   c. The nutrient composition of banked donor milk is comparable to preterm human milk.
   d. Premature infants who receive donor milk demonstrate similar rates of weight gain as those who are fed premature formula.

ANSWER

1. **a.** Donors are screened for infectious risk and the milk is also heat pasteurized to avoid bacterial and viral contamination. Pasteurization reduces some of the nutritional and immunologic properties of human milk, such as various immune cells, IgA, and lactoferrin, and completely destroys milk lipase. Future research should be directed at optimizing pasteurization to preserve the beneficial properties of human milk.

   Human milk banks usually obtain milk from donors who delivered term infants; consequently, the protein content of donor milk is lower than that obtained from women who have delivered prematurely. Macronutrient content of pooled donor milk has been evaluated, with some investigators reporting average protein content less

than 1 g/dL and energy content less than 15 kcal/ounce in samples analyzed. Similarly, although pasteurization did not alter fatty acid levels in donor milk, the content of DHA and ARA were lower than what previously has been reported in human milk (Valentine et al, 2010).

A randomized trial of donor human milk versus preterm formula as substitutes for mothers' own milk in the feeding of extremely premature infants found lower rates of weight gain in infants fed donor milk; a substantial number of infants who received donor human milk in this study were switched to premature formula because of poor weight gain (Schanler et al, 2005). Future studies are needed to define more clearly the potential role of banked human milk in infants whose mothers are unable to provide their own milk.

Fortification of Human Milk

CASE STUDY 5

EB tolerates advancement of enteral feeds by 20 mL/kg/day. At 9 days of age, she is receiving 100 mL/kg/day of her mother's own milk. After regaining her birth weight at 6 days of age, she has gained approximately 10 grams per day.

EXERCISE 5

QUESTIONS

1. Which of the following alterations should be made to her feeding regimen?
   a. Add an additional source of protein to feedings.
   b. Add a multicomponent human milk fortifier (HMF).
   c. Change to premature formula.
   d. No changes are required; weight gain is adequate for a premature infant.

2. Which of the following nutrients do HMFs supply?
   a. Protein, primarily whey based
   b. A balanced source of calories from protein, carbohydrate, and lipid
   c. Calcium and phosphorus
   d. Sodium, zinc, and vitamins

ANSWERS

1. **b**.

2. All of the responses are correct. Preterm human milk provides insufficient quantities of protein, energy, sodium, phosphate, and calcium to meet the estimated needs of the

preterm infant. In an effort to meet needs for growth and to avoid osteopenia, a number of multicomponent HMFs are available for in-hospital use.

Options for fortification of human milk include bovine and human milk-based products. Given the potential risk of infectious complications, the use of powdered products should be avoided. There are significant differences in protein content between the two liquid bovine HMFs that are currently available in the United States (difference of 1 g/dL protein between the two products). The human milk–based product provides considerably less protein.

A multicenter randomized clinical trial compared the new liquid HMF and standard powder HMF in preterm infants with birth weight ≤1250 grams receiving expressed and/or donor human milk. Achieved weight and linear growth rate were significantly higher in infants randomized to receive the liquid HMF with no difference in the number of days to achieve full enteral feedings or in the incidence of feeding intolerance (Moya et al, 2012). The human milk–based fortifier (Prolacta) was evaluated in a randomized clinical trial. In this trial, an exclusive human milk diet was compared to mother's own milk fortified with bovine HMF and preterm formula. The investigators found no difference in the primary outcome of duration of PN, but did suggest that the incidence of NEC or death was higher in the group of infants who received the bovine fortifier than in the exclusive human milk group (Sullivan et al, 2010).

Although many clinicians delay the addition of HMF until the infant is tolerating full-volume enteral feedings, some experts suggest that fortification of human milk can be introduced at much lower volumes (>50 mL/kg/day) in an effort to minimize nutrient deficits and to optimize postnatal growth (Senterre et al, 2011). As a strategy for fortification of human milk is implemented, it is important to take into consideration the alterations in protein content that take place as lactation progresses in order to ensure that requirements are met.

A systematic review has evaluated outcomes associated with multicomponent fortification of human milk. Fortifiers included in the analysis provided protein, calcium, phosphate, and carbohydrate, as well as vitamins and trace minerals. The reviewers concluded that the use of multicomponent fortifiers is associated with short-term improvements in weight gain, linear growth, and head circumference growth. The data were insufficient to evaluate the effect of fortifiers on long-term growth outcomes and neurodevelopment (Kuschel et al, 2004).

Preterm Formula

CASE STUDY 6

EG is a former 29-week gestation female whose birth weight was 1250 grams. She is now 3 weeks of age and mom's milk supply is not adequate, despite excellent support from a lactation counselor. The medical student asks what types of formulas are available for premature infants.

EXERCISE 6

QUESTION

1. Which of the following statements regarding premature infant formulas are true?
   a. Like human milk, lactose is the exclusive source of carbohydrate in premature formulas.
   b. In contrast to formulas designed for term infants, premature formulas supply 40% to 50% of the total lipid content as medium chain triglycerides.
   c. The protein composition of premature formulas is predominantly casein based.
   d. The protein content of premature formula is similar to fortified human milk.
   e. The calcium and phosphorus content of premature formulas is lower than that of term formula.

ANSWER

1. **b** and **d**. Lactose is the only source of carbohydrate in both term and preterm human milk. The carbohydrate content of premature formulas, on the other hand, is a blend of 40% to 50% lactose and 50% to 60% glucose polymers (such as corn syrup solids). Premature infants have low levels of intestinal lactase activity; consequently, the reduced lactose content of premature formulas theoretically enhances digestion. Glucose polymers are easily digested by alpha-glucosidase enzymes (sucrase, isomaltase, maltase, glucoamylase); these enzymes, in contrast to lactase, are abundant in the small intestine of premature infants and approximate adult levels much sooner.

   Human milk supplies approximately 50% of total calories from fat. Preterm formulas contain medium-chain triglycerides (MCT) in order to compensate for low levels of intestinal lipase and bile salts in premature infants. In addition, most formulas are now supplemented with docosahexaenoic (DHA) and arachidonic (ARA) acids, and long-chain polyunsaturated fatty acids similar to those found in human milk, which are thought to be important for brain and retinal development.

The protein content of premature formulas is higher than term formulas. Standard preterm formulas supply 3 g/100 kcal and the newer "high protein" preterm formulas supply 3.3 to 3.6 g/100 kcal. In order to meet the recommended protein intake in infants weighing <1 kg, the higher protein content formulas are necessary. Patterned after human milk, premature formulas are whey-predominant. Soy-based formulas are not routinely recommended for the premature infant because they contain significantly less phosphorus and may result in metabolic bone disease; in addition, the phytates in soy formulas can interfere with iron absorption.

A comparison of protein intake with different enteral feedings is shown in Table 7-2. Although most clinicians focus on enteral intake in terms of volume (mL/kg/day) or caloric intake (kcal/kg/day), it is equally important to consider protein intake when caring for ELBW infants. Inadequate protein intake is associated with poor growth and with adverse neurodevelopmental outcomes.

MONITORING GROWTH AND OUTCOMES

Classification of Intrauterine Growth

CASE STUDY 7

AL and ML are twin boys delivered at 26 weeks' gestation to a 26-year-old primigravida whose pregnancy was complicated by twin-twin transfusion syndrome status post–laser ablation. Delivery was via emergent cesarean birth for breech presentation and variable fetal heart rate decelerations in twin A. Anthropometric parameters of the infants at birth were as follows:

> *Twin A: weight – 800 grams; length 32 cm; head circumference 23.5 cm*

> *Twin B: weight – 860 grams; length 34.5 cm; head circumference 24 cm*

The mother asks if her infants weigh more or less than you would have expected for twins born at 26 weeks.

EXERCISE 7

QUESTIONS

1. Which of the following is the best answer to her question?
   a. Both infants are SGA (small for gestational age).
   b. Both infants are AGA (appropriate for gestational age).
   c. Twin B is LGA (large for gestational age).
   d. Given the 60-gram difference in birth weight, the twins are considered discordant.

2. Which of the following answers best represents the percentage of VLBW infants who are identified as being SGA at birth?
   a. 90%
   b. 74%
   c. 22%
   d. 10%

ANSWER

1. **b.** The medical student on rounds is somewhat surprised that an infant who weighs less than 1000 grams at birth is not automatically considered to have experienced intrauterine growth restriction (IUGR).

2. **c.** Although IUGR is more frequent in multiple gestations, both infants are AGA. It is important to recognize that not all premature infants are SGA at birth. Large multicenter studies have reported that approximately 22% of VLBW and 17% of ELBW infants are SGA at the time of birth. Small for gestational age is a term used to describe an infant whose weight is less than the 10th percentile for a given gestational age.

   A recent cohort study of infants born at <27 weeks' gestation found that SGA infants had higher mortality and were more likely to have postnatal growth failure, prolonged mechanical

TABLE 7-2	**Comparison of Protein Intake with Enteral Feedings at 150 mL/kg/day**
	Protein (g/kg/day)
Recommended intake for <1000 g	4.0-4.5
Donor human milk (assume 0.7-1 g/dL)	1.05-1.5
Preterm human milk (assume 1.4-1.6 g/dL)	2.1-2.4
Preterm human milk + HMF (24 kcal/oz)	3.5-4.5
"High protein" preterm formula (24 kcal/oz)	4.0-4.3
Preterm formula (24 kcal/oz)	3.6
Postdischarge formula (22 kcal/oz)	3.1
Term formula	2.1

ventilation, and postnatal steroid use compared with non-SGA infants. Furthermore, an increased risk of death or neurodevelopmental impairment was also observed in SGA infants (De Jesus et al, 2013). At 18 to 22 months' CA, significantly more children born SGA than AGA will fall below the 10th percentile for weight, length, and head circumference.

Postnatal Growth Failure: Incidence and Etiology

Postnatal growth failure is a common complication of extreme prematurity. Although only 17% of ELBW infants are SGA at the time of birth, by 36 weeks' postmenstrual age (PMA), the vast majority of these infants will have experienced suboptimal growth. In the most recent (2003 to 2007) cohort reported by the NICHD Neonatal Research Network, 79% of the VLBW infants had weight less than the 10th percentile at 36 weeks' PMA (Stoll et al, 2010). Observational studies have shown that differences in nutritional practices, particularly differences in protein intake, account for the largest difference in growth among premature infants.

EXERCISE 8

QUESTION

1. Which of the following neonatal factors are associated with postnatal growth failure in ELBW infants?
   a. Male gender
   b. Need for respiratory support at 28 days
   c. Necrotizing enterocolitis
   d. All of the above

ANSWER

1. **d.** The correct response is all of the above. While the risk of postnatal growth failure is inversely related to birth weight and gestational age, there are also many neonatal factors associated with poor in-hospital growth of premature infants, including duration of mechanical ventilation, use of postnatal steroids, severe intracranial hemorrhage/periventricular leukomalacia, and NEC. Many of the morbidities that are associated with slow growth velocity, such as NEC, also affect the provision of nutritional support and the utilization of nutrients supplied.

   There are a number of growth charts available for assessment of postnatal growth. Options to monitor growth include postnatal curves that utilize longitudinal data of actual growth over time and intrauterine curves that use cross-sectional data of fetal growth. The Fenton and Olsen

curves are commonly used intrauterine curves to monitor growth in many NICUs. The Olsen curves represent a large sample of infants from the United States and include weight, length, and head circumference-for-age curves from 23 to 41 weeks' gestation.

Consequences of Postnatal Growth Failure

CASE STUDY 8

EG is a former 25-week gestation female who is now 11 weeks of age. At the time of birth, her weight, length, and head circumference were all at the 50th percentile for gestational age. She regained her birth weight at 10 days of age and achieved full enteral feeds at 26 days of age. At 36 weeks' PMA, both her weight and weight–length ratio are less than the 10th percentile.

EXERCISE 9

QUESTION

1. Which of the following statements regarding her growth is true?
   a. Although EG is SGA at 36 weeks' CA, she will more than likely experience "catch-up" growth and be AGA when she is 18 months' CA.
   b. EG's growth has been suboptimal, but this will not impact her neurodevelopmental outcome.

ANSWER

1. Neither statement is true. In general, once an extremely premature infant regains birth weight, the rate of weight gain typically follows the rate of intrauterine growth. However, at 36 weeks' PMA, a significant percentage of these infants remain less than the 10th percentile according to the reference data for fetal growth. The obvious question is whether failure to grow in the NICU is associated with longer-term growth failure and/or neurodevelopmental deficits. At 18 to 22 months CA, 40% of ELBW infants still weigh less than the 10th percentile. As the rate of in-hospital weight gain of ELBW infants increases, the incidence of cerebral palsy, Bayley Mental Developmental Index (MDI) and Psychomotor Developmental Index (PDI) <70, abnormal neurologic exam, neurodevelopmental impairment, and need for rehospitalization decrease. The unacceptably high incidence of postnatal growth failure underscores the urgent need to improve outcomes and reduce complications in VLBW infants with optimal nutritional practices.

SPECIAL CONSIDERATIONS

Bronchopulmonary Dysplasia (BPD)

CASE STUDY 9

EM is a 580-gram, 24 weeks' gestation male who was delivered by precipitous vaginal birth to a mother with suspected chorioamnionitis. The infant was intubated and received three doses of surfactant. On day 2, owing to increasing respiratory support and $PaCO_2$ retention, the infant's ventilator strategy was changed from conventional mechanical ventilation to high frequency oscillatory ventilation. By 3 days of age, EM was receiving PN infusing at 160 mL/kg/day that provided 3.5 g/kg/day amino acids, 4 g/kg/day lipid, and 12.8 g/kg/day carbohydrate (total of 94 kcal/kg/day). On day 4, a patent ductus arteriosus (PDA) was suspected and the infant was fluid restricted to 130 mL/kg/day and given a course of indomethacin. The following day an echocardiogram (ECHO) revealed a closed PDA; however, there was no improvement in his respiratory status. As a result, EM was started on a trial of furosemide. Enteral nutrition was begun by day 7 and over the next few weeks his enteral feedings were slowly advanced to achieve full enteral nutrition at a restricted volume of 130 mL/kg/day of mother's milk and HMF (providing ≈104 kcal/kg/day). At 28 weeks of gestation, EM's weight is 760 grams, which according to the 2013 Fenton Growth Curve is at the 9th percentile for his PMA.

EXERCISE 10

QUESTION

1. An appropriate next step in managing EM's nutrition may include:
   a. Continue current management. EM's energy needs are being met and growth failure is inevitable in this critically ill neonate. EM just needs time for the nutritional supports to begin to demonstrate good growth.
   b. Increase total daily kilocalories by introducing high calorie preterm formula for 2 to 3 feedings per day.
   c. Check and correct any electrolyte abnormalities.
   d. Work with neonatal dietitian to increase fortification of mother's milk to supply 27 or 30 calories/ounce to provide a greater amount of total daily calories.

ANSWER

1. Statements **c** and **d** should be considered to optimize EM's nutrition and growth. The approach

to an infant with evolving BPD or established BPD is not unlike the approach or recommendations for the critically ill neonate. However, the clinician must be cognizant of the nutritional ramifications of bedside medical practices and nutritional strategies that are prescribed to infants with evolving severe lung disease. Such practices as fluid restriction, diuretic delivery, and provision of postnatal steroids will impact overall nutritional delivery and resultant growth.

During the first few days of life macronutrient recommendations can be achieved with PN. This was easily accomplished in EM's case; however, after reducing the total volume of PN with fluid restriction, the total kcals/kg/day delivered decreased from 94 to 85 and total daily carbohydrate fell from 12.8 g/kg to 10.4 g/kg. EM was already receiving the maximum recommended daily protein and lipid amounts; thus to provide more calories the glucose infusion rate (GIR) should be increased as long as euglycemia can be maintained. Simply returning the total carbohydrate delivery to 13 g/kg/day, similar to the amount the infant was receiving prior to fluid restriction, would return total energy to 94 kcal/kg/day. In this scenario, the GIR prior to fluid restriction was 8.3 mg/kg/min and following the fluid restriction and a compensatory increase in dextrose delivery the GIR was 9.0 mg/kg/min. Therefore, it is anticipated that the infant will tolerate these adjustments.

The approach to initiation and advancement of enteral feedings for an infant with persistent or evolving lung disease should not be different from other premature infants; although it is possible that critically ill infants may demonstrate a greater degree of enteral feeding intolerance, taking longer to achieve full enteral feedings. More important, however, is the knowledge that there are no established or proven contraindications to enteral feedings in the critically ill premature infant with lung disease.

Infants with severe lung disease require more energy to sustain growth compared to infants without BPD and may require up to 120 to 150+ kcal/kg/day in the chronic, convalescent phase. If the infant is fluid restricted and/or receiving diuretics or steroids, careful attention must be paid to closely following electrolyte values and growth. Electrolyte derangements should be corrected and protein and total energy needs must be met, especially during fluid restriction and diuretic therapy. At full enteral feedings using fortified breast milk with an estimated caloric density of 24 calories per ounce, EM is only receiving 104 kcal/kg/day; thus providing additional calories to meet his total energy needs is warranted.

Vitamin D and iron delivery should also parallel the recommendations for other preterm infants. For infants <1000 grams, providing 5000 international units of vitamin A (IM) three times per week for 4 weeks has been shown to reduce the incidence of BPD; however due to manufacturing limitations this option it is not currently available.

POSTDISCHARGE NUTRITION

Postdischarge Nutrition in the Breastfed Infant

The benefits of mother's own milk are well established. The use of human milk in the NICU and the need for fortification to meet the specific needs of the preterm infant during the NICU hospitalization have been discussed in a previous case.

In preparation for discharge from the NICU to home, continued fortification of breast milk still may be necessary and different strategies from those used as an in-patient need to be implemented because continued fortification with HMF as an out-patient is not currently an option. Commercial HMFs are typically recommended for in-hospital use only.

The decision to fortify breast milk after discharge is based on the growth patterns observed while in the NICU and whether the discharge weight is within acceptable range for the infant's PMA. It is recommended that intrauterine growth restricted infants and infants who developed extrauterine growth restriction while in the hospital be discharged with additional calories to optimize their growth potential. The number of additional calories to add should be individualized based on the infant's growth patterns. Evidence for using a postdischarge formula (PDF) versus a standard term formula is inconsistent. Furthermore, there are insufficient data to decide if calorie supplementation is best offered mixed in with expressed breast milk or provided as separate formula feedings. Ideally, strategies that minimize disruption of breast milk feedings should be implemented.

Changing the in-hospital diet to the discharge diet is recommended a few days prior to discharge to assess for feeding tolerance and growth, provide discharge teaching to the family, and to allow time to change the diet if the nutritional goals are not being met. Data are limited on the optimal duration of breast milk feedings specifically for the former preterm infant. Currently for term infants the AAP recommends exclusive breastfeeding for a minimum of 6 months. This may be a challenge for preterm infants because the duration of exclusive breastfeeding is less for preterm infants compared to term infants. Lactation support during the NICU hospitalization and extended into the postdischarge period may improve breastfeeding rates.

Postdischarge Nutrition in the Formula-Fed Infant

CASE STUDY 10

TE is a former 29-week premature infant whose clinical course was complicated by mild RDS. He received two doses of surfactant and was mechanically ventilated for less than 72 hours. He weaned from nasal cannula (NC) oxygen to room air at 32 weeks' corrected gestational age. He has had no episodes of apnea or bradycardia for 3 to 4 weeks. He is now 37 weeks' corrected gestational age and is taking all feeds orally with 24 calorie/ounce premature formula and has been demonstrating excellent weight gain. TE's mother is no longer expressing human milk. The social worker informs you that TE will qualify for assistance from the food assistance program.

EXERCISE 11

QUESTION

1. Which formula would be most appropriate for TE's discharge needs?
   a. Standard term formula (20 calorie/ounce)
   b. Standard premature formula (24 calorie/ounce)
   c. Elemental formula
   d. Transitional/postdischarge premature formula (22 calorie/ounce)

ANSWER

1. Either **a** or **d** may be acceptable depending on the infant's growth patterns and current weight for PMA. The evidence is mixed for routinely using a standard formula or an enriched transitional formula (also referred to as a "postdischarge formula" [PDF]) for all preterm infants after discharge. A recent Cochrane Systemic Review found no consistent evidence to recommend PDFs. In fact, the continued use of preterm formulas may achieve better growth outcomes; however, this is not currently an option in the United States. Theoretically, there may be some benefit to using an enriched, transitional care formula in the most vulnerable group of infants who were born growth restricted or were less than the 10th percentile for PMA in one or more anthropometric measures at discharge

(extrauterine growth restriction) as these may be indicators of acquired and ongoing nutritional deficits. Use of a PDF may help meet these additional nutritional needs. If a PDF is used it should continue until 40 to 52 weeks PMA for optimal nutrient exposure during a critical growth period. Preterm infants who are not less than the 10th percentile for PMA but require additional calories to maintain an appropriate growth velocity are likely able to meet their nutrient goals with a standard term formula.

Iron and Vitamin Supplementation

Preterm infants should be supplemented with 400 international units of vitamin D for the first year of life. For the formula-fed infant, supplementation should be continued until the daily intake of formula exceeds 1000 mL per day. Once this volume is exceeded the daily requirement for vitamin D can be achieved with formula alone. Supplementation for the breastfed infant should continue throughout the first year of life.

Without iron supplementation, the preterm infant is at risk for iron deficiency and its associated complications. Specific recommendations for iron deficiency vary among pediatric organizations. Although all experts agree that supplementation should continue throughout the first year of life, the recommendations differ, with the minimum being 2 mg/kg/day. This amount may be achieved with formula if the infant is predominantly formula fed; otherwise the infant should receive iron supplementation either as stand-alone iron drops or as part of a multivitamin preparation.

Although concerns have been raised regarding premature infants' increased risk of adult-onset hypertension and metabolic syndrome, this remains controversial and the risk is likely not uniform for all preterm infants. Those infants with intrauterine or extrauterine growth restriction may be at greater risk. In contrast, there is sufficient evidence to demonstrate a greater risk of poor long-term neurodevelopment than of later adult-onset disease secondary to poor growth during the first 18 months of life. Thus, unless new evidence suggests the contrary, growth during infancy should be closely monitored and supported to achieve growth patterns that are within appropriate ranges for the infant's PMA using standard growth curves.

Future studies are needed to more clearly define the nutrient requirements of preterm infants—both during their initial hospitalization and postdischarge thereafter in order to minimize complications and optimize growth and neurodevelopment. The optimal rate of catch-up growth for this high-risk population has yet to be defined.

Postdischarge Nutrition in the Late-Preterm Infant

CASE STUDY 11

GR is a 2550-gram, 35{2/7} weeks' gestation female born by vaginal delivery to a 32-year-old primiparous mother. At 48 hours of age, the infant is being assessed for discharge to home. She is now 2346 grams, down 8% from birth weight. GR has 2 to 3 wet diapers per 24 hours and she breastfeeds every 2 hours; however, her mother is unsure whether she is producing milk. The physical examination is entirely normal.

EXERCISE 12

QUESTION

1. Nutritional management and discharge planning should include:
   a. An outpatient visit within 48 hours after discharge by pediatrician
   b. Access to a lactation consultant
   c. Close monitoring of growth every 2 to 4 weeks
   d. Iron supplementation
   e. Vitamin D supplementation

ANSWER

1. All of the above should be arranged to optimize nutrition and minimize the readmission risk in this late-preterm infant. Much of our attention in nutrition and growth in the preterm infant has been focused on the lower gestational age infants (<34 weeks of gestation). However, increasing attention is being placed on evaluating the medical needs and outcomes of the late-preterm infant (34{0/7} to 36{6/7} weeks of gestation), a gestational age category representing more than 70% of all preterm infants. The data demonstrate that these infants, when compared to term infants, are at increased risk for transitional medical issues such as hypothermia, hypoglycemia, hyperbilirubinemia, respiratory distress, and poor feeding. Some of these issues may not be evident until after discharge, accounting for a high incidence of readmissions in this gestational age group. As a result, late-preterm infants warrant specific medical monitoring and nutritional practices that optimize their growth and outcomes.

When compared to term infants, late-preterm infants are at increased risk for altered brain development, particularly reduced gray matter volume. This may account for the increased risk of impaired long-term neurodevelopmental outcomes in this population compared to healthy, term infants. Although the link between poor postnatal growth and neurodevelopmental status has not been made in the late-preterm infant, it is a plausible hypothesis given the strength of this association in more infants with greater degrees of prematurity.

Appropriate establishment of enteral feedings in the late-preterm infant should be monitored closely during the early postnatal period. This can be done in the newborn nursery; however, some hospitals have established guidelines to perform such monitoring in the special care nursery or NICU, especially for infants less than 36 weeks' gestation. When these infants are monitored in the NICU there is a greater likelihood their mothers will initiate and sustain breastfeeding.

As with all newborns, breast milk is the preferred diet. It is critical to have appropriate lactation support for the mother because of an increased risk of transitional difficulties in establishing breastfeeding in this population both in the hospital and after discharge. Difficulties in feeding may not be evident until after discharge from the hospital and thus can possibly be missed unless there is regular contact with a health professional. Additionally, late-preterm infants are at risk for poor growth compared to term infants. If growth is not being adequately maintained, additional calorie supplementation should be considered.

If the family chooses formula as the primary diet, a standard term formula can be used. However, if growth is inadequate, an enriched transitional care formula providing 22 calories/ounce can be used as a nutritional strategy to optimize growth. Recommendations for iron and vitamin D for the late-preterm infant are the same as previously described above.

SUGGESTED READINGS

Adamkin DH: Postdischarge nutritional therapy, *J Perinatol* 26(Suppl 1):S27–S30, 2006. discussion S31–S33.

Aggett PJ, Agostoni C, Axelsson I, et al: Feeding preterm infants after hospital discharge: a commentary by the ESPGHAN Committee on Nutrition, *J Pediatr Gastroenterol Nutr* 42(5):596–603, 2006.

Agostoni C, Braegger C, Decsi T, et al: Breast-feeding: a commentary by the ESPGHAN Committee on Nutrition, *J Pediatr Gastroenterol Nutr* 49(1):112–125, 2009.

Agostoni C, Buonocore G, Carnielli VP, et al: Enteral nutrient supply for preterm infants: commentary from the European Society of Paediatric Gastroenterology, Hepatology and Nutrition Committee on Nutrition, *J Pediatr Gastroenterol Nutr* 50(1):85–91, 2010.

Allen J, Zwerdling R, Ehrenkranz R, et al: Statement on the care of the child with chronic lung disease of infancy and childhood, *Am J Respir Crit Care Med* 168(3):356–396, 2003.

American Academy of Pediatrics, Section on Breastfeeding: Breastfeeding and the use of human milk, *Pediatrics* 129(3): e827–e841, 2012.

Arslanoglu S, Moro GE, Ziegler EE, The WAPM Working Group on Nutrition: Optimization of human milk fortification for preterm infants: new concepts and recommendations, *J Perinat Med* 38(3):233–238, 2010.

Bernstein IM, Horbar JD, Badger GJ, Ohlsson A, Golan A: Morbidity and mortality among very-low-birth-weight neonates with intrauterine growth restriction. The Vermont Oxford Network, *Am J Obstet Gynecol* 182(1 Pt 1):198–206, 2000.

Biniwale MA, Ehrenkranz RA: The role of nutrition in the prevention and management of bronchopulmonary dysplasia, *Semin Perinatol* 30(4):200–208, 2006.

Bombell S, McGuire W: Early trophic feeding for very low birth weight infants, *Cochrane Database Syst Rev* (3):CD000504, 2009.

Callen J, Pinelli J: A review of the literature examining the benefits and challenges, incidence and duration, and barriers to breastfeeding in preterm infants, *Adv Neonatal Care* 5(2):72–88, 2005. quiz 89–92.

Carlson SJ: Current nutrition management of infants with chronic lung disease, *Nutr Clin Pract* 19(6):581–586, 2004.

Clyman R, Wickremasinghe A, Jhaveri N, et al: Enteral feeding during indomethacin and ibuprofen treatment of a patent ductus arteriosus, *J Pediatr* 163(2):406–411, 2013. e404.

Colaizy TT, Morriss FH: Positive effect of NICU admission on breastfeeding of preterm US infants in 2000 to 2003, *J Perinatol* 28(7):505–510, 2008.

Corpeleijn WE, Kouwenhoven SM, Paap MC, et al: Intake of own mother's milk during the first days of life is associated with decreased morbidity and mortality in very low birth weight infants during the first 60 days of life, *Neonatology* 102(4):276–281, 2012.

Dall'Agnola A, Beghini L: Post-discharge supplementation of vitamins and minerals for preterm neonates, *Early Hum Dev*. 85(10 Suppl):S27–S29, 2009.

De Jesus LC, Pappas A, Shankaran S, et al: Outcomes of small for gestational age infants born at <27 weeks' gestation, *J Pediatr* 163(1):55–60, 2013. e51-e53.

Ehrenkranz RA: Early nutritional support and outcomes in ELBW infants, *Early Hum Dev* 86(Suppl 1):21–25, 2010.

Ehrenkranz RA, Das A, Wrage LA, et al: Early nutrition mediates the influence of severity of illness on extremely LBW infants, *Pediatr Res* 69(6):522–529, 2011.

Fallon EM, Nehra D, Potemkin AK, et al: A.S.P.E.N. clinical guidelines: nutrition support of neonatal patients at risk for necrotizing enterocolitis, *JPEN J Parenter Enteral Nutr* 36(5):506–523, 2012.

Goyal NK, Fiks AG, Lorch SA: Persistence of underweight status among late preterm infants, *Arch Pediatr Adolesc Med* 166(5):424–430, 2012.

Greer FR: Post-discharge nutrition: what does the evidence support? *Semin Perinatol* 31(2):89–95, 2007.

Havranek T, Johanboeke P, Madramootoo C, Carver JD: Umbilical artery catheters do not affect intestinal blood flow responses to minimal enteral feedings, *J Perinatol* 27(6):375–379, 2007.

Hay Jr WW: Strategies for feeding the preterm infant, *Neonatology* 94(4):245–254, 2008.

Klingenberg C, Embleton ND, Jacobs SE, O'Connell LA, Kuschel CA: Enteral feeding practices in very preterm infants: an international survey, *Arch Dis Child Fetal Neonatal Ed* 97(1):F56–F61, 2012.

Kuschel CA, Harding JE: Multicomponent fortified human milk for promoting growth in preterm infants, *Cochrane Database Syst Rev* (1):CD000343, 2004.

Lapillonne A, Griffin IJ: Feeding preterm infants today for later metabolic and cardiovascular outcomes, *J Pediatr* 162(Suppl 3):S7–S16, 2013.

Lapillonne A, O'Connor DL, Wang D, Rigo J: Nutritional recommendations for the late-preterm infant and the preterm infant after hospital discharge, *J Pediatr* 162(Suppl 3):S90–S100, 2013.

Leaf A, Dorling J, Kempley S, et al: Early or delayed enteral feeding for preterm growth-restricted infants: a randomized trial, *Pediatrics* 129(5):e1260–e1268, 2012.

Morgan J, Bombell S, McGuire W: Early trophic feeding versus enteral fasting for very preterm or very low birth weight infants, *Cochrane Database Syst Rev* 3:CD000504, 2013.

Morgan J, Young L, McGuire W: Slow advancement of enteral feed volumes to prevent necrotising enterocolitis in very low birth weight infants, *Cochrane Database Syst Rev* 3:CD001241, 2013.

Morgan J, Young L, McGuire W: Delayed introduction of progressive enteral feeds to prevent necrotising enterocolitis in very low birth weight infants, *Cochrane Database Syst Rev* 5:CD001970, 2013.

Mosqueda E, Sapiegiene L, Glynn L, Wilson-Costello D, Weiss M: The early use of minimal enteral nutrition in extremely low birth weight newborns, *J Perinatol* 28(4):264–269, 2008.

Moya F, Sisk PM, Walsh KR, Berseth CL: A new liquid human milk fortifier and linear growth in preterm infants, *Pediatrics* 130(4):e928–e935, 2012.

Munakata S, Okada T, Okahashi A, et al: Gray matter volumetric MRI differences late-preterm and term infants, *Brain Dev.* 35(1):10–16, 2013.

Neu J: Gastrointestinal development and meeting the nutritional needs of premature infants, *Am J Clin Nutr* 85(2):629S–634S, 2007.

Niinikoski H, Stoll B, Guan X, et al: Onset of small intestinal atrophy is associated with reduced intestinal blood flow in TPN-fed neonatal piglets, *J Nutr* 134(6):1467–1474, 2004.

O'Connor DL, Jacobs J, Hall R, et al: Growth and development of premature infants fed predominantly human milk, predominantly premature infant formula, or a combination of human milk and premature formula, *J Pediatr Gastroenterol Nutr* 37(4):437–446, 2003.

O'Connor DL, Unger S: Post-discharge nutrition of the breastfed preterm infant, *Semin Fetal Neonatal Med*, May 21, 2013.

Patole SK, de Klerk N: Impact of standardised feeding regimens on incidence of neonatal necrotising enterocolitis: a systematic review and meta-analysis of observational studies, *Arch Dis Child Fetal Neonatal Ed* 90(2):F147–F151, 2005.

Premer DM, Georgieff MK: Nutrition for ill neonates, *Pediatr Rev.* 20(9):e56–e62, 1999.

Ramel SE, Demerath EW, Gray HL, Younge N, Boys C, Georgieff MK: The relationship of poor linear growth velocity with neonatal illness and two-year neurodevelopment in preterm infants, *Neonatology* 102(1):19–24, 2012.

Sallakh-Niknezhad A, Bashar-Hashemi F, Satarzadeh N, Ghojazadeh M, Sahnazarli G: Early versus late trophic feeding in very low birth weight preterm infants, *Iran J Pediatr* 22(2):171–176, 2012.

Schanler RJ, Lau C, Hurst NM, Smith EO: Randomized trial of donor human milk versus preterm formula as substitutes for mothers' own milk in the feeding of extremely premature infants, *Pediatrics* 116(2):400–406, 2005.

Senterre T, Rigo J: Optimizing early nutritional support based on recent recommendations in VLBW infants and postnatal growth restriction, *J Pediatr Gastroenterol Nutr* 53(5):536–542, 2011.

Sisk P, Quandt S, Parson N, Tucker J: Breast milk expression and maintenance in mothers of very low birth weight infants: supports and barriers, *J Hum Lact* 26(4):368–375, 2010.

Stoll BJ, Hansen N, Fanaroff AA, et al: Late-onset sepsis in very low birth weight neonates: the experience of the NICHD Neonatal Research Network, *Pediatrics* 110(2 Pt 1):285–291, 2002.

Stoll BJ, Hansen NI, Bell EF, et al: Neonatal outcomes of extremely preterm infants from the NICHD Neonatal Research Network, *Pediatrics* 126(3):443–456, 2010.

Sullivan S, Schanler RJ, Kim JH, et al: An exclusively human milk-based diet is associated with a lower rate of necrotizing enterocolitis than a diet of human milk and bovine milk-based products, *J Pediatr* 156(4):562–567, 2010. e561.

Tudehope DI: Human milk and the nutritional needs of preterm infants, *J Pediatr* 162(Suppl 3):S17–S25, 2013.

Tudehope DI, Page D, Gilroy M: Infant formulas for preterm infants: in-hospital and post-discharge, *J Paediatr Child Health* 48(9):768–776, 2012.

Tyson JE, Wright LL, Oh W, et al: Vitamin A supplementation for extremely-low-birth-weight infants. National Institute of Child Health and Human Development Neonatal Research Network, *N Engl J Med* 340(25):1962–1968, 1999.

Valentine CJ, Morrow G, Fernandez S, et al: Docosahexaenoic acid and amino acid contents in pasteurized donor milk are low for preterm infants, *J Pediatr* 157(6):906–910, 2010.

Vohr BR, Poindexter BB, Dusick AM, et al: Beneficial effects of breast milk in the neonatal intensive care unit on the developmental outcome of extremely low birth weight infants at 18 months of age, *Pediatrics* 118(1):e115–e123, 2006.

Vohr BR, Poindexter BB, Dusick AM, et al: Persistent beneficial effects of breast milk ingested in the neonatal intensive care unit on outcomes of extremely low birth weight infants at 30 months of age, *Pediatrics* 120(4):e953–e959, 2007.

Wagner CL, Greer FR: American Academy of Pediatrics Section on Breastfeeding, American Academy of Pediatrics Committee on Nutrition. Prevention of rickets and vitamin D deficiency in infants, children, and adolescents, *Pediatrics* 122(5):1142–1152, 2008.

Wemhoner A, Ortner D, Tschirch E, Strasak A, Rudiger M: Nutrition of preterm infants in relation to bronchopulmonary dysplasia, *BMC Pulm Med* 11:7, 2011.

Worrell LA, Thorp JW, Tucker R, et al: The effects of the introduction of a high-nutrient transitional formula on growth and development of very-low-birth-weight infants, *J Perinatol* 22(2):112–119, 2002.

Woythaler MA, McCormick MC, Smith VC: Late preterm infants have worse 24-month neurodevelopmental outcomes than term infants, *Pediatrics* 127(3):e622–e629, 2011.

Young L, Morgan J, McCormick FM, McGuire W: Nutrient-enriched formula versus standard term formula for preterm infants following hospital discharge, *Cochrane Database Syst Rev* 3:CD004696, 2012.

CHAPTER 8

ANEMIA

Robin Kjerstin Ohls, MD

The newborn period marks a time when red blood cell (RBC) indices vary remarkably from indices of children and adults. Determining the etiology of anemia in an infant becomes a challenge requiring sufficient knowledge of both normal and abnormal blood values. Anemia is defined as an inability of the circulating RBCs (erythrocytes) to meet the oxygen demands of the tissues. In this sense, many of the conditions affecting newborn erythropoiesis represent early alterations from "normal" values, but do not represent true anemia. The importance of discovering the etiology surrounding an infant's altered hemoglobin or other RBC parameter lies in potentially preventing a future anemic state, where the immediate action of an erythrocyte transfusion might be required. Thus it is critical to gather information beyond the hemoglobin or hematocrit in order to define a pathologic state.

Anemia can occur at various times in the neonatal period, and is the result of one (or a combination) of three main causes: hemorrhage of red cells (either internal or external to the body), increased destruction of red cells (hemolysis), or inadequate production of red cells. Severe anemia presenting in the first hours of life likely represents acute hemorrhage or significant hemolysis owing to isoimmunization. Anemia presenting after the first day or two of life may be because of multiple reasons, including new or continued blood loss, immune-mediated hemolysis, or nonimmune hemolysis. The task for the clinician is to decipher the evidence in order to prevent a further drop in red cell concentration, if possible, and to treat the anemia appropriately.

CASE STUDY 1

Baby girl A is a term appropriate for gestational age (AGA) infant born to a 30-year-old B+, AST negative, gravida 1 African American mother via spontaneous vaginal delivery at 39 weeks' gestation. The mother had prolonged rupture of membranes and received intrapartum antibiotics. Birth weight was 3210 grams; Apgar scores were 9 and 9 at 1 and 5 minutes, respectively. A screening complete blood count (CBC) was obtained in the newborn nursery, which showed hematocrit 44%, hemoglobin 14.9 g/dL, RBC 4.79×10^6/mL, mean corpuscular volume (MCV) 92 fL, mean corpuscular hemoglobin (MCH) 31 pg, mean corpuscular hemoglobin concentration (MCHC) 33.8 g/dL, and red cell distribution width (RDW) 12.8%. The peripheral smear was remarkable for mild poikilocytosis.

EXERCISE 1

QUESTIONS

1. Which of the infant's RBC indices are abnormal, if any?

2. Which of the following would be helpful in working up the infant's hematologic abnormalities?
   a. Information on maternal iron intake during pregnancy
   b. Detailed family history
   c. Maternal Kleihauer-Betke (KB) test
   d. Neonatal blood type and direct Coombs test
   e. Neonatal hemoglobin electrophoresis

ANSWERS

1. The infant has low mean corpuscular volume (MCV), a low mean corpuscular hemoglobin (MCH), and hemoglobin/hematocrit that is greater than 1 standard deviation below the average for a term infant.

2. **b** and **c**. The differential of a low MCV in the newborn period includes iron deficiency secondary to fetal maternal hemorrhage or into a twin (not applicable in this case), or alpha thalassemia trait. Obtaining detailed parent and family information regarding a history of anemia, transfusions, or abnormal RBC indices in either parent or first-degree relative is helpful in identifying inherited anemias such as red cell membrane defects, red cell enzyme defects, or alpha thalassemia. Neonatal hemoglobin electrophoresis is a part of newborn screening, but would not be helpful in identifying alpha thalassemia trait in the infant.

CASE STUDY 1 (continued)

A maternal KB test was negative. Further informa-tion from the family revealed a history of microcytic anemia in the maternal grandmother, two maternal aunts, and in the mother herself. The father was also of African American descent, but did not know of red cell abnormalities in his family, and was never evaluated himself. A CBC was sent on the father, which revealed an MCV of 72 fL and MCH of 26 pg. A presumptive diagnosis of alpha thalassemia trait was made, and the family was referred to a pediat-ric hematologist following discharge.

FETAL ERYTHROPOIESIS AND ADAPTATION TO EXTRAUTERINE LIFE

Erythropoiesis *in utero* is controlled by ery-throid growth factors produced solely by the fetus. Erythropoietin (Epo) is the primary regu-lator of erythropoiesis in adults and appears to be the controlling factor for fetal erythropoi-esis. Epo does not cross the placenta in humans, and stimulation of maternal Epo production does not result in stimulation of fetal red cell production.

Epo concentrations in the fetus gradually increase until birth. Elevated Epo concentra-tions in fetal blood and/or amniotic fluid may indicate fetal hypoxia; and although Epo may have a protective role for some fetal cells, such as neurons, placental, hepatic, and intestinal villous cells, it might also be a marker for poor neurodevelopmental outcome on the basis of severe or chronic hypoxia. Serum Epo concen-trations at birth normally range 5 to 100 mU/mL. Epo concentrations range in healthy adults range from 0 to 25 mU/mL, whereas serum Epo

concentrations in anemic, nonuremic adults range from 300 to 400 mU/mL.

RED BLOOD CELL INDICES IN THE FETUS AND NEONATE

Red Blood Cell Concentrations and Hematocrit

RBC indices vary during gestation, and continue to do so through the first year of life. Table 8-1 shows changes in red cell indices during ges-tation. The RBC value generally reflects the hemoglobin and hematocrit, and is useful in determining the absolute reticulocyte count, or ARC (RBC × % retics = ARC).

In parallel with increasing RBC concentra-tions, hematocrits increase from 30% to 40% during the second trimester, and continue to increase to term values over the latter part of the third trimester (Figure 8-1, *A*). Term hematocrits range from 50% to 63%, with some variability caused by delayed clamping of the umbilical cord (Jopling et al., 2009). Values are also dependent on the sampling site. Capillary hematocrits may measure 9 to 12 hematocrit points higher than venous or arterial samples.

Hemoglobin

Hemoglobin concentrations gradually rise during gestation (Figure 8-1, *B*). At 10 weeks' gestation, the average hemoglobin is approxi-mately 9 g/dL. Hemoglobin concentrations continue to increase during gestation, are rel-atively constant over the last 6 to 8 weeks of gestation, and at term are approximately 16 to 17 g/dL. At birth there may be a 1 to 2 g/dL rise in hemoglobin as a result of transfusion

TABLE 8-1	**Red Blood Cell Values During Gestation**								
Age (weeks)	Hemoglo-bin (g/dL)	Hema-tocrit (%)	RBCs (× 10⁶/μL)	Mean Cell Volume (fL)	Mean Cor-puscular Hemoglo-bin (pg)	Mean Corpuscular Hemoglobin Concentra-tion (g/dL)	Nucleated RBCs (% of RBCs)	Reticu-locytes (%)	Diameter (microns)
12	8.0-10.0	33	1.5	180	60	34	5.0-8.0	40	10.5
16	10.0	35	2.0	140	45	33	2.0-4.0	10-25	9.5
20	11.0	37	2.5	135	44	33	1.0	10-20	9
24	14.0	40	3.5	128	38	31	1.0	5-10	8.8
28	14.5	45	4.0	120	40	31	0.5	5-10	8.7
34	15.0	47	4.4	118	38	32	0.2	3-10	8.3

Modified from Oski FA: Normal blood values in the newborn period. In Oski FA, Naiman JL, editors: Hematologic prob-lems in the newborn, *3rd ed, Philadelphia, PA, 1982, Saunders, p 4.*

of placental blood at delivery. An increase in hemoglobin by 2 hours of postnatal life occurs in most infants, owing to a decrease in plasma volume.

In term infants, improved oxygenation after birth results in significantly decreased erythrocyte production, reflecting a natural adaptation to the extrauterine environment. The continued fall in hemoglobin concentration over the next several weeks (Figure 8-2, *B*) results from: (1) decreased red cell production; (2) a shortened red cell life span of the fetal erythrocyte; and (3) plasma dilution and an increase in blood volume related to growth. The nadir of hemoglobin concentration in full-term infants is seen at approximately 4 to 8 weeks with an average hemoglobin concentration of 11.2 g/dL, and a lower range of normal of 9 g/dL.

This nadir is called *physiologic anemia*. By 6 months the average term infant has a hemoglobin concentration of 12.1 g/dL. Table 8-2 shows changes in red cell indices over the first 6 months of life.

The average decline in the hemoglobin of preterm infants weighing less than 1500 grams is significantly different from that of term infants (Figure 8-2, *D*). This is due in part to phlebotomy losses that often occur, as well as the effects of transfusions on endogenous erythropoiesis. Such infants reach a nadir of hemoglobin that averages 8 g/dL at 4 to 8 weeks of age. Infants born small for gestational age, infants of diabetic mothers, infants of mothers who smoke, and infants born at higher altitudes tend to have a higher hemoglobin concentration at birth.

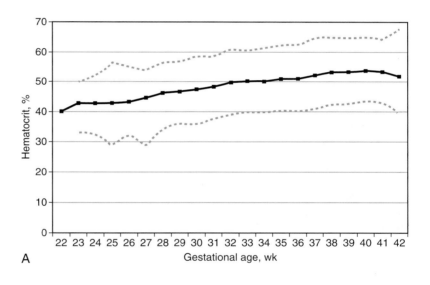

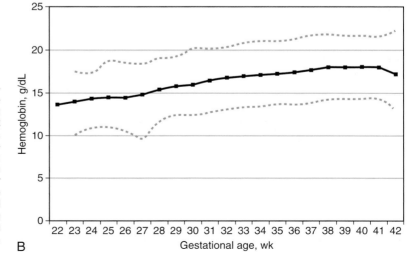

FIGURE 8-1 ■ Changes in hematocrit (*upper panel*) and hemoglobin (*lower panel*) following premature delivery from 22 weeks' gestation through term. The lines represent the 5th percentile, the mean, and the 95th percentile reference range. (From Jopling J, Henry E, Wiedmeier SE, Christensen RD: Reference ranges for hematocrit and blood hemoglobin concentration during the neonatal period: data from a multihospital healthcare system, *Pediatrics* 123:e333-337, 2000.)

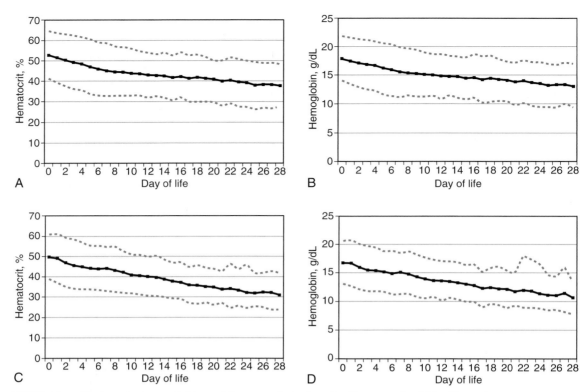

FIGURE 8-2 ■ **Changes in hemoglobin and hematocrit during the first month of life.** The reference ranges are shown for hematocrit (**A** and **C**) (*N* = 41,957 patients) and blood hemoglobin (**B** and **D**) (*N* = 39,559 patients) during the 28 days after birth. Values were divided into 2 groups (**A/B** and **C/D**) on the basis of gestational age at delivery. Patients were excluded when their diagnosis included abruption, placenta previa, or fetal anemia or when a blood transfusion was given. Analysis was not possible for patients <29 weeks' gestation because virtually all of these had repeated phlebotomy and erythrocyte transfusions. **A** and **B**, Late preterm and term infants (35 to 42 weeks' gestation). **C** and **D**, Preterm infants (29 to 34 weeks' gestation). (From Jopling J, Henry E, Wiedmeier SE, Christensen RD: Reference ranges for hematocrit and blood hemoglobin concentration during the neonatal period: data from a multi-hospital healthcare system. *Pediatrics* 123:e333-337, 2009.)

TABLE 8-2　Postnatal Changes in RBC Values over 6 Months

RBC Parameters	Days			Weeks			Months		
	1	3	7	2	4	2	3	4	6
Hemoglobin (g/dL)									
Mean	19.4	18.6	18.7	17.6	13.9	11.2	11.4	12	12.1
±2 SD	17.2	16.5	16.5	13.9	10.6	9.3	9.5	10.7	10.4
(N)	(78)	(66)	(78)	(275)	(272)	(271)	(73)	(123)	(114)
Mean Copuscular Volume (fL)									
$\bar{x}$	114	110	108	106	101	92	88	84	77
±2 SD	101-128	104-116	102-114	88-125	90-112	83-107	78-98	74-95	67-87
(N)	(59)	(47)	(66)	(232)	(240)	(241)	(60)	(123)	(114)
Mean Corpuscular Hemoglobin (pg)									
$\bar{x}$	36.6	36.7	36.2	33.6	32.5	30.4	30.4	28.1	26.4
(N)	(59)	(47)	(66)	(232)	(240)	(241)	(60)	(123)	(114)
Mean Corpuscular Hemoglobin Concentration (g/dL)									
$\bar{x}$	33.0	33.1	33.9	31.7	32.1	32.0	34.6	33.3	34.2
(N)	(78)	(66)	(78)	(275)	(272)	(271)	(73)	(123)	(114)

Modified from Guest GM, Brown EW: Erythrocytes and hemoglobin of the blood in infancy and childhood. III. Factors in variability, statistical studies, Am J Dis Child 93:486-509, 1957; Saarinen UM, Siimes MA: Developmental changes in red blood cell counts and indices of infants after exclusion of iron deficiency by laboratory criteria and continuous iron supplementation, J Pediatr 92:412-416, 1978; Matoth Y, Zaizov R, Varsano I: Postnatal changes in some red cell parameters, Acta Paediatr Scand 60:317-323, 1971.

Mean Corpuscular Volume

The size of the red cell gradually decreases during development. The mean corpuscular volume (MCV) is greater than 180 fL in the embryo, falls to 130 to 140 fL by midgestation, and decreases to 115 fL by the end of pregnancy (MCV values below the fifth percentile are seen in neonates with α-thalassemia trait or hereditary spherocytosis. A low MCV at birth caused by fetal iron deficiency is less common, but this can occur with chronic fetomaternal hemorrhage (FMH) or twin-to-twin transfusion syndrome. By 1 year of age, the MCV reaches an average of 82 fL. Figure 8-3, *A* demonstrates the changes in MCV observed from 22 through 42 weeks' gestation. The MCV of preterm infants declines quickly after birth, and the postpartum changes in MCV appear to be related to chronologic age rather than postconceptional age.

Mean Corpuscular Hemoglobin Concentration

The mean corpuscular hemoglobin concentration (MCHC) remains relatively constant from approximately 32 weeks' gestation through adulthood, averaging 33 to 34 g/dL (Figure 8-3, *B*). Increases in MCHC reflect distortions of RBC volume that cause compression of hemoglobin into a smaller space. Disorders such as hereditary spherocytosis, ABO incompatibility, or microangiopathic hemolytic anemia will show elevated MCHCs, as the surface area of the RBC decreases while the hemoglobin concentration remains stable.

Mean Corpuscular Hemoglobin

The mean corpuscular hemoglobin (MCH) reflects the average amount of hemoglobin in circulating erythrocytes, measured in pg/cell (Figure 8-3, *C*), and ranges 34 to 36 pg around the time of delivery.

Red Cell Distribution Width

The red cell distribution width (RDW) reflects the variation in RBC size. A more heterogeneous red cell population will be reflected by a "wider" (greater) RDW. Because immature cells are larger than older red cells, an infant with active erythropoiesis will have an elevated RDW.

Reticulocyte Count

Active erythropoiesis occurs *in utero*, and reticulocyte counts are elevated at birth. Infants born at term generally have reticulocyte counts in the range of 3% to 7% (ARC 150,000 to 400,000/μL). Infants born prematurely will have higher reticulocyte counts, generally between 6% and 10%. Erythropoiesis decreases significantly after birth, such that the reticulocyte count drops to 1% by 1 week of life. Reticulocyte counts will increase following the physiologic nadir (around 4 to 8 weeks of life) when erythropoiesis becomes active.

Shape, Deformability, and Life Span

Just as there is much variation in the size of newborn RBCs, there is much variation in shape. Irregularly shaped cells are present in much greater numbers in the peripheral blood of newborn infants as compared with those of adults. Target cells, acanthocytes, puckered immature erythrocytes, stomatocytes, siderocytes, and other irregular projections may normally be found.

Red cell deformability is principally governed by three factors: the surface-area/volume relationship of the RBC, the viscosity of the cytoplasm of the cell, and intrinsic red cell membrane rigidity. Red cell deformability appears to be an important determinant of red cell life span *in vivo*. The removal of an RBC from the circulation is thought to be a consequence of declining deformability, making the red cell susceptible to sequestration in the spleen and other organs where it must negotiate extraordinarily narrow passages. In addition, red cell deformability directly influences blood flow in the peripheral circulation. Finally, whole blood viscosity is affected by red cell deformability, which in turn affects peripheral vascular resistance and cardiac workload.

The densest neonatal RBCs (representing the oldest cells in the circulation) lose more volume than adult RBCs, have a higher MCHC, and are less deformable than the oldest RBCs seen in adults. Red cells from newborns have a shorter red cell survival than red cells from children and adults. The life span of term neonatal red cells is estimated to be 60 to 80 days with use of the ^{51}Cr method and 45 to 70 days using [59]Fe. Fetal studies using [^{14}C] cyanate-labeled red cells in sheep revealed an increase in mean red cell life span from 35 to 107 days as the fetal age increased from 97 days (midgestation) to 136 days (term).

HEMORRHAGE

Hemorrhage is a common cause of anemia in neonates. Blood loss can occur prior to birth or during delivery, can be associated with maternal hemorrhage or obstetrical accidents, or can be caused by internal hemorrhage or recurrent phlebotomy losses after birth. Maternal factors that increase the incidence of hemorrhage include

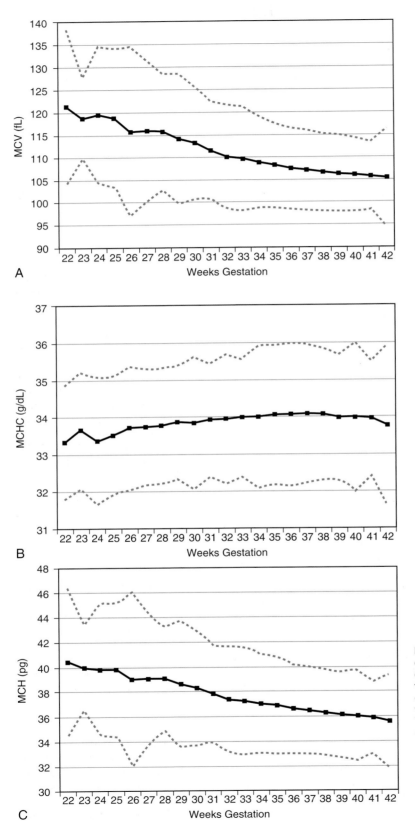

FIGURE 8-3 ■ **Erythrocyte mean corpuscular volume (MCV), mean corpuscular hemoglobin concentration (MCHC), and mean corpuscular hemoglobin (MCH) from 22 weeks' gestation through term.** The lines represent the 5th percentile, the mean, and the 95th percentile reference range. (From Christensen RD, Jopling J, Henry E, Wiedmeier SE: The erythrocyte indices of neonates, defined using data from over 12,000 patients in a multihospital healthcare system, *J Perinatol* 28:24-28, 2008.)

BOX 8-1 | Causes of Hemorrhage in the Perinatal Period

A. Prior to delivery
1. Chronic and/or acute twin-to-twin transfusion syndrome
2. Chronic and/or acute fetal-maternal hemorrhage
3. Hemorrhage into amniotic fluid following periumbilical blood sampling (PUBS)
4. Traumatic amniocentesis
5. Maternal trauma
6. Trauma following external cephalic version

B. During delivery
1. Placental abruption
2. Placenta previa
3. Vasa previa
4. Trauma or incision of placenta during cesarean section

5. Ruptured normal or abnormal (varices, aneurysms) umbilical cord
6. Cord or placental hematoma
7. Velamentous insertion of the cord
8. Nuchal cord

C. During or following delivery
1. Subgaleal hemorrhage
2. Cephalohematoma
3. Intraventricular/intracranial hemorrhage (prematurity, trauma, isoimmune thrombocytopenia)
4. Hemorrhage associated with DIC/sepsis
5. Organ trauma (liver, spleen, adrenal, renal)
6. Pulmonary hemorrhage
7. Iatrogenic blood loss (phlebotomy, central line accidents, arterial line accidents)

third trimester bleeding with placenta previa, placental abruption, vasa previa, emergency cesarean section, twin gestation, amniocentesis, and percutaneous umbilical blood sampling (PUBs).

The clinical manifestations of hemorrhage at birth depend on the extent and duration of blood loss. When significant acute blood loss has occurred, the infant will be limp, pale, unresponsive, and require immediate volume expansion and (likely) a rapid transfusion. Although the hemoglobin may be in the normal range initially, or may be low, it will fall within hours after birth. Internal hemorrhage should be suspected when a 24- to 48-hour newborn has evidence of hypovolemic shock without signs of external blood loss.

As many as one fourth of newborns admitted to neonatal intensive care units (NICUs) experience a decrease in their red cell volume owing to hemorrhage. Hemorrhagic anemia in the newborn period can be divided into three general categories (Box 8-1): prenatal hemorrhage from the fetus into the maternal circulation or into a twin; hemorrhage caused by obstetrical accidents of the placenta or cord around the time of delivery; and hemorrhage caused by trauma, sepsis/disseminated intravascular coagulation (DIC), or phlebotomy loss. Severe hemorrhage will produce pallor and shock, and should be recognized immediately in order to prevent significant organ damage or death.

BLOOD VOLUME

The placenta and umbilical cord contain 75 to 125 mL of blood at term, or approximately a quarter to a third of the fetal blood volume. Umbilical arteries constrict shortly after birth,

but the umbilical vein remains dilated. The neonatal blood volume can be 50% higher in infants who experience delayed cord clamping (or cord milking) than in infants who have their cord clamped immediately after birth.

Preterm infants have slightly larger blood volumes (89 to 105 mL/kg) owing to an increased plasma volume. At 30 weeks' gestation, half of the approximately 120 mL/kg total blood volume of the fetoplacental circulation is in the fetus. Preterm infants commonly experience rapid cord clamping resulting in a decreased blood volume. Higher hematocrit, decreased transfusion requirements, and decreased incidence of intracranial hemorrhage (ICH) were reported in studies randomizing infants to delayed cord clamping or cord milking (stripping the umbilical cord from the placenta toward the infant two to four times before clamping the cord).

CASE STUDY 2

Baby boy B is a term newborn male born to a 22-year-old gravida 2 Hispanic mother. Maternal labs: blood type AB positive, antibody screen negative, and other serologies negative. Delivery was via a repeat cesarean section that occurred at 39 weeks' gestation. The infant required "blow-by" oxygen and positive pressure ventilation for 30 seconds before spontaneous respirations occurred. Apgar scores were 6 at 1 minute and 7 at 5 minutes. The birth weight was 2710 grams. On physical examination at 2 hours of age, heart rate was 178 bpm, respiratory rate 64, temperature 36.9° C, and blood pressure 51/31 mmHg. The infant was pale and in moderate respiratory distress. Oxygen saturation was 98% on 35% oxygen by oxyhood. The cardiac examination revealed a capillary refill of 3 to 4 seconds, a 2/6 systolic ejection murmur over the lower left sternal border, a liver edge 3.5 cm below the right costal margin, and decreased pulses. The rest of the physical examination was normal.

EXERCISE 2

QUESTIONS

1. Which of the following diagnoses would be consistent with this clinical picture?
   a. Perinatal hypoxic injury
   b. Septic shock
   c. Acute hemorrhage
   d. Congenital heart disease
   e. All of the above

2. What is the first step in management of this infant?
   a. Transfuse with 10 mL/kg type O negative packed RBCs.
   b. Obtain a blood gas analysis for acid–base and ventilation status.
   c. Intubate and provide 100% oxygen.
   d. Administer prostaglandins.
   e. Begin phototherapy.

ANSWERS

1. **e**. Any of these diagnoses may present in similar fashion in the immediate newborn period as a pale infant with respiratory distress.

2. **b**. Determining the infant's ability to ventilate and the adequacy of overall circulation via acid–base status will be the most helpful of these choices in order to rapidly determine appropriate care. An immediate transfusion is not indicated without knowing the infant's circulatory status. Intubation may be required if the infant is not ventilating adequately. Administering prostaglandins prior to other testing is not recommended. Phototherapy is not indicated at this time until a bilirubin determination is made or knowledge of hemolytic disease is obtained.

CASE STUDY 2 (continued)

A spun hematocrit was 16% and the CBC demonstrated hematocrit 14.8%, hemoglobin 5.0 g/dL, MCV 94 fL, MCHC 32 g/dL, and RDW 21%. The capillary blood gas shows the following: pH 7.10, PCO_2 32 mmHg, PO_2 41 mmHg, bicarbonate 8, and base deficit 16. Further maternal information was gathered. The mother noted decreased fetal movement during the last 2 days prior to birth. External monitoring prior to cesarean section showed a sinusoidal pattern. There was no evidence of abruption or trauma to the placenta or cord.

EXERCISE 3

QUESTION

1. Which of the following maternal laboratory tests would be helpful?
   a. Repeat antibody screen
   b. Maternal CBC and RBC indices
   c. KB test
   d. Group B *Streptococcus* (GBS) status
   e. Maternal liver function tests

ANSWER

1. **c**. A KB test to search for evidence of fetal hemorrhage into the maternal circulation would be the most helpful in determining the cause of this infant's anemia. In this case, the KB test was positive for fetal cells in the maternal circulation. This infant's anemia was the result of chronic, severe FMH. Calculations to determine the extent of FMH are provided in the next section.

FETOMATERNAL HEMORRHAGE

Fetal contamination of the maternal circulation can occur prior to delivery. Up to 75% of pregnancies are associated with less than 1 mL of fetomaternal hemorrhage (FMH), whereas one pregnancy in 400 is associated with a fetal transplacental bleed of 30 mL or greater, and one pregnancy in 2000 is associated with a fetal transplacental hemorrhage of 100 mL or more. Severe FMH occurs in one in 1000 deliveries, and has been associated with decreased fetal movements and a fetal sinusoidal heart rate (SHR) pattern (Kosasa et al., 1993).

Following FMH, the overall risk of Rh immunization occurring in an Rh-incompatible pregnancy is 16% if the fetus is Rh positive, ABO compatible with its mother. This risk decreases to 1.5% if the fetus is Rh positive, ABO incompatible. Fetal transfer of cells to the mother occurs during abortions as well (about a 2% incidence of such transfer with spontaneous abortion and a 4% to 5% rate if induced).

Because fetal hemoglobin is resistant to acid-elution, cells containing fetal hemoglobin (Hgb F) can be distinguished from cells containing adult hemoglobin (HGB A). The Kleihauer Betke (KB) stain of peripheral maternal blood utilizes this characteristic of fetal hemoglobin to detect fetal cells in the maternal circulation. Peripheral smears of maternal blood stained in this fashion will reveal "ghost-like" cells of maternal origin (previously containing adult hemoglobin), and pink fetal cells, still containing fetal hemoglobin, which have resisted elution (Figure 8-4). Results from mothers with increased fetal hemoglobin synthesis (i.e., sickle cell disease, thalassemia, and hereditary persistence of fetal hemoglobin) are less reliable. Diagnosis of FMH may also be missed with ABO incompatibility, as fetal cells are rapidly cleared from the maternal circulation by maternal anti-A or anti-B antibodies. An example of how to estimate fetal blood loss based on the results of a KB stain follows:

- Information to gather: maternal weight, maternal hematocrit, infant weight, KB stain results
- Assume: average maternal blood volume is 75 mL/kg at term (normal adult blood volume = 60 mL/kg); average fetal-placental blood volume is 120 mL/kg at term
- **Example:** A mother's KB stain result is reported as 2%. This means that 2% of the red cells on the mother's peripheral smear

contain HgbF. If the mother weighs 75 kg and her hematocrit is 32%, then her red cell volume can be calculated as:

75 kg (weight) × 0.32 (hematocrit) × 75 mL/kg (blood volume) = 1800 mL (red cell volume)

- If 2% of this red cell volume is fetal, then the estimated fetal red cell mass transferred into the maternal circulation is 1800 mL × 0.02 = 36 mL.
- If the infant weighs 3 kg and had a prehemorrhage hematocrit of 45%, then the fetoplacental red cell volume can be calculated as 3 kg × 0.45 × 120 mL/kg = 162 mL.
- The infant would therefore have hemorrhaged 36 of 162 mL, or 22%, of its red cell volume into the maternal circulation. This would be considered a mild to moderate FMH. The infant might exhibit signs of volume loss if the hemorrhage occurred acutely.

Infants in whom a significant acute hemorrhage is suspected need rapid evaluation and treatment. The infant with massive hemorrhage will present with pallor and tachypnea, but may not have an oxygen requirement. Hemoglobin concentrations can be extremely low at birth, between 4 and 6 grams/dL. A significant metabolic acidosis is often present as a result of hypoperfusion. Other causes of pallor in the newborn period do occur, and can be ruled out once the infant is stable. Infants with asphyxia and infants with chronic anemia owing to hemolysis can also present with pallor. These diagnoses can be distinguished from acute hemorrhage based on differences in clinical signs and symptoms (Table 8-3).

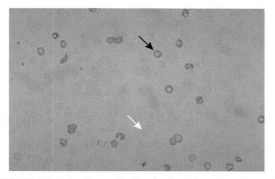

FIGURE 8-4 ■ Kleihaur Betke (KB) stain of maternal blood. Dark cells (*upper arrow*) contain fetal hemoglobin, whereas clear or "ghost" cells (*lower arrow*) contain adult hemoglobin.

TABLE 8-3 Differential Diagnosis of the Pale Newborn

Affected Organ System	Severe Acute Hemorrhage	Hemolysis	Asphyxia
Neurologic	Normal or hyper-alert/hyper-irritable ("catecholamine response")	Normal	Abnormal transition period, hypotonic, decreased arousal state, seizures in first days of life
Respiratory	Tachypnea, minimal or no O₂ requirement	Normal	Respiratory distress, O₂ requirement
Cardiovascular	Tachycardia, hypotension	May vary from normal to presence of congestive heart failure and hydrops, depending on degree of anemia	Normal to bradycardia
Hematologic	Drop in hematocrit/hemoglobin	Anemic from birth Hepatosplenomegaly Jaundice Positive Coombs test	Hematocrit/hemoglobin remains stable over time; may develop thrombocytopenia and DIC from hypoxic injury to marrow

TWIN-TO-TWIN TRANSFUSION SYNDROME

Twin-to-twin transfusion syndrome (TTS) is a complication of monochorionic twin gestations, occurring in 5% to 30% of these pregnancies. The perinatal mortality rate can be as high as 70% to 100%, depending on severity and timing of presentation.

Acute TTS generally results in twins of similar size, but with hemoglobin concentrations that vary by more than 5 grams/dL. In the chronic form of TTS, one twin becomes progressively anemic and growth retarded, whereas the recipient twin becomes polycythemic, macrosomic, and sometimes hypertensive. Both infants can develop hydrops fetalis; the donor twin becomes hydropic from profound anemia, whereas the recipient twin becomes hydropic from congestive heart failure and hypervolemia. Because of significant differences in blood volume, renal blood flow, and urine output, the donor twin experiences oligohydramnios, whereas the recipient twin experiences polyhydramnios.

The diagnosis of chronic TTS can be made by serial prenatal ultrasounds measuring cardiomegaly, discordant amniotic fluid production, fetal growth discrepancy of greater than 20%, and by measuring hemoglobin differences of greater than 5 g/dL between infants. After birth the donor twin often requires transfusions and can also experience neutropenia, hydrops from severe anemia, growth restriction, congestive heart failure, and hypoglycemia. The recipient twin is often sicker, and can suffer from hypertrophic cardiomyopathy, congestive heart failure, polycythemia, hyperviscosity, respiratory difficulties, hypocalcemia, and hypoglycemia. The risk of antenatally acquired neurologic cerebral lesions is 20% to 30% in both twins, and the incidence of neurologic morbidities following the intrauterine death of one of the fetuses averages 20% to 25%. Morbidities include multiple cerebral infarctions, hypoperfusion syndromes from hypotension, and periventricular leukomalacia. Long-term neurologic follow up is indicated for all TTS survivors.

Current evidence suggests the best treatment for significant TTS involves laser ablation of bridging vessels. Alternative treatments consist of close monitoring, reduction amniocenteses to decrease uterine stretch and prolong the pregnancy, selective feticide, or septostomy. A randomized study comparing laser ablation with amnioreduction in mothers randomized before 26 weeks' gestation was concluded early because of a significant benefit in the laser group (Senat et al., 2004). Infants in the laser group had a 76% survival rate of at least one twin at 28 days, compared to 56% survival in the amnioreduction group. Infants in the laser group had a lower incidence of cystic periventricular leukomalacia (6% vs. 14%, $p = 0.02$) and were more likely to be free of neurologic complications at 6 months of age (52% vs. 31%, $p = 0.003$). Randomized trials continue to identify timing of laser therapy for TTS in order to achieve improved outcomes for both twins.

OBSTETRIC COMPLICATIONS

Obstetric complications can be a significant source of blood loss, and include placenta previa and placental abruption, incision or tearing of the placenta during cesarean section, and cord avulsion of normal or abnormal umbilical cords. In addition, newborns may experience significant blood loss back into the placenta (fetoplacental hemorrhage). Moreover, placental anomalies including multilobed placenta and placental chorioangiomas may be a source of hemorrhage during the perinatal period.

Placenta Abruption and Placenta Previa

Placental abruption involves premature separation of the placenta from the uterus, and occurs in 3 to 6 per 1000 live births. Severe fetal growth restriction, prolonged rupture of membranes, chorioamnionitis, hypertension (chronic or pregnancy-induced), cigarette smoking, advanced maternal age, and male fetal gender are potential risk factors for placental abruption. The incidence increases with decreasing gestation, and mortality ranges 0.8 to 2 per 1000 births, which equates to 15% to 20% of deliveries in which significant abruption occurs.

Placenta previa occurs when part or all of the placenta overlies the cervical os. Women with a history of a previous cesarean birth and increased parity are at increased risk of having a pregnancy complicated by placenta previa. In addition, current cigarette smoking is associated with a 2- to 4-fold increased risk of placenta previa.

The need for postnatal transfusions in the infant is generally associated with the combined volume of maternal and fetal hemorrhage. Whenever there is evidence of placental abruption, placenta previa, or unusual vaginal bleeding, the infant's hemoglobin should be measured at birth and again at 12 to 24 hours. A KB stain should also be performed on maternal blood to determine if fetal-maternal hemorrhage occurred. Monitoring mothers with a history of second or third trimester bleeding with Doppler flow ultrasound may decrease the incidence of anemia and fetal loss in newborns, by anticipating fetal hemorrhage associated with placental abnormalities.

Fetoplacental Hemorrhage

Blood loss into the placenta is a common etiology for a low hematocrit in neonates. As mentioned previously, a large residual volume of blood remains in the placenta, and blood primarily flows in the direction of gravity after birth. Fetoplacental blood flow can occur when the infant is held above the placenta after birth, and for this reason infants born by cesarean section have smaller blood volumes than those born vaginally. In addition, infants can lose 10% to 20% of their total blood volume when born with a tight nuchal cord. Tight nuchal cords allow blood to be pumped through umbilical arteries while constricting flow through the umbilical vein.

CASE STUDY 3

Baby boy M is a term, large for gestation male born to a 32-year-old gravida 1 white mother with gestational diabetes. The delivery required vacuum assistance for the last 15 minutes prior to birth. The infant was pale and gasping at birth, and had a significant caput succedaneum. He received routine drying, stimulation, and some "blow-by" oxygen. Apgar scores were 7 at 1 minute and 8 at 5 minutes. His respirations were 70, heart rate 180 bpm, and blood pressure was 55/29 mmHg. He was taken to the newborn nursery. Birth weight was 3965 grams and oxygen saturation on room air was 95%. At 80 minutes of life his respirations were 65, his heart rate was 190 bpm, and blood pressure was 44/22 mmHg. He was pale, not jaundiced, and appeared in distress. The cardiac examination was significant for tachycardia; pulses were weak but symmetrical, and the abdominal examination was normal.

EXERCISE 4

QUESTIONS

1. What is the differential diagnosis for this infant?

2. What labs would you obtain to help determine the diagnosis?

ANSWERS

1. The differential diagnosis for a pale infant includes acute hemorrhage, hypoxic ischemic encephalopathy (HIE), hemolytic disease, congenital heart disease, and septic shock.

2. A CBC with differential will identify a low hemoglobin/hematocrit, and may give evidence for infection or HIE. A blood gas will determine acid–base status.

CASE STUDY 3 (continued)

A CBC was obtained that showed hematocrit 28%, hemoglobin 9.7 g/dL, MCV 105 fL, MCHC 32.5 g/dL, RDW 13.2%, NRBCs 8/100 WBCs, and platelets 89,000/mL. Baby M was quickly transferred to the NICU where an umbilical venous catheter was placed and 20 mL/kg of normal saline rapidly administered. A blood gas was obtained, which showed pH 7.22, P_{CO_2} 36 mmHg, P_{O_2} 47 mmHg, bicarbonate 12, and base deficit 14.

EXERCISE 5

QUESTION

1. What additional studies would be helpful in the ongoing care of this infant?
   a. Chemistry panel
   b. Liver function studies
   c. Coagulation studies
   d. Head computed tomography (CT) scan
   e. Abdominal ultrasound

ANSWER

1. **c.** This infant shows evidence of significant acute blood loss and hypovolemic shock owing to a subgaleal hemorrhage. Table 8-6, later in this chapter, provides a differential diagnosis for pallor in the neonate. Any cause of acute prepartum or intrapartum hemorrhage can present with a similar clinical picture and should be distinguishable from the causes of chronic blood loss. Because subgaleal hemorrhages can result in the infant's entire blood volume accumulating in the subgaleal space, this potentially life-threatening event must be recognized immediately so that shock and possible ensuing DIC can be treated effectively.

BIRTH TRAUMA

Subgaleal Hemorrhage

Blood loss into the subgaleal space can occur during difficult deliveries requiring instrument assistance, such as face presentation, occiput posterior presentation, or shoulder dystocia. Subgaleal hematomas are potentially life-threatening events, and must be recognized as early as possible to prevent significant morbidity or mortality. These hematomas occur when emissary or "bridging" veins are torn. Blood accumulates into a large potential space between the galea aponeurotica (the epicranial aponeurosis) and the periosteum of the skull. The subgaleal space extends from the orbital ridge to the base of the skull, and can easily accommodate greater than 85 mL/kg of blood, an infant's entire blood volume.

Subgaleal hematomas may form because of preexisting risk factors (such as coagulopathy or asphyxia), but vacuum extraction itself predisposes an infant toward subgaleal bleeding. The presence of a ballotable fluid collection in dependent regions of the infant's head—coupled with signs of hypovolemia in a neonate—raises the possibility of subgaleal bleeding. Treatment of symptomatic infants requires restoration of blood volume and control of bleeding. Exsanguination owing to subgaleal hemorrhage has been reported, and mortality is high if the hemorrhage goes unrecognized. A formula predicting the volume of blood loss has been developed: for every 1 centimeter increase in head circumference that occurs, 38 mL of blood has been lost.

Limiting the frequency and duration of vacuum assistance in high-risk infants may decrease the incidence of subgaleal hematomas. It is important to remember that delivery by cesarean section does not preclude the use of vacuum or forceps, and significant hemorrhage can still occur via this route of delivery.

Internal Hemorrhage

Anemia appearing after the first 24 hours of life in an infant without jaundice may result from internal hemorrhage. In addition to birth trauma causing visible hemorrhages such as cephalohematomas, excessive bruising, and subgaleal hemorrhages, internal hemorrhage can occur following a traumatic delivery. Breech deliveries may be associated with renal, adrenal, or splenic hemorrhage into the retroperitoneal space. Delivery of large infants, such as infants born to diabetic mothers, may also result in organ damage and hemorrhage. Infants with overwhelming sepsis may develop DIC and hemorrhage into liver, adrenal glands, and lungs.

Adrenal Hemorrhage

Adrenal hemorrhage may result in anemia, but may also result in circulatory collapse owing to the loss of organ function. The reported incidence of adrenal hemorrhage is 1.7 per 1000 births. Adrenal hemorrhage can be caused by trauma; however, infectious etiologies resulting in DIC and hemorrhage have also been reported.

Adrenal hemorrhage can also affect surrounding organs, resulting in intestinal obstruction and kidney dysfunction. Diagnosis can be made using ultrasonography, where calcifications or cystic masses are noted. Adrenal hemorrhage can be distinguished from renal vein thrombosis by ultrasound, in that renal vein thrombosis generally results in a solid mass. Infants with renal vein thrombosis may have gross or microscopic hematuria, and may also develop renal failure and hypertension.

Hepatic, Splenic, and Other Soft Tissue Hemorrhages

Hepatic or splenic rupture can result from birth trauma or as a result of distention caused by extramedullary hematopoiesis, such as that seen in erythroblastosis fetalis. Abdominal distension and discoloration, scrotal swelling, and pallor are clinical signs of splenic rupture, but may also be seen with adrenal hemorrhage or hepatic rupture. Other less common causes of hemorrhage in the newborn include hemangiomas of the gastrointestinal tract, vascular malformations of the skin, and hemorrhage into soft tumors such as giant sacrococcygeal teratomas.

DIC/Sepsis

Hemorrhage associated with overwhelming sepsis can occur owing to DIC and consumption of clotting factors in the neonate. Infections caused by group B *Streptococcus* (GBS), *Escherichia coli* (*E. coli*), and other organisms can progress to septic shock and DIC. Viral pathogens such as cytomegalovirus (CMV), toxoplasmosis, herpes simplex, and others may cause a hemolytic anemia, but may also be a cause of overwhelming sepsis and DIC.

Hemorrhage Due to Abnormal Clotting Mechanisms or Iatrogenic Causes

Infants may develop a hemorrhagic anemia due to abnormalities in hemostasis. Male infants with Factor VIII or IX deficiency may bleed excessively following circumcision, and infants with Factor XIII deficiency may have continual oozing of blood from the umbilical stump. These infants require further evaluation of their bleeding.

Infants with central umbilical lines are at risk for external hemorrhage from accidental blood loss. Lines should be monitored constantly to make sure that connections do not become displaced, as exsanguination can occur. Preterm infants can also develop anemia caused by excessive phlebotomy losses, which can exceed 10% of the infant's total blood volume per day.

DIAGNOSIS AND MANAGEMENT OF HEMORRHAGE

The diagnosis of hemorrhage in the newborn can at times be difficult. Infants can present with a spectrum of clinical characteristics, depending on the degree of hypovolemia and anemia, and depending on the timing of blood loss. Table 8-4 describes the differences seen in acute versus chronic blood loss. Infants with acute hemorrhage will be pale and tachycardic. They may be neurologically normal, hyperalert, or may appear lethargic. Infants who present with hypotension have generally experienced significant blood loss, and are at risk for shock and death. Infants are often tachypneic from the metabolic acidosis seen with underperfusion. Hemoglobin concentrations may initially be normal, then drop in the first 6 to 8 hours of life. RBC morphology shows typical normochromic, macrocytic newborn cells.

Rapid resuscitative measures can be lifesaving for infants with a significant acute hemorrhage. In a newborn with extreme pallor, resuscitative measures include establishing rapid intravenous access. Volume resuscitation with available fluid, generally normal saline, can be given even if the etiology of the pallor has not yet been determined, because some infants present with both anemia and asphyxia (such as infants born following placental abruption). Using packed red blood cells (PRBCs) as an initial volume expander without knowing the etiology of pallor might result in transfusing an infant with a normal hematocrit, possibly leading to transfusion associated circulatory overload (TACO) or transfusion related acute lung injury (TRALI). Infants with acute blood loss will often show dramatic improvement, whereas those with ongoing internal hemorrhage, DIC, subgaleal hemorrhage, or asphyxiated infants may remain limp and unresponsive.

Once the diagnosis of hypovolemia owing to acute blood loss has been established, repeat boluses can be given as needed, and type O negative PRBCs can be infused over 30 minutes. Infants with acute blood loss (unlike those with chronic blood loss) have lost platelets and plasma clotting factors along with the loss of red cells. Further resuscitative measures should therefore include evaluation of the infant's bleeding status and replacement with fresh frozen plasma and platelets as needed.

Infants who are anemic at birth from chronic blood loss may be asymptomatic (Table 8-4). Their hemoglobin concentration will be low, and the peripheral smear often reveals microcytic, hypochromic cells indicating iron deficiency. Infants with significant chronic blood loss (such as the donor twin in TTS) may present in congestive heart failure and hydrops. Therapy

---

TABLE 8-4   Acute Versus Chronic Blood Loss in the Neonate

	Acute Blood Loss	Chronic Blood Loss
Clinical characteristics		
General appearance	Pale, hyperalert, "stunned" gaze	Pale, normal neurologic exam
Cardiovascular	Tachycardic, weak pulses, low blood pressure	Normal, rarely may have congestive heart failure with hepatomegaly, normal or increase blood pressure
Respiratory	Tachypneic, no oxygen requirement	Normal, rarely may be tachypneic with an oxygen requirement if congestive heart failure is present
Hematologic		
Hemoglobin	May be normal, drops over 24 hours	Low at birth
Morphology	Macrocytic normochromic (normal)	Microcytic hypochromic anemia
Iron	Normal to low iron at birth, depending on volume of blood loss	Low iron at birth
Course	Promptly treat hypovolemia, may need rapid volume expansion to prevent shock, DIC, and death	Usually uneventful hospital course, may need treatment for congestive heart failure and hydrops
Treatment	Volume expansion with isotonic fluid and PRBCs, FFP, and platelets; iron therapy later; Epo therapy may be appropriate to enhance erythropoiesis	Iron therapy PRBC transfusion rarely needed Epo therapy may be appropriate to enhance erythropoiesis

includes supporting cardiac function with pressors and diuretics as needed.

Iron therapy is indicated for both groups of infants. Infants suffering acute blood loss will receive iron in the form of transfused blood if they are transfused, but generally the replacement does not equal the amount of iron lost. Infants who have experienced chronic blood loss are iron deficient at birth, and replacement therapy should start immediately at 6 mg/kg/day of ferrous sulfate. The administration of Epo to enhance erythropoiesis may be appropriate for some of these infants, especially those born prematurely.

HEMOLYSIS

CASE STUDY 4

Baby girl A is a preterm AGA infant born to a 30-year-old gravida 4 white mother via spontaneous vaginal delivery at 34 weeks' gestation, following preterm premature rupture of membranes. The mother received intrapartum antibiotics. Apgar scores were 7 at 1 minute and 9 at 5 minutes. Birth weight was 2240 grams. A CBC with differential showed hematocrit 38%, hemoglobin 12.9 g/dL, RBC 3.79 × 10⁶/μL, MCV 110 fL, MCHC 35.8 g/dL, RDW 18.8%, and nucleated red blood cells (NRBCs) 12/100 white blood cells (WBCs). The peripheral smear was remarkable for moderate spherocytosis, poikilocytosis, and anisocytosis. On physical examination the following morning, the heart rate was 152 bpm, the respiratory rate was 40 and unlabored, the temperature was 36.9° C, and the blood pressure was 63/40 mmHg. The infant was pink, slightly jaundiced, and in no distress. She had a normal cardiac examination, no hepatosplenomegaly, and was normal neurologically. A total bilirubin obtained at 24 hours of life was 14.2 mg/dL with a direct component of 0.3 mg/dL. A repeat spun hematocrit was 36%.

EXERCISE 6

QUESTIONS

1. Which of the following laboratory values would be helpful in establishing a diagnosis?
   a. Coombs test
   b. Maternal blood type
   c. Maternal antibody screening test
   d. Osmotic fragility test
   e. **b** and **c**
   f. **a**, **b**, and **c**

2. Which of the general categories of hemorrhage, hemolysis, or hypoproliferative disorder would be most likely, and which would be least likely?

ANSWERS

1. **f.** Maternal blood type, antibody screening test, and a direct Coombs test on neonatal blood will assist in the diagnosis of hemolytic disease. The presence of spherocytes on the peripheral smear may be caused by immune-mediated hemolysis or may represent congenital spherocytosis. However, an osmotic fragility test would not be performed until the presence or absence of immune-mediated hemolysis is determined, and until the infant reaches a period without significant active hemolysis. In this case, the mother was type O positive, antibody screening test negative, and the infant was type A positive, direct Coombs test positive. This infant has one of the most common diagnoses for hemolytic disease: ABO incompatibility resulting in immune-mediated hemolysis, elevated bilirubin, and a decrease in hematocrit.

2. Hemolysis is most likely, given the rapid elevation in bilirubin and the mild decrease in hematocrit. A hypoproliferative disorder would be less likely, given the elevated RDW, which reflects a wide range of blood cell sizes and thus new RBC production.

Hemolytic anemia is commonly seen in the newborn period, and can be caused by a variety of factors both intrinsic and extrinsic to the RBC. Regardless of etiology, the fundamental characteristic of all hemolytic anemias is a reduction in the lifespan of RBCs. The average life span for a neonatal RBC is 60 to 90 days, approximately one-half to two-thirds that of an adult RBC. Remarkably shorter red cell life spans (35 to 50 days) are found with increasing prematurity. The shortened red cell life span of the preterm and term neonate may be explained by some of the characteristics specific to newborn RBCs. These include a rapid decline in intracellular enzyme activity and ATP, loss of membrane surface area, decreased levels of intracellular carnitine, and increased mechanical fragility and susceptibility to oxidative stress.

Hemolysis in the newborn period is most commonly marked by jaundice, and may also be associated with hepatosplenomegaly. Common causes of hemolysis in the newborn period are listed in Table 8-5. Hemolysis can be classified into three general categories: immune-mediated hemolysis, congenital defects of the red cell, and acquired defects of the red cell.

ISOIMMUNE HEMOLYTIC ANEMIAS

Red cell antigens in the ABO, MN, Rh, Kell, Duffy, and Vel systems are well developed in early intrauterine life. They are easily

TABLE 8-5 Causes of Hemolysis in the Newborn Period

A. Immune-mediated
  Rh incompatibility (anti-D antibody)
  ABO incompatibility
  Minor blood group incompatibility: c, C, e, G, Fya
    (Duffy), Kell group, Jka, MNS, Vw
  Drug-induced (penicillin, alpha-methyl DOPA,
    cephalothin)
  Maternal autoimmune hemolytic anemia
B. Infection
  Bacterial sepsis (*Escherichia coli*, Group B
    Streptococcus)
  Parvovirus B-19 (can present with hydrops
    fetalis)
  Congenital syphilis
  Congenital malaria
  Congenital TORCH infections (Toxoplasmosis,
    Cytomegalovirus, Rubella, disseminated
    Herpes)
  Other congenital viral infections
C. Disseminated intravascular coagulation
D. Hereditary erythrocyte membrane disorders
  Spherocytosis
  Elliptocytosis
  Stomatocytosis
  Pyropoikilocytosis
  Other membrane disorders

E. Congenital erythrocyte enzyme defects
  Glucose-6-phosphate dehydrogenase (G6PD)
    deficiency
  Pyruvate kinase (PK) deficiency
  Hexokinase deficiency
  Glucose phosphate isomerase deficiency
  Pyrimidine 5' nucleotidase deficiency
F. Hemoglobin defects
  Alpha thalassemia syndromes
  Gamma thalassemia syndromes
  Alpha and gamma chain structural anomalies
G. Macro- and microangiopathic hemolysis
  Cavernous hemangiomas
  Arteriovenous malformations
  Renal artery stenosis or thrombosis
  Other large vessel thrombi
  Severe coarctation of the aorta
  Severe valvular stenoses
H. Other causes
  Galactosemia
  Lysosomal storage diseases
  Prolonged metabolic acidosis from metabolic dis-
    ease (amino acid and organic acid disorders)
  Transfusion reactions
  Thrombocytopenia-absent radius syndrome
  Drug-induced hemolysis (valproic acid)

demonstrated in the fifth to seventh gestational week and remain constant through the remainder of intrauterine development. A and B antigens are present early *in utero*, however antibody production occurs much later. By 30 to 34 weeks' gestation, however, about 50% of infants will have some measurable anti-A or anti-B antibodies. The fetal production of such antibodies is not related to maternal ABO blood type. Intrauterine exposure to gram-negative organisms whose antigens are chemically related to those of blood groups A and B is a potent stimulus for the development of these antibodies.

RH AND ABO ISOIMMUNIZATION

Isoimmunization owing to maternal anti-D antibody is one of the most common forms of immune-mediated hemolysis. Severe hemolysis can lead to hydrops and fetal demise. With the development of RhoGAM the incidence of severe Rh hemolytic disease has decreased dramatically. In fetuses severely affected with Rh hemolytic disease, ultrasound-guided intravascular intrauterine transfusions can treat anemia and reverse hydrops. Infants with Rh hemolytic disease often have an early (congenital) anemia owing to hemolysis, and can develop a "late" (age 1 to 3 months) anemia owing to diminished erythrocyte production.

Isoimmunization owing to ABO incompatibility is the most common cause of hemolytic disease in the newborn period. ABO incompatibility represents a spectrum of hemolytic disease in newborns, ranging from infants with little or no evidence of erythrocyte sensitization, but evidence of hemolysis, to infants with severe hemolytic disease in which erythrocyte sensitization is markedly present. ABO incompatibility can occur during a first pregnancy, as well as during subsequent pregnancies. Unlike Rh disease, there is no way to predict severity for ABO incompatibility in subsequent pregnancies. Table 8-6 compares the laboratory and clinical aspects of Rh isoimmune hemolytic anemia and ABO isoimmune hemolytic anemia.

OTHER ISOIMMUNE ANEMIAS

Anti-Kell anemic fetuses have lower reticulocyte counts and total serum bilirubin levels than do comparable anti-D anemic fetuses. The level of hemolysis caused by anti-Kell antibodies is less than that caused by anti-D antibodies, but fetal erythropoiesis appears blunted, suggesting that Kell sensitization results in suppression of fetal erythropoiesis as well as hemolysis (Vaughn et al., 1998). Fetuses with anti-Kell hemolytic anemia may therefore benefit from fetal blood sampling

TABLE 8-6 Comparison of Rh and ABO Incompatibility

	Rh	ABO
Blood group setup		
Mother	Negative	O
Infant	Positive	A or B
Type of antibody	Incomplete (IgG)	Immune (IgG)
Clinical aspects		
Occurrence in firstborn	5%	40%-50%
Predictable severity in subsequent pregnancies	Usually	No
Stillbirth or hydrops	Frequent	Rare
Severe anemia	Frequent	Rare
Degree of jaundice	+++	+
Hepatosplenomegaly	+++	+
Laboratory findings		
Direct Coombs test (infant)	+	(+) or O
Maternal antibodies	Always present	Not clear-cut
Spherocytes	0	+
Treatment		
Need for antenatal measures	Yes	No
Value of phototherapy	Limited	Great
Exchange transfusion		
Frequency	Approx. 67%	Approx. 1%
Donor blood type	Rh-negative	Rh same as infant
	Group-specific, when possible	Group O only
Incidence of late anemia	Common	Rare

Modified from Naiman JL: Erythroblastosis fetalis. In Oski FA, Naiman JL, editors: Hematologic problems in the newborn, 3rd ed, Philadelphia, PA, 1982, Saunders, p 333.

rather than amniotic fluid analysis, which might underestimate the degree of anemia.

Extremely high titers of anti-C antibody have been associated with neonatal hemolysis, however routine screening of titers is not warranted, because antibody titers do not accurately reflect the severity of hemolytic disease.

Rhesus and Kell antigen status can be determined by deoxyribonucleic acid (DNA) studies, and molecular biology techniques such as polymerase chain reaction (PCR) have been used recently to determine fetal blood type. These methods may represent an advance in the clinical management of Rh and Kell isoimmunization in the future.

CASE STUDY 5

Baby girl A is a 35-week AGA infant born to a 30-year-old, B–, AST negative, gravida 1 mother via spontaneous vaginal delivery. RhoGAM was administered at 28 weeks during the pregnancy. The mother developed preterm labor, had premature rupture of membranes, and received intrapartum antibiotics prior to vaginal delivery. Birth weight was 2610 grams, Apgar scores were 9 and 9 at 1 and 5 minutes, respectively. A screening CBC was obtained that showed hematocrit 38%, hemoglobin 13.9 g/dL, RBC 3.79 × 10⁶/mL, MCV 104 fL, MCH 36 pg, MCHC 34.8 g/dL, and RDW 19.8%. The peripheral smear showed moderate anisocytosis and spherocytosis.

EXERCISE 7

QUESTIONS

1. What are common reasons for the infant's abnormal RBC indices?

2. Which of the following would be helpful in working up the infant's hematologic abnormalities?
   a. Information on maternal iron intake during pregnancy
   b. Detailed family history
   c. Maternal KB test
   d. Neonatal blood type and direct Coombs test
   e. Neonatal hemoglobin electrophoresis

ANSWERS

1. The infant has mildly decreased MCV, a high MCHC, an increased RDW, and a decreased hemoglobin/hematocrit for a preterm infant. The differential involves causes of hemolytic disease, such as ABO incompatibility and congenital spherocytosis, as microspherocytes can be present on the peripheral smear in both cases.

2. **b** and **d**. Obtaining detailed parent and family information regarding a history of anemia, transfusions, or abnormal RBC indices in either parent or first-degree relative is helpful in identifying inherited anemias such as red cell membrane defects, red cell enzyme defects, or alpha thalassemia. Chronic hemorrhage owing to FMH would result in a low MCHC, and would not be part of the differential. The neonatal blood type should be obtained to identify ABO incompatibility

CASE STUDY 5 (continued)

The infant's blood type was B positive, direct Coombs negative. Further maternal information revealed a history of splenectomy in a maternal

aunt, and mild anemia in the mother. A diagnosis of congenital spherocytosis was considered and a pediatric hematologist was consulted. The hematologist advised an osmotic fragility test be performed between 2 to 4 months of age.

CONGENITAL RBC DEFECTS

Congenital defects of the red cell include enzymatic defects, membrane defects, and defects of hemoglobin synthesis. Enzyme defects such as glucose-6-phosphate dehydrogenase (G6PD) deficiency, pyruvate kinase deficiency, hexokinase deficiency, and glucose phosphate isomerase deficiency may present with hemolytic anemia in the first week of life.

Membrane defects such as hereditary spherocytosis, hereditary elliptocytosis, and other hereditary disorders of the red cell cytoskeleton may also cause hemolysis in the newborn period. Neonatal red cell membranes deform more to a given shear force than do adult red cell membranes, resulting in greater susceptibility of neonatal cells to yield and fragment. These mechanical properties lead to accelerated membrane loss and a decreased lifespan in normal newborns. The red cells of infants with membrane abnormalities have even shorter lifespans.

Hereditary spherocytosis is a congenital defect in membrane deformability caused by various defects in erythrocyte membrane proteins such as spectrin, ankyrin, band 3, and protein 4.2. A diagnosis of hereditary spherocytosis is made by determining the red cell osmotic fragility. Neonatal red cells have an increased osmotic resistance when compared to adults. When an osmotic fragility test is obtained in a neonate, neonatal reference values should be used. In addition, erythrocytes in other hemolytic states such as ABO incompatibility may demonstrate a similar abnormality in osmotic fragility, therefore further testing may be necessary to distinguish these two disorders. The increased osmotic fragility of hereditary spherocytosis (but not ABO incompatibility) can be reduced by the addition of glucose.

Disorders of hemoglobin synthesis can also lead to increased hemolysis. Alpha thalassemia trait is an important diagnosis to make in the newborn period. This abnormality of alpha chain production is common in African American and Asian populations. These newborns may benefit from an initial evaluation of their RBC indices to look for microcytosis, in order to detect the presence of the α-thalassemia trait. Because the differential diagnosis of microcytosis at this age is limited, the newborn period is the best time to establish the diagnosis. Beyond a few months of life, iron deficiency becomes a more common cause of microcytosis. Hemoglobin electrophoresis in the α-thalassemia trait is normal, although some studies have reported minor increases in Bart's hemoglobin (2% to 8%) that is transiently present in neonates and detectable in many newborn screening laboratories. Molecular biologic techniques are being evaluated; however, it remains easiest to make this diagnosis by the observation of a low MCV (<95 fL) in the newborn period.

The α-thalassemia syndromes are gene deletion disorders, involving up to four genes. Four genes are necessary to make the total complement of α-globin. Twenty-eight percent of African American children and adults lack a single gene. This condition is known as the silent carrier state of α-thalassemia. The silent carrier state is not detectable by any routine laboratory study. A two-gene deletion state, seen in about 3% of African Americans, is known as α-thalassemia trait. A three-gene deletion disorder is known as hemoglobin H disease. Hemoglobin H disease results in the production of large quantities of γ-chains (compared to α-globin chains) leading to the formation of Bart's hemoglobin. The four-gene deletion state causes hydrops fetalis and is incompatible with life.

Unlike α-thalassemia, β-thalassemia trait does not produce abnormalities in red cell indices at birth because β-globin chain production is not sufficiently developed in comparison to γ-globin chain production. Structural β-globin chain defects (such as sickle-cell anemia) do not normally present at birth. β-thalassemia trait can be diagnosed in the older infant or child by an elevation of hemoglobin A_2 and/or hemoglobin F on electrophoresis assays.

ACQUIRED RBC DEFECTS

Infection, drugs, or toxins may cause acquired hemolytic anemias. In addition, vascular pathology such as arteriovenous malformations, cavernous hemangiomas, and vascular thromboses can result in a hemolytic process.

Infection and DIC

Infants with viral or bacterial sepsis can develop a hemolytic anemia. Sepsis caused by bacteria such as GBS and *E. coli* may result in hemolysis, DIC, and hemorrhage. Infants are often jaundiced and have hepatosplenomegaly, although the degree of hyperbilirubinemia does not always correlate with the degree of anemia. Infants may have an elevated direct bilirubin as well owing to hepatitis. Some bacteria such as *E. coli* will produce hemolytic endotoxins, which result in increased red cell destruction, often associated with a microangiopathic process.

Congenital viral infections caused by CMV, toxoplasmosis, rubella, and herpes simplex may also be associated with a hemolytic anemia, and are a cause of nonimmune hydrops. Box 8-2 reviews some of the more common causes of nonimmune hydrops. Congenital syphilis may present with hemolytic anemia despite negative testing in the mother in the face of overwhelming infection.

Fetal and neonatal infection with parvovirus B19 can cause severe anemia, hydrops, and fetal demise. The infant generally presents with a hypoplastic anemia, but hemolysis can occur as well. The virus replicates exclusively in erythroid progenitor cells. Thus, in infants with an underlying hemolytic disorder, infection with parvovirus B19 can result in aplastic anemia. *In utero* transfusions for hydropic fetuses have been investigated, but are not successful in all patients. Treatment with intravenous immunoglobulin (IVIG) during aplastic crises leads to resolution of the anemia.

Other infections associated with neonatal anemia include malaria and human immunodeficiency virus (HIV). Congenital malaria may occur in endemic urban areas where imported cases of malaria are increasing. Congenital HIV infection can be asymptomatic in newborns. Infants born to mothers on zidovudine may have a hypoplastic anemia caused by side effects of the drug.

IMPAIRED RBC PRODUCTION

Impaired erythrocyte production can result from a variety of causes. Lack of an appropriate or sufficient marrow environment for growth, as seen in osteopetrosis, can cause decreased red cell production. Lack of specific substrates or their carriers, such as iron, folate, vitamin B_{12}, or transcobalamin II deficiency, can lead to deficient production. Lack of specific red cell growth factor activity, such as decreased Epo production seen in anemia of prematurity or abnormalities in Epo receptors seen in Diamond-Blackfan syndrome, can also lead to hypoproliferative anemia.

| **BOX 8-2** | **Nonimmune Hydrops Fetalis: Causes and Associations** |

Cardiovascular
  Tachyarrhythmias: paroxysmal supraventricular tachycardia, atrial flutter
  Congenital heart disease
  Premature closure of foramen ovale
  Cardiomyopathy
  Large arteriovenous malformation
  Bradyarrhythmias: heart block
  Fibroelastosis
  Tuberous sclerosis
Chromosomal/genetic
  Trisomy 21, 18, 13
  XO
  Noonan syndrome
  Multiple pterygium syndrome
  Lysosomal storage disease
  Achondroplasia
  E trisomy
  Gaucher disease
  Niemann-Pick disease
  Microdeletions
  Pena-Shokeir syndrome
  Arthrogryposis
Hematologic
  Homozygous α-thalassemia
  Chronic fetomaternal transfusion
  Twin-to-twin transfusion (recipient or donor)
  Severe nonimmune mediated anemia (see rest of this chapter)
Thoracic/pulmonary
  Cystic adenomatoid malformation of lung
  Pulmonary lymphangiectasia

Pulmonary hypoplasia (diaphragmatic hernia)
Intra-thoracic tumors (hamartoma, mediastinal tumor)
Thoracic skeletal dysplasias
Infectious
  Parvovirus B19
  Cytomegalovirus
  Syphilis
  Herpes simplex virus
  Toxoplasmosis
  Listeria
  Influenza
  Leptospirosis
  Varicella
  Adenovirus
  Enterovirus
  Chagas disease
  Congential hepatitis
Miscellaneous
  Meconium peritonitis
  Adrenal neuroblastoma
  Sacrococcygeal teratoma
  Small bowel volvulus
  Congenital nephrosis
  Renal vein thrombosis
  Placental anomalies
Maternal
  Systemic lupus erythematosus
  Hyperparathyroidism
  Diabetes mellitus
  Toxemia
Idiopathic

CASE STUDY 6

Baby boy H is a term AGA male born at 37 weeks' gestation by elective repeat cesarean section to a 29-year-old gravida 3 white mother. Birth weight was 2910 grams, Apgar scores were 6 and 8 at 1 and 5 minutes, respectively. Because of ongoing respiratory distress, the infant was admitted to the NICU for evaluation. A chest x-ray revealed normal lung fields and no bony abnormalities. Blood cultures were obtained and a CBC showed hematocrit 28%; hemoglobin 9.1 g/dL; WBC 9.8 × 10³/μL; differential 34 neutrophils, 4 bands, 47 lymphocytes, 12 monocytes, 2 eosinophils, and 1 basophil; platelets 214 × 10³/μL; MCV 88 fL; MCHC 30.4 g/dL; and RDW 17.2%. The infant's respiratory distress resolved over the next 4 hours.

EXERCISE 8

QUESTIONS

1. What are the common nutritional deficiencies associated with this infant's RBC indices?

2. What immediate treatments are required?

ANSWERS

1. The infant has a hypochromic, microcytic anemia. Possible nutritional deficiencies include iron and copper. Both folate and B_{12} deficiency result in a megaloblastic anemia, and would not fit this clinical picture.

2. The infant does not show signs of acute anemia, therefore an immediate transfusion of PRBCs is not necessary. The infant can be treated conservatively with nutritional supplementation. The lack of bony abnormalities, the normal neutrophil count, and the fact that the infant is a term newborn make copper deficiency less likely. Iron deficiency owing to chronic fetal blood loss is the most common cause of microcytic hypochromic anemia at birth.

NUTRITIONAL DEFICIENCIES CAUSING ANEMIA

With the exception of iron deficiency anemia in newborns with prolonged hemorrhage, hypoproliferative anemias caused by nutritional deficiencies rarely present in term newborns. In preterm infants, however, nutritional deficiency anemias do occur, although they generally do not become evident until after the first weeks of life. Deficiencies of iron, folate, B_{12}, vitamin E, and copper have been described, and can lead to varying degrees of anemia.

Iron deficiency anemia can occur at various times during the newborn period in both term and preterm infants. Following chronic FMH or TTS, term and preterm infants can present with iron deficiency anemia manifested by hypochromic, microcytic red cells on a peripheral smear and a low hematocrit. Because 75% to 80% of the total body iron is stored in hemoglobin, infants born with decreased red cell volumes have decreased iron stores. Preterm infants will develop an iron-deficient state even more rapidly, given their relatively smaller total blood volumes and greater phlebotomy losses. As blood cells are destroyed, the iron from hemoglobin is recycled, becoming available for future erythropoiesis. Without adequate initial red cell volumes, the iron for new hemoglobin production is lacking, and iron deficiency anemia ensues. Thus, the initial hemoglobin concentration significantly impacts the ability of preterm infants to maintain normal hematologic indices during growth.

The use of Epo to prevent and treat anemia in preterm infants has added a new level of complexity in determining the iron requirements of preterm infants. Numerous studies of preterm infants receiving Epo have shown evidence of iron deficiency when iron supplementation is not adequate. Iron has been administered both parenterally and enterally in published studies, ranging from 3 to 7 mg/kg/week parenterally and 2 to 40 mg/kg/day orally in clinical studies. No evidence of hemolysis was noted in either of the two Epo trials in which the greatest amounts of supplemental iron were used, and the most recent studies continue to show decreased ferritin concentrations in Epo recipients despite both parenteral and enteral iron dosing. Further evaluation is required to determine the optimal dose and route of administration of iron in these preterm infants.

Vitamin E is an antioxidant, inhibiting peroxidation of polyunsaturated fatty acids (PUFAs) present in the lipid bilayers of all cell membranes. Because vitamin E is transferred across the placenta to the greatest degree in the last trimester, preterm infants are born with lower stores than term infants. Unlike other nutritional deficiency anemias, vitamin E deficiency does not result in a hypoproliferative anemia, but rather a hemolytic anemia, owing to the functions of the compound. Vitamin E-deficient, hemolytic anemia has largely disappeared because of improvements in preterm infant formulas containing lower concentrations of PUFAs and adequate vitamin E supplementation. Infants with severe fat malabsorption require greater vitamin E supplementation. In addition, vitamin E requirements are likely increased in preterm infants receiving increased iron supplementation, because iron promotes oxidation of cellular membranes and also inhibits intestinal absorption of vitamin E. Preterm infants receiving Epo require greater iron supplementation, and should therefore receive vitamin E supplementation as well. The optimal dose of vitamin E in preterm infants receiving Epo has not been determined, but oral doses in recent studies ranged 15 to 25 IU per day. Investigators evaluating the use of higher doses of vitamin E (50 IU per day) did not show evidence of increased erythropoiesis (Pathak et al., 2003).

Folate is stored in the fetal liver late in gestation, and infants can become deficient if born prematurely. Infants fed diets low in folate, those with malabsorption, and infants receiving goat's milk or milk that has been boiled are at risk for becoming folate deficient. Red cell folate concentrations represent total body folate stores, whereas serum folate concentrations reflect recent folate intake. Both serum and RBC folate concentrations are greater in preterm and term infants than in adults. RBC folate concentrations decrease rapidly after birth, and are generally lower than adult concentrations by 1 to 3 months of life. Folate deficiency results in a megaloblastic anemia, with MCV generally greater than 110 fL. Preterm infants with lower folate stores need supplementation in situations where erythropoiesis is increased, such as infants with hemolytic anemia or infants receiving Epo. General requirements for term and preterm infants are 25 to 50 μg orally per day, which require separate supplementation as folate is not a component of preterm multivitamin preparations.

Vitamin B_{12} (or cobalamin) must be obtained through dietary intake because only microorganisms are able to synthesize the compound. B_{12} is actively transported across the placenta and stored in the fetal liver. B_{12} deficiency is rare in preterm infants, but can sometimes be seen in breastfed infants of vegetarian mothers who are B_{12} deficient, or in infants with gastrointestinal abnormalities such as short gut syndrome, necrotizing enterocolitis (NEC), or post-NEC stenoses. The hematologic characteristics of B_{12} deficiency anemia are similar to those seen in folate deficiency anemia. Erythroid hyperplasia and a decreased myeloid to erythroid ratio (M:E) is present in the range of 2:1 to 1:1. Megaloblastic proerythroblasts have a shortened survival, and remaining cells have an increased MCV. Reticulocytosis occurs rapidly with B_{12} supplementation.

Copper deficiency anemia may occur in some specific situations where supplemental copper is not given: low birth-weight premature infants fed milk only, protracted total parenteral nutrition without trace mineral supplements,

and chronic diarrhea with severe malnutrition. Severe neutropenia generally precedes the onset of sideroblastic, hypochromic anemia. Serum iron concentrations are usually low, but iron therapy is ineffective in resolving the anemia. The diagnosis is established by low serum copper concentrations, the presence of fractures or periosteal reaction on radiographs, and a dramatic reticulocytosis in response to copper therapy. The recommended intake of copper for term infants is 0.4 to 0.6 mg per day.

CASE STUDY 7

Baby girl E is a 32-day-old former 900-gram infant born at 27 weeks' gestation to a 17-year-old gravida 1 now para 1 mother with preterm labor and premature rupture of membranes. The initial hematocrit was 42%, and the rest of the CBC and RBC indices were within normal limits. The infant received 14 days of mechanical ventilation and is currently on nasal cannula oxygen. She is receiving full gavage feedings. Her spun hematocrit today is 24%.

A central CBC shows hematocrit 22%, hemoglobin 7.4 g/dL, MCV 92 fL, MCHC 33.0 g/dL, RDW 12.8%, and NRBCs 0/100 WBCs. An uncorrected reticulocyte count is 1.0%, with an absolute reticulocyte count of 30,000 cells/μL. The peripheral smear shows mild anisocytosis and poikilocytosis.

EXERCISE 9

QUESTIONS

True or false?

1. This anemia can be rapidly corrected with iron supplementation.

2. This disorder is rare in preterm infants.

3. The RBC indices show active erythropoiesis.

4. This anemia results from inadequate production of erythropoietin.

ANSWERS

1. **False**. The anemia of prematurity does not respond to nutritional supplementation alone, but requires the addition of erythropoiesis-stimulating agents (ESAs) to stimulate red cell production.

2. **False**. The anemia of prematurity is the most common anemia seen in preterm infants.

3. **False**. An absolute reticulocyte count of 30,000 cells/μL reflects minimal erythropoietic activity.

4. **True**. This normocytic, normochromic, hypoproliferative anemia involves inadequate Epo

production despite signs of anemia. Clinical studies administering recombinant Epo to preterm infants to treat the anemia of prematurity have resulted in reduced transfusion requirements. Preterm, otherwise healthy infants receiving 400 units/kg three times per week will increase their reticulocyte counts within 3 to 7 days, and will generally maintain or increase hematocrits by 7 to 14 days. Supplemental iron (6 mg/kg/day) is important to provide optimal substrate for new RBC production.

THE ANEMIA OF PREMATURITY

In preterm infants, adaptive mechanisms to the extrauterine environment are incomplete. Epo concentrations in anemic preterm infants are still significantly lower than those found in adults, given the degree of their anemia. This normocytic, normochromic anemia, termed the "anemia of prematurity," is the most common anemia seen in infants ≤32 weeks' gestation. The anemia of prematurity is not responsive to the addition of iron, folate, or vitamin E. Some infants may be asymptomatic, whereas others demonstrate signs of anemia, which are alleviated by transfusion. These signs include tachycardia, increased episodes of apnea and bradycardia, poor weight gain, an increased oxygen requirement, and elevated serum lactate concentrations that decrease following transfusion.

Infants with the anemia of prematurity have a decreased ability to increase serum Epo concentrations, despite diminished "available oxygen" to tissues and the appearance of signs of anemia. However, marrow erythroid progenitors are highly sensitive to Epo, and concentrations of other erythropoietic growth factors responsible for erythrocyte production appear to be normal.

The molecular and cellular mechanisms responsible for the anemia of prematurity remain undefined. Possible explanations include the transition from fetal to adult hemoglobin, shortened erythrocyte survival, and hemodilution associated with a rapidly increasing body mass. It is unknown whether preterm infants rely on Epo produced by the liver (the source of Epo *in utero*), or that produced by the kidney, or a combination of the two. The anemia of prematurity likely involves a delay in shifting the anatomic site of Epo production from liver to kidney, and represents an inability of extremely low birth weight (ELBW) infants to prematurely alter gene expression in the kidney in response to the extrauterine environment.

Given the risks of transfusions, such as transmission of hepatitis, CMV, and HIV, possible development of graft-versus-host disease, and potential increase in morbidities associated with prematurity such as NEC and ICH, treatment of the anemia of prematurity using ESAs might be cost effective. In a recent study in preterm infants 500 to 1250 grams birth weight, ESA recipients received half the number of transfusions and were exposed to half the donors as infants in the placebo group (Ohls et al., 2013). Instituting more rigorous and standardized transfusion criteria, diminishing the volume of blood lost through phlebotomy, and judicious use of ESAs will have the greatest impact in decreasing transfusion requirements in both term and preterm infants.

CONGENITAL ANEMIAS

Congenital syndromes may primarily diminish or inhibit red cell production, or may secondarily alter the red cell mass through chronic blood loss or hemolysis. Table 8-7 lists genetic disorders associated with anemia in the newborn. The most common syndromes are summarized.

Diamond-Blackfan Anemia

Diamond-Blackfan anemia (DBA) consists of a group of congenital pure RBC aplasias diagnosed generally within the first year of life. The syndrome represents a phenotypic expression of multiple genotypic abnormalities affecting erythropoiesis. Up to 25% of patients are anemic at birth. Hydrops fetalis associated with severe anemia has been reported, but is rare. The majority of cases are sporadic, but 10% to 15% of cases are familial, and more cases of autosomal dominant (AD) inheritance have recently been reported.

Physical abnormalities are present in about one third of DBA patients. Abnormalities include short stature, triphalangeal or duplicated thumbs, cleft palate, ocular anomalies, short or webbed neck, and congenital heart disease. Patients can be profoundly anemic and reticulocytopenic; however, other cell lineages are normal in number and function. The bone marrow reflects hypoproliferative erythropoiesis, showing a very low number of erythropoietic precursors and a reduction of erythroid progenitor cells. Proliferation and differentiation of the other lineages are normal. Many patients respond clinically to corticosteroids, and some develop hematologic remissions (both spontaneous and following corticosteroid therapy).

TABLE 8-7   **Genetic Disorders Associated with Anemia**

Syndrome	Genetic Characteristics	Hematologic Phenotype
Diamond Blackfan anemia	Autosomal recessive (AR); sporadic mutations and autosomal dominant (AD) inheritance have been described	Steroid responsive hypoplastic anemia, often macrocytic after 5 months of age
Schwachman Diamond syndrome	AR, owing to mutations in Schwachman Bodian Diamond Syndrome (SBDS) gene, chromosome 7q11	Neutropenia most common, anemia and thrombocytopenia can occur
Fanconi pancytopenia	AR, thought to be caused by abnormalities in multiple genes (at least 5 genetic subtypes have been identified)	Steroid responsive hypoplastic anemia, reticulocytopenia, some macrocytic RBCs, shortened RBC lifespan Cells are hypersensitive to DNA cross-linking agents
Aase syndrome	AR , possible AD	Steroid responsive hypoplastic anemia that improves with age
Pearson's syndrome	Mitochondrial DNA abnormalities, X-linked or AR	Hypoplastic sideroblastic anemia unresponsive to pyridoxine
Osteopetrosis	AR, caused by defective resorption of immature bone	Hypoplastic anemia owing to marrow compression
Congenital dyserythropoietic anemias (CDA)	AR	Type I: megaloblastoid erythroid hyperplasia and nuclear chromatin bridges between cells Type II: erythroblastic multinuclearity and positive acidified serum test results (HEMPAS) Type III: erythroblastic multinuclearity and macrocytosis
Peutz Jeghers syndrome	AD	Iron deficiency anemia from chronic blood loss
Dyskeratosis congenita	X-linked recessive, locus on Xq28 some cases with AD inheritance	Hypoplastic anemia usually presenting between 5 to 15 years of age
X-linked α-thalassemia/mental retardation (ATR-X and ATR-16) syndromes	ATR-X: X-linked recessive, mapped to Xq13.3 ATR-16: mapped to 16p13.3, deletions of α-globin locus	ATR-X: hypochromic, microcytic anemia; mild form of hemoglobin H disease ATR-16: more significant hemoglobin H disease and anemia are present
Pearson syndrome	Mitochondrial DNA abnormalities, X-linked or AR	Hypoplastic sideroblastic anemia unresponsive to pyridoxine
Thrombocytopenia-absent radius syndrome (TAR)	Autosomal recessive (AR)	Hemorrhagic anemia, possibly hypoplastic anemia as well
Osler hemorrhagic telangiectasia syndrome	AD, mapped to 9q33-34	Hemorrhagic anemia

Shwachman-Diamond Syndrome

Shwachman-Diamond syndrome (SDS) is an autosomal recessive marrow failure syndrome that occurs as a result of genetic abnormalities in the Shwachman-Bodian-Diamond syndrome (SBDS) gene, a regulator of ribosomal assembly. Neutropenia is the most common hematopoietic abnormality occurring in almost all patients, with predisposition to development of myelodysplastic syndrome and acute myeloid leukemia. Hypoplastic anemia occurs in up to 80% of patients with SDS. Exocrine pancreatic insufficiency is the other prominent clinical component of this disorder. Skeletal abnormalities can occur, including abnormalities in thoracic size and shape. In addition the brain, liver, kidneys, teeth, and immune system can be affected. Patients require pancreatic enzyme replacement and consistent surveillance for cytopenias and myelodysplasia or leukemia.

Fanconi Anemia

Fanconi anemia (FA) is an autosomal recessive disorder characterized by marrow failure and congenital anomalies, including abnormalities in skin pigmentation, gastrointestinal anomalies, renal anomalies, and upper limb anomalies. Approximately one-third of patients have no obvious congenital anomalies. Most patients present in early childhood, but newborns with FA have been reported, usually when obvious congenital anomalies are present. Patients generally have a steroid responsive hypoplastic anemia, reticulocytopenia, macrocytic RBCs on peripheral smear, and shortened RBC lifespan. A significant percentage of patients will develop myelodysplastic syndrome or acute myelogenous leukemia later in life. Treatment of FA is similar to that for DBA, and marrow transplantation has been successful.

GUIDELINES FOR ERYTHROCYTE TRANSFUSIONS

CASE STUDY 8

Baby girl L is a preterm AGA female born at 26 weeks' gestation to a 24-year-old gravida 3 mother. The pregnancy was complicated by preterm labor and preterm premature rupture of membranes (PPROM). The mother informed her perinatologist that she and her husband were Jehovah's Witnesses, and opposed transfusions for herself and her infant. You are asked to consult on this case and counsel the family.

The mother develops a fever overnight and preterm labor is augmented. Vaginal delivery occurs the next morning. Following your consultation with the family and perinatologists, a plan for cord milking was put into place. The infant delivered vaginally and the umbilical cord was milked four times while the infant was held slightly below the level of the placenta. The infant was handed to the resuscitation team, dried, and stimulated. The birth weight was 770 grams and the infant's Apgar scores were 6 and 8 at 1 and 5 minutes, respectively. Umbilical cord blood was collected sterilely for type and screen, CBC with differential, umbilical cord gas, and blood culture. The infant was brought to the NICU and placed on continuous positive airway pressure (CPAP). Central lines were placed.

EXERCISE 10

QUESTION

1. With respect to the infant's hematologic status, what are treatment options you can implement to diminish the infant's need for transfusions?

ANSWER

1. The infant can be started immediately on Epo, by adding it to protein-containing IV fluid at a dose of 200 units/kg/day. Microsampling devices can be used so that phlebotomy losses are minimized.

CASE STUDY 8 (continued)

The initial CBC showed hematocrit 56%, hemoglobin 18.7 g/dL, WBC $9.8 \times 10^3/\mu L$, platelets $178 \times 10^3/\mu L$, MCV 119 fL, MCHC 33.4 g/dL, and RDW 14.2%. Parenteral nutrition was ordered and included 200 units/kg Epo. Initial arterial blood gas was 7.34/38/67/22/2. The infant was placed on Hudson prong CPAP of 5 cm H_2O. Trophic feedings were initiated the following morning.

EXERCISE 11

QUESTION

1. Which of the following measures would benefit the infant in terms of improving her chances of remaining transfusion free?
   a. Maintaining central venous access until after she has reached full volume feedings
   b. Supplementing with parenteral iron while she is receiving trophic feedings
   c. Ordering bedside hemoglobin measures every day to follow adequacy of Epo administration
   d. Continuing subcutaneous (SC) Epo administration after IV access is no longer available.

ANSWER

1. **b** and **d**. Supplementing the infant with parenteral iron until she is on adequate volume feedings to tolerate oral iron supplements, and continuing Epo administration 400 units/kg SC three times weekly will support erythropoiesis. Removing central lines, especially central arterial lines, and ordering labs on an as-needed basis will help to minimize phlebotomy losses. Daily hemoglobin or hematocrit is unnecessary. A reticulocyte count can be measured after 10 to 14 days of Epo therapy to assure active erythropoiesis.

CASE STUDY 8 (continued)

The infant weans to one-half liter per minute (LPM) nasal canula oxygen and 25% to 30% oxygen after 1 week, and achieves full volume feedings by Day 14 of age. All central lines have been discontinued and current weight is 840 grams. Blood cultures and a CBC are obtained at night following an increase in apnea and bradycardia: hematocrit 37%; hemoglobin 12.7 g/dL; WBC $11.4 \times 10^3/\mu L$; platelets $110 \times 10^3/\mu L$; MCV 102 fL; differential 44 neutrophils, 2 bands, 37 lymphocytes, 8 monocytes, 1 metamyelocyte, 7 eosinophils, and 2 basophils. The infant is started on antibiotics for suspected sepsis.

EXERCISE 12

QUESTION

1. Management of the infant includes which of the following?
   a. Obtain a court order in case the infant is septic and a transfusion is needed.
   b. Stop Epo and iron.
   c. Follow blood cultures and continue antibiotics.
   d. Obtain a blood gas and monitor for additional signs of infection.
   e. Repeat the CBC the following day.

ANSWER

1. **c** and **d**. Current information suggests the infant is not in need of immediate increase in oxygen delivery to tissues, although a blood gas will provide better evidence regarding ventilation and circulation. Epo and iron can be continued, as there is no evidence for neutropenia. Aside from mild thrombocytopenia there are no abnormalities in the CBC that would require repeating.

CASE STUDY 8 (continued)

Four weeks have passed. Sepsis was ruled out and antibiotics stopped after 48 hours. The infant is now growing well on 24 calorie EBM, currently weighs 1360 grams, and has a mild oxygen requirement with occasional apnea and bradycardia for which she continues to receive caffeine. She remains on SC Epo, oral vitamin E, folate, and iron. A bedside hemoglobin of 12.2 g/dL is obtained. Her first eye exam shows immature vessels, zone 2, and no evidence of ROP.

EXERCISE 13

QUESTIONS

1. Should Epo be discontinued?
2. What other labs are needed at this time?

ANSWERS

1. Epo can be continued through 35 weeks' corrected gestation, or longer if infants are on significant respiratory support with hemoglobin in a range that might put them at risk for transfusion. This infant has a minimal oxygen requirement and an adequate hemoglobin.

2. Serum ferritin can serve as an indirect measure of iron sufficiency, and infants administered Epo on oral iron supplements often require additional supplementation.

CASE STUDY 8 (continued)

A serum ferritin was sent and was 87 mg/dL. Her iron dosing was increased by 50% to 8 mg/kg oral iron, and a serum ferritin repeated. At 36 weeks' corrected age she now weighs 1980 grams and is stable on room air. She has avoided transfusions and total phlebotomy losses were calculated to be 27 mL, or 35 mL/kg based on body weight. Her CBC, reticulocyte count and ferritin were measured at 36 weeks: hematocrit 34%, hemoglobin 11.8 g/dL, WBC 11.4 × $10^3/\mu L$, platelets 110 × $10^3/\mu L$, MCV 98 fL, RBC 3.09 × $10^6/\mu L$, retic count 7.6%, and ferritin 114 mg/dL.

EXERCISE 14

QUESTIONS

1. What is her absolute reticulocyte count?
2. How should her Epo and vitamin supplements be managed?

ANSWERS

1. The absolute reticulocyte count can be calculated: RBC × % retic = 3.09 × $10^6/\mu L$ × 0.076 = 235 × $10^3/\mu L$, reflecting active erythropoiesis.

2. SC Epo can be discontinued, but oral iron supplements should be continued at 2 to 4 mg/kg. This can be supplied as ferrous sulfate, or in the form of an iron fortified multivitamin for this infant.

Guidelines for administering an erythrocyte transfusion differ in term and preterm infants, and differ depending on the etiology and duration of blood loss. Regardless of etiology, an infant should never be transfused based on hemoglobin alone. Factors such as heart rate, blood pressure, oxygen requirements, neurologic status, metabolic status, and hemoglobin concentration should all be considered in order to determine the immediate need for erythrocytes.

Indications for transfusions in preterm infants have been gradually changing in the past decade, primarily owing to clinical studies of Epo administration in this population. Instituting strict transfusion guidelines has resulted in a decreased number of transfusions administered to preterm infants. Transfusion guidelines in conjunction with decreasing phlebotomy losses instituting Epo therapy form the triad of measures that have all impacted neonatal transfusion therapy. Instituting transfusion guidelines is most beneficial to preterm infants in a practical sense, because guidelines can be implemented in NICUs throughout the world, without additional cost and without obtaining new medications. An example of specific

TABLE 8-8   Transfusion Guidelines for Preterm Infants

(HCT VALUES IN %, HGB VALUES IN G/DL)

Hematocrit/ Hemoglobin	Ventilator Requirements and/or Signs	Transfusion Volume
Hct ≤30/Hgb ≤10	Infants requiring **moderate or significant mechanical ventilation** (MAP >8 cm H_2O **and** FiO_2 >40%)	15 mL/kg PRBCs over 2-4 hours
Hct 24-27/Hgb 8-9	Infants requiring **minimal mechanical ventilation** (any mechanical ventilation, or CPAP >6 cm H_2O **and** FiO_2 ≤40%)	15 mL/kg PRBCs over 2-4 hours
Hct 22-24/Hgb 7-8	Infants on supplemental oxygen who are **not requiring mechanical ventilation**, and **one or more** of the following is present: • ≥24 hours of tachycardia (HR >180) or tachypnea (RR >80) • An increased oxygen requirement from the previous 48 hours • An elevated lactate concentration (≥2.5 mEq/L) • Weight gain <10 grams/kg/day over the previous 4 days while receiving ≥110 kcal/kg/day • An increase in the episodes of apnea and bradycardia (>9 episodes in a 24-hour period or ≥2 episodes in 24 hours requiring bag-mask ventilation) while receiving therapeutic doses of methylxanthines • Undergoing significant surgery	20 mL/kg PRBCs over 2-4 hours (divide into 2 10 mL/kg volumes if fluid sensitive)
Hct ≤21/Hgb ≤7	Infants **without any signs** and an absolute reticulocyte count <100,000 cells/μL (RBC × % uncorrected reticulocytes).	20 mL/kg PRBCs over 2-4 hours (divide into 2 10 mL/kg volumes if fluid sensitive)

transfusion criteria for preterm infants is presented in Table 8-8.

Caregivers will need to determine their group's level of comfort in following specific transfusion criteria; however, general guidelines can still be used. Phlebotomy losses should be minimized to the greatest extent possible without compromising patient care. Hemoglobin or hematocrit values should be determined at birth, then followed at 1- to 4-week intervals during hospitalization (as determined by the infant's level of wellness). During the first week of life, replacing the volume of blood with an alternative isotonic colloid or crystalloid may benefit ELBW infants in maintaining adequate intravascular volume. Earlier studies have shown equivalent improvement in diminishing apnea of prematurity with volume expansion using normal saline, 5% albumin, or packed cells. Supplementation with iron as soon as possible (intravenously if available) will prevent iron deficiency and maintain adequate iron stores. Finally, optimizing nutrition and ensuring adequate vitamin and mineral supplements will improve RBC production and decrease red cell destruction, whether or not the infant is receiving Epo.

Two studies evaluating specific transfusion strategies have reported conflicting results. Bell and colleagues randomized 100 preterm infants to a liberal versus restrictive transfusion strategy (Bell et al., 2005). Those investigators reported an increase in serious ICH and PVL in those infants randomized to a lower transfusion threshold (Any grade ICH: 17/51 in the liberal transfusion group versus 14/49 in the restrictive transfusion group; Grade 4 ICH or PVL: 0/51 liberal versus 6/49 restrictive). Despite these findings, follow up at 8 to 12 years of age revealed improved magnetic resonance imaging (MRI) and developmental measures in the restrictive group. Kirpalani and colleagues randomized 451 infants to low or high threshold hemoglobin strategies (Kirpalani et al., 2006). Infants in the low threshold group (hemoglobins were allowed to drop lower before transfusion) did not have an increase in neurologic morbidities (12.6% with ultrasound-identified brain injury in the low threshold group compared to 16% in the high threshold group). Follow up of PINT study subjects showed no differences in neurodevelopmental disabilities between groups (94 of 208 low threshold, 82 of 213 high threshold), but post hoc analysis revealed a greater number of subjects with mental developmental index <80 in the restrictive group (70 of 156 low threshold, 56 of 165 high threshold) (White et al., 2009). Investigators from these two important studies have teamed up to perform a comprehensive multicenter transfusion study (TOP Trial) in order to determine 2-year neurodevelopmental

| **BOX 8-3** | **Measures to Increase Red Cell Mass and Reduce Transfusions** |

1. Discuss delayed cord clamping or cord milking with the obstetric team and document the plan in the mother's chart. The infant should be held at or below the placenta for 30 to 60 seconds prior to cord clamping. Alternatively, the cord can be milked from placenta to infant 2 to 4 times prior to clamping. Both of these procedures will increase red cell mass.
2. Initial labs can be drawn off the umbilical cord (type and screen, CBC, blood culture).
3. Initiate erythropoietin (Epo) treatment during the first day of life. Administer a subcutaneous injection of 400 units/kg Epo, or add 200 units/kg into a protein-containing intravenous (IV) solution (such as a 5% dextrose solution with 2% amino acids, or total parenteral nutrition [TPN]), to run over 4 to 24 hours.
4. Administer parenteral iron, 3 to 5 mg/kg once a week or 0.5 mg/kg/day (added to TPN or administered via IV solution over 4 to 6 hours) until the infant is tolerating adequate volume feedings, then administer oral iron at 6 mg/kg/day, along with folate and Vitamin E.
5. Use in-line blood sampling or micro sampling devices (such as the I-Stat) to decrease the volume needed for each lab.
6. Remove central lines as soon as possible.
7. Order labs judiciously (for example, avoid "blood gas every 6 hours" orders), and reconsider the need for "standard" or "routine" labs, such as weekly CBCs, daily blood gases, or daily chemistry panels.
8. Monitor phlebotomy losses daily.
9. Communicate the lowest hemoglobin or hematocrit that will be tolerated for a variety of typical clinical scenarios such as: (1) infant is on 100% oxygen, significant ventilator support, blood pressure support, and has a metabolic acidosis; (2) infant is on minimal ventilator support or CPAP; (3) infant is receiving enteral feeds and requiring oxygen; (4) infant is on full feeds, growing well, no oxygen support. Consider these scenarios when the infant is less than 2 weeks of age, 2 to 4 weeks of age, or greater than 4 weeks of age.

outcomes of infants randomized to liberal versus restrictive transfusion strategies.

When Families Oppose Transfusions

When a family has indicated they are opposed to neonatal transfusions and a premature birth is anticipated, an action plan can be created to optimize the infant's chances of avoiding transfusion. Without plans to optimize red cell mass, a majority (85% to 90%) of ELBW infants receive transfusions. However, the percentage of ELBW infants remaining untransfused can be improved to 40% to 50%, through the use of such measures as delayed cord clamping or cord milking, using umbilical cord blood for initial labs, immediate red cell growth factor and iron therapy, judicious laboratory testing using micro sampling, and a restrictive transfusion policy. These measures can be identified and a plan created prenatally with the family, allowing the neonatologists to establish a relationship with the family and discuss their NICU transfusion thresholds and minimize the need for last-minute court orders to transfuse. Box 8-3 summarizes these measures. Evidence that a specific transfusion will be "lifesaving" is difficult to identify unless it is administered in response to a significant acute hemorrhage. Stable ELBW infants with an initially normal hemoglobin will often tolerate a gradual decrease in hemoglobin (in the range of 0.25 to 0.4 g/dL/day), and transfusing based on hemoglobin alone is not warranted. Currently there is no definitive evidence

to suggest that neurodevelopmental outcomes will improve when transfusions are administered at any specific hemoglobin trigger. In fact, there is retrospective evidence that morbidities specific to preterm infants (such as worsening ICH or the development of NEC) might occur following transfusion. Both of these associations need further study in prospective, randomized controlled trials in order to identify a causal relationship.

DIFFERENTIAL DIAGNOSIS AND MANAGEMENT OF ANEMIA

The diagnosis of anemia in the newborn period often requires rapid investigation and laboratory evaluation. Infants presenting in shock from their anemia have most likely suffered massive hemorrhage, and patient stabilization is of utmost importance to avoid organ damage and death. The "ABCs" of newborn resuscitation should be followed. Once the infant is stable, information can be gathered to help determine the cause of anemia and determine a treatment plan. If circulation has been restored and cardiac output optimized, there is really only one management choice for an infant requiring an immediate need for increased oxygen delivery to tissues, and that is to administer a red cell transfusion. If the infant is not in need of immediate increase in oxygen delivery to tissues, treatment options can be considered.

One example of a diagnostic and management approach to anemia is shown in Figure 8-5.

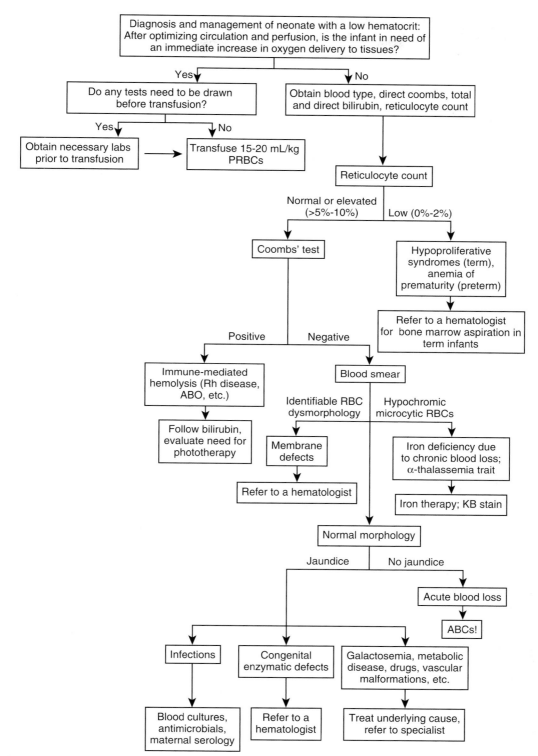

FIGURE 8-5 ■ Diagnostic approach to an infant with abnormal hematocrit. *KB stain,* Kleihauer-Betke stain; *RBC,* red blood cell.

A thorough maternal history should be obtained, and should include information on vaginal bleeding, trauma, infection or exposure to infected individuals, and any prescribed or nonprescribed drug use (including herbs or dietary supplements) during the pregnancy. The timing of presentation of anemia is important to note. Infants with significant acute blood loss before or during delivery may be anemic and hypovolemic at birth, whereas infants with chronic FMH, TTS, or hemolysis from isoimmunization may not be symptomatic for 24 to 48 hours. Infants with internal trauma and hemorrhage (adrenal, renal, splenic, or hepatic) may not become symptomatic for 48 to 72 hours, then may rapidly decompensate. The initial laboratory evaluation of the anemic infant includes a CBC with RBC indices and peripheral smear, a reticulocyte count, a direct Coombs test, and a bilirubin if jaundice is evident. In addition a KB stain of maternal blood is helpful in identifying fetal cells in the maternal circulation. With minimal lab tests, a thorough history, and a physical exam, most causes of anemia in the newborn period can be determined.

A working knowledge of the various therapies is required in order to determine the best treatment strategy for each infant. Would the infant benefit from specific growth factors, such as Epo or darbepoetin in order to increase red cell mass, or other growth factors such as GM-CSF or stem cell factor? Does s/he require nutritional support with iron, vitamin E, folate, or B_{12}? Will the infant require repeated erythrocyte transfusions and therefore be at increased risk for iron overload? Are steroids or IVIG indicated? Will a bone marrow transplant give the infant the best chance for long-term survival? Although a few infants with anemia presenting in the newborn period go undiagnosed despite vigorous evaluation, most newborn anemias can be diagnosed and treated successfully.

Acknowledgments

I wish to thank Cynthia Suniga for her assistance in manuscript preparation and Bob Jordan for his review and guidance regarding families who oppose transfusions.

SUGGESTED READINGS

Abkowitz JL, Sabo KM, Nakamoto B, et al.: Diamond-Blackfan anemia: in vitro response of erythroid progenitors to the ligand for c-kit, *Blood* 78(9):2198–2202, 1991.

Alter BP: Fanconi's anaemia and its variability, *Br J Haematol* 85(1):9–14, 1993.

Baer VL, Lambert DK, Henry E, Snow GL, Christensen RD: Red blood cell transfusion of preterm neonates with a Grade 1 intraventricular hemorrhage is associated with extension to a Grade 3 or 4 hemorrhage, *Transfusion* 51:1933–1999, 2011.

Bechensteen AG, Hågå P, Halvorsen S, et al.: Erythropoietin, protein, and iron supplementation and the prevention of anaemia of prematurity, *Arch Dis Child* 69:19–23, 1993.

Bell EF, Strauss RG, Widness JA, et al.: Liberal versus restrictive guidelines for red blood cell transfusion in preterm infants, *Pediatrics* 115:1685, 2005.

Benirschke K: Obstetrically important lesions of the umbilical cord, *J Reprod Med* 39(4):262–272, 1994.

Berkowitz K, Baxi L, Fox HE: False-negative syphilis screening: the prozone phenomenon, nonimmune hydrops, and diagnosis of syphilis during pregnancy, *Am J Obstet Gynecol* 163(3):975–977, 1990.

Bifano EM, Smith F, Borer J: Relationship between determinants of oxygen delivery and respiratory abnormalities in preterm infants with anemia, *J Pediatr* 120:292–296, 1992.

Bohler T, et al.: Mechanical fragility of erythrocyte membrane in neonates and adults, *Pediatr Res* 32:92–96, 1992.

Brown KE, Young NS: Parvovirus B19 infection and hematopoiesis, *Blood Rev* 9:176–182, 1995.

Bussel JB: Immune thrombocytopenia in pregnancy: autoimmune and alloimmune, *J Reprod Immunol* 37(1):35–61, 1997.

Bussel JB, Zabusky MR, Berkowitz RL, et al.: Fetal alloimmune thrombocytopenia, *N Engl J Med* 337(1):22–26, 1997.

Chadwick LM, Pemberton PJ, Kurinczuk JJ: Neonatal subgaleal haematoma: associated risk factors, complications and outcome, *J Paediatr Child Health* 32(3):228–232, 1996.

Charles JM, Key LL: Developmental spectrum of children with congenital osteopetrosis, *J Pediatr* 132(2):371–374, 1998.

Christensen RD: Association between red blood cell transfusions and necrotizing enterocolitis, *J Pediatr* 158:349–350, 2011.

Christensen RD, Lambert DK, Baer VL, et al.: Postponing or eliminating red blood cell transfusions of very low birth weight neonates by obtaining all baseline laboratory blood tests from otherwise discarded fetal blood in the placenta, *Transfusion* 51:253–258, 2011.

Church MW, Crossland WJ, Holmes PA, et al.: Effects of prenatal cocaine on hearing, vision, growth, and behavior, *Ann N Y Acad Sci* 846:12–28, 1998.

Crowther C, Middleton P: Anti-D administration after childbirth for preventing Rhesus alloimmunisation, *Cochrane Database Syst Rev* (2):CD000021, 2000.

Davis LE, Widness JA, Brace RA: Renal and placental secretion of erythropoietin during anemia or hypoxia in the ovine fetus, *Am J Obstet Gynecol* 189:1764–1770, 2003.

Deans A, Jauniaux E: Prenatal diagnosis and outcome of subamniotic hematomas, *Ultrasound Obstet Gynecol* 11:319–323, 1998.

Dennis LG, Winkler CL: Twin-to-twin transfusion syndrome: aggressive therapeutic amniocentesis, *Am J Obstet Gynecol* 177(2):342–347, 1997.

Dianzani I, Garelli E, Crescenzio N, et al.: Diamond-Blackfan anemia: expansion of erythroid progenitors in vitro by IL-9, but exclusion of a significant pathogenetic role for the IL-9 gene and the hematopoietic gene cluster on chromosome 5q, *Exp Hematol* 25(12):1270–1277, 1997.

Dianzani I, Garelli E, Ramenghi U: Diamond-Blackfan anemia: a congenital defect in erythropoiesis, *Haematologica* 81(6):560–572, 1996.

Dror Y, Donadieu J, Koglmeier J, et al.: Draft consensus guidelines for diagnosis and treatment of Shwachman-Diamond syndrome, *Ann N Y Acad Sci* 1242:40–55, 2011.

Erslev AJ, Wilson J, Caro J: Erythropoietin titers in anemic, nonuremic patients, *J Lab Clin Med* 109:429–433, 1987.

Felc Z: Ultrasound in screening for neonatal adrenal hemorrhage, *Am J Perinatol* 12(5):363–636, 1995.

Friel AK, Andrews WL, Hall MS, et al.: Intravenous iron administration to very-low-birth-weight newborns receiving total and partial parenteral nutrition, *J Parenteral Enteral Nutr* 19:114–118, 1995.

Gallagher PG, Ehrenkranz RA: Nutritional anemias in infancy, *Clin Perinatol* 22:671–692, 1995.

Geifman-Holtzman O, Wojtowycz M, Kosmos E, et al.: Female alloimmunization with antibodies known to cause hemolytic disease, *Obstet Gynecol* 89:272–275, 1997.

Gerritsen EJ, Vossen JM, van Loo IH, et al.: Autosomal recessive osteopetrosis: variability of findings at diagnosis and during the natural course, *Pediatrics* 93(2):247–253, 1994.

Gojic V, van't Veer-Korthof ET, Bosch LJ, et al.: Congenital hypoplastic anemia: another example of autosomal dominant transmission, *Am J Med Genet* 50(1):87–89, 1994.

Izraeli S, Ben-Sira L, Harell D, et al.: Lactic acid as a predictor for erythrocyte transfusion in healthy preterm infants with the anemia of prematurity, *J Pediatr* 122:629–631, 1993.

Jopling J, Henry E, Wiedmeier SE, Christensen RD: Reference ranges for hematocrit and blood hemoglobin concentration during the neonatal period: data from a multihospital health care system, *Pediatrics* 123:e333–337, 2009.

Keyes WG, Donohue PK, Spivak JL, et al.: Assessing the need for transfusion of premature infants and the role of hematocrit, clinical signs, and erythropoietin level, *Pediatrics* 84:412–417, 1989.

Kirpalani H, Whyte R, Andersen C, et al.: The Premature Infants in Need of Transfusion Study (PINT): a randomized trial of a low versus high transfusion threshold for extremely low birth weight infants, *Pediatrics* 149:301–307, 2006.

Kleihauer E, et al.: Demonstration of fetal hemoglobin in the erythrocytes of the blood of a newborn, *Klin Wochenschr* 35:637, 1957.

Kosasa TS, Ebesugawa I, Nakayama RT, et al.: Massive fetomaternal hemorrhage preceded by decreased fetal movement and a nonreactive fetal heart rate pattern, *Obstet Gynecol* 82:711–714, 1993.

Levine Z, Sherer DM, Jacobs A, et al.: Nonimmune hydrops fetalis due to congenital syphilis associated with negative intrapartum maternal serology screening, *Am J Perinatol* 15(4):233–236, 1998.

Linderkamp O, Nelle M, Kraus M, Zilow EP: The effect of early and late cord-clamping on blood viscosity and other hemorheological parameters in full-term neonates, *Acta Paediatr* 81:745–750, 1992.

Lipitz S, Many A, Mitrani-Rosenbaum S, et al.: Obstetric outcome after RhD and Kell testing, *Hum Reprod* 13(6):1472–1475, 1998.

Lopriore E, Vandenbussche FP, Tiersma ES, et al.: Twin-to-twin transfusion syndrome: new perspectives, *J Pediatr* 127:675–680, 1995.

McLennan AC, Chitty LS, Rissik J, et al.: Prenatal diagnosis of Blackfan-Diamond syndrome: case report and review of the literature, *Prenat Diagn* 16(4):349–353, 1996.

McMahon MJ, Li R, Schenck AP, et al.: Previous cesarean birth. A risk factor for placenta previa? *J Reprod Med* 42(7):409–412, 1997.

Miller ST, Desai N, Pass KA, Rao SP: A fast hemoglobin variant on newborn screening is associated with alpha-thalassemia trait, *Clin Pediatr* 36:75–78, 1997.

Moise Jr KJ, Dorman K, Lamvu G, et al.: A randomized trial of amnioreduction versus septostomy in the treatment of twin-twin transfusion syndrome, *Am J Obstet Gynecol* 193(3):701–707, 2005.

Ohls RK: Erythropoietin to prevent and treat the anemia of prematurity, *Curr Opin Pediatr* 11:108–114, 1999.

Ohls RK, Christensen RD, Kamath-Rayne BD, et al.: A randomized, masked, placebo controlled study of darbepoetin administered to preterm infants, *Pediatrics* 132:e119–127, 2013.

Ohls RK, Veerman MW, Christensen RD: Pharmacokinetics and effectiveness of recombinant erythropoietin administered to preterm infants by continuous infusion in parenteral nutrition solution, *J Pediatr* 128:518–523, 1996.

Oski FA: The erythrocyte and its disorders. In Oski FA, Nathan DG, editors: *Hematology of infancy and childhood*, Philadelphia, PA, 1993, Saunders, pp 18–43.

Pathak A, Roth P, Piscitelli J, Johnson L: Effects of vitamin E supplementation during erythropoietin treatment of the anaemia of prematurity, *Arch Dis Child Fetal Neonatal Ed* 88(4):F324–328, 2003.

Perel Y, Butenandt O, Carrere A, et al.: Oesophageal atresia, VACTERL association: Fanconi's anaemia related spectrum of anomalies, *Arch Dis Child* 78(4):375–376, 1998.

Pollak A, Hayde M, Hayn M, et al.: Effect of intravenous iron supplementation on erythropoiesis in erythropoietin-treated premature infants, *Pediatrics* 107:78–85, 2001.

Rasmussen S, Irgens LM, Bergsjo P, et al.: Perinatal mortality and case fatality after placental abruption in Norway 1967-1991, *Acta Obstet Gynecol Scand* 75(3):229–234, 1996.

Roberts D, Neilson JP, Kilby M, Gates S: Interventions for the treatment of twin-twin transfusion syndrome, *Cochrane Database Syst Rev* (1):CD002073, 2008. http://dx.doi.org/10.1002/14651858.CD002073.pub2.

Rogers BB, Bloom SL, Buchanan GR: Autosomal dominantly inherited Diamond-Blackfan anemia resulting in nonimmune hydrops, *Obstet Gynecol* 89(5, pt 2):805–807, 1997.

Senat MV, Deprest J, Boulvain M, Paupe A, Winer N, Ville Y: Endoscopic laser surgery versus serial amnioreduction for severe twin-to-twin transfusion syndrome, *N Engl J Med* 351(2):136–144, 2004.

Shalev H, Tamary H, Shaft D, et al.: Neonatal manifestations of congenital dyserythropoietic anemia type I, *J Pediatr* 131(1, pt 1):95–97, 1997.

Sieff C, Guinan E: In vitro enhancement of erythropoiesis by steel factor in Diamond-Blackfan anemia and treatment of other congenital cytopenias with recombinant interleukin 3/granulocyte-macrophage colony stimulating factor, *Stem Cells* 11:113–122, 1993.

Stahl MM, Neiderud J, Vinge E: Thrombocytopenic purpura and anemia in a breast-fed infant whose mother was treated with valproic acid, *J Pediatr* 130:1001–1003, 1997.

Teng FY, Sayre JW: Vacuum extraction: does duration predict scalp injury? *Obstet Gynecol* 89(2):281–285, 1997.

Thorp JA, Poskin MF, McKenzie DR, et al.: Perinatal factors predicting severe intracranial hemorrhage, *Am J Perinatol* 14:631–636, 1997.

Toivanen B, Hirvonen T: Iso- and heteroagglutinins in human fetal and neonatal sera, *Scand J Haematol* 6:42, 1969.

Van Dijk BA, Dooren MC, Overbeeke MA: Red cell antibodies in pregnancy: there is no 'critical titre', *Transfus Med* 5(3):199–202, 1995.

Van Heteren CF, Nijhuis JG, Semmekrot BA, et al.: Risk for surviving twin after fetal death of co-twin in twin-twin transfusion syndrome, *Obstet Gynecol* 92(2):215–219, 1998.

Vaughan JI, Manning M, Warwick RM, et al.: Inhibition of erythroid progenitor cells by anti-Kell antibodies in fetal alloimmune anemia, *N Engl J Med* 338:798–803, 1998.

Verma U, Tejani N, Klein S, et al.: Obstetric antecedents of intraventricular hemorrhage and periventricular leukomalacia in the low-birth-weight neonate, *Am J Obstet Gynecol* 176:275–281, 1997.

Vogel H, Kornman M, Ledet SC, et al.: Congenital parvovirus infection, *Pediatr Pathol Lab Med* 17(6):903–912, 1997.

Wardrop CA, Holland BM: The roles and vital importance of placental blood to the newborn infant, *J Perinat Med* 23:139–143, 1995.

Weiner CP, Widness JA: Decreased fetal erythropoiesis and hemolysis in Kell hemolytic anemia, *Am J Obstet Gynecol* 174:547–551, 1996.

Whyte RK, Kirpalani H, Asztalos EV, et al.: PINTOS Study Group. Neurodevelopmental outcome of extremely low birth weight infants randomly assigned to restrictive or liberal hemoglobin thresholds for blood transfusion, *Pediatrics* 123:207–213, 2009.

Zinkham WH, Oski FA: Henna: a potential cause of oxidative hemolysis and neonatal hyperbilirubinemia, *Pediatrics* 97:707–709, 1996.

CHAPTER 9

RESPIRATORY DISTRESS SYNDROME

Alain Cuna, MD • **Waldemar A. Carlo, MD**

Respiratory distress syndrome (RDS) is a common lung disorder that mostly affects preterm infants. RDS is caused by insufficient surfactant production and structural immaturity of the lungs leading to alveolar collapse. Clinically, RDS presents soon after birth with tachypnea, nasal flaring, grunting, retractions, hypercapnia, and/or an oxygen need. If untreated, the natural history of RDS is clinical worsening followed by recovery in 3 to 5 days as adequate surfactant production occurs. Research in the prevention and treatment of this disease has led to major improvements in the care of preterm infants with RDS and increased survival. However, RDS remains an important cause of morbidity and mortality especially in the most immature infants. This chapter reviews the most current evidence-based management of RDS, including prevention, delivery room stabilization, respiratory management, and supportive care.

CASE STUDY 1

A 30-year-old gravida 2, para 1 mother presents to the local community hospital at 25 weeks' gestation because of leaking vaginal fluid and menstrual-like cramping since earlier that day. Her past medical history is pertinent for gestational diabetes and chronic hypertension. She also had a previous preterm delivery at 27 weeks' gestation.

EXERCISE 1

QUESTIONS

1. Which of the following is the highest risk factor that predisposes this infant to develop respiratory distress syndrome (RDS)?
   a. Prematurity
   b. Premature rupture of membranes
   c. Preterm labor
   d. Maternal diabetes
   e. Maternal hypertension

2. What prenatal interventions will have a large effect on preventing or reducing the severity of RDS in this case?
   a. Tocolytic therapy
   b. Antenatal steroids
   c. Antibiotic therapy
   d. a and b
   e. a, b, and c

ANSWERS

1. **a**.

2. **b**.

RISK FACTORS AND PATHOPHYSIOLOGY OF RDS

Prematurity is the main risk factor for RDS. Other risk factors associated with RDS include maternal diabetes, multiple gestation, elective cesarean delivery without labor, Caucasian race, male sex, precipitous delivery, and perinatal asphyxia. Factors associated with decreased risk for RDS include chronic hypertension, preeclampsia, chorioamnionitis, and prolonged rupture of membranes.

This preterm infant was born during the late canalicular to early saccular stage of lung development, which corresponds to the period when respiratory bronchioles capable of gas exchange and type II alveolar cells capable of surfactant production are just beginning to develop (Burri, 1984). The combination of immature airways and inadequate surfactant production prevents preterm lungs from maintaining an adequate functional residual capacity (FRC), leading to alveolar atelectasis, hypoventilation, and ventilation–perfusion mismatch.

EFFECTIVE PRENATAL CARE FOR DECREASING RDS

Prevention of Preterm Delivery

An effective way of decreasing the risk and severity of RDS is prevention of preterm delivery. However, therapies for prevention of preterm birth have limited effectiveness. Mothers at risk for preterm delivery should be closely managed as high-risk pregnancies. Risk factors for preterm delivery include previous preterm delivery, short cervix, history of certain surgical procedures on the uterus or cervix, multiple gestation, smoking, substance abuse, and poor nutrition. Care should also be exercised in performing elective caesarean delivery without labor for late preterm infants (34 to 36 weeks' gestation) because the risk of RDS is increased in this population compared to term infants (Ramachandrappa & Jain, 2008).

Antenatal Steroids for Pharmacologic Acceleration of Fetal Lung Maturity

For mothers who go into preterm labor and are at risk for preterm delivery, several interventions are available to decrease the risk for RDS. The most studied and most effective intervention is administration of antenatal corticosteroids. Corticosteroids given during pregnancy cross the placenta and promote accelerated maturity of the fetal lung. The most recent Cochrane metaanalysis of antenatal steroids for fetal acceleration of lung maturity showed that antenatal steroids significantly reduce the incidence of RDS (RR 0.66, 95% CI 0.59-0.73) as well as overall neonatal mortality in preterm infants (RR 0.69, 95% CI 0.58-0.81) (Roberts & Dalziel, 2006). Other benefits include decreased incidences of intraventricular hemorrhage (RR 0.54, 95% CI 0.43-0.69), necrotizing enterocolitis (RR 0.46, 95% CI 0.29-0.74), early onset sepsis (RR 0.56, 95% CI 0.38-0.85), and developmental delay (RR 0.49, 95% CI 0.24-1.00) without an increased risk of maternal infection or death. Current recommendations call for administration of antenatal steroids to women between 24 and 34 weeks of gestation who are at risk of preterm delivery. However, a recent large prospective multicenter cohort study showed that antenatal steroids also benefit preterm infants born as early as 23 weeks' gestation, with decreased death (OR 0.49, 95% CI 0.39-0.61), severe intraventricular hemorrhage (OR 0.59, 95% CI 0.40-0.87), and death or neurodevelopmental impairment at 18 to 22 months (OR 0.58, 95% CI 0.42-0.80).

Thus, antenatal steroids should be considered for infants who may be born as early as 23 weeks' gestation (Carlo et al., 2011).

Transfer to Tertiary Facility

Transfer to a facility with proper equipment and skilled personnel experienced in taking care of preterm infants is important. Survival and long-term outcomes are better for infants born in referral centers (Phibbs et al., 2007; Lasswell et al., 2010).

Tocolytic Therapy

Although tocolytic therapy to delay preterm delivery have not been shown to improve neonatal outcomes, short-term use may be considered to allow completion of antenatal corticosteroids as well as transfer of the mother to a tertiary facility (Haas et al., 2012). Among the available drugs for tocolysis, indomethacin compared to placebo provides the highest probability of delivery being delayed by 48 hours (OR 5.39, 95% CI 2.14 to 12.34). However, some observational studies have raised concern that indomethacin tocolysis is associated with increased incidences of necrotizing enterocolitis (NEC), patent ductus arteriosus (PDA), and intraventricular hemorrhage (IVH) (Doyle et al., 2005; Sood et al., 2011). Magnesium sulfate is another tocolytic agent that is effective in delaying preterm delivery by >48 hours and has the added benefit of reducing the incidence of cerebral palsy (Doyle et al., 2009).

Fetal Surveillance

Close monitoring of a fetus at risk for preterm delivery is also essential because perinatal asphyxia is associated with an increased incidence and severity of RDS. Tools for antepartum surveillance of fetal well-being include nonstress test, contraction stress test, biophysical profile, and Doppler velocimetry of fetal umbilical artery blood flow. During labor, continuous electronic fetal heart rate (HR) monitoring and fetal scalp pH analysis are used to determine how well the fetus is tolerating labor.

CASE STUDY 2

A 22-year-old woman was transferred to the regional perinatal center because of preterm labor at 24 weeks' gestation after receiving a dose of betamethasone as well as magnesium sulfate. Upon admission to the labor and delivery floor, her cervix was noted to be 3 cm dilated. Magnesium sulfate was continued, and she was able to receive the second dose of betamethasone. However, she continued to have uterine contractions with progressive cervical dilation. The neonatal intensive care unit (NICU) team was called and preparations were made for the imminent vaginal delivery of a preterm infant at 24 weeks' gestation.

EXERCISE 2

QUESTION

1. Which of the following are appropriate delivery room stabilization measures for this 24-week preterm infant?
   a. Delayed cord clamping
   b. Use of radiant warmer, preheated blankets, and hat
   c. Placing infant inside plastic bag without drying
   d. a and b
   e. a, b, and c

ANSWER

1. **e**.

DELIVERY ROOM STABILIZATION

Optimal delivery room resuscitation is important in decreasing neonatal morbidity and mortality including RDS. The most recent guidelines on neonatal resuscitation released by the American Heart Association, the European Resuscitation Council, and the International Liaison Committee on Resuscitation for delivery room stabilization should be followed (Kattwinkel et al., 2010).

Delayed Cord Clamping

Delayed clamping of the umbilical cord following delivery allows for blood flow from the placenta to the infant to continue, resulting in an increase in blood volume, which may in turn improve outcomes for preterm infants. A Cochrane metaanalysis of randomized controlled trials (15 studies, 738 infants) of early versus delayed cord clamping in preterm infants showed that delayed cord clamping decreases blood transfusions for anemia (RR 0.61, 95% CI 0.46-0.81), IVH (RR 0.59, 95% CI 0.41-0.85), and NEC (RR 0.62, 95% CI 0.43-0.90) (Rabe et al., 2012).

Thermoregulation

Thermoregulation is important during the first days after birth because both hypothermia and hyperthermia are associated with increased neonatal morbidity and mortality (McCall et al., 2010).

In preparing for the delivery of a preterm infant, the delivery room temperature should be set at 26 to 28° C (79 to 82° F) and the radiant warmer turned on to maximum power (Kent et al., 2008). Warm blankets and a hat should also be available. For preterm infants less than 32 weeks' gestation, additional interventions are recommended to prevent hypothermia. Placing the preterm infant immediately in a plastic bag without drying decreases evaporative heat loss, while still allowing delivery of heat from the radiant warmer (Vohra et al., 2004). An additional exothermic mattress may also be used (Singh et al., 2010), but caution should be exercised because its combined use with the other interventions above may increase the risk of hyperthermia (McCarthy et al., 2012). The overall goal is to maintain normal body temperature and avoid both hypothermia and hyperthermia.

Ventilation

The most important step in newborn stabilization at birth is establishment of effective ventilation. Due to their immature airways and surfactant deficiency, preterm infants have difficulty in preventing alveolar collapse and establishing an adequate FRC. Preterm infants frequently need support to establish adequate ventilation. A quick assessment of an infant's need for respiratory support requires evaluation of the HR and respiratory effort. If the HR is less than 100 beats per minute or if the infant is apneic or gasping, positive pressure ventilation using a bag-mask or T-piece is needed. Care should be exercised with the inflation pressures because use of excessive tidal volumes is associated with lung injury (Hillman et al., 2007). Inadequate pressure administration leads to ineffective ventilation and is also harmful. Typically, applied inflation pressures can be lowered quickly following establishment of adequate FRC.

Oxygenation

Optimal management of oxygenation is also important as both inadequate and excessive oxygenation are potentially harmful to newborn infants. Metaanalyses of trials show that resuscitation with 100% oxygen increased mortality compared to room air resuscitation in term and late-preterm babies (Saugstad et al., 2008). Though few studies have been performed in preterm infants, there is evidence that 100% oxygen is not needed for resuscitation of most preterm infants. Thus, current guidelines recommend titrating supplemental oxygen using a blender to target the normal gradual increase in oxygen saturations following birth (80% to 85% at 5 minutes, >85% at 10 minutes) (Kamlin et al., 2006).

CASE STUDY 3

A preterm male infant at 25 weeks' gestation was delivered vaginally. After 60 seconds of delayed cord clamping, he was received in a warm blanket and immediately placed under a radiant warmer and inside a plastic bag without drying. A quick assessment revealed poor respiratory effort and HR <100 despite gentle stimulation. Positive pressure ventilation was initiated using a bag-mask device with appropriate pressures, and a pulse oximeter was placed on his right hand to allow targeted administration of oxygen. At 3 minutes, he had spontaneous breathing with a HR >100 beats per minute.

EXERCISE 3

QUESTION

1. Which of the following is the most appropriate next step in the management of this infant?
   a. Continue positive pressure ventilation via bag-mask device
   b. Intubate and administer surfactant
   c. Provide continuous positive airway pressure (CPAP)

ANSWER

1. **c**.

INTUBATION AND SURFACTANT ADMINISTRATION VERSUS CPAP INITIATED AT BIRTH

Surfactant therapy is one of the major advances in neonatology that has significantly improved the outcomes of preterm infants. Following determination that surfactant therapy was effective in the treatment of established RDS, a number of clinical trials were designed to determine the optimal timing of surfactant therapy. Strategies for timing of surfactant include prophylactic and selective therapy (in babies with established RDS). In prophylactic therapy, surfactant is routinely administered at birth to prevent at-risk preterm infants from developing RDS; whereas in selective therapy, surfactant is administered as treatment once the infant has symptomatic evidence of RDS.

In early clinical trials comparing prophylactic with selective surfactant therapy, prophylactic surfactant therapy led to better outcomes including decreased air leak syndromes and mortality (Soll & Morley, 2001). These trials led to the widespread

practice of routine intubation and surfactant administration in the delivery room. These first surfactant trials were done at a time when CPAP for stabilization in the delivery room was not widely practiced. However, it is now known that intubation and ventilation of preterm infants without surfactant administration can result in lung injury. Thus, the control groups in the surfactant trials may have been exposed to an injurious ventilation strategy. Subsequently, multiple observational studies and small, randomized controlled trials have demonstrated the benefits of CPAP instead of intubation and surfactant administration.

Recent large trials reflecting the current practice of early stabilization with CPAP have demonstrated that early CPAP with later selective surfactant therapy actually leads to better outcomes when compared to prophylactic therapy, including decreased mortality and risk of bronchopulmonary dysplasia (BPD) at 36 weeks (Rojas-Reyes, Morley, & Soll, 2012). The largest trial to date—the Surfactant, Positive Pressure, and Pulse Oximetry Randomized Trial (SUPPORT) conducted by the National Institute of Child Health and Human Development (NICHD) Neonatal Research Network—enrolled 1316 preterm infants between 24 to 27⅞ weeks and showed that early CPAP administration initiated in the delivery room resulted in decreased mortality among 24 to 25 weeks' gestation infants (RR 0.74, 95% CI 0.57,0.98, p = 0.03). In infants 24 to 27 weeks' gestation there was a trend toward decreased death or BPD at 36 weeks (RR 0.91, 95% CI 0.83, 1.01, p = 0.07) (Finer et al., 2010).

A similar trial by the Vermont Oxford Network Delivery Room Management Trial (VON DRM Trial) also tested the strategy of CPAP application with delayed surfactant administration (Dunn et al., 2011). The metaanalysis of these two trials showed that prophylactic administration of surfactant compared with stabilization with CPAP and selective surfactant administration resulted in a higher risk of death or BPD (RR 1.12, 95% CI, 1.02-1.24, p<0.05).

Thus, the most current evidence supports the strategy of early CPAP, initiated at birth, with rescue surfactant therapy if indicated (Committee on Fetus and Newborn [COFN], 2014). That strategy appears to be superior to prophylactic intubation, surfactant administration, and ventilation in preterm infants.

CASE STUDY 4

A 27-week female infant was delivered vaginally owing to preterm labor. At birth, she had spontaneous breathing with a HR >100. She was supported by early application of CPAP, and oxygen was titrated to target oxygen saturations. By 10 minutes, she was on 40% oxygen to keep oxygen saturations above 85%. Upon admission to the NICU, her oxygen saturations are now 99% on CPAP at 40% oxygen.

EXERCISE 4

QUESTION

1. What target oxygen saturation range would you select for this infant?
   a. 85 to 95%
   b. 85 to 89%
   c. 91 to 95%
   d. 96 to 99%

ANSWER

1. **c**.

OXYGENATION TARGETS

Supplemental oxygen is an important therapy in neonatal care that is known to have important benefits but can also cause serious harm. A Cochrane metaanalysis in 2009 of restricted versus liberal oxygen exposure concluded that there was insufficient data to determine the optimal target range for maintaining blood oxygen levels in preterm infants (Askie, Henderson-Smart, & Ko, 2009). Since then, several large multicenter randomized trials assessed the effect of targeting lower oxygen saturations (85% to 89%) versus higher oxygen saturations (91% to 95%) on neonatal outcomes.

In the SUPPORT trial, targeting lower oxygen saturations of 85% to 89% decreased severe ROP but increased the risk of mortality (Carlo et al., 2010). A similar study, the Benefits of Oxygen Saturation Targeting (BOOST) II trial, also compared the effects of lower versus higher target oxygen saturation ranges (Stenson et al., 2013). This study was stopped before enrollment was completed because the interim analysis showed that, similar to SUPPORT, targeting lower oxygen saturations led to a significant increased risk of mortality. In contrast, the Canadian Oxygen Trial (COT) showed only a trend for increased death in infants randomized to the lower oxygen saturation group (Schmidt et al., 2013). Targeting lower oxygen saturations decreased severe ROP but did not reduce blindness in infants. Based on the current best evidence, it appears prudent to target higher oxygen saturations (90% to 95%) for preterm infants receiving supplemental oxygen therapy.

CASE STUDY 5

A preterm infant born at 27 weeks' gestation with birth weight of 900 grams is admitted to the NICU on nasal CPAP. His initial chest x-ray demonstrated low lung volumes with air bronchograms and a fine granular lung pattern. Over the past hour his work of breathing has increased and his oxygen requirement has risen from 30% to 60% to maintain oxygen saturation values between 90% and 95%. The arterial blood gas shows pH of 7.15, P_{CO_2} of 76 mmHg, P_{O_2} of 35 mmHg, and HCO_3 of 14 mEq/L.

EXERCISE 5

QUESTIONS

1. Which of the following is the next step in the management of this infant?
   a. Continue on CPAP.
   b. Switch to high flow nasal cannula.
   c. Intubate and administer surfactant.
   d. Briefly administer positive pressure ventilation via bag-mask device then place back on CPAP.

2. Which of the following statements is true regarding surfactant?
   a. Synthetic surfactant is superior to natural surfactant.
   b. A single dose of surfactant is as effective as multiple doses of surfactant.
   c. Earlier administration of surfactant therapy is superior to late surfactant therapy.

ANSWERS

1. **c**.

2. **c**.

INDICATIONS FOR INTUBATION AND SURFACTANT ADMINISTRATION

Although early initiation of CPAP at birth is a safe and effective form of respiratory support for preterm infants with RDS, CPAP does not completely eliminate the need for intubation, surfactant administration, and mechanical ventilation. Indeed, the majority of extremely preterm infants eventually require intubation and subsequent mechanical ventilation. At birth, indications for intubation and assisted ventilation should follow current guidelines from the Neonatal Resuscitation Program (NRP). For spontaneously breathing extremely preterm infants, CPAP should be administered initially, and their respiratory status followed closely. Infants with continued worsening blood gases despite CPAP application should be intubated for surfactant administration and assisted ventilation. In the SUPPORT trial, the criteria for intubation for an infant on CPAP included the following: (1) FiO_2 >50% to meet target oxygen saturations, (2) $PaCO_2$ >65 mmHg, or (3) hemodynamic instability (poor perfusion, low blood pressure). In more mature preterm infants (birthweight ≥1250 grams) with mild to moderate RDS, intubation and early surfactant do not improve outcomes (Escobedo et al., 2004).

SURFACTANT THERAPY

Surfactant therapy is one of the most important advances in neonatal care that has significantly reduced mortality of preterm infants with RDS. Numerous clinical trials have shown that surfactant therapy decreases mortality, air leak syndromes, and the combined outcome of BPD or death in treated infants (Seger & Soll, 2009). Subsequently, many randomized clinical trials have been completed to delineate optimal treatment strategies, including the type of surfactant, dose of surfactant, route of administration, and timing of therapy.

Type of Surfactant: Natural Versus Synthetic

The two main types of surfactant are synthetic (protein-free) and natural (derived from animal lungs and containing proteins). A Cochrane review of randomized clinical trials comparing use of natural versus synthetic surfactant shows that treatment with natural surfactants results in faster reduction of inspired oxygen and ventilator pressures and, more importantly, natural surfactants result in fewer deaths and fewer pneumothoraces than protein-free surfactants (Soll & Blanco, 2001).

A new generation of synthetic surfactant that has surfactant protein analogues has become available, with Lucinactant receiving U.S. Food and Drug Administration (FDA) approval in 2012. Results of studies comparing Lucinactant with animal-derived natural surfactants demonstrated equivalent clinical outcomes (Pfister, Soll, & Wiswell, 2007).

Dosing of Surfactant: Single Versus Multiple

A single dose versus multiple doses of surfactant has been studied in randomized clinical trials, and a Cochrane metaanalysis showed that treatment with multiple doses of surfactant reduced

pneumothoraces. Furthermore, there was a trend to reduced mortality in treated infants. Studies of higher versus lower dose of surfactant of poractant alfa showed that a dose of 200 mg/kg versus 100 mg/kg resulted in better oxygenation, less need for repeat doses, and fewer deaths in treated infants (Cogo et al., 2009; Singh, Hawley, & Viswanathan, 2011).

Timing of Therapy: Early Versus Late

Surfactant therapy for established RDS can be classified as early (within 2 hours after birth) and late. In a Cochrane metaanalysis of trials comparing early versus late selective surfactant therapy, earlier surfactant treatment for RDS decreased air leak syndromes, death, and BPD in treated infants (Bahadue & Soll, 2012).

Method of Administration

Most clinical trials of surfactant therapy tested surfactant by bolus administration directly into the trachea via an endotracheal tube, followed by a variable period of mechanical ventilation until low ventilator settings were achieved and extubation was attempted. Because of concerns of lung injury from prolonged mechanical ventilation, trials have been conducted to evaluate a different approach that involves intubation, early surfactant administration, and *brief* ventilation (less than 1 hour) followed by prompt extubation of the infant to nasal CPAP. This technique, also known as INSURE (INtubate – SURfactant – Extubate to CPAP), has been shown in randomized trials to result in decreased mechanical ventilation, air leak syndromes, and BPD in treated infants (Stevens et al., 2007; Rojas et al., 2009).

Another method of surfactant administration that avoids intubation and mechanical ventilation is the delivery of surfactant via a thin catheter temporarily placed in the trachea under direct visualization with laryngoscopy. A randomized multicenter trial using this novel approach compared to standard intervention demonstrated fewer days on mechanical ventilation without differences in mortality or other adverse events in treated infants (Göpel et al., 2011).

CASE STUDY 6

A preterm male infant is delivered at 29 weeks by vaginal delivery to a 30-year-old mother. Her pregnancy was complicated by preterm rupture of membranes for 3 weeks. She received 2 doses of betamethasone prior to delivery. At delivery, the infant was limp, apneic, with a HR <100 despite prolonged effective bag-mask ventilation. He was *intubated, given surfactant in the delivery room, and admitted to the NICU. On physical examination, he weighs 1100 grams and vital signs are stable. He is tachypneic with subcostal retractions and is requiring 35% oxygen to maintain his target oxygen saturations.*

EXERCISE 6

QUESTIONS

1. Which of the following are other possible causes of this infant's respiratory failure besides RDS?
   a. Pneumonia/infection
   b. Pneumothorax
   c. Congenital lung malformation
   d. Critical congenital heart disease
   e. All of the above

2. Which of the following would you include in the initial evaluation of this infant?
   a. Arterial blood gas
   b. Chest x-ray
   c. Complete blood count
   d. Blood culture
   e. All of the above

ANSWERS

1. **e**.

2. **e**.

DIFFERENTIAL DIAGNOSIS OF RDS

Though RDS is by far the most common cause of respiratory distress in preterm infants during the immediate newborn period, other diagnoses should be considered. The differential diagnosis may include pneumonia/infection, pneumothorax, persistent pulmonary hypertension of the newborn, congenital lung malformations, and critical congenital heart disease.

Pneumonia/Infection

It is difficult to distinguish RDS from pneumonia and early onset sepsis in the immediate newborn period. Signs of respiratory distress are similar between the two, and chest x-ray findings can be identical. Risk factors that are more suggestive of pneumonia and early onset sepsis include maternal fever, prolonged rupture of membranes, intrapartum antibiotic treatment for clinical chorioamnionitis, and colonization with group B *Streptococcus* (Puopolo et al., 2011). In contrast, preterm delivery owing to maternal indications, such as preeclampsia and abruptio placenta, is associated with decreased risk for pneumonia/infection. Nevertheless, it is prudent to do a screening workup for sepsis and empirically start broad-spectrum antibiotic (e.g., ampicillin and gentamicin) in an infant who presents with respiratory distress in the immediate newborn period.

Transient Tachypnea of the Newborn

Distinguishing transient tachypnea of the newborn (TTN) from RDS is important. TTN is more often seen in term or late preterm infants delivered by caesarean section without labor secondary to delay in reabsorption of fetal lung fluid. Classic signs include tachypnea, retractions, and cyanosis requiring modest oxygen supplementation. The chest x-ray typically reveals normal to high lung volumes, hazy lungs with fluid in the intralobar fissures, and occasionally pleural effusions. Infants with TTN rarely need ventilator support and recover rapidly over 1 to 4 days, usually with just supportive treatment.

Pneumothorax

Risk factors for development of pneumothorax include underlying lung diseases (such as RDS, meconium aspiration, pulmonary hypoplasia, congenital lobar emphysema) and excessive inflation pressures delivered via bag-mask, T-piece, or mechanical ventilator. Signs suggestive of a pneumothorax include respiratory distress, asymmetric chest wall movement, and decreased breath sounds on affected side. Positive bedside transillumination may identify a pneumothorax, but a chest x-ray is usually needed for definitive diagnosis.

Persistent Pulmonary Hypertension of the Newborn

During transition from fetal to postnatal life, there is rapid decline of pulmonary vascular resistance as the lungs expand with air. In persistent pulmonary hypertension of the newborn (PPHN), pulmonary vascular resistance remains elevated, hampering blood flow to the lungs and resulting in profound hypoxemia. PPHN is more often seen in term and post-term infants although preterm infants are also at risk. Predisposing factors include perinatal asphyxia, early-onset sepsis, severe RDS, and meconium aspiration syndrome. Clinical signs include differential oxygenation of preductal and postductal blood, severe cyanosis, tachypnea, grunting, flaring, retractions, and shock. In idiopathic PPHN, the chest x-ray typically shows minimal lung disease with decreased pulmonary vascular markings. The chest x-ray in infants with PPHN secondary to other disorders reflects the underlying pathology (e.g., patchy infiltrates in infants with pneumonia or meconium aspiration syndrome). The diagnosis of PPHN is made clinically and confirmed by echocardiography.

Congenital Lung Malformations

A number of congenital lung malformations may also present with respiratory distress in the newborn period, although the majority of diagnoses are now detected prenatally with ultrasound. Examples include diaphragmatic hernia, congenital cystic adenomatoid malformation, bronchopulmonary sequestration, bronchogenic cyst, and lobar emphysema. A chest x-ray is the most helpful study in ruling in or out these conditions.

Critical Congenital Heart Disease

Critical congenital heart diseases typically present with cyanosis unresponsive to oxygen with no signs of increased work of breathing, but may present with signs of left heart failure depending on the specific type of congenital heart defect. The majority of infants with critical congenital heart diseases are now detected by prenatal ultrasound; however, total anomalous pulmonary venous return with obstructed pulmonary veins is known to be difficult to detect prenatally and is also difficult to differentiate from RDS postnatally. The diagnosis is made by echocardiography, though an abnormal cardiac silhouette is present on the chest x-ray in many infants.

INITIAL DIAGNOSTIC EVALUATION IN RDS

Chest X-ray

The signs of respiratory distress are nonspecific and do not generally point to a definitive etiology. Following a thorough history and physical examination, the chest x-ray is probably the single most helpful diagnostic test and should be part of the initial evaluation of any newborn infant with respiratory symptoms. In RDS, the three characteristic radiographic features are low lung volumes, diffuse fine granular lung pattern, and air bronchograms.

Arterial Blood Gas

The results of an arterial blood gas include the pH and the partial pressures of arterial carbon dioxide ($PaCO_2$) and oxygen (PaO_2) and provide information critical to make an assessment of gas exchange. In infants with RDS, the blood gases typically show low PaO_2, high $PaCO_2$, and mixed respiratory and metabolic acidosis. The blood gas results help determine how the infant's lungs are functioning and whether more or less respiratory support is needed.

Sepsis Work-Up

Because pneumonia/sepsis and RDS present similarly in the newborn period, a sepsis workup should be included in the initial evaluation of most infants with persistent respiratory distress. This includes a complete blood count (CBC) and a blood culture. The blood culture is the gold standard for sepsis, and results should be followed until it shows no growth for at least 48 hours. In the meantime, it is prudent to treat with empiric antibiotics. Urinary tract infections are uncommon at birth and a urine culture is not indicated in the evaluation of early onset sepsis. Likewise, the incidence of meningitis is low in healthy-appearing infants or infants with RDS, and a lumbar puncture may not be necessary (Eldadah et al., 1987). However, if the blood culture is positive or if the clinical picture strongly suggests bacterial sepsis, a lumbar puncture should be performed (Polin et al., 2012).

Echocardiography

Echocardiography is reserved for infants with persistent hypoxemia despite intubation and surfactant therapy or those who have pre- and post-ductal differences in oxygenation to rule out cardiac involvement or PPHN.

CASE STUDY 7

A preterm infant born at 28 weeks and weighing 1000 grams was admitted to the NICU. She was intubated in the delivery room due to persistent poor respiratory effort and received surfactant. Upon admission, the respiratory therapist asks for ventilator settings to transfer the patient to a stable ventilation mode.

EXERCISE 7

QUESTIONS

1. Which of the following ventilator settings would you start with?
   a. Rate of 30 breaths per minute (bpm), inspiratory time of 0.8 seconds, peak inspiratory

pressure (PIP) of 20 cm H_2O with an exhaled tidal volume of 8 mL/kg

b. Rate of 50 bpm, inspiratory time of 0.3 seconds, PIP of 15 cm H_2O with an exhaled tidal volume of 4 mL/kg

2. What positive end expiratory pressure (PEEP) would you use?
   a. PEEP of 4 cm H_2O
   b. PEEP of 8 cm H_2O

3. An hour following intubation, surfactant administration, and mechanical ventilation, the repeat blood gas shows pH of 7.18, Pco_2 of 72 mmHg, Po_2 of 40 mmHg, and HCO_3 of 15 mEq/L. Current ventilator settings are rate of 50 bpm, PIP of 15 cm H_2O, inspiratory time of 0.30 seconds, and PEEP of 4 cm H_2O. Which of the following ventilator changes is the most appropriate?
   a. Increase in rate
   b. Increase in PIP
   c. Increase in PEEP
   d. Increase in inspiratory time

4. Four hours after the ventilator changes have been made, the repeat blood gas now shows a pH of 7.45, Pco_2 of 32 mmHg, Po_2 of 80 mmHg, and HCO_3 of 20 mEq/L. Current ventilator settings are rate of 70 bpm, PIP of 15 cm H_2O, inspiratory time of 0.30 seconds, and PEEP of 4 cm H_2O. Which of the following ventilator changes is most appropriate?
   a. Decrease in rate
   b. Decrease in PIP
   c. Decrease in PEEP
   d. Decrease in inspiratory time

5. At 36 hours, she remains on the ventilator with current settings as follows: rate of 15 bpm, PIP of 12 cm H_2O, PEEP of 4 cm H_2O, and Fio_2 of 30%. Her blood gas shows pH of 7.32, Pco_2 of 48 mmHg, Po_2 of 60 mmHg, and HCO_3 of 21 mEq/L. Which of the following is the most appropriate next step in her management?
   a. Maintain on mechanical ventilation
   b. Extubate to nasal cannula
   c. Extubate to nasal CPAP

ANSWERS

1. **b**.

2. **a**.

3. **a**.

4. **b**.

5. **c**.

MECHANICAL VENTILATION STRATEGIES IN RDS

Although mechanical ventilation is necessary and life-saving for many preterm infants with RDS, it is known to cause lung injury and may lead to complications including air leak syndromes and BPD. Knowledge of proper management of preterm infants on mechanical ventilation is important, with the goal of promoting adequate gas exchange while preventing or minimizing lung injury.

Low Peak Inspiratory Pressure

Inspiratory pressures used should be the lowest possible to maintain adequate gas exchange but minimize volutrauma. Adequacy of peak inspiratory pressure (PIP) or tidal volume can be determined initially by assessing chest rise, which should be minimal. Alternatively, exhaled tidal volume as measured by the ventilator may also be used, and ideally should be no more than 4 to 6 mL/kg body weight. Subsequent changes in PIP can be based on blood gases.

Moderate Positive End Expiratory Pressure

Adequate positive end expiratory pressure (PEEP) should also be used to prevent alveolar collapse, improve FRC, and enhance ventilation–perfusion matching. A PEEP of 4 to 5 cm H_2O is usually adequate to achieve this goal in infants with RDS. Low PEEP causes alveolar collapse at the end of expiration, which increases lung injury from atelectotrauma (repeated collapse and reexpansion of alveoli). High PEEP leads to overdistention of alveoli, which may decrease venous return and preload, thus decreasing cardiac output.

Fast Ventilator Rate and Short Inspiratory Time

Preterm infants with RDS tolerate fast ventilatory rates ($\geq$60 breaths per minute) because their respiratory system has low compliance and low resistance and thus a short time constant (compliance × resistance). The use of fast ventilator rates and short inspiratory times results in a decrease in air leak syndromes and a trend for lower mortality when compared to slow rates and long inspiratory times (Greenough, 2008).

Permissive Hypercapnia and Avoidance of Hypocapnia

Infants on assisted ventilation require frequent assessment of CO_2 levels with the goal of allowing permissive hypercapnia and avoiding hypocapnia. Permissive hypercapnia is a lung protective strategy aimed at reducing ventilator associated lung injury by allowing mild hypercapnia instead of targeting normocapnia. Permissive hypercapnia is part of the early CPAP strategy discussed earlier. Clinical trials of permissive hypercapnia have demonstrated that it is safe and effective, resulting in earlier extubation and a reduced need for mechanical ventilation (Ryu, Haddad, & Carlo, 2012). Avoidance of hypocapnia is likewise important, as it is associated with increased risk for BPD and periventricular leukomalacia (Erickson et al., 2002; Okumura et al., 2001).

The two main ventilator settings that control CO_2 elimination are rate and PIP/tidal volume. When P_{CO_2} is elevated, increasing the rate is preferable to increasing PIP/tidal volume to minimize lung injury. Likewise, when P_{CO_2} is low, it is preferable to wean the PIP/tidal volume first before weaning the rate.

Extubation

Rapid weaning and subsequent extubation are essential to minimize lung injury in preterm infants with RDS and may be attempted once the neonate is breathing spontaneously and is able to maintain an acceptable P_{CO_2} (<65 mmHg with a pH >7.20) while receiving minimal ventilator support (rate of ≤20 bpm, low PIP/tidal volume, and F_{iO_2} ≤50%) (Finer et al., 2010). Several strategies to facilitate extubation have been evaluated in Cochrane metaanalyses. Extubation from low ventilator rates improves the chances of a successful extubation compared to extubation from endotracheal CPAP and is recommended (Davis & Henderson-Smart, 2001). Extubation to nasal CPAP with or without augmented intermittent positive pressure ventilation is also effective in preventing extubation failure (Davis & Henderson-Smart, 2003; Davis, Lemyre, & de Paoli, 2001). Methylxanthines, such as caffeine, increase the respiratory drive and reduce extubation failure (Henderson-Smart & Davis, 2003).

CASE STUDY 8

You are called for a prenatal consult of a 31-year-old mother with preterm labor at 24 weeks' gestation. She has lost two pregnancies at gestational ages of 18 weeks and 19 weeks owing to an incompetent cervix. You talk with her about the risks and possible course of a preterm infant born at 24 week' gestation, including immature lungs and RDS. You explain the importance of antenatal steroids for acceleration of lung maturity, delivery room stabilization including CPAP, intubation with surfactant administration

and mechanical ventilation, and oxygen administration. She asks what other medications or interventions can help with her infant's lung disease.

EXERCISE 8

QUESTIONS

1. Which of the following pharmacologic adjunct(s) decrease the incidence of BPD?
   a. Vitamin A supplementation given intramuscularly to help with lung development
   b. Caffeine citrate started soon after birth to decrease apnea and facilitate extubation
   c. Inhaled nitric oxide (iNO) for preterm infants on the ventilator to improve oxygenation
   d. a and b
   e. a, b, and c

2. Besides meticulous respiratory management, which of the following non-respiratory interventions help in RDS?
   a. Servo-controlled regulation of temperature with a skin setting of 36.0° to 36.5° C
   b. Fluid intake to prevent weight loss during the first week
   c. Delaying enteral feedings until the infant is extubated
   d. All of the above

ANSWERS

1. **d**.

2. **a**.

PHARMACOLOGIC ADJUNCTS

Vitamin A

Vitamin A is a fat-soluble micronutrient important for the differentiation, orderly growth, and maintenance of respiratory epithelial cells. Preterm infants are born with low plasma vitamin A levels because fetal accretion occurs mostly in the third trimester. Preterm infants with lower levels of vitamin A are more likely to develop BPD, and clinical trials have demonstrated that vitamin A supplementation results in a modest but significant decrease in risk of BPD (Darlow & Graham, 2011). In the NICHD multicenter trial of vitamin A supplementation, the calculated number of extremely low birth weight infants who needed treatment to prevent one infant from developing BPD was only 14 to 15 (Tyson et al., 1999). The standard regimen of vitamin A supplementation (5000 international units intramuscularly given three times a week for 4 weeks) is recommended (Ambalavanan et al., 2003).

Caffeine

Methylxanthines such as caffeine are among the most commonly used drugs in neonatology. Methylxanthines are potent respiratory stimulants that reduce apnea, facilitate weaning from the ventilator, and decrease reintubation. In a large international randomized study that compared short- and long-term effects of caffeine versus placebo, preterm infants treated with caffeine had shorter duration of CPAP and mechanical ventilation and were less likely to develop BPD compared to preterm infants treated with a placebo (Schmidt, Roberts, Davis, 2006). In addition, infants treated with caffeine had better survival without increased neurodevelopmental disability (Schmidt et al., 2007).

Inhaled Nitric Oxide

Inhaled nitric oxide (iNO), a potent selective pulmonary vasodilator, is an established therapy for term and near-term infants with hypoxic respiratory failure. In term infants with PPHN, iNO improves oxygenation and reduces the need for extracorporeal membrane oxygenation. Preterm infants may also benefit from iNO by several potential mechanisms, including better matching of ventilation and perfusion, decreased need for oxygen and subsequent oxidant stress, and improved lung growth by stimulating angiogenesis and alveolarization. Because of heterogeneity, a Cochrane review of iNO for respiratory failure in preterm infants grouped clinical trials into three categories based on entry criteria: (1) routine use of iNO in intubated preterm infants, (2) early use of iNO as rescue therapy for very ill preterm infants, and (3) late use of iNO as rescue therapy in preterm infants at risk of BPD. In each of these three categories the use of iNO did not reduce mortality or BPD in preterm infants (Barrington & Finer, 2010). Thus, based on available evidence, the use of iNO is not recommended for early-routine, early-rescue, or later-rescue therapy in preterm infants who require respiratory support.

Postnatal Steroids

Inflammation is a major contributor to the progressive lung injury seen in mechanically ventilated preterm infants with RDS. Because of its powerful antiinflammatory effect, steroid use has been studied in ventilator-dependent preterm infants to prevent or treat BPD. Although randomized trials showed that postnatal steroids result in a rapid improvement in lung function, facilitate weaning from the ventilator, decrease the incidence of BPD, and reduce mortality, its use is associated with an increased risk of gastrointestinal bleeding, hypertension, hyperglycemia, and, most concerning, poor neurodevelopmental outcome. A Cochrane review of trials using early postnatal steroid therapy (≤7 days of life) concluded that benefits from early steroid therapy may not outweigh its potential adverse outcomes (Halliday, Ehrenkranz, & Doyle, 2009a). In contrast, the most recent Cochrane review of late postnatal steroids for BPD (>7 days of life), demonstrated benefits including decreased death and BPD, but without an increased risk for adverse long-term neurodevelopmental outcomes (Halliday, Ehrenkranz, & Doyle, 2009b). Based on current evidence, the American Academy of Pediatrics (AAP) admonishes clinicians to consider late postnatal steroids only for preterm infants at very high risk of developing BPD (i.e., prolonged high ventilator and oxygen support for first 1 to 2 weeks of age), using individual clinical judgment along with discussion with the parents in balancing possible risks and benefits of postnatal steroid therapy (Watterberg et al., 2010).

NON-RESPIRATORY MANAGEMENT

Thermoregulation

Preterm infants are dependent on external measures for maintaining normal body temperature because of increased radiant heat loss as well as decreased mechanisms for heat production and conservation. Following measures to maintain normothermia at birth, the preterm infant should be transported to the NICU in a heated incubator. A prewarmed incubator with humidity set at 80% should be prepared. Servo-control of the incubator temperature to maintain anterior abdominal skin temperature at 36 to 36.5° C decreases the risk of death and is recommended (Sinclair, 2002). Frequent assessment is required as technical difficulties may inadvertently lead to incorrect temperature control (i.e., skin temperature probe reads falsely low because it is displaced or falsely high because of infant/object laying over it).

Fluid Management

Preterm infants are at risk for dehydration from high insensible water loss because of thinner, more permeable skin and an inability of the immature kidney to concentrate the urine. However, liberal fluid intake in the first few days after birth may increase the risks of PDA, NEC, and BPD (Bell & Accaregui, 2008; Oh et al., 2005). Thus, careful fluid balance is important, with the goal of cautious restriction of fluid intake to meet physiologic needs without causing dehydration. Total fluid intake is initially started at 80 mL/kg/day in the first day and increased by increments of ~10 mL/kg/day to reach a goal of 120 to 140 mL/kg/day. Daily assessment of weight loss, urine output, and serum sodium levels should be used for individualized management of fluid intake. The goal is to allow gradual weight loss of about 10% to 15% of birth weight (the most immature infants have the highest percentage weight loss) over 10 days, while maintaining urine output between 1 to 3 mL/kg/day and serum sodium levels between 130 to 150 mEq/L.

Nutrition

Nutrition is an essential part of the care of any infant, especially those born prematurely. The goal is to allow for growth that mirrors intrauterine growth rates without adverse effects. Nutrition should begin immediately after birth with continuous infusion of glucose at 4 to 6 mg/kg/minute and amino acids at 1 to 2 g/kg/day. Enteral feedings should also be initiated soon after birth with trophic feeds, also called minimal enteral nutrition. Trophic feedings are generally started at a volume of ~20 mL/kg/day, preferably using human breast milk. Delaying enteral feeds to decrease risk of NEC is unfounded and is associated with increased risk for late-onset sepsis (Morgan, Bombell, & McGuire 2013; McClure & Newell, 2000).

CASE STUDY 9

A preterm infant born at 30 weeks' gestation with birth weight of 1250 grams is now 10 days old and remains on CPAP with PEEP of 5 cm H2O and FiO2 of 35%. His echocardiogram reveals a small to moderate PDA.

EXERCISE 9

QUESTION

1. Which of the following is the most appropriate next step in the management of this infant?
   a. Continued observation
   b. Indomethacin for PDA closure
   c. PDA ligation

ANSWER

1. **a**.

PATENT DUCTUS ARTERIOSUS AND RDS

In utero, the ductus arteriosus allows blood from the right ventricle to bypass the fluid-filled lungs and flow into the systemic circulation. Over the first hours or days after birth, there is usually spontaneous closure of the ductus arteriosus, especially in term infants. In preterm infants, however, the ductus arteriosus may remain open for longer periods of time. As pulmonary vascular resistance falls, shunting occurs through the PDA from the systemic to pulmonary circulation, resulting in increased pulmonary blood flow and decreased systemic blood flow. Increased pulmonary blood flow through the immature pulmonary vascular bed may lead to adverse pulmonary consequences including pulmonary edema, alteration in lung mechanics and gas exchange, and abnormal development of the pulmonary vasculature. Likewise, decreased systemic blood flow from "ductal stealing" may cause hemodynamic consequences including decreased perfusion to the kidneys, gastrointestinal tract, and the brain. Numerous studies have associated PDA with poor neonatal outcomes including worsening RDS, BPD, NEC, pulmonary hemorrhage, renal impairment, cerebral palsy, and death (Benitz, 2010).

However, randomized controlled trials of different strategies for closure of the PDA using either pharmacologic (indomethacin or ibuprofen) or surgical intervention do not show improvement in major outcomes. Although interventions were effective in closing the PDA, metaanalyses from Cochrane reviews found no evidence of any long-term benefit associated with PDA closure (Fowlie, Davis, & McGuire, 2010; Mosalli & Alfaleh, 2008; Ohlsson, Walia, & Shah, 2008). The lack of long-term benefit, the potential harm associated with interventions used for PDA closure, and the high rate of spontaneous closure have encouraged clinicians to take a more restrictive approach to pharmacologic or surgical closure of the PDA. Current evidence supports a more conservative, individualized approach to PDA closure. Infants with birth weight >1000 grams have a high rate of spontaneous closure and rarely require treatment (Nemerofsky et al., 2008). For infants with birth weight <1000 grams, the rate of spontaneous closure is decreased, and treatment may be needed for those with signs of pulmonary and hemodynamic compromise including persistent or increased ventilator support, hypotension, heart failure, or renal impairment (Koch et al., 2006). In one study, a more conservative approach to treating PDA was associated with less NEC without increased rates of death, BPD, or IVH (Jhaveri, Moon-Grady, & Clyman, 2010).

CASE STUDY 10

A 3-day-old preterm infant born at 25 weeks' gestation remains on the ventilator for RDS. She was initially managed with early CPAP in the delivery room, but subsequently required intubation and surfactant. She received three doses of surfactant and had been weaning on the ventilator when she suddenly experienced an acute deterioration in her respiratory status. On examination she is tachypneic with nasal flaring and retractions. Her oxygen saturation is 60% despite receiving 100% FiO$_2$.

EXERCISE 10

QUESTION

1. Which of the following could be causing this infants' sudden respiratory decompensation?
   a. Pneumothorax
   b. Endotracheal tube obstruction
   c. Pulmonary hemorrhage
   d. a and b
   e. a, b, and c

ANSWER

1. **e.**

COMPLICATIONS OF RDS

Pneumothorax

Pneumothorax is a common complication of preterm infants with RDS, especially in those receiving mechanical ventilation. A pneumothorax is caused by rupture of overdistended alveoli with the escaped air collecting in the pleural space. A major risk factor is severe lung disease requiring the use of high PIP, high tidal volume, high PEEP, prolonged inspiratory times, inadequate expiratory times, and high flow rates. Patient-ventilator asynchrony also increases the risk of a pneumothorax. Sudden worsening of respiratory status should always raise concern for a pneumothorax, especially in infants receiving high levels of CPAP or ventilator support. Treatment includes needle thoracentesis and/or chest tube insertion. Ventilated preterm infants with a pneumothorax who are on lower ventilator settings and receiving only moderate concentrations of inspired oxygen may also be managed expectantly without chest tube placement

(Litmanovitz & Carlo, 2008). Management strategies that decrease the risk of pneumothorax include avoidance of high PIP and PEEP, use of faster rates (≥60 bpm) and shorter inspiratory times (<0.5 seconds), prompt administration of surfactant following intubation, and rapid weaning from the ventilator (Kamlin & Davis, 2004; Greenough et al., 2008).

Pulmonary Hemorrhage

Pulmonary hemorrhage is another serious complication in preterm infants with RDS that occurs during the first days after birth when pulmonary vascular resistance falls, resulting in increased pulmonary blood flow through the PDA and an exaggerated hemorrhagic pulmonary edema. Risk factors include prematurity, mechanical ventilation, surfactant therapy, PDA, sepsis, and coagulopathy. The usual clinical picture is a ventilated preterm infant with RDS who suddenly presents with frank blood or blood-tinged secretions from the trachea, along with a marked clinical deterioration (hypoxia, hypercapnia, hypotension, and bradycardia). Treatment is mainly supportive and may include increased ventilator support, blood transfusion, inotropes for blood pressure support, correction of coagulopathy if present, and antibiotics for possible sepsis. The mortality rate is >50% and survivors have an increased risk of BPD and poor neurodevelopmental outcome.

Bronchopulmonary Dysplasia

BPD complicates the course of RDS in some preterm infants. With advances in neonatal care including the routine use of antenatal steroids, surfactant therapy, and gentler ventilation, preterm infants similar to those described in the original paper now rarely develop the classic variety of BPD. Instead, a "new" BPD characterized by arrest in alveolar lung development now affects many preterm infants with RDS and remains a major cause of morbidity and mortality. The pathogenesis of BPD is multifactorial. In addition to immature lungs, other contributing factors include antenatal infection/inflammation, mechanical ventilation, oxygen toxicity, excessive fluid administration, and poor nutrition.

CONCLUSION

The highest levels of evidence available, including meta-analysis, have been reviewed in this chapter, with focus on interventions that reduce

TABLE 9-1 **Interventions That Reduce Negative Outcomes in Preterm Infants with RDS**

Intervention	Effects	RR	95% CI
Antenatal steroids for accelerating fetal lung maturity (Roberts & Dalziel, 2006)	Reduced:		
	- Death	0.69	0.58-0.81
	- RDS	0.66	0.59-0.73
	- IVH	0.54	0.43-0.69
	- Early onset sepsis	0.56	0.38-0.85
	- NEC	0.46	0.29-0.74
Delayed vs. immediate cord clamping (Rabe et al., 2012)	Reduced:		
	- Transfusion for anemia	0.61	0.46-0.81
	- IVH	0.59	0.41-0.85
	- NEC	0.62	0.43-0.90
Surfactant for treatment of RDS (natural) (Seger & Soll, 2009)	Reduced:		
	- Death	0.68	0.57-0.82
	- Pneumothorax	0.42	0.34-0.52
	- BPD or death	0.83	0.77-0.90
Natural vs. synthetic surfactant (Soll & Blanco, 2001)	Reduced:		
	- Death	0.63	0.53-0.75
	- Pneumothorax	0.86	0.76-0.98
Multiple vs. single doses of surfactant (Soll & Ozek, 2009)	Reduced pneumothorax	0.51	0.30-0.88
	Trend towards reduced death	0.63	0.39-1.02
Early vs. delayed surfactant (Bahadue & Soll, 2012)	Reduced:		
	- Death	0.84	0.74-0.95
	- BPD	0.69	0.55-0.86
	- BPD or death	0.83	0.75-0.94
	- Pneumothorax	0.69	0.59-0.82
Faster ventilator rate (≥60 bpm) vs. slower ventilator rate (<60 bpm) (Greenough et al., 2008)	Reduced pneumothorax	0.69	0.51-0.93
Vitamin A (Darlow & Graham, 2011)	Reduced:		
	- BPD	0.93	0.88-0.99
	- BPD or death	0.87	0.77-0.98
Caffeine (Schmidt et al., 2006)	Reduced BPD	0.63	0.52-0.76

negative outcomes in preterm infants with RDS (Table 9-1). Interventions that may be promising but require further evaluation (Table 9-2) and interventions that may be harmful (Table 9-3) have also been addressed. Management of the preterm infant with RDS begins with good prenatal care, including administration of antenatal steroids to mothers at risk for preterm birth. Proper stabilization at birth is also important, with emphasis on early initiation of CPAP for infants who breathe spontaneously following resuscitation. Postnatal respiratory management includes close monitoring to evaluate the need for intubation and surfactant therapy and meticulous management of mechanical ventilation. Supportive care is equally important, including attention to thermoregulation, cautious administration of fluids, aggressive nutritional support, and infection control.

TABLE 9-2 **Interventions That May Be Promising but Require Further Evaluation**

Intervention	Effects	RR	95% CI
21% vs. 100% oxygen resuscitation (term and near-term infants) (Saugstad et al., 2008)	Reduced death	0.69	0.54-0.88
Late postnatal steroids (Halliday, Ehrenkranz, & Doyle, 2009)	Reduced BPD or death	0.72	0.61-0.85
	No increase in CP	1.14	0.79-1.64

TABLE 9-3 Interventions That May Be Harmful in Preterm Infants with RDS

Intervention	Effects	RR	95% CI
Prophylactic surfactant vs CPAP at birth and selective surfactant (Rojas-Reyes, Morley, & Soll, 2012; COFN, 2014)	Increased BPD or death	1.12	1.02-1.24
Lower (85%-89%) versus higher (91%-95%) oxygen saturations			
- SUPPORT (Carlo et al., 2010)	Increased death	1.27	1.01-1.60
- BOOST II (Stenson et al., 2013)	Increased death	1.45	1.15-1.84
- COT (Schmidt et al., 2013)	Trend toward increased death	1.11	0.80-1.54
Early postnatal steroids (Halliday, Ehrenkranz, & Doyle, 2009)	Reduced BPD	0.79	0.71-0.88
	Increased CP	1.45	1.08-1.98

SUGGESTED READINGS

Alfaleh K, Smyth JA, Roberts RS, et al: Prevention and 18-month outcomes of serious pulmonary hemorrhage in extremely low birth weight infants: results from the trial of indomethacin prophylaxis in preterms, *Pediatrics* 121(2):e233–e238, 2008.

Ambalavanan N, Wu TJ, Tyson JE, et al: A comparison of three vitamin A dosing regimens in extremely-low-birth-weight infants, *J Pediatr* 142(6):656–661, 2003.

Arul N, Konduri GG: Inhaled nitric oxide for preterm neonates, *Clin Perinatol* 36(1):43–61, 2009.

Askie LM, Henderson-Smart DJ, Ko H: Restricted versus liberal oxygen exposure for preventing morbidity and mortality in preterm or low birth weight infants, *Cochrane Database Syst Rev* (1):CD001077, 2009.

Bahadue FL, Soll R: Early versus delayed selective surfactant treatment for neonatal respiratory distress syndrome, *Cochrane Database Syst Rev* 11:CD001456, 2012.

Bancalari E, Claure N: Oxygenation targets and outcomes in premature infants, *JAMA* 309(20):2161–2162, 2013.

Barrington KJ, Finer N: Inhaled nitric oxide for respiratory failure in preterm infants, *Cochrane Database Syst Rev* (12):CD000509, 2010.

Bell EF, Acarregui MJ: Restricted versus liberal water intake for preventing morbidity and mortality in preterm infants, *Cochrane Database Syst Rev* (1):CD000503, 2008.

Benitz WE: Treatment of persistent patent ductus arteriosus in preterm infants: time to accept the null hypothesis? *J Perinatol* 30(4):241–252, 2010.

Burri PH: Fetal and postnatal development of the lung, *Annu Rev Physiol* 46:617–628, 1984.

Carlo WA, Finer NN, Walsh MC, et al: Target ranges of oxygen saturation in extremely preterm infants, *N Engl J Med* 362(21):1959–1969, 2010.

Carlo WA, McDonald SA, Fanaroff AA, et al: Association of antenatal corticosteroids with mortality and neurodevelopmental outcomes among infants born at 22 to 25 weeks' gestation, *JAMA* 306(21):2348–2358, 2011.

Cogo PE, Facco M, Simonato M, et al: Dosing of porcine surfactant: effect on kinetics and gas exchange in respiratory distress syndrome, *Pediatrics* 124(5):e950–e957, 2009.

Cole FS, Alleyne C, Barks JD, et al: NIH Consensus Development Conference statement: inhaled nitric-oxide therapy for premature infants, *Pediatrics* 127(2):363–369, 2011.

Committee on Fetus and Newborn (COFN): Respiratory support in preterm infants at birth. *Pediatrics* 133(1):171-174, 2014.

Darlow BA, Graham PJ: Vitamin A supplementation to prevent mortality and short- and long-term morbidity in very low birthweight infants, *Cochrane Database Syst Rev* (10):CD000501, 2011.

Davis PG, Henderson-Smart DJ: Extubation from low-rate intermittent positive airways pressure versus extubation after a trial of endotracheal continuous positive airways pressure in intubated preterm infants, *Cochrane Database Syst Rev* (4):CD001078, 2001.

Davis PG, Henderson-Smart DJ: Nasal continuous positive airways pressure immediately after extubation for preventing morbidity in preterm infants, *Cochrane Database Syst Rev* (2):CD000143, 2003.

Davis PG, Lemyre B, de Paoli AG: Nasal intermittent positive pressure ventilation (NIPPV) versus nasal continuous positive airway pressure (NCPAP) for preterm neonates after extubation, *Cochrane Database Syst Rev* (3):CD003212, 2001.

Doyle LW, Crowther CA, Middleton P, Marret S, Rouse D: Magnesium sulphate for women at risk of preterm birth for neuroprotection of the fetus, *Cochrane Database Syst Rev* (1):CD004661, 2009.

Doyle NM, Gardner MO, Wells L, Qualls C, Papile LA: Outcome of very low birth weight infants exposed to antenatal indomethacin for tocolysis, *J Perinatol* 25(5):336–340, 2005.

Dunn MS, Kaempf J, de Klerk A, et al: Randomized trial comparing 3 approaches to the initial respiratory management of preterm neonates, *Pediatrics* 128(5):e1069–e1076, 2011.

Eldadah M, Frenkel LD, Hiatt IM, Hegyi T: Evaluation of routine lumbar punctures in newborn infants with respiratory distress syndrome, *Pediatr Infect Dis J* 6(3):243–246, 1987.

Erickson SJ, Grauaug A, Gurrin L, Swaminathan M: Hypocarbia in the ventilated preterm infant and its effect on intraventricular haemorrhage and bronchopulmonary dysplasia, *J Paediatr Child Health* 38(6):560–562, 2002.

Escobedo MB, Gunkel JH, Kennedy KA, et al: Early surfactant for neonates with mild to moderate respiratory distress syndrome: a multicenter, randomized trial, *J Pediatr* 144(6):804–808, 2004.

Finer N, Leone T: Oxygen saturation monitoring for the preterm infant: the evidence basis for current practice, *Pediatr Res* 65(4):375–380, 2009.

Finer NN, Barrington KJ: Nitric oxide for respiratory failure in infants born at or near term, *Cochrane Database Syst Rev* (4):CD000399, 2006.

Finer NN, Carlo WA, Walsh MC, et al: Early CPAP versus surfactant in extremely preterm infants, *N Engl J Med* 362(21):1970–1979, 2010.

Fowlie PW, Davis PG, McGuire W: Prophylactic intravenous indomethacin for preventing mortality and morbidity in preterm infants, *Cochrane Database Syst Rev* (7):CD000174, 2010.

Göpel W, Kribs A, Ziegler A, et al: Avoidance of mechanical ventilation by surfactant treatment of spontaneously breathing preterm infants (AMV): an open-label, randomised, controlled trial, *Lancet* 378(9803):1627–1634, 2011.

Greenough A, Dimitriou G, Prendergast M, Milner AD: Synchronized mechanical ventilation for respiratory support in newborn infants, *Cochrane Database Syst Rev* (1):CD000456, 2008.

Haas DM, Caldwell DM, Kirkpatrick P, McIntosh JJ, Welton NJ: Tocolytic therapy for preterm delivery: systematic review and network meta-analysis, *BMJ* 345:e6226, 2012.

Halliday HL: Surfactants: past, present and future, *J Perinatol* 28(suppl 1):S47–S56, 2008.

Halliday HL, Ehrenkranz RA, Doyle LW: Early (<8 days) postnatal corticosteroids for preventing chronic lung disease in preterm infants, *Cochrane Database Syst Rev* (1):CD001146, 2009.

Halliday HL, Ehrenkranz RA, Doyle LW: Late (>7 days) postnatal corticosteroids for chronic lung disease in preterm infants, *Cochrane Database Syst Rev* (1):CD001145, 2009.

Henderson-Smart DJ, Davis PG: Prophylactic methylxanthines for extubation in preterm infants, *Cochrane Database Syst Rev* (1):CD000139, 2003.

Hillman NH, Moss TJ, Kallapur SG, et al: Brief, large tidal volume ventilation initiates lung injury and a systemic response in fetal sheep, *Am J Respir Crit Care Med* 176(6):575–581, 2007.

Jhaveri N, Moon-Grady A, Clyman RI: Early surgical ligation versus a conservative approach for management of patent ductus arteriosus that fails to close after indomethacin treatment, *J Pediatr* 157(3):381–387, 2010. 387.e381.

Jobe AJ: The new BPD: an arrest of lung development, *Pediatr Res* 46(6):641–643, 1999.

Kamlin C, Davis PG: Long versus short inspiratory times in neonates receiving mechanical ventilation, *Cochrane Database Syst Rev* (4):CD004503, 2004.

Kamlin CO, O'Donnell CP, Davis PG, Morley CJ: Oxygen saturation in healthy infants immediately after birth, *J Pediatr* 148(5):585–589, 2006.

Kattwinkel J, Perlman JM, Aziz K, et al: Neonatal resuscitation: 2010 American Heart Association Guidelines for Cardiopulmonary Resuscitation and Emergency Cardiovascular Care, *Pediatrics* 126(5):e1400–e1413, 2010.

Kent AL, Williams J: Increasing ambient operating theatre temperature and wrapping in polyethylene improves admission temperature in premature infants, *J Paediatr Child Health* 44(6):325–331, 2008.

Koch J, Hensley G, Roy L, Brown S, Ramaciotti C, Rosenfeld CR: Prevalence of spontaneous closure of the ductus arteriosus in neonates at a birth weight of 1000 grams or less, *Pediatrics* 117(4):1113–1121, 2006.

Laptook AR, Salhab W, Bhaskar B, Network NR: Admission temperature of low birth weight infants: predictors and associated morbidities, *Pediatrics* 119(3):e643–e649, 2007.

Lasswell SM, Barfield WD, Rochat RW, Blackmon L: Perinatal regionalization for very-low-birth-weight and very preterm infants: a meta-analysis, *JAMA* 304(9):992–1000, 2010.

Litmanovitz I, Carlo WA: Expectant management of pneumothorax in ventilated neonates, *Pediatrics* 122(5):e975–e979, 2008.

McCall EM, Alderdice F, Halliday HL, Jenkins JG, Vohra S: Interventions to prevent hypothermia at birth in preterm and/or low birthweight infants, *Cochrane Database Syst Rev* (3):CD004210, 2010.

McCarthy LK, Hensey CC, O'Donnell CP: In vitro effect of exothermic mattresses on temperature in the delivery room, *Resuscitation* 83(10):e201–e202, 2012.

McClure RJ, Newell SJ: Randomised controlled study of clinical outcome following trophic feeding, *Arch Dis Child Fetal Neonatal Ed* 82(1):F29–F33, 2000.

Morgan J, Bombell S, McGuire W: Early trophic feeding versus enteral fasting for very preterm or very low birth weight infants, *Cochrane Database Syst Rev* 3:CD000504, 2013.

Mosalli R, Alfaleh K: Prophylactic surgical ligation of patent ductus arteriosus for prevention of mortality and morbidity in extremely low birth weight infants, *Cochrane Database Syst Rev* (1):CD006181, 2008.

Nemerofsky SL, Parravicini E, Bateman D, Kleinman C, Polin RA, Lorenz JM: The ductus arteriosus rarely requires treatment in infants >1000 grams, *Am J Perinatol* 25(10):661–666, 2008.

Northway WH, Rosan RC, Porter DY: Pulmonary disease following respirator therapy of hyaline-membrane disease. Bronchopulmonary dysplasia, *N Engl J Med* 276(7):357–368, 1967.

Oh W, Poindexter BB, Perritt R, et al: Association between fluid intake and weight loss during the first ten days of life and risk of bronchopulmonary dysplasia in extremely low birth weight infants, *J Pediatr* 147(6):786–790, 2005.

Ohlsson A, Walia R, Shah S: Ibuprofen for the treatment of patent ductus arteriosus in preterm and/or low birth weight infants, *Cochrane Database Syst Rev* (1):CD003481, 2008.

Okumura A, Hayakawa F, Kato T, et al: Hypocarbia in preterm infants with periventricular leukomalacia: the relation between hypocarbia and mechanical ventilation, *Pediatrics* 107(3):469–475, 2001.

Perlman JM: Hyperthermia in the delivery: potential impact on neonatal mortality and morbidity, *Clin Perinatol* 33(1):55–63, 2006. vi.

Pfister RH, Soll RF, Wiswell T: Protein containing synthetic surfactant versus animal derived surfactant extract for the prevention and treatment of respiratory distress syndrome, *Cochrane Database Syst Rev* (4):CD006069, 2007.

Phibbs CS, Baker LC, Caughey AB, Danielsen B, Schmitt SK, Phibbs RH: Level and volume of neonatal intensive care and mortality in very-low-birth-weight infants, *N Engl J Med* 356(21):2165–2175, 2007.

Polin RA, Bateman D: Oxygen-saturation targets in preterm infants, *N Engl J Med* 368(22):2141–2142, 2013.

Polin RA, CoFa Newborn: Management of neonates with suspected or proven early-onset bacterial sepsis, *Pediatrics* 129(5):1006–1015, 2012.

Puopolo KM, Draper D, Wi S, et al: Estimating the probability of neonatal early-onset infection on the basis of maternal risk factors, *Pediatrics* 128(5):e1155–e1163, 2011.

Rabe H, Diaz-Rossello JL, Duley L, Dowswell T: Effect of timing of umbilical cord clamping and other strategies to influence placental transfusion at preterm birth on maternal and infant outcomes, *Cochrane Database Syst Rev* 8:CD003248, 2012.

Ramachandrappa A, Jain L: Elective cesarean section: its impact on neonatal respiratory outcome, *Clin Perinatol* 35(2):373–393, 2008. vii.

Rautava L, Eskelinen J, Häkkinen U, Lehtonen L, Group PPIS: 5-year morbidity among very preterm infants in relation to level of hospital care, *JAMA Pediatr* 167(1):40–46, 2013.

Roberts D, Dalziel S: Antenatal corticosteroids for accelerating fetal lung maturation for women at risk of preterm birth, *Cochrane Database Syst Rev* (3):CD004454, 2006.

Rojas MA, Lozano JM, Rojas MX, et al: Very early surfactant without mandatory ventilation in premature infants treated with early continuous positive airway pressure: a randomized, controlled trial, *Pediatrics* 123(1):137–142, 2009.

Rojas-Reyes MX, Morley CJ, Soll R: Prophylactic versus selective use of surfactant in preventing morbidity and mortality in preterm infants, *Cochrane Database Syst Rev* 3:CD000510, 2012.

Ryu J, Haddad G, Carlo WA: Clinical effectiveness and safety of permissive hypercapnia, *Clin Perinatol* 39(3):603–612, 2012.

Saugstad OD, Ramji S, Soll RF, Vento M: Resuscitation of newborn infants with 21% or 100% oxygen: an updated systematic review and meta-analysis, *Neonatology* 94(3):176–182, 2008.

Schmidt B, Roberts RS, Davis P, et al: Caffeine therapy for apnea of prematurity, *N Engl J Med* 354(20):2112–2121, 2006.

Schmidt B, Roberts RS, Davis P, et al: Long-term effects of caffeine therapy for apnea of prematurity, *N Engl J Med* 357(19):1893–1902, 2007.

Schmidt B, Whyte RK, Asztalos EV, et al: Effects of targeting higher vs lower arterial oxygen saturations on death or disability in extremely preterm infants: a randomized clinical trial, *JAMA* 309(20):2111–2120, 2013.

Seger N, Soll R: Animal derived surfactant extract for treatment of respiratory distress syndrome, *Cochrane Database Syst Rev* (2):CD007836, 2009.

Sinclair JC: Servo-control for maintaining abdominal skin temperature at 36C in low birth weight infants, *Cochrane Database Syst Rev* (1):CD001074, 2002.

Singh A, Duckett J, Newton T, Watkinson M: Improving neonatal unit admission temperatures in preterm babies: exothermic mattresses, polythene bags or a traditional approach? *J Perinatol* 30(1):45–49, 2010.

Singh N, Hawley KL, Viswanathan K: Efficacy of porcine versus bovine surfactants for preterm newborns with respiratory distress syndrome: systematic review and meta-analysis, *Pediatrics* 128(6):e1588–e1595, 2011.

Soll R, Ozek E: Multiple versus single doses of exogenous surfactant for the prevention or treatment of neonatal respiratory distress syndrome, *Cochrane Database Syst Rev* (1):CD000141, 2009.

Soll RF, Blanco F: Natural surfactant extract versus synthetic surfactant for neonatal respiratory distress syndrome, *Cochrane Database Syst Rev* (2):CD000144, 2001.

Soll RF, Morley CJ: Prophylactic versus selective use of surfactant in preventing morbidity and mortality in preterm infants, *Cochrane Database Syst Rev* (2):CD000510, 2001.

Sood BG, Lulic-Botica M, Holzhausen KA, et al: The risk of necrotizing enterocolitis after indomethacin tocolysis, *Pediatrics* 128(1):e54–e62, 2011.

Stenson BJ, Tarnow-Mordi WO, Darlow BA, et al: Oxygen saturation and outcomes in preterm infants, *N Engl J Med* 368(22):2094–2104, 2013.

Stevens TP, Harrington EW, Blennow M, Soll RF: Early surfactant administration with brief ventilation vs. selective surfactant and continued mechanical ventilation for preterm infants with or at risk for respiratory distress syndrome, *Cochrane Database Syst Rev* (4):CD003063, 2007.

Tyson JE, Wright LL, Oh W, et al: Vitamin A supplementation for extremely-low-birth-weight infants. National Institute of Child Health and Human Development Neonatal Research Network, *N Engl J Med* 340(25):1962–1968, 1999.

Vohra S, Roberts RS, Zhang B, Janes M, Schmidt B: Heat Loss Prevention (HeLP) in the delivery room: A randomized controlled trial of polyethylene occlusive skin wrapping in very preterm infants, *J Pediatr* 145(6):750–753, 2004.

Watterberg KL: Newborn AAoPCoFa. Policy statement—postnatal corticosteroids to prevent or treat bronchopulmonary dysplasia, *Pediatrics* 126(4):800–808, 2010.

CHAPTER 10

PRINCIPLES OF MECHANICAL VENTILATION

Steven M. Donn, MD • Sunil K. Sinha, MD, PhD

Mechanical ventilation is used to provide partial or total assistance to the newborn with respiratory compromise or failure. It can support pulmonary gas exchange and the work of breathing when pulmonary, neurologic, or systemic conditions prevent this from happening normally. Respiratory support (beyond simple supplemental oxygen) ranges from the most minimally invasive, continuous positive airway pressure (CPAP), to the most invasive, extracorporeal membrane oxygenation (ECMO). In between are conventional (tidal) and high-frequency (nontidal) ventilation. Terminology used to describe noninvasive forms of respiratory support is not standardized and can be confusing. This chapter will focus on the principles of conventional mechanical ventilation (CMV) and high-frequency ventilation (HFV), which includes high-frequency jet ventilation (HFJV) and high-frequency oscillatory ventilation (HFOV).

MECHANISMS OF RESPIRATORY FAILURE

Respiratory failure results when there is inadequate pulmonary gas exchange to provide sufficient oxygenation of the blood and removal of carbon dioxide, usually referred to as alveolar hypoventilation. Respiratory failure is usually classified on whether its cause is extrinsic (extrapulmonary) or intrinsic (pulmonary). Examples of these are listed in Box 10-1. Infants may have more than one mechanism, such as a premature infant with severe respiratory distress syndrome complicated by apnea.

Extrinsic respiratory failure generally occurs because there is a limitation of gas flow into or out of the lungs. This can result, for example, from a compression of the airways or from inadequate respiratory drive. Intrinsic respiratory failure results from pathology related to lung parenchyma (such as pneumonia) or pulmonary vasculature (such as persistent pulmonary hypertension of the newborn, PPHN). Parenchymal lung disease may impede gas exchange at the alveolar-capillary level. Increased pulmonary vascular resistance (PVR) may restrict pulmonary blood flow and result in ventilation/perfusion mismatch (often referred to as intrapulmonary shunting) and extrapulmonary shunting through the foramen ovale and/or patent ductus arteriosus (PDA).

BOX 10-1	Causes of Neonatal Respiratory Failure

EXTRAPULMONARY (EXTRINSIC)

Neurologic
Central (e.g., brainstem injury)
Peripheral (e.g., phrenic nerve palsy)
Drug-induced (e.g., maternal anesthesia or analgesia, hypermagnesemia)
Airway malformation or obstruction (e.g., tracheal stenosis)
Right-to-left shunting (e.g., persistent pulmonary hypertension of the newborn)
Altered oxygen-carrying capacity (e.g., methemoglobinemia)
Cyanotic congenital heart disease
Inadequate inspired oxygen (e.g., high altitude)

PULMONARY (INTRINSIC)

Lung malformations (e.g., CPAM)
Diminished surface area (e.g., pulmonary hypoplasia)
Surfactant deficiency (e.g., respiratory distress syndrome)
Inflammation
Pneumonia
Meconium aspiration
Air leaks
Pneumothorax
Pulmonary interstitial emphysema
Pulmonary edema (e.g., congestive heart failure)
Diffusion abnormalities (e.g., alveolar capillary dysplasia)
Bronchopulmonary dysplasia

CPAM, Congenital pulmonary adenomatoid malformation.

CASE STUDY 1

Baby A was born at 25 weeks of gestation weighing 650 grams. Although the mother was not in labor, delivery had to be expedited by emergency cesarean section because of worsening preeclampsia despite treatment with antihypertensive drugs and intravenous magnesium sulfate. The baby was flaccid and unresponsive at birth and required positive pressure breaths and external cardiac compression for two minutes. He was transferred to the neonatal unit.

EXERCISE 1

QUESTIONS

1. As a part of his early respiratory management for RDS, which of the following forms of respiratory support would you consider appropriate?
   a. Nasal CPAP
   b. Nasal intermittent positive pressure ventilation (NIPPV)
   c. High flow nasal cannula (HFNC)
   d. Bilevel positive airway pressure (BiPAP)
   e. Intubation and mechanical ventilation

2. Which of the following factors should be considered important in making the choice of respiratory support for management of early RDS?
   a. Baby's gestational age and birth weight
   b. Baby's condition at birth and requirement of resuscitation
   c. Inability to maintain oxygen saturation above 90% in room air
   d. Baby's endurance and central drive for spontaneous breathing
   e. All of the above

ANSWERS

1. **e.** Because the baby was flaccid and unresponsive at birth, any form of support dependent upon spontaneous breathing is not likely to succeed. This baby may be depressed as a consequence of intrauterine hypoxia and/or the effects of maternal magnesium sulfate therapy. The proper initial support should be provided by intubation and mechanical ventilation.

2. **e.** All of these factors should be taken into consideration when deciding upon the level of support to provide.

CASE STUDY 1 (continued)

A decision was made to initiate mechanical ventilation and to give exogenous surfactant. Umbilical arterial and venous catheters were placed. A chest radiograph done at 4 hours of age showed a bilateral ground glass appearance. The baby needed an FiO_2 of 0.5 to maintain oxygen saturation between 90% and 95%. An arterial blood gas at this time showed normal PaO_2 and PCO_2.

EXERCISE 2

QUESTIONS

1. What modality of ventilation would you choose and why?
   a. Time cycled, pressure-limited ventilation
   b. Volume-targeted ventilation
   c. Pressure control ventilation
   d. High-frequency ventilation

2. How would you choose your initial ventilator settings?
   a. Set the peak inspiratory pressure (PIP) at an arbitrary setting based on your experience.
   b. Set the PIP according to desired tidal volume delivery.
   c. Manually ventilate the baby with a T-piece and see what kind of pressure is required to achieve sufficient chest wall movement.

3. What is your target tidal volume delivery in this baby with RDS?
   a. 4 to 6 mL/kg
   b. 6 to 8 mL/kg
   c. 8 to 10 mL/kg

ANSWERS

1. The choice of modality of ventilation depends upon a number of factors, including which ventilator is at one's disposal, level of experience and comfort with particular modalities, goals of mechanical ventilation, and the underlying pathophysiology. The best available evidence does not clearly define one brand of ventilator or one modality of ventilation as being clearly superior. Different manufacturers use various names for similar features of ventilation, which makes it all the more confusing. What is important is an understanding of the underlying principles, the factors that affect oxygenation and ventilation, and a vision of what one is trying to accomplish with mechanical ventilation. However, neither intermittent mandatory ventilation (IMV) nor synchronized intermittent mandatory ventilation (SIMV) is a good mode for a baby with acute respiratory dysfunction, as spontaneous breaths are supported only by positive end expiratory pressure (PEEP), which is generally inadequate.

2. **a, b.** This is the "art" of mechanical ventilation. Choosing the initial ventilator settings should be done with specific goals in mind. The target tidal volumes (discussed later) will depend upon both

the disease state and a need to avoid overinflation and excessive volume delivery (volutrauma). Choosing the initial ventilator settings should focus on specific ventilation and oxygenation goals, paying particular attention to mean airway pressure, tidal volume, and minute ventilation, as well as the patient's responses.

Most present-day ventilators incorporate real-time pulmonary graphics and breath-to-breath data displays, which assist in choosing or modifying the settings. An understanding of both waveforms (flow, pressure, and volume) and "loops" (pressure-volume and flow-volume) can enable the clinician to better define the pathophysiology and assess the patient–ventilator interactions. Adjusting the ventilator depends upon a thorough understanding of the relationship between the ventilator variables and the patient.

3. **a.** Based on the best available evidence, the tidal volume target for an infant of this size should be in the 4 to 6 mL/kg range to avoid lung injury while providing adequate ventilation.

VENTILATOR VARIABLES

Oxygen Concentration

The fraction of inspired oxygen (FiO_2) refers to the percentage of oxygen in the gas delivered to the patient. It ranges from 21% (room air) to 100% (pure oxygen). A blender, either external to the ventilator or within it, is used to adjust the concentration. Oxygen is warmed and humidified by an external device to about 37° C. before it reaches the airway. The temperature of the delivered gas can be adjusted to prevent excessive condensation in the ventilator circuit or endotracheal tube.

Pressure

The peak inspiratory pressure (PIP) refers to the highest pressure delivered during inspiration. It is set during pressure-targeted ventilation and is variable during volume-targeted ventilation. The baseline pressure is the lowest pressure reached during expiration, and is referred to as positive end-expiratory pressure (PEEP). The mean airway pressure (mean PAW) is the average pressure delivered to the airway during a ventilator cycle. It is represented graphically as the area under the pressure waveform.

Volume

Delivered gas volumes are set during volume-targeted ventilation, and pressure is allowed to vary. During pressure-targeted ventilation, tidal volume is displayed on machines capable of measuring it, and some devices display both inspired and expired tidal volumes, percentage leak, and minute ventilation.

Flow

Flow is the time rate of volume delivery. During continuous flow ventilation, the patient has a source of fresh gas flowing through the ventilator circuit (bias flow) from which to breathe. Circuit flow rate is set by the clinician. It should be high enough so that the desired PIP is reached during inspiration but not so high that it results in turbulence, inadvertent PEEP, or gas trapping. If it is set too low, it may result in air hunger and increased work of breathing for the patient. Inappropriate flow has been referred to as rheotrauma.

Some ventilatory modalities use variable inspiratory flow, proportional to patient effort (see below), and others use a demand flow system, in which the patient must "open" a valve to initiate inspiratory flow.

Rate

For IMV and SIMV, the clinician chooses the frequency of mandatory breaths to be delivered to the patient, irrespective of spontaneous breaths. For assist-control (A/C) ventilation, the clinician chooses the control rate, which is a true backup rate. This determines the minimum number of breaths the baby will receive as a safety net in the event of apnea or inadequate patient effort.

Cycle

The respiratory cycle consists of inspiratory and expiratory phases. During inspiration, gas flows into the airway under positive pressure. During expiration, gas flows passively from the airway, dependent upon the elastic recoil of the lungs (except during HFOV, where exhalation is active, with gas being withdrawn from the airway). Between inspiration and expiration, and between expiration and inspiration, there is a zero flow state. The cycling mechanism is the way in which the switchover from inspiration to expiration and expiration to inspiration occurs.

Most ventilatory modes use time as the cycling mechanism, and thus discrete inspiratory and expiratory times (and/or inspiratory/expiratory ratios) can be selected. Cycling can also be accomplished by changes in airway flow (inspiration ends when airway flow declines to a preselected percentage of peak flow) or by changes in inspired volume. However, true volume cycling cannot occur if uncuffed endotracheal tubes are used because of leaks around the endotracheal tube.

Mode

The clinician selects the mode of ventilation. They include IMV, SIMV, A/C, and pressure support ventilation (PSV). Newer ventilators also offer hybrid or combined modes, such as SIMV/PSV or volume assured pressure support (VAPS).

Assist Sensitivity

For ventilators offering patient-triggered ventilation, assist sensitivity refers to the triggering threshold, usually in liters per minute (LPM) for flow triggers and cm H_2O for pressure triggers.

The lower the assist sensitivity, the easier it is for the patient to trigger the ventilator, although the risk of autotriggering increases.

Rise Time

This feature, available on some ventilators, modifies the slope of the inspiratory pressure waveform. It is a semiquantitative variable, for which "1" may represent the steepest (most aggressive) slope, "5" may represent an intermediate slope, and "9" may represent the gentlest slope. This also varies among ventilators. If set too low (too steep), pressure overshoot may occur, and if set too high (not steep enough), there may be inadequate hysteresis and lung inflation. This is demonstrated in Figure 10-1.

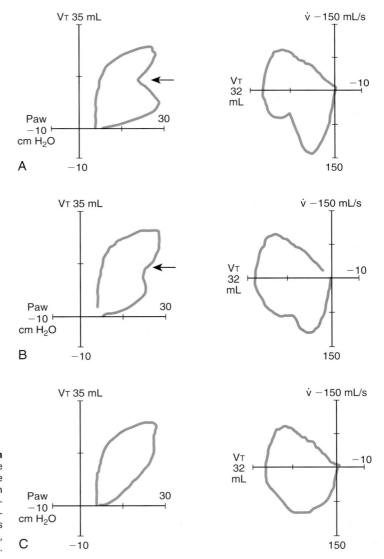

FIGURE 10-1 ■ **Effect of rise time on pressure-volume relationship. A,** Rise time of 1 produces the steepest slope of the inspiratory pressure waveform and results in significant pressure overshoot (*arrow*). **B,** A more moderate setting, 3, results in less overshoot but is still too high. **C,** The gentlest setting, 7, results in a normal degree of hysteresis.

CASE STUDY 1 (continued)

You decided to choose initial ventilator settings of PIP 16, PEEP 4, rate 50, and inspiratory time 0.3 seconds. On review, you find that oxygen saturation is 80% to 85% despite FiO_2 of 0.5 and poor peripheral perfusion (capillary refill time 5 seconds).

EXERCISE 3

QUESTIONS

1. What adjustments of the ventilator settings will you make to improve oxygenation?
    a. Increase PIP from 16 to 18.
    b. Increase PEEP from 4 to 6.
    c. Increase inspiratory time from 0.3 to 0.5 seconds.
    d. Increase the ventilator rate from 50 to 60 per minute.

ANSWER

1. **b.** Given the foregoing findings, increasing the PEEP is the most effective way to improve oxygenation in this patient. Although all of the preceding measures will increase the mean airway pressure, increasing the PEEP would be the most effective approach.

    Adjusting settings on a ventilator requires familiarity with the device and the patient. For example, the initial chest x-ray may demonstrate poor expansion, but by the time you review the chest x-ray and examine the patient again, the oxygen saturation may have improved. *Never respond solely to the findings on a chest radiograph, blood gas analysis, or pulmonary graphics without examining the patient.* Even if the results of a blood gas analysis are good, it does not mean that the ventilator settings are ideal or that the pressure should not be weaned.

OXYGENATION

The primary determinants of oxygenation are the fraction of inspired oxygen (FiO_2) and the mean airway pressure. Increasing the amount of oxygen delivered to the alveoli may help to overcome diffusion gradients and improve the delivery of oxygen to the capillary blood. Raising the mean airway pressure recruits collapsed alveoli, thus increasing the pulmonary surface area available for gas exchange. Neither of these is without risk. High concentrations of oxygen may result in tissue injury through the generation of free radicals; excessive pressure may be

detrimental, contributing to hyperinflation, dead space ventilation, and increased PVR, which can impair venous return, cardiac output, and pulmonary blood flow.

There are several ways to increase mean airway pressure. Raising the PEEP has a direct 1:1 relationship in increasing the mean airway pressure. Thus, a 1.0 cm H_2O increase in PEEP raises the mean airway pressure by 1.0 cm H_2O. Increasing the PIP by 1.0 cm H_2O will also increase the mean airway pressure but to a much lesser extent.

Increasing the inspiratory time will raise the mean pressure by increasing the duration of positive pressure. Increasing the ventilator rate may also have a small impact on increasing the mean airway pressure by decreasing time spent in expiration as well as having more cycles in the same interval of time. Mean airway pressure during HFOV is set directly and represents a static inflation value. Because the mean airway pressure is represented by the area under the curve of the pressure waveform for the entire respiratory cycle, maneuvers that increase the area under the curve increase the mean pressure. These effects are represented in Figure 10-2.

CASE STUDY 1 (continued)

Six hours later, this infant still requires 50% oxygen with abnormal arterial blood gases showing a PaO_2 of 60 torr, PCO_2 of 70 torr, and pH of 7.10.

EXERCISE 4

QUESTION

1. What adjustments in ventilator settings will you make to improve the arterial blood gases?
    a. Increase the PEEP.
    b. Increase the inspiratory time.
    c. Increase the ventilator rate.
    d. Increase the PIP.
    e. Increase the tidal volume.

ANSWER

1. **c, d, e.** Increasing the ventilator rate, PIP, and tidal volume should all result in improved ventilation. Again, making proper ventilator changes requires a review of all aspects of respiratory management. Sometimes it is appropriate to make no changes at all in the ventilator settings but to suction the endotracheal tube or reposition the infant. Always make sure that when the carbon dioxide level is elevated the problem is not related to a mechanical problem, such as plugging of the endotracheal tube with

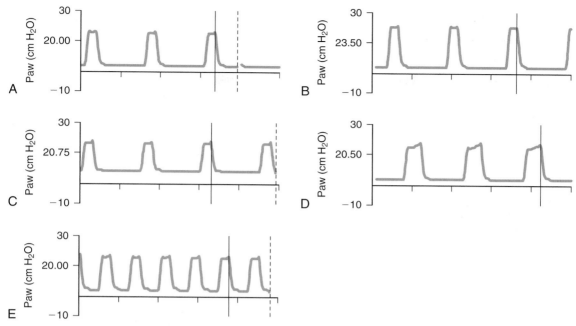

FIGURE 10-2 ■ **Changes that affect mean airway pressure, shown here as the area under the pressure waveform. A,** Initial settings, peak pressure 20 cm H_2O, end expiratory pressure 3 cm H_2O, inspiratory time 0.25 second. **B,** Peak pressure increased to 24 cm H_2O. **C,** End expiratory pressure increased to 6 cm H_2O. **D,** Inspiratory time increased to 0.4 second. **E,** Rate increased.

mucus, inadvertent extubation, kinking of the endotracheal tube, crying or agitation, stacking of breaths, or an air leak.

EXERCISE 5

QUESTION

1. Following adjustments of the ventilator, the Pco_2 has declined from 70 to 50 torr but the baby is still requiring an Fio_2 of 0.7 to maintain oxygen saturation of 85% and Pao_2 of 40 torr. What investigations should you undertake?
   a. Repeat chest radiograph
   b. Simultaneous pre- and postductal oximetry
   c. Complete blood count and hematocrit
   d. Echocardiography
   e. Cranial ultrasound

ANSWER

1. **a**, **b**, and **d**. Lack of improvement in oxygenation with improved Pco_2 indicates abnormality of mechanisms that control oxygenation. Normal Pco_2 after changes of ventilator settings suggests that tidal volume delivery is adequate and the problem may be related to inadequate perfusion, or there may be a developing right-to-left shunt. Simultaneous measurements of preductal (right hand) and postductal site (left foot) is a good bedside test to detect the presence

of right-to-left ductal shunt if this shows a difference in oxygen saturation of more than 10% to 15%. This, however, requires confirmation by echocardiography.

VENTILATION

Ventilation refers to the removal of carbon dioxide. Carbon dioxide removal during CMV can be calculated as the product of the frequency and tidal volume (f × V_T). Thus, maneuvers that increase either the ventilator rate or the tidal volume will increase CO_2 removal. V_T is reflected by the difference between the PIP and PEEP, also referred to as amplitude, or ΔP. Amplitude may be increased by raising the PIP, lowering the PEEP, or doing both. During HFV, CO_2 removal is proportional to f × $(V_T)^2$ and small changes in amplitude can have a profound effect on ventilation.

During HFOV, amplitude is adjusted directly, whereas during HFJV it is controlled the same way as it is during CMV, by adjusting to the difference between PIP and PEEP. Ventilation is also affected by the expiratory time (T_e), because the lung needs sufficient time to empty after being filled. This is determined by the respiratory time constant, the product of resistance and compliance. Generally, a length of time equal to three to five time constants is necessary

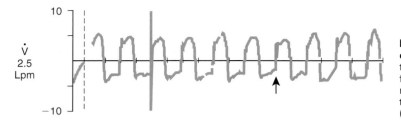

FIGURE 10-3 ■ **Flow waveform demonstrating gas trapping.** Note that the expiratory portion of the waveform (the area below the baseline) never returns to the baseline before the subsequent breath begins (arrow). *LPM,* Liters per minute.

to achieve 95% emptying. As an example, lung disorders that are characterized by low compliance, such as RDS, will fill (and empty) faster than normal lungs (0.10 to 0.12 sec) and have a shorter time constant. Failure to appreciate this may result in gas trapping and inadvertent PEEP, increasing the risk of pulmonary air leaks. Gas trapping can be easily recognized by looking at the flow waveform on pulmonary graphics. The expiratory portion fails to reach the baseline (zero flow state) before the initiation of the subsequent breath. This is shown in Figure 10-3.

Modes of Ventilation

Modes describe the way in which mechanical ventilators deliver positive pressure. There are four modes of ventilation used in newborn infants: IMV, SIMV, A/C, and PSV.

IMV has been used for more than four decades to treat newborn infants with respiratory failure. The most common application is time cycled, pressure-limited IMV, in which the clinician chooses a peak pressure limit, inspiratory time or inspiratory:expiratory ratio, and ventilator rate, and regular mechanical breaths are delivered to the baby. In between these breaths, the baby may breathe spontaneously from fresh gas flowing continuously through the ventilator circuit, but these breaths are supported only by PEEP and may be ineffective if pulmonary compliance or patient effort is low. Moreover, the baby's spontaneous effort maybe asynchronous with the mechanical breaths, and the delivered tidal volumes may fluctuate widely.

Asynchronous ventilation can result in inefficient gas exchange, increased work of breathing, and a higher need for sedatives, and has been associated with an increased risk of pneumothorax and intraventricular hemorrhage. Achieving synchrony during IMV can be challenging and may require the use of sedatives, higher ventilator rates or pressures (to "capture" the infant), or even the use of skeletal muscle relaxants in refractory cases (but this is often associated with adverse systemic effects).

SIMV attempts to synchronize the onset of the mandatory breaths with the onset of spontaneous breaths and is thus a form of patient-triggered ventilation (PTV). Again, the clinician chooses the mandatory breath rate and the baby is free to breathe spontaneously. However, when the ventilator is ready to cycle, it will wait for a few milliseconds before or after its "scheduled" onset of inspiration, looking for patient effort. If this occurs, the ventilator will cycle in response to the patient "trigger," and inspiratory synchrony is achieved. The trigger signal is a measure of spontaneous effort, most commonly a change in airway flow or pressure, although changes in abdominal or thoracic impedance have been used in the past. As in IMV, spontaneous breaths that do not trigger mechanical breaths are supported only by PEEP.

A/C ventilation was introduced into neonatal use in the early 1990s. In this mode of ventilation, every spontaneous breath that exceeds the trigger threshold results in the delivery of a mechanical breath synchronized to the onset of respiration. The baby thus controls the rate of ventilator cycling, provided that spontaneous breathing exceeds the control rate. In this mode, there is a mandatory minimum set rate. Synchrony can be enhanced even further if flow cycling is used. With flow cycling, changes in airway flow are used not only to trigger inspiration, but to trigger expiration as well. It does this by arbitrarily terminating inspiration when inspiratory flow has declined to a small fraction—but not zero—of peak inspiratory flow. This is indicative of the patient's nearing the end of his/her own inspiratory phase. It is also a safeguard against inversion of the inspiratory:expiratory ratio if the infant becomes tachypneic, because inspiration will end at a percentage of peak flow, rather than after a preset time. In the latter case, the faster the infant breaths, the shorter the expiratory time. Additionally, flow cycling affords the infant the chance to set the inspiratory time and rate.

PSV may be used to overcome the shortcomings of unsupported spontaneous breathing during SIMV. It is a "spontaneous" mode applied to spontaneous breaths and provides an inspiratory pressure "boost" to overcome the increased work of breathing created by both the underlying disease process and the imposed work of breathing created by the narrow lumen endotracheal tube, ventilator circuit, and demand valve of the ventilator (if one is used). PSV is pressure- and time-limited but flow-cycled. It can be adjusted to provide a fully supported (e.g., full tidal volume) breath, referred to as PS_{max}, or a partially supported breath during weaning. PS_{min} represents the minimal amount of pressure needed to overcome the imposed work of breathing, estimated to be about 3 to 4 mL/kg in term infants. If PSV is used, it is reasonable to use a low SIMV rate. If PSV is successful, the synchrony developed between baby and ventilator will not be interrupted by excessive mandatory breaths.

CASE STUDY 1 (continued)

After adjustments of ventilator settings and provision of hemodynamic support, the baby's general condition has improved. He is still receiving time cycled, pressure-limited, assist-control ventilation and a decision is made to commence weaning.

EXERCISE 6

QUESTIONS

1. What parameters are likely to predict a baby's readiness for weaning and extubation?
   a. Rapid shallow breathing
   b. Minute ventilation of more than 240 mL/kg/min
   c. Generating good tidal volume with spontaneous breathing
   d. Maintaining PaO_2 of 60 at a PEEP <8 cm H_2O

2. What steps would you take to wean him from assist-control?
   a. Decrease the rate
   b. Decrease the PIP
   c. Decrease the PEEP
   d. Decrease the tidal volume delivery below 4 mL/kg

ANSWERS

1. **b** and **c.** Various indices have been used in clinical practice to assess a patient's readiness for extubation but none of them have complete accuracy. Fast and shallow breathing is associated with failure to extubate. Another simple bedside test is to assess the baby's own respiratory effort and measure the tidal volume of spontaneous breaths, giving a good predictive value for readiness for extubation.

2. **b.** The best choice would be to decrease the PIP. Because the baby is being managed in assist-control, weaning the ventilator rate will not affect ventilation as long as the baby is breathing

above the control rate. Decreasing the PEEP will increase the amplitude (V_T) and increase ventilation. Decreasing the inspiratory time will allow more time for expiration and result in increased ventilation, but the shorter inspiratory time may not be tolerated. A tidal volume below 4 mL/kg is undesirable because it is likely to result in atelectasis especially in premature infants.

Pressure-Targeted Ventilation

In pressure-targeted ventilation, the inspiratory pressure is set by the clinician, usually by adjusting a pressure limit. The mechanical breaths will not exceed this limit. However, the delivered tidal volume will depend upon the patient's compliance and to a lesser extent resistance. At the same pressure, more tidal volume will be delivered at a higher compliance than at a lower one. This has important clinical implications. For instance, compliance generally improves after exogenous surfactant treatment. If the inspiratory pressure is not decreased, tidal volume delivery will increase, thus increasing the probability of lung injury.

Three major ventilator modalities utilize pressure-targeted ventilation: time or flow cycled, pressure-limited ventilation; pressure control (PC) ventilation; and PSV. Time or flow cycled, pressure-limited ventilation has been described previously. Its major advantage is its ease of use. Delivered breaths are all at the same pressure. Pressure-limited ventilation may be used in IMV, SIMV, and A/C ventilation modes.

PC ventilation is a newer pressure-targeted modality. In PC ventilation, the inspiratory time is usually fixed; that is, it is time cycled. Inspiratory flow is rapid and is variable, depending upon the patient's inspiratory effort. The harder the baby "pulls," the greater is the flow rate. PC also has a rapidly rising (accelerating-decelerating) pressure waveform. Its theoretical advantage is that this quickly pressurizes the ventilator circuit and delivers gas flow to the baby, enhancing diffusion and alveolar inflation.

Most ventilators offering PC also have an adjustable rise time, which affects the slope of the inspiratory pressure waveform. If the rise time, a qualitative parameter, is set too low, there will be inadequate hysteresis on the pressure-volume loop. If it is set too high, pressure overshoot may occur, as demonstrated in Figure 10-1. Pressure control may benefit babies who have high airway resistance because of the more rapid flow rate during inspiration. It can also be delivered as IMV, SIMV, or A/C ventilation.

Pressure support was described earlier. It, too, is pressure targeted, and is time limited and

TABLE 10-1 **A Comparison of Pressure-Targeted Modalities**

Parameter	Pressure Limited	Pressure Control	Pressure Support
Flow	Fixed	Variable	Variable
Cycle	Time or flow	Time or flow	Flow (time limited)
Limit	Pressure	Pressure	Pressure

flow cycled. Tidal volume delivery depends upon patient compliance. Table 10-1 lists the differences and the similarities among these three modalities.

Volume-Targeted Ventilation

In contrast to pressure-targeted ventilation, volume-targeted ventilation enables the clinician to choose a desired volume of gas to be delivered (referred to as V_{del}) and allows the pressure required to deliver this volume to vary. For safety reasons, pressure may be limited, but this negates the whole philosophy of volume targeting, as fixed pressure may not achieve the target tidal volume. Because cuffed endotracheal tubes are not used in newborn infants, the term "volume cycling" should not be applied to this form of ventilation, since there is almost always a degree of gas leak around the endotracheal tube. It is preferable to think of this as "volume-targeted," "volume-limited," or "volume-controlled" ventilation. A unique feature of volume-targeted ventilation is its auto-weaning capability. As compliance improves, the pressure required to deliver an equivalent volume of gas decreases, and the ventilator automatically responds by weaning the pressure. Conversely, a decrease in compliance results in an automatic increase in pressure to deliver the desired tidal volume.

Clinicians using volume-targeted ventilation should choose a device that measures the tidal volume at the proximal airway. When the lungs are stiff, there may be considerable compression of gas volume within the ventilator circuit, and it is critical to know exactly how much volume is being delivered to the patient. In addition, clinicians need to be aware of the minimal tidal volume the machine is capable of delivering to avoid overinflation in extremely low birth weight babies.

During volume-targeted ventilation, inspiratory time is a function of the gas flow rate. The higher the flow rate is, the shorter will be inspiratory time. The inspiratory time should be checked each time there is a change in ventilator parameters. Volume-targeted ventilation also differs from pressure-targeted ventilation

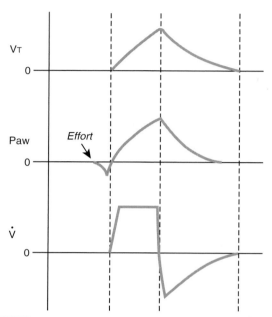

FIGURE 10-4 ■ **Characteristics of volume-targeted ventilation.** On the top is the volume waveform. Note that peak volume delivery occurs at the end of inspiration. In the middle is the "shark's fin" pressure waveform. On the bottom is the "square" flow waveform, which differs from the more sinusoidal pattern in pressure-targeted ventilation.

by delivering flow in a "square waveform" and delivering pressure in a "shark's fin waveform," resulting in a slower ramping of pressure and the delivery of maximal volume and pressure at the end of inspiration (Figure 10-4). Newer devices allow the optional use of a decelerating flow waveform but the merits of this have yet to be explored.

Volume-targeted ventilation may be applied in IMV, SIMV, and A/C ventilation, and may be combined in SIMV with PSV. Recent advances have enabled hybrid forms of ventilation, such as pressure-regulated volume control and volume guarantee, and volume-assured pressure support, in which a targeted volume is delivered within a single breath by transitioning a pressure-targeted breath to a volume-targeted breath by extending flow in inspiration, and increasing pressure, if necessary.

CASE STUDY 1 (continued)

Unfortunately, this infant failed a trial of extubation and had to be reintubated because of marked deterioration in gas exchange. A later chest radiograph showed significant pulmonary interstitial emphysema in both lungs and required escalation of ventilatory support with high PIP and mean airway pressure of 14 cm H_2O. In view of this, a decision was made to switch to high-frequency ventilation using an oscillator (HFOV).

EXERCISE 7

QUESTIONS

1. What will your initial settings be on high-frequency oscillatory ventilation?
   a. Mean airway pressure of 14
   b. FiO_2 of 0.8
   c. Amplitude (Delta P) 30
   d. I:E ratio of 50%
   e. Rate 15 Hz

2. Despite being switched onto HFOV, there is no improvement in the baby's oxygenation. Which of the following actions would you take?
   a. Increase the FiO_2 to 1.0.
   b. Increase the mean airway pressure in small increments.
   c. Increase the amplitude.
   d. Decrease the I:E ratio to 33%.

3. Oxygenation has now improved but $PaCO_2$ still remains high at 75 torr. Which of the following adjustments in the ventilatory settings are appropriate in this situation?
   a. Increase frequency to 20 Hz.
   b. Decrease frequency to 8 Hz.
   c. Increase the amplitude.
   d. Increase the mean airway pressure.

ANSWERS

1. **a** and **c**. In high-frequency ventilation, mean airway pressure controls the oxygenation and amplitude controls CO_2 elimination.

2. **b**. The poor response in oxygenation may be secondary to inadequate opening pressure, and thus raising mean airway pressure by small increments is the preferred method. Reaching the appropriate pressure is indicated by improvement in oxygenation.

3. **b** and **c**. Increasing the amplitude or decreasing the rate will probably result in improved ventilation, although adjusting the amplitude is usually the preferred choice. Although it may be counterintuitive, increasing the frequency may

further attenuate gas flow and total cycle time and therefore decrease patient ventilation (see the following discussion).

High-Frequency Ventilation

High-frequency ventilation delivers extremely small tidal volumes (less than anatomic dead space) at extremely rapid rates. The two major forms of HFV are HFJV and HFOV. HFJV uses a pulsatile, high-velocity flow to deliver gas, but it involves passive exhalation. HFOV uses a piston-driven diaphragm, which delivers gas to the airway and also actively withdraws it (active exhalation). Tidal volumes are slightly larger during HFJV, and ventilator rates are faster during HFOV, typically 8 to 15 Hz. HFJV has been shown to be superior to conventional ventilation in the management of air leaks, and HFOV may result in less chronic lung disease less than conventional SIMV.

The principles of management are similar to CMV; mean airway pressure determines oxygenation and amplitude determines ventilation. HFJV is applied in tandem with a conventional ventilator to provide PEEP and sigh breaths, whereas HFOV (in the United States) is used alone. During HFV, most clinicians choose to keep the ventilator frequency constant and adjust other parameters to affect carbon dioxide removal.

Weaning from HFV tends to be a personal preference. Some clinicians will extubate a baby directly from HFV, and others prefer to transition to CMV first.

There are some strategies to be considered when choosing the initial ventilator settings. It may depend upon one's familiarity with the device and whether it is used as a rescue therapy or as a primary mode of ventilation. Of course, it will also depend upon the disease state. If a baby is given surfactant in the delivery room and then placed on the oscillator, the settings will likely be initially lower than in the baby who is initially placed on the oscillator and then given surfactant. It is crucial, however, that once the baby is placed on the oscillator, the clinician does not leave the bedside, particularly if the baby has recently received surfactant. There can be a rapid improvement in compliance over just a few minutes. Utilization of noninvasive monitoring methods, such as pulse oximetry and transcutaneous carbon dioxide monitoring, is useful in making frequent necessary adjustments and avoiding overshooting the desired goals. The physical examination is also important in assessing the settings on the oscillator. Assessment of "chest wiggle" takes experience but allows for some fine-tuning of the settings. Many clinicians will obtain a chest radiograph 30 to 60 minutes after initially placing the baby on the oscillator to assess lung expansion. It may be useful to obtain a follow up film 2 to 3 hours later to reassess expansion. Proper use of the oscillator depends on integrating the findings of the physical examination, chest radiograph, and blood gas analysis.

MATCHING STRATEGY WITH PATHOPHYSIOLOGY

Although considerable controversy still exists over the "best" ventilator mode or modality, the major changes brought about by the new technology enable the clinician to customize management for the individual patient and to develop strategies that match specific pathophysiologic states. This is an important element in maximizing outcomes and minimizing complications. The following brief review of the major respiratory disorders afflicting the newborn will illustrate this.

RESPIRATORY DISTRESS SYNDROME

RDS is the primary respiratory disorder of the preterm infant. Its pathophysiology is related to both anatomic and biochemical abnormalities of the immature lung. The more premature the baby, the greater are these problems. Anatomic problems result from decreased alveolarization, underdeveloped airways, and in extreme cases, an increased distance from the terminal breathing unit to the adjacent capillary. The biochemical abnormality is the absence or reduction of pulmonary surfactant, leading to an increase in alveolar surface tension and a tendency toward progressive atelectasis. RDS has been referred to as a low lung volume disease.

Although the advent of exogenous surfactant therapy has radically altered the disease process, infants with severe disease are generally treated with mechanical ventilation. The infant with RDS, at least prior to surfactant administration, has diminished pulmonary compliance (ranging from 0.1 to 1.0 mL/cm H_2O/kg; normal lungs have a compliance of 3 to 5 mL/cm H_2O/kg) and increased resistance (100 cm H_2O/L/sec or higher; normal is 25 to 50 cm H_2O/L/sec). Ventilatory strategies should be designed to achieve normal inflation and lung volumes and to overcome the tendency of alveoli to collapse. Use sufficient PEEP to overcome the need for high opening pressure, and adequate PIP to ensure reasonable tidal volumes (4 to 6 mL/kg). Careful attention must be paid to rapid changes in compliance after surfactant administration. These changes may be manifested by increases in chest excursions, higher delivered tidal volumes, hyperinflation on radiography or pulmonary graphics, or hypocapnia on blood gas analysis.

The incidence of pulmonary air leaks (pneumothorax and pulmonary interstitial emphysema) has been markedly reduced in the exogenous surfactant era, but they still occur, more so with extreme prematurity. Therefore, avoidance of gas trapping, inadvertent PEEP, and prolonged inspiratory times are all warranted in this population (Figure 10-3). Treatment of air leaks may be facilitated by HFV, especially for pulmonary interstitial emphysema.

MECONIUM ASPIRATION SYNDROME

Intrauterine passage of meconium occurs in about 30% of term infants and in up to 40% of postterm infants. It may be aspirated prior to birth or during/after delivery and can lead to significant pulmonary disease. Meconium contains bile salts, which inactivate surfactant. It can also cause airway obstruction, leading to gas trapping, hyperinflation, and air leaks. It may progress to chemical pneumonitis, with resultant ventilation/perfusion mismatch, and ultimately PPHN (see below). It may even interfere with gas diffusion at the alveolar level. Because of the tendency for gas trapping and hyperinflation, meconium aspiration syndrome (MAS) should be thought of as a high lung volume disease.

Ventilatory management is directed at maintaining reasonable gas exchange without contributing to the risks of hyperinflation, gas trapping, and air leaks. This involves the use of shorter inspiratory times, slower ventilator rates, and lower flow rates. Monitoring pulmonary waveforms for evidence of gas trapping (Figure 10-3), and observing pulmonary mechanics for evidence of hyperinflation are strongly recommended. Even greater care is necessary if the disease is patchy and not homogeneous.

PERSISTENT PULMONARY HYPERTENSION OF THE NEWBORN

PPHN is generally a disorder of the term infant. It is a condition characterized by maintenance of elevated PVR, leading to right-to-left shunting of blood, profound hypoxemia, and metabolic acidosis. PPHN may occur as a primary process, believed to result from excessive muscularization of the pulmonary arterioles, or it may be secondary to a number of processes that affect either lung parenchyma (such as pneumonia or asphyxia), pulmonary vasculature (such as chronic intrauterine hypoxia), or both (such as congenital diaphragmatic hernia or pulmonary hypoplasia).

The pathophysiology of the disorder centers around abnormally elevated PVR and suprasystemic pulmonary arterial pressure. This causes shunting of blood away from the lung, creating a venous admixture, ultimately resulting in profound hypoxemia. This leads to acidosis, further constricting pulmonary vessels and impairing myocardial contractility, systemic blood pressure, and pulmonary blood flow. Thus, a vicious circle is established. For several decades, the management of PPHN was highly controversial. Two strategies evolved. The first, deliberate hyperventilation, sought to take advantage of the pulmonary vasodilating effects of hyperoxia, hypocapnia, and extreme alkalosis. The second, referred to as conservative or gentle ventilation, sought to minimize the contributory effects of high intrathoracic pressure to increased PVR, and it promoted the acceptance of marginal gas exchange until remodeling of the pulmonary vasculature had been accomplished. Unfortunately, no direct randomized controlled trials were ever performed, and ventilator management tended to be based on personal or institutional preferences.

The introduction of inhaled nitric oxide (iNO), a selective pulmonary vasodilator, significantly altered the approach to PPHN. iNO has been shown to be effective in reversing the hypoxemic respiratory failure associated with PPHN. It is administered directly into the inspiratory limb of the ventilator circuit and delivered to the alveolus, where it diffuses into the capillaries and results in vascular relaxation. iNO has also been shown to work best when the lungs are optimally inflated, often using HFOV. Whatever strategy is adopted, care must be taken to avoid situations that contribute to increased PVR,

including high peak and mean airway pressures, overdistention of the lung (Figure 10-5), and inadvertent PEEP, especially if rapid ventilator rates are used and there is inadequate time for lung emptying. In addition, weaning needs to be accomplished very slowly; small changes in FiO_2 or $PaCO_2$ can have profound effects on PaO_2. In addition, clinicians need to recognize "transition disease," usually around the fourth postnatal day, when pulmonary vasoreactivity begins to diminish, and the effects of hyperoxia, hyperventilation, and alkalosis are less apparent.

CASE STUDY 2

A full-term newborn with meconium aspiration syndrome requires intubation and ventilation but then develops features of persistent pulmonary hypertension of the newborn (PPHN).

EXERCISE 8

QUESTION

1. Which of the following options would you consider?
   a. PEEP of 8 cm H_2O
   b. Tidal volume delivery >8 mL/kg
   c. Hyperventilation to achieve respiratory alkalosis
   d. Change to high-frequency ventilation
   e. Start dopamine and/or dobutamine infusion

ANSWER

1. **d** and **e.** The excess of distending pressure either in the form of excessive PEEP or increased tidal volume is only likely to produce a further rise in intrathoracic pressure and promote further right-to-left shunting (Figure 10-6). A poor hemodynamic status from reduced cardiac output is also detrimental because it will facilitate right-to-left shunting from increased gradients between the pulmonary and systemic circulations. Hyperventilation to achieve respiratory alkalosis is not desirable because hypocarbia may contribute to ischemic brain injury.

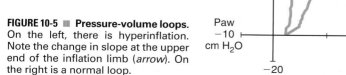
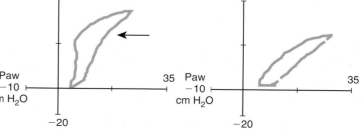

FIGURE 10-5 ■ **Pressure-volume loops.** On the left, there is hyperinflation. Note the change in slope at the upper end of the inflation limb (*arrow*). On the right is a normal loop.

EXERCISE 9

QUESTION

1. Despite intervention, this baby continues to deteriorate with poor oxygenation. A repeat echocardiogram shows increased pulmonary resistance with worsening right-to-left shunting. A decision is made to start inhaled nitric oxide. Which of the following actions will you take?
   a. Start at 5 parts per million (PPM) and stop after an hour if there is no improvement.
   b. Start at 20 PPM and reduce the dose according to response.
   c. Perform lung lavage with dilute surfactant.
   d. Combine inhaled nitric oxide therapy with HFOV.
   e. Refer for ECMO.

ANSWER

1. **b**, **c**, **d**, and **e.** The use of echocardiography to assess pulmonary hypertension must be done with caution. Echocardiograms can identify whether there is evidence of increased PVR, but it is up to the clinician to determine the cause. Hyperinflation of the lungs from excessive HFOV can increase PVR, worsen oxygenation, and decrease cardiac output (as noted in this case).

   For PPHN, iNO at 20 ppm seems to be the optimal and safe initial dose. Most babies will respond to this dose, often within 15 minutes with an increase in PaO_2 and a decrease in ductal shunting. Babies not responding within an hour should be discussed with an ECMO center. Do not delay referral to an ECMO center waiting for a late response.

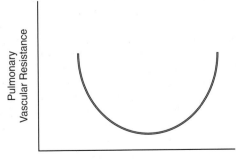

FIGURE 10-6 ■ **Relationship between lung volume and pulmonary vascular resistance.** When lung volume is low, such as in RDS, or when it is high, such as in meconium aspiration syndrome, pulmonary vascular pressure is elevated, leading to higher pulmonary arterial pressure than when the lung is ventilated at functional residual capacity.

BRONCHOPULMONARY DYSPLASIA (CHRONIC LUNG DISEASE)

CASE STUDY 3

A baby was born at 23%/₇ weeks' gestation and required treatment for RDS. He is now 28 days old and still dependent on time cycled pressure-limited ventilation, requiring a PIP of 18 and PEEP of 6 cm H_2O with an inspiratory time of 0.35 seconds. Blood gases show a pH of 7.26, PCO_2 of 55 torr and oxygen saturation between 88% to 92% in FiO_2 of 0.45. A chest x-ray shows a hazy appearance with some cystic areas.

EXERCISE 10

QUESTION

1. What are the likely causes of this child's ventilatory dependence?
   a. Respiratory distress syndrome
   b. Pulmonary edema secondary to a PDA
   c. Evolving bronchopulmonary dysplasia (BPD)
   d. Ventilator associated pneumonia
   e. Hypoplastic lungs

ANSWER

1. **c.** An x-ray at 4 weeks of age with these findings in a chronically ventilated baby is most likely evolving BPD. A similar picture can be seen in babies with acquired pneumonia of bacterial, viral, or fungal origin and should be considered in the differential diagnosis. Another cause for this clinical presentation could be congestive heart failure from a PDA or excess fluid retention. Such babies require thorough investigation including sepsis screening, echocardiography, and pulmonary mechanics testing.

CASE STUDY 3 (continued)

This baby was started on empirical treatment with antibiotics. He was given caffeine citrate and attempts were made to wean him from mechanical ventilation, but without success.

EXERCISE 11

QUESTION

1. Which of the following ventilator strategies would you select?
   a. Volume-targeted ventilation; maintain a tidal volume 4 to 6 mL/kg
   b. Continue on time cycled pressure-limited ventilation with a higher PEEP

c. Tolerate higher pCO$_2$ and reduce PIP
d. Change to PSV
e. Initiate high-frequency ventilation
f. Extubate to NIPPV

ANSWER

1. Babies with evolving BPD have deranged pulmonary mechanics and gas exchange. Various forms of mechanical ventilation may be suitable for such cases. For example, PSV or PC ventilation may offer some advantages. PSV augments spontaneous breathing and provides synchronization with mechanically delivered breaths. Although noninvasive forms of ventilation increasingly are being used to treat BPD, under the impression that this minimizes lung injury, this has not been confirmed in large clinical trials. Nonetheless, it may provide an alternative for babies who can be extubated successfully and who have regular respiratory drive.

Bronchopulmonary dysplasia (BPD) is a chronic lung disorder affecting newborn infants who have undergone mechanical ventilation. BPD was originally attributed to the combined effects of exposure to high concentrations of oxygen and positive pressure ventilation over time. Affected infants displayed the histopathologic changes of inflammation, fibrosis, and vascular smooth muscle hypertrophy, with radiographic findings of alternating areas of hyperinflation and atelectasis, producing the "honeycomb" lung appearance. Infants with the "new BPD" are likely to be much more premature and not exposed to a severe a degree of mechanical ventilation. Radiographs show a hazy to granular pattern with diminished lung volumes, and histopathologic examination of the lungs shows much less inflammation and fibrosis, but fewer and larger alveoli.

BPD is thought to result from a combination of factors. Infants with BPD are delivered before adequate alveolarization of the lung has occurred, and this process is further interrupted by an entity referred to as ventilator-induced lung injury (VILI). VILI is multifactorial, and is related to barotrauma (excessive pressure), volutrauma (excessive volume), atelectotrauma (damage resulting from the continuous opening and closing of lung units), biotrauma (injury resulting from infection and inflammation), and rheotrauma (abnormal airway gas flow; excessive flow causes turbulence, gas trapping, and inadvertent PEEP, and inadequate flow causes air hunger and increased work of breathing). BPD has been defined in many different ways, most centering around a prolonged oxygen dependency. Infants who require long-term mechanical ventilation for BPD are often difficult to manage.

First, it must be recognized that BPD affects not only lung parenchyma but also the airways. Airway resistance may be significantly elevated. If so, a modality offering variable inspiratory flow—such as pressure control or pressure support—may be beneficial. Second, the expectation for the degree of gas exchange needs to be revised from parameters targeted during RDS. Tolerance of a higher PaCO$_2$ (and perhaps a slightly lower PaO$_2$) and careful attention to other complications such as pulmonary edema, pulmonary hypertension, and cor pulmonale may help guide ventilator management. The clinician must remember that the lungs of these babies are still undergoing alveolarization and the damaging effects of mechanical ventilation must be minimized.

WEANING AND EXTUBATION

Weaning is the process by which the work of breathing is transferred from the mechanical ventilator to the patient. Prior to extubation, a baby must demonstrate reliable respiratory drive, adequate pulmonary gas exchange, and minimal distress. It is probably best to start weaning by first decreasing the parameter that is potentially the most injurious to the patient. For a premature infant receiving a high concentration of inspired oxygen, decreasing the oxygen may be the primary objective. For a term infant with meconium aspiration syndrome requiring high oxygen concentrations and high pressures, decreasing the pressure first may be important to prevent gas trapping, decrease intrathoracic pressure and PVR, and avoid chronic lung injury.

Weaning tends to be a style more than a science. Infants receiving IMV or SIMV are traditionally weaned by reduction in the ventilator rate, while keeping PIP constant or lowering it slowly. Some clinicians prefer to add PSV to the spontaneous breaths to overcome the imposed work of breathing, followed by a further reduction in the mandatory rate. In assist-control ventilation, the PIP is weaned first; weaning the control rate will have no effect as long as the baby is breathing above the control rate. In volume-targeted ventilation, weaning is more straightforward, depending upon the mode, as the ventilator will automatically reduce the pressure.

Babies should be considered ready for extubation when they have been weaned to low ventilator support, exhibit good respiratory drive, and can maintain oxygenation and minute ventilation. The latter may be utilized as an objective measure for readiness for extubation. Postextubation management is still controversial. Some centers use methylxanthine therapy in the periextubation period to stimulate breathing and improve diaphragmatic contractility. Others prefer to use some form of distending pressure after extubation, such as nasal CPAP or high flow nasal cannula to maintain upper airway patency and overcome airway resistance.

CONCLUSION

Respiratory failure in the newborn infant may result from numerous causes. Present-day mechanical ventilation offers the clinician a variety of options to approach this problem. Decisions as to which type, mode, and modality of ventilation to choose should be based on an understanding of not only how the ventilator functions, but also on the underlying lung disease and how the individual baby responds to the settings chosen. Careful assessment of the baby through physical examination, laboratory results, and real-time monitoring will dictate the adjustments necessary to achieve adequate gas exchange and to minimize lung injury.

SUGGESTED READINGS

Bunnell JB: General concepts of high-frequency ventilation. In Donn SM, Sinha SK, editors: *Manual of neonatal respiratory care*, 3rd ed, New York, 2012, Springer, pp 301–318.

Cannon ML, Cornell J, Tripp-Hamel DS, et al.: Tidal volumes for ventilated infants should be determined with a pneumotachometer placed at the endotracheal tube, *Am J Respir Care* 162:2109–2112, 2000.

Carlo WA, Ambalavanan N, Chatburn RL: Basic principles of mechanical ventilation. In Donn SM, Sinha SK, editors: *Manual of neonatal respiratory care*, 3rd ed, New York, 2012, Springer, pp 73–85.

Clark RH: High-frequency oscillatory ventilation In: Donn SM. In Sinha SK, editor: *Manual of neonatal respiratory care*, 3rd ed, New York, 2012, Springer, pp 327–340.

Coalson JJ: Pathology of the new bronchopulmonary dysplasia, *Semin Neonatol.* 8:73–82, 2003.

Courtney SC, Durand DJ, Asselin JM, et al.: High frequency oscillatory ventilation versus conventional mechanical ventilation for very-low-birth weight infants, *N Engl J Med.* 347:643–652, 2002.

Donn SM: Pressure control ventilation. In Donn SM, Sinha SK, editors: *Manual of neonatal respiratory care*, 3rd ed, New York, 2012, Springer, pp 281–283.

Donn SM, Nicks JJ, Becker MA: Flow-synchronized ventilation of preterm infants with respiratory distress syndrome, *J Perinatol* 14:90–94, 1994.

Donn SM, Sinha SK: Assisted ventilation and its complications. In Martin RJ, Fanaroff AA, Walsh ML, editors: *Neonatal perinatal medicine: diseases of the fetus and infant*, 8th ed, St. Louis, MO, 2011, Elsevier/Mosby, pp 1116–1140.

Donn SM, Sinha SK: Controversies in patient triggered ventilation, *Clin Perinatol.* 25:49–61, 1998.

Donn SM, Sinha SK: Minimising ventilator induced lung injury in preterm infants, *Arch Dis Child Fetal Neonatal Ed* 91(3):F226–230, 2006.

Donn SM, Sinha SK: Newer modes of mechanical ventilation for the neonate, *Curr Opin Pediatr.* 13:99–103, 2001.

Donn SM, Sinha SK: Newer techniques of mechanical ventilation: an overview, *Semin Neonatol.* 7:401–407, 2002.

Donn SM, Sinha SK: Respiratory distress syndrome. In Donn SM, Sinha SK, editors: *Manual of neonatal respiratory care*, 3rd ed, New York, 2012, Springer, pp 523–532.

Gillespie LM, White SD, Sinha SK, Donn SM: Usefulness of the minute ventilation test in predicting successful extubation in newborn infants: A randomized controlled trial, *J Perinatol.* 23:205–207, 2003.

Greenough A, Milner AD: Mechanisms of respiratory failure. In Donn SM, Sinha SK, editors: *Manual of neonatal respiratory care*, 3rd ed, New York, 2012, Springer, pp 513–516.

Hagus CK, Donn SM: Pulmonary graphics: basics of clinical application. In Donn SM, editor: *Neonatal and pediatric pulmonary graphics: principles and clinical applications*, Armonk, New York, 1998, Futura Publishing, pp 28–81.

Keszler M: High-frequency jet ventilation and the Bunnell Life Pulse high-frequency jet ventilator. In Donn SM, Sinha SK, editors: *Manual of neonatal respiratory care*, 3rd ed, New York, 2012, Springer, pp 319–326.

Keszler M, Donn SM, Bucciarelli RL, et al.: Multicenter-controlled trial comparing high-frequency jet ventilation and conventional mechanical ventilation in newborn infants with pulmonary interstitial emphysema, *J Pediatr.* 119:85–93, 1991.

Kinsella JP, Neish SR, Abman SH: Low-dose inhalational nitric oxide in persistent pulmonary hypertension of the newborn, *Lancet.* 340:819–820, 1992.

Lacaze-Masmonteil T: Exogenous surfactant therapy: newer developments, *Semin Neonatol* 8:433–440, 2003.

Nicks JJ, Becker MA, Donn SM: Bronchopulmonarydysplasia: response to pressure support ventilation, *J Perinatol* 14:495–497, 1994.

Northway Jr WH, Rosan RC, Porter DY: Pulmonary disease following respiratory therapy for hyaline membrane disease—bronchopulmonary dysplasia, *N Engl J Med* 276:357–368, 1967.

Peckham GS, Fox WW: Physiological factors affecting pulmonary artery pressures in infants with persistent pulmonary hypertension, *J Pediatr* 93:1005–1110, 1978.

Perlman JM, McMenamin JP, Volpe JJ: Fluctuating cerebral blood flow velocity in respiratory distress syndrome: relationship to subsequent development of intraventricular hemorrhage, *N Engl J Med.* 309:204–209, 1983.

Philip AGS: Oxygen plus pressure plus time: the etiology of bronchopulmonary dysplasia, *Pediatrics* 55:44–48, 1975.

Roberts JD, Fineman JR, Morin III FC, et al.: Inhaled nitric oxide and persistent pulmonary hypertension of the newborn, *N Engl J Med* 336:605–610, 1997.

Singh J: Sinha SK, Clarke P, Donn SM. Mechanical Ventilation of very low birth weight infants: is volume or pressure a better target variable? *J Pediatr* 149:308–313, 2006.

Sinha IP, Sinha SK: Alternative therapies for respiratory distress syndrome in preterm infants, *Res Rep Neonatol* 1:67–75, 2011.

Sinha SK, Donn SM: Difficult extubation in babies receiving assisted mechanical ventilation, *Arch Dis Child Educ Pract Ed* 91(2):42–46, 2006.

Sinha SK, Donn SM: Volume-targeted ventilation. In Goldsmith JP, Karotkin EH, editors: *Assisted ventilation of the neonate*, 5th ed, St. Louis, MO, 2011, Saunders, pp 186–199.

Walsh MC, Stork EK: Persistent pulmonary hypertension of the newborn: rational therapy based on pathophysiology, *Clin Perinatol* 28:609–627, 2001.

Wilson Jr BJ, Becker MA, Linton ME, Donn SM: Spontaneous minute ventilation predicts readiness for extubation in mechanically ventilated preterm infants, *J Perinatol* 18:436–439, 1998.

Wiswell TE: Meconium aspiration syndrome. In Donn SM, Sinha SK, editors: *Manual of neonatal respiratory care*, 3rd ed, New York, 2012, Springer, pp 555–564.

Wung JT, James LS, Kilchevsky E, et al.: Management of infants with severe respiratory failure and persistence of the fetal circulation without hyper-ventilation, *Pediatrics* 76:488–493, 1985.

CHAPTER 11

BRONCHOPULMONARY DYSPLASIA

Ben-Hur Johnson, MD • Bernard Thébaud, MD, PhD

Bronchopulmonary dysplasia (BPD) is a chronic lung disease characterized by lung inflammation, abnormal lung growth, and abnormal development of the alveoli and pulmonary vasculature in premature infants. Clinically, the disease will manifest as a need for supplementary oxygen at 36 weeks' postmenstrual age (PMA) and in many patients with long-term impairment of pulmonary function, persisting into adolescence and early adulthood (Walsh et al., 2004).

In 1967 Northway and colleagues described for the first time the clinical, radiologic, and pathologic features of BPD in 32 preterm infants with a mean gestational age of 34 weeks (Northway et al., 1967). The course of the disease evolved over four stages of radiographic and clinical changes. A chest radiograph with increased density owing to fibrosis, areas of lung collapse alternating with hyperinflation, and emphysema characterized the most severe form. Northway and colleagues hypothesized that BPD resulted from the combined effects of pulmonary oxygen toxicity and mechanical ventilation on the healing process of infants with severe respiratory distress syndrome (RDS). At the time of Northway's original description, most premature infants with BPD weighed more than 1500 grams at birth and received aggressive mechanical ventilation. They exhibited a severe form of chronic lung disease ("old" BPD) with the radiologic features described above. However, improvements in perinatal and neonatal care including the use of antenatal steroids and surfactant have allowed the survival of a population of infants with greater degrees of prematurity, but who exhibit a milder form of chronic lung disease ("new" BPD). "New" BPD is characterized by impaired lung growth (Jobe & Bancalari, 2001), and while milder than the "old" BPD, the long-term consequences of this early interference with normal lung development will unravel in the affected patients over the next decades (Mosca et al., 2011).

EPIDEMIOLOGY

The reported incidence of BPD varies broadly, but the National Institute of Child Health and Human Development (NICHD) Neonatal Network reports that BPD is diagnosed at the time of discharge from the neonatal intensive care unit (NICU) in 25% to 35% of very low birth weight (VLBW) infants (those born with a birth weight below 1500 grams) (Walsh et al., 2004); with infants born at 22 to 26 weeks at higher risk. Mortality rates of babies below 1500 grams have decreased substantially parallel to better obstetrical care, use of antenatal steroids, early surfactant treatment for RDS, and advanced respiratory support strategies; however, there is still divergence in opinion on whether the incidence of BPD has decreased in association with these improvements in perinatal care. In a large study by Stoll and colleagues (Stoll et al., 2010) at the NICHD Neonatal Network of infants born between 22 to 28 weeks during 2003 to 2007, the incidence of BPD increased from 42% to 68% over the 5-year study period. A similar trend has been described in the Canadian Neonatal Network in which the incidence of BPD over the past 10 years had increased by 10% (Shah et al., 2012). In contrast, a study of a large national database revealed a 4.3% annual decrease in the incidence of BPD between 1993 and 2006 (Stroustrup & Trasande, 2010). This decrease in the incidence of BPD was associated with an increased use of noninvasive respiratory support but also with a concomitant increase in cost and days of hospitalization. Thus, there is still a discrepancy in the literature regarding the incidence of BPD and many authors believe this might be related to the definition of the disease, the different protocols for the use of oxygen at 36 weeks' PMA, to variations in the use of postnatal steroids, and to a plateau in survival that may have been reached among extremely preterm infants.

CASE STUDY 1

A 32-year-old mother in her second pregnancy is admitted to her local hospital after premature rupture of membranes at 26 weeks' gestation associated with mild contractions. She has been healthy and this was an uneventful pregnancy until 20 weeks' gestation when she developed increased blood pressure believed to be gestational hypertension. An ultrasound at 24 weeks' gestation showed decreased fetal growth with an estimated fetal weight more consistent with 20 weeks' gestation. Her prenatal screening tests revealed the following data: hepatitis B negative, human immunodeficiency virus (HIV) negative, Venereal Disease Research Laboratory (VDRL) test negative, blood group B positive, and group B Streptococcus (GBS) status unknown.

EXERCISE 1

QUESTIONS

1. At this point, the antenatal management of this pregnant patient can be optimized by providing which of the following?
   a. Glucocorticoids to accelerate lung maturation in the fetus
   b. Antibiotics to prevent maternal and fetal sepsis
   c. Transfer to a hospital with a level 3 NICU center
   d. All of the above

2. If this infant is delivered, what are potential risk factors for developing BPD?
   a. Gestational age
   b. Premature rupture of the membranes
   c. High blood pressure
   d. Unknown GBS status

ANSWERS

1. **d**.

2. **a**.

DIAGNOSTIC CRITERIA

The initial clinical definition of BPD in the early 1980s was based on the need of supplemental oxygen on Day 28 of age along with chest radiograph abnormalities (Bancalari et al., 1979). This definition allowed an infant to carry the diagnosis of BPD without undergoing lung biopsy and histologic confirmation. However, validation of the definition was nearly impossible because of three issues: (1) the need of supplemental oxygen at 28 days of life was completely at the discretion

of the physician and not supported by any quantitative physiologic assessment; (2) there was lack of consensus on the optimal arterial oxygen level for these infants (saturation levels considered as acceptable varied on an individual- or institutional-basis, ranging from 84% to 96%; Ellsbury et al., 2002); and (3) this definition was appropriate for identifying those infants less than 30 weeks' gestation with risk of poor pulmonary outcome, but lost sensitivity as gestational age decreased.

In the late 1980s Shennan and colleagues revised this definition of BPD by extending oxygen dependence to 36 weeks' PMA (Shennan et al., 1988). With this new criterion the positive predictive value of the definition increased from 38% to 63%, with a prediction of normal pulmonary outcome of 90% in those infants not receiving oxygen at 36 weeks' PMA. The definition gained wide acceptance and has been validated by other authors. This new definition has been used to identify BPD as one of the most significant predictors of abnormal pulmonary function and neurodevelopmental impairment in infancy and early childhood, even with the strict criterion for infants at lower gestational age who require longer periods of supplemental oxygen to be diagnosed with BPD.

In 2000, a workshop on BPD from the NICHD (Jobe & Bancalari, 2001) led to a refined definition, which maintained the oxygen dependency for ≥28 days and at 36 weeks' PMA, but added oxygen concentration and degree of support needed, to define the severity of the lung injury (Table 11-1). Outcome was graded into mild, moderate, and severe BPD. Neonates born at <32 weeks' gestation are assessed at 36 weeks' PMA or discharge home, whichever comes first; those born at ≥32 weeks' gestation are assessed at >28 days, but <56 days, or discharge home, whichever comes first. This definition was validated and identified a spectrum of risk for adverse pulmonary and neurodevelopmental outcomes in early infancy more accurately than previous definitions (Ehrenkranz et al., 2005).

In an attempt to overcome the physician's individual assessment to define the need of supplemental oxygen, Walsh and co-workers presented a physiologic definition of BPD (Table 11-2) with set weaning criteria based on oxygen saturation (Walsh et al., 2003). Infants requiring >30% oxygen, mechanical ventilation, or continuous positive airway pressure (CPAP), were labeled as having BPD with no need of saturation testing. Infants requiring <30% oxygen were challenged with a stepwise reduction to room air; those who failed were diagnosed as having BPD. Infants in room air were assumed not to have BPD. The physiologic definition detected a group of infants receiving supplemental oxygen for indications not related to pulmonary disease,

TABLE 11-1 Definition of Bronchopulmonary Dysplasia from the NICHD Workshop on BPD

Gestational Age	<32 weeks	≥32 weeks
Time point of assessment	36 weeks' PMA or discharge to home, whichever comes first	>28 days, but <56 days' postnatal age or discharge home, whichever comes first
	Treatment with oxygen >21% for at least 28 days **plus**	
Mild BPD	Breathing room air at 36 weeks' PMA or discharge, whichever comes first	Breathing room air by 56 days' postnatal age or discharge, whichever comes first
Moderate BPD	Need* for <30% oxygen at 36 weeks' PMA or discharge, whichever comes first	Need* for <30% oxygen at 56 days' postnatal age or discharge, whichever comes first
Severe BPD	Need* for ≥30% oxygen and/or positive pressure (PPV/NCPAP) at 36 weeks' PMA or discharge, whichever comes first	Need* for ≥30% oxygen and/or positive pressure (PPV/NCPAP) at 56 days' postnatal age or discharge, whichever comes first

Modified from Jobe AH, Bancalari E. Bronchopulmonary dysplasia, Am J Resp Crit Care Med 163:1723-1729, 2001.
BPD, Bronchopulmonary dysplasia; NCPAP, nasal continuous positive airway pressure; PPV, positive pressure ventilation; PMA, postmenstrual age.
*A physiologic test confirming that the oxygen requirement at the assessment time point remains to be defined. BPD usually develops in neonates being treated with oxygen and positive pressure ventilation for respiratory failure, most commonly respiratory distress syndrome. Persistence of clinical features of respiratory disease (tachypnea, retractions, rales) are considered common to the broad description of BPD and have not been included in the diagnostic criteria describing the severity of BPD. Infants treated with oxygen >21% and/or positive pressure for nonrespiratory disease (e.g., central apnea, diaphragmatic paralysis) do not have BPD unless they also develop parenchymal lung disease and exhibit clinical features of respiratory distress. A day of treatment with oxygen >21% means that the infant received oxygen >21% for more than 12 hours on that day. Treatment with oxygen >21% and/or positive pressure at 36 weeks' PMA, or at 56 days' postnatal age or discharge, should not reflect an "acute" event, but should rather reflect the infant's usual daily therapy for several days preceding and following 36 weeks' PMA, 56 days' postnatal age, or discharge.

TABLE 11-2 Physiologic Definition of Bronchopulmonary Dysplasia

Oxygen			<30%		>30% or PPV/CPAP
Stepwise Challenge to Room Air			YES		NO
Oxygen Saturation	<80%	80%-87%	88%-95%	≥96%	
Monitoring	1 min	5 min	15 min	60 min	
Outcome	Failed	Failed	Passed	Passed	
BPD	YES	YES	NO	NO	YES

BPD, Bronchopulmonary dysplasia; PPV, positive pressure ventilation, CPAP, continuous positive airway pressure; PMA, postmenstrual age; Min, minute.
Infants at 36 weeks' PMA requiring concentrations of oxygen above 30%, and/or mechanical ventilation or NCPAP, were defined as having BPD without a challenge test to room air. Infants at the same PMA in room air were considered not having BPD. Those newborns requiring less than 30% oxygen were challenged to a stepwise reduction of oxygen (by 2% steps every 10 minutes) until reaching room air, with continuous monitoring of oxygen saturations and heart rate. In this study Walsh and co-workers defined as the lowest acceptable saturation a value of 88%.

and when compared to the clinical definition of BPD using supplemental oxygen requirement as the only criterion, the number of babies diagnosed with BPD dropped from 31% to 25%.

RADIOLOGIC FEATURES OF BPD

The chest x-ray was central in the initial description of BPD by Northway, a radiologist at Stanford University. The classic radiologic features included: coarse interstitial densities scattered with cystlike areas, hyperinflation, lung cysts, and emphysema (Figure 11-1). In later stages, linear densities secondary to fibrosis developed in the lung.

Infants with the new form of BPD generally exhibit a milder respiratory course and have less severe abnormalities on the chest radiograph (Figure 11-2). The main radiographic finding

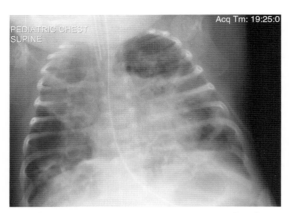

FIGURE 11-1 ■ "Old" bronchopulmonary dysplasia. Chest x-ray of an ex-28⅞ weeks' gestation infant, now 38 weeks corrected, with severe bronchopulmonary dysplasia. There are patchy airspace opacities consistent with atelectasis, alternating with areas of cystic lucencies and lung overinflation. Coarse lung markings are also present, secondary to fibrosis.

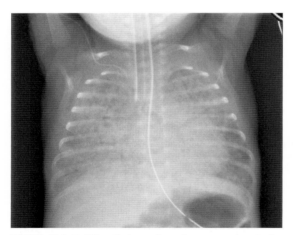

FIGURE 11-2 ■ "New" bronchopulmonary dysplasia. Anterior-posterior chest x-ray of an ex-25⅞ weeks' infant, now 6 weeks old and still requiring mechanical ventilation. Notice the pulmonary hyperinflation with bilateral homogenous interstitial pattern.

in "new" BPD is a diffuse haziness, associated sometimes with pulmonary hyperinflation.

In most cases there is poor reliability of the plain chest x-ray to correlate radiologic features of BPD to clinical status or respiratory outcome (Moya et al., 2001). In the older individual, abnormal chest computed tomography (CT) scans demonstrate a better correlation with poor pulmonary function and clinical course (Mahut et al., 2007; Wong et al., 2008). The CT scan is a more sensitive test (Wilson, 2010), but its use is limited to the follow up of infants with radiographic abnormalities during adolescence and adulthood.

ETIOLOGY

The etiology of BPD is multifactorial (Figure 11-3), combining several risk factors including lung immaturity, mechanical ventilation, oxidative stress, and inflammation (Sosenko et al., 2012). A genetic susceptibility is also being considered. Each is briefly reviewed below.

Immaturity and Lung Development

Improvements in perinatal care have allowed the survival of more immature infants. BPD occurs now in infants born at less than 28 weeks' PMA. Many of these extremely preterm infants who develop BPD do not exhibit signs of RDS at birth and many of them have not required mechanical ventilation or supplemental oxygen. The increased vulnerability of the most immature preterm infants, especially those between 23 to 26 weeks, might be explained by the extreme immaturity of their lungs.

Even in the absence of antenatal inflammation, extreme preterm birth interferes with normal lung growth (Hjalmarson & Sandberg, 2002). Extremely immature infants are born at the late canalicular stage of lung development (Figure 11-4), just when the airways become juxtaposed to the blood vessels and before alveolar saccules emerge. Many of the interventions to maintain adequate gas exchange in these infants also interfere with the normal process of lung development inducing an arrest in alveolar and lung vascular growth, characteristic features in the "new" BPD (Jobe, 1999).

Insights into the molecular mechanisms that control normal lung development have revealed the crucial interaction between epithelium and mesenchyme and the role of transcription factors, growth factors, and the extracellular matrix (Fox & Post, 2009). Members of the fibroblast growth factors family (FGF-7, FGF-9, FGF-10), platelet-derived growth factor (PDGF), bone morphogenetic proteins (BMP-4, BMP-5, BMP-7), genes from the Sprouty family, sonic hedgehog transcripts, insulin-like growth factors (IGF-I and IGF-II), and retinoic acid regulate cell to cell interactions. More recently the role of the pulmonary vasculature and vascular growth factors (including vascular endothelial growth factor [VEGF], hypoxia inducible factor [HIF], and Angiopoietin 1) has been recognized in actively contributing to alveolar development and the maintenance of alveolar structures throughout postnatal life (Thébaud & Abman, 2007). Although many of the above-named growth factors have been investigated in animal models of BPD, none of these discoveries has yet led to novel therapies to prevent

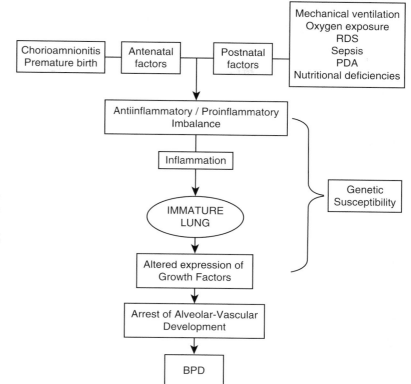

FIGURE 11-3 ■ Pathophysiology of BPD. Bronchopulmonary dysplasia is a multifactorial disease. Prenatal and postnatal factors may affect the proinflammatory/antiinflammatory balance in a genetically predisposed infant. All these factors may alter the expression of growth factors and impede normal lung development, resulting in the characteristic changes of inhibition or arrest of alveologenesis and vascular development. *RDS,* Respiratory distress syndrome; *PDA,* patent ductus arteriosus; *BPD,* bronchopulmonary dysplasia.

lung injury and promote normal lung growth in the vulnerable prematurely born human neonate.

Hyperoxia and Oxidative Stress

The role of hyperoxia in the pathogenesis of BPD was well identified by Northway and colleagues in 1967 (Northway et al., 1967) and has been confirmed in multiple animal models (Tanswell & Jankov, 2003). Free radicals are highly reactive and unstable molecules with unpaired electrons that tend to donate or abstract electrons from other biologic substrates altering the structure of proteins, lipids, and ultimately damaging cellular function. Reactive oxygen species (ROS) and reactive nitrogen species (RNS) are generated in the preterm infant when transitioning from the relative hypoxemic *in utero* environment to relative hyperoxia at birth. ROS are also released by neutrophils and macrophages at sites of inflammation from chorioamnionitis and mechanical ventilation (Auten & White, 2009). Evidence suggests an oxidant/antioxidant imbalance in premature infants at risk for BPD, confirmed by a plasmatic antioxidant profile with low levels of glutathione peroxidase, vitamin E, selenium, copper, and zinc (Gitto et al., 2002). The lung is protected against ROS mainly by antioxidant enzymes that

are developmentally regulated, including superoxide dismutase, glutathione peroxidase, glucose-6-phosphate dehydrogenase, and catalase. Animal studies suggest that antioxidant enzymes activities are very low until the final 15% to 20% of gestation with a dramatic rise up to 500% at the end of gestation (Frank & Sosenko, 1991). Thus, the premature infant may have a lower baseline antioxidant enzyme protective capacity than the full term infant, and at the same time an inability to increase this activity in response to hyperoxia. In preterm baboons exposed to 100% O_2, a catalytic antioxidant, metalloporphyrin AEOL 10113, has been shown to attenuate lung injury (Chang & Crapo, 2003); nevertheless, strategies aimed at reducing oxygen exposure and increasing antioxidant capacity in infants at risk of developing BPD have had mixed long-term results: although there was no difference in the incidence of BPD at 36 weeks between placebo and CuZnSOD-treated infants, there was a reduction in asthma-like symptoms and need for medications in CuZn-SOD-treated infants at 1 year (Davis et al., 2003).

Inflammation

It is suggested that inflammation contributes to the pathogenesis of BPD. Several animal and

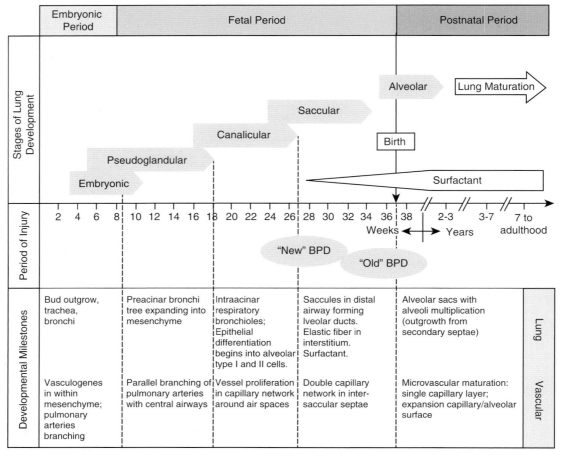

FIGURE 11-4 ■ Stages of lung development. (Modified from Wu S. Molecular bases for lung development, injury, and repair. In Bancalari E, Polin RA, editors: *The newborn lung: neonatology questions and controversies*, 2nd ed, Philadelphia, PA, 2012, Saunders, pp 3-27.)

clinical studies have demonstrated a large number of inflammatory cells and increased levels of proinflammatory cytokines and chemokines in the lung (Johnson et al., 2009) and in bronchoalveolar lavage (BAL) of infants with BPD (Ogden et al., 1983); whereas others have proved that the presence of inflammatory mediators—such as IL-8, antiinflammatory IL-10, and granulocyte colony stimulating factor in the serum of infants on Day 1 of life—predicted the risk of BPD (Paananen et al., 2009). High postnatal serum concentrations of IL-1β, IL-6, IL-8, and IL-10 from Days 0 to 3 of life have also been associated with the development of BPD or death in infants <1000 grams (Ambalavanan et al., 2009).

Prenatal and Postnatal Infection

Evidence suggests the possibility that antenatal exposure of the immature lung to inflammation during chorioamnionitis or postnatal exposure from early onset sepsis or nosocomial infection may increase the risk of acute lung damage and BPD (Thomas & Speer, 2011; Watterberg et al., 1996). There is a strong association between chorioamnionitis, preterm labor (PTL), and preterm premature rupture of membranes (PPROM) (Goldenberg et al., 2008). Intrauterine infection is present in 70% of deliveries before 28 weeks' gestation, but only in 15% of deliveries at 34 to 36 weeks. *Ureaplasma* spp. are the most frequently isolated microorganisms inside the amniotic cavity during pregnancy and in conjunction with *Mycoplasma hominis* have been associated with PTL and PPROM. *Ureaplasma urealyticum* (*Uu*) may trigger *in utero* inflammation, and has been isolated from the respiratory tract of infants who develop BPD (even without clinical or laboratory signs of infection). In animal studies *Uu* contributes to early fibrosis and altered developmental signaling in the immature lung.

Beeton and co-workers (Beeton et al., 2011) analyzed gastric and BAL samples from term and preterm infants to identify prenatal and postnatal microbial infection. The presence of 16S rRNA genes and *Ureaplasma* spp. in cultures of gastric and lung fluid was significantly associated with the development of BPD. These samples were collected before and after Day 3 of life, confirming early and postnatal infection, and this microbial presence also was accompanied by a peak in the concentration of IL-6 and IL-8 in BAL fluid, confirming inflammation secondary to microbial infection and not simple colonization. Although there is clear evidence with this and other studies for a strong association between perinatal *Ureaplasma* infection and BPD, the prophylactic use of erythromycin in ventilated infants has not decreased the incidence of BPD.

Whether chorioamnionitis is a risk factor for BPD remains controversial. Animal models and clinical studies suggest that antenatal infection contributes to lung maturation, but subsequently may increase the risk of developing BPD (Jobe, 2012). Fetal sheep exposed to proinflammatory cytokines *in utero* show enhanced lung maturation superior to steroid-induced surfactant production (Kuypers et al., 2012). Ammari and colleagues (Ammari et al., 2005) observed that infants exposed to chorioamnionitis experienced a reduced incidence of RDS: 31% of infants born at 23 to 25 weeks and 78% born at 26 to 28 weeks did not require surfactant or mechanical ventilation, indicating that these infants had more mature lung function for their gestational age. Conversely, a multicenter study from the Canadian Neonatal Network noted that clinical chorioamnionitis was associated with increased risk for severe intraventricular hemorrhage (IVH) and early onset sepsis, but not respiratory outcomes (Soraisham et al., 2009). In the Alabama Preterm Birth Study (Andrews et al., 2006), a prospective study following 446 consecutive deliveries of singletons <32 weeks' gestation, exposure to histologic chorioamnionitis was associated with neonatal systemic inflammatory response, but BPD was not increased in these infants. Similarly Lahra and colleagues (2009) and Van Marter (2002) concluded that the incidence of BPD was reduced by antenatal infection/inflammation.

Genetics

There is growing evidence that genetic susceptibility may contribute to the risk of BPD. Studies of premature monozygotic twins suggest that 53% of the variance in liability of BPD is attributable to genetic factors after adjusting for major covariates such as gender, birth weight, and RDS (Bhandari & Gruen, 2006). Identifying

the high-risk genes has been more challenging. Most candidate genes examined for a potential role in BPD are genes encoding surfactant proteins, innate immunity, antioxidant defenses, and proteins involved in regulating mechanisms of vascular and lung remodeling (Lavoie & Dubé, 2010). More studies exploring genetic susceptibility are ongoing (Somaschini et al., 2012).

PREVENTION AND THERAPIES FOR BPD

Despite breakthrough therapies and incremental improvements in the management of extreme premature infants, before and after birth, there is no specific U.S. Food and Drug Administration (FDA) approved intervention for BPD. Postnatal dexamethasone had the most striking benefit, but is associated with important adverse effects and fine-tuning its use seems to be one of the most promising avenues for the prevention of BPD. A brief overview of other interventions is provided below.

EXERCISE 2
QUESTION

1. Which of the following interventions are evidence-based therapies for prevention of BPD?
   a. Diuretics
   b. Prophylactic indomethacin
   c. Fluid restriction
   d. Vitamin A
   e. Caffeine
   f. Inhaled nitric oxide
   g. Surfactant
   h. Antenatal steroids
   i. Postnatal steroids
   j. Antioxidants

ANSWER

1. **d**, **e**, and **i**.

Antenatal Interventions

Prevention of Preterm Birth

Preterm birth is the most important cause of perinatal and neonatal mortality and its prevention is considered the single most effective way to decrease neonatal morbidities including BPD (Lockwood & Kuczynski, 2001). Preterm birth is a clinical syndrome arising from activation of many maternal and fetal processes that result in a dysregulation of the immune system and exaggeration of inflammatory processes (Romero et al., 2006). Optimal management of preterm birth includes the use of regionalization of care, antenatal maternal transfer to tertiary care units, progesterone, antibiotics, and tocolytic drugs; however, delayed delivery may not always be associated with improved neonatal outcomes (Dodd et al., 2006).

Antenatal Glucocorticoids

Liggins and Howie's breakthrough observation brought the most effective intervention for the prevention of RDS: antenatal administration of a course of glucocorticoids in women between 24 and 34 weeks' gestation with imminent risk of preterm birth (Liggins & Howie, 1972). Antenatal glucocorticoids significantly reduce RDS and neonatal mortality, but have not affected the incidence of BPD (Crowley, 2000).

Postnatal Interventions

Postnatal Glucocorticoids

In a double blind, crossover randomized clinical trial Mammel and colleagues were the first investigators to show that administration of dexamethasone improved lung function and hastened weaning from the ventilator in infants with BPD (Mammel et al., 1983). In the late 1980s Cummings and colleagues randomized 36 preterm infants at high risk of BPD who were still requiring mechanical ventilation and oxygen at 14 days of age, to treatment with an 18-day or 42-day tapering course of parenteral dexamethasone (Cummings et al., 1989). The 42-day course group showed faster weaning from mechanical ventilation and supplemental oxygen, and improved neurodevelopmental outcome with no clinical side effects from the treatment.

Subsequent studies confirmed the beneficial effects of glucocorticoids on pulmonary outcomes, and metaanalyses of randomized controlled trials (RCTs) have provided a better picture of the various dosing regimens proposed. Three different time frames have been examined: (1) early treatment with steroids (within 96 hours of life); (2) moderately early treatment (7 to 14 days of life); and (3) late treatment (more than 3 weeks of life). Early treatment with dexamethasone has significant benefits, including earlier extubation and a decreased risk of BPD at 28 days and 36 weeks' PMA, and death or BPD at 28 days and 36 weeks' PMA. It is also associated with lower incidences of PDA and retinopathy of prematurity (ROP). However, early treatment

with glucocorticoids is associated with serious side effects including gastrointestinal bleeding and perforation, hypertrophic cardiomyopathy, hyperglycemia, hypertension, and growth failure. Importantly, an increased risk of adverse neurologic outcome including cerebral palsy (CP) was also found (Halliday et al., 2008). Thus the severe side effects outweigh the benefits of the early use of dexamethasone for the prevention of BPD.

When glucocorticoids are used between 7 and 14 days of life, pulmonary outcomes are similar to those observed with early treatment; steroids facilitate early extubation and reduce the incidence of BPD and death at 28 days or 36 weeks' PMA (Halliday et al., 2003); side effects remain a concern during this time frame. In babies treated after 3 weeks of life (late treatment) a metaanalysis of 19 trials (Halliday et al., 2003) described a reduction of BPD at 28 days and 36 weeks, and a reduction in the combined outcome of BPD or death. Furthermore, a reduction in the need for supplemental oxygen at the time of discharge home was evident. The risk of CP or death was not significantly increased in the group of infants treated with glucocorticoids after 3 weeks of age, but not all studies reported long-term outcomes.

This concern over the potential neurodevelopmental harm associated with the use of systemic glucocorticoids has restricted their use for the prevention or treatment of BPD. Glucocorticoids are now limited to those infants who cannot be weaned off mechanical ventilation; lower doses and shorter duration are generally recommended. The likelihood that an infant will develop BPD may determine whether dexamethasone improves or worsens neurodevelopmental outcomes. In a study, Doyle and colleagues have shown that glucocorticoids increase the risk for death or BPD in infants with low risk for BPD, but they improves outcomes in infants with higher risk (Doyle et al., 2005). Determining the optimal steroid, dose, route, and timing to decrease the risk of BPD without increasing the risk for neurodevelopmental sequelae in ventilated preterm infants remains worthwhile for exploring in well-designed RCTs (Onland et al., 2009).

Caffeine

Caffeine, a member of the family of methylxanthines, is used for the treatment of apnea of prematurity. A large RCT was performed to evaluate the short- and long-term benefits of caffeine in very preterm infants (Schmidt et al., 2006). A secondary analysis of the data showed a significant reduction of BPD at 36 weeks' PMA in the group of infants receiving caffeine, with the authors speculating that this reduction in BPD in the group treated with caffeine might have been explained by the shorter exposure to positive pressure ventilation in comparison to the placebo group. Caffeine therapy also reduced the rates of CP and cognitive delay at 18 months of age but not at 5 years (Schmidt et al., 2012).

Treatment of Patent Ductus Arteriosus and Fluid Restriction

About 65% of VLBW infants develop a PDA that when hemodynamically significant and occurring after the first week of life has been associated with an increased risk of BPD (Rojas et al., 1995). Its role as a risk factor for BPD may be explained by the pulmonary edema and increased pulmonary flow from the systemic-to-pulmonary shunting associated with prolonged exposure to mechanical ventilation. However, approaches to prevent or treat the hemodynamically significant PDA have not been shown to reduce the incidence of BPD.

The trial of indomethacin prophylaxis in VLBW infants (Schmidt et al., 2001) showed that indomethacin started on the first day life, before the onset of a hemodynamically significant PDA, reduces the frequency of PDA but does not reduce the incidence of BPD. Other investigators reported that treatment of PDA with ibuprofen did not reduce the risk for BPD (Shah et al., 2006). In contrast, Kabra and colleagues (Kabra et al., 2007) compared two groups of infants with a hemodynamically significant PDA who were treated medically or with surgical ligation and suggested that surgical PDA ligation may be associated with an increased risk of BPD. Other studies have reached a similar conclusion (Chrone et al., 2007; Mirea et al., 2012). These discrepancies may be explained by the duration of ductal patency and time of exposure to increased pulmonary blood flow (Bancalari et al., 2005).

Many neonatologists try to overcome the potential effects of PDA-associated pulmonary edema with fluid restriction to physiologic requirements. A Cochrane review demonstrated that although the incidence of PDA is reduced by fluid restriction, the incidence of BPD is unaffected by restricted fluid administration alone (Bell & Acarregui, 2008). Similarly, the use of diuretics in established BPD has only shown short-term improvement in pulmonary function and oxygen requirements, but no significant effect on the incidence of the disease (Brion & Primhak, 2000; Brion et al., 2002).

Vitamin A

Preterm infants have low vitamin A status at birth and this has been associated with an increased risk of developing BPD (Shenai, 1999). Vitamin A exerts pleiotropic effects on lung development and repair including lung maturation, epithelial repair, antioxidant and antiinflammatory properties (Guimaraes et al., 2012). A recent metaanalysis of nine trials evaluating vitamin A supplementation in VLBW infants showed a reduction in death and oxygen requirements at 1 month of age and a trend toward a reduction of BPD. Follow up of these infants up to 18 to 22 months corrected age showed no effects on neurodevelopmental outcomes (Darlow & Graham, 2011). Only intramuscular doses were evaluated and this has contributed to hampering wide acceptance of vitamin A therapy (Kaplan et al., 2010).

Antioxidants

Exogenously administered superoxide dismutase (SOD) has been tested in clinical trials to prevent BPD in preterm infants (Suresh et al., 2001). Two RCTs showed no benefit. A trial examining intratracheal recombinant human (r-h) CuZn-SOD did not reduce the incidence of BPD, but at 1 year follow up, significantly fewer infants in the r-h CuZnSOD had respiratory illness severe enough to require bronchodilators and/or corticosteroids (Davis et al., 2003).

CASE STUDY 1 (continued)

Two hours after admission, the mother is transferred to a tertiary care center after receiving a first injection of betamethasone and antibiotics. In view of her risk of delivering an extremely premature baby, the neonatology fellow is called to counsel the parents regarding issues relevant for the baby and outcomes including mortality and long-term disabilities. Shortly after arrival, the mother develops fever and has more contractions. Because of a suspicion of chorioamnionitis, a decision is made to let her progress to spontaneous vaginal delivery. At that time she is started on magnesium sulfate and receives a second dose of betamethasone. Four hours later a 635-gram male infant is born. He has poor respiratory effort and a heart rate of 90. Resuscitation includes bag ventilation and mask with 40% oxygen with improvement in heart rate, color, and initiation of regular spontaneous respirations. Apgar scores are 2, 6, and 8 at 1, 5, and 10 minutes, respectively. At 15 minutes of life, the baby requires 30% oxygen to maintain saturations at 95% with minor work of breathing.

EXERCISE 3

QUESTION

1. At this point, how would you manage this baby?
   a. Intubate and ventilate in conventional mode with FiO_2 to maintain O_2 saturations at 98%.
   b. Provide CPAP with an FiO_2 of 30% to maintain saturations at 95% and monitor the respiratory status.
   c. Intubate, administer surfactant, and provide mechanical ventilation for 2 weeks to allow the baby to grow.
   d. Intubate and use high-frequency oscillatory ventilation to achieve O_2 saturations of 95%.

ANSWER

1. **b**.

Mechanical Ventilation

Although technologic improvements have brought better-performing ventilators into the NICU, the only effective way to prevent BPD is to avoid mechanical ventilation. More recently, the focus has shifted to changes in delivery room practices as a strategy to prevent lung injury. Indeed, in the last two decades many observational studies have reported decreased rates of BPD in babies with RDS treated with early CPAP instead of mechanical ventilation with intubation. Well-designed RCTs such as the COIN (Morley et al., 2008) and the SUPPORT trial (Finer et al., 2010), in which close to 2000 infants between 24 and 27 weeks' PMA were randomized to early CPAP versus intubation and surfactant, found no significant differences between groups in composite outcome of death or BPD, but a trend toward improved outcomes. However, in these studies less than 50% of infants born before 28 weeks required mechanical ventilation. Further studies—aiming at optimizing the combined use of limiting mechanical ventilation and oxygen exposure—are warranted.

In some circumstances (no antenatal steroids, severe RDS) mechanical ventilation will not be avoidable. Under the term of "gentle ventilation," several investigators have attempted to decrease lung injury by using low tidal volumes. Permissive hypercapnia accepts higher $PaCO_2$ ($PaCO_2$ >55 mmHg) to allow ventilation with lower tidal volumes avoiding lung overdistention; nevertheless, some randomized controlled trials have failed to demonstrate a reduction in BPD with the use of permissive hypercapnia (Thome & Ambalavanan, 2009).

High frequency ventilation (HFV), whereby small tidal volumes are delivered at frequencies above 240/minute (depending on the ventilator design), is another approach for gentle ventilation. Although animal studies have confirmed lung protective effects of HFV, RCTs and metaanalysis in humans have shown no benefits of HFV when compared to conventional ventilation in preventing BPD. These conflicting results might be explained by variance in the ventilation strategies used for HFV, the timing when HFV was started, and the different type of ventilators and technology used (Cools et al., 2009; Henderson-Smart, 2009). These trials highlight the importance of understanding the underlying pathophysiology of RDS and using a ventilator skillfully.

Nitric Oxide

Inhaled nitric oxide (iNO) is a selective pulmonary vasodilator and FDA approved for the treatment of hypoxic respiratory failure and persistent pulmonary hypertension (PH) in term and near-term infants. iNO reduces the combined outcome of need for extracorporeal membrane oxygenation (ECMO) and death (Clark et al., 2000). Experimental studies show that iNO has antiinflammatory effects; it reduces ventilation-induced lung injury in preterm lambs and promotes alveolar and lung vascular growth in neonatal rodents (Thébaud & Abman, 2007).

Several RCTs have evaluated the effect of iNO in preterm infants (Soll, 2012), but a recent National Institutes of Health panel (Cole et al., 2011) concluded that iNO is of no benefit in reducing the incidence of BPD.

CASE STUDY 1 (continued)

After respiratory stabilization, intravascular catheters are inserted in the umbilical vein and umbilical artery, blood cultures are drawn, and antibiotics and total parenteral nutrition are initiated. The baby is admitted to the level 3 NICU for further management. At 3 hours of life, oxygen requirements increase to 45% with increased subcostal retractions. The baby is intubated and receives exogenous surfactant. The early course is uncomplicated and extubation occurs at 24 hours of life to nasal CPAP and 25% to 30% oxygen. At the same time a patent ductus arteriosus was found but not considered hemodynamically significant.

On Day 15 of life, the baby is reintubated for prolonged episodes of apneas and increased oxygen requirements. He is diagnosed with a central line–associated blood stream infection and treated with antibiotics for 10 days. On the third day of antibiotic therapy the ductus arteriosus reopens and requires surgical ligation. At 4 weeks of life, the baby remains on a high-frequency oscillator with FiO₂ requirements fluctuating between 60% and 80%; there are recurrent episodes of bradycardia and desaturation. Following a 5-day course of dexamethasone, the baby is finally extubated to nCPAP, and by the 36th week postconceptual age requires 30% oxygen. Four weeks later, the infant transitions to nasal cannula oxygen. He is finally discharged home 2 weeks later with supplemental oxygen. The head ultrasound demonstrates a resolving grade 2 IVH.

EXERCISE 4

QUESTIONS

1. According to the definition of the workshop on BPD from the NICHD, how would you grade the severity of this infant's BPD?
   a. Severe BPD
   b. Mild BPD
   c. Moderate BPD
   d. No BPD

2. What are the potential postnatal risk factors of developing BPD in this baby?
   a. Apnea and bradycardia
   b. Patent ductus arteriosus
   c. Nosocomial infection
   d. Grade 2 intraventricular hemorrhage

ANSWERS

1. **a**.

2. **b** and **c**.

LONG-TERM OUTCOMES IN PATIENTS WITH BPD

Pulmonary Outcomes

Most of the information available about the pulmonary outcomes of children who have had BPD comes from survivors in the presurfactant era with the "old" form of the disease. Information from children and young adults who were treated with antenatal glucocorticoids and postnatal surfactant are just beginning to emerge.

BPD increases the need for hospital readmissions during early childhood for respiratory illness, and is frequently associated with severe respiratory syncytial virus (RSV) infection (Smith et al., 2004). Follow up studies demonstrate that pulmonary function and compliance tends to improve over time; nevertheless, evaluation of forced expiratory flows (FEV) in

survivors during the first 3 years of life show frequently significant limitation of the airflow, probably reflecting deterioration of airway function (Baraldi & Filippone, 2007). In many cases, this limitation persists beyond childhood into adolescence and young adulthood, and is associated with cough and recurrent wheezing in an asthma-like picture with air trapping and abnormal chest radiographs (Bhandari & Panitch, 2006). The percentage of predicted FEV may also be decreased in extremely preterm infants without BPD, reflecting the consequences of preterm birth on the very immature lung (Kotecha et al., 2013). Moreover, the degree of airflow limitation in the first years of life seems to predict pulmonary function in later life, allocating to this group a higher risk of developing obstructive pulmonary disease (Broström et al., 2010). These trends seem to be consistent with the results of large cohort studies such as EPICURE (Fawke et al., 2010).

More recently, case reports of young adults born in the postsurfactant era are emerging, suggesting persistent alveolar growth impairment (Cutz & Chiasson, 2008) or early-onset emphysema (Wong et al., 2008). Longitudinal studies of large cohorts of extremely premature infants born in recent years are crucial to better understand the long-term respiratory outcome of this population.

Pulmonary Vascular Disease

Abnormalities in vascular development are important components of BPD. In many cases, these alterations are severe enough to lead to PH and cor pulmonale. The signs can be subtle and manifest only as prolonged oxygen dependency, impaired gas exchange, and decreased exercise intolerance.

The incidence of PH in preterm infants with the "new" BPD was unknown until recently. Current studies suggest that the overall incidence is close to 25%, reaching 50% in infants with severe BPD (Mourani & Abman, 2013). Although the echocardiogram is the most commonly used modality to make the diagnosis of PH, it is not entirely reliable. For example, tricuspid regurgitation is present in only 30% to 60% of infants with BPD and PH.

PH significantly worsens the outcome of BPD and increases the risk of death (48% mortality 2 years after the diagnosis of PH) (Berkelhamer et al., 2013). The risk factors are not well understood yet but fetal growth restriction appears as a significant predictor of PH. Further studies in large cohorts will provide better insights into the incidence and management of PH in this patient population.

Neurodevelopmental Outcomes

The neurologic outcome in BPD survivors includes cognitive, behavioral, and educational problems (Anderson & Doyle, 2006). BPD is an independent risk factor for adverse neurodevelopmental outcome. Using the physiologic definition of BPD, Natarajan and colleagues found lower head circumferences, moderate to severe CP, and reduced cognitive (12.8% vs. 4.6%) and language scores in ELBW infants with BPD compared to those without BPD (Natarajan et al., 2012). Others have reported lower intelligence quotients in children with BPD than in VLBW infants without BPD. Similarly, these children also display more attention impairment, have more delays in expressive and receptive language, and score lower in tests of visual and special perception when compared to their match controls. Additionally, they experience more frequent behavioral disorders such as attention-deficit/hyperactivity (ADHD). Early intervention such as those described in chronic care models using interdisciplinary care teams—including occupational therapists and physical therapists—addressing neurobehavioral skills, protocol-based guidance of interventions, and comprehensive care extending to outpatient care after discharge seem to improve the neurodevelopmental outcome of these infants (Shepherd et al., 2012).

CONCLUSION

Neonatology is a relatively young discipline that has experienced remarkable changes over the last 20 years. A better understanding of newborn physiology coupled with technologic advances and extensive clinical investigation has produced new treatments and modalities of care, resulting in a steady decrease in neonatal mortality. Major breakthroughs include the discovery of antenatal steroids and postnatal surfactant. These have allowed health care teams to push back the limits of viability every 5 to 10 years, so that neonatologists have needed to adjust to an ever more immature patient population with more vulnerable lungs, making the task of preventing BPD ever more challenging. Education, regionalization of care, avoidance of mechanical ventilation, and more judicious use of oxygen when all combined are likely to result in further incremental improvements in survival and morbidity. Further progress will be achieved through a better understanding of the mechanisms that regulate lung development and how these mechanisms are perturbed in BPD in order to develop novel therapeutic strategies. Through recent strides in stem cell biology, cell-based therapies have emerged as a promising intervention to prevent/repair lung damage in extremely premature infants (Alphonse et al., 2011/2012). Carefully conducted human trials over the next decade may unravel their therapeutic potential.

SUGGESTED READINGS

Alphonse RS, Rajabali S, Thebaud B: Lung injury in preterm neonates: the role and therapeutic potential of stem cells, *Antioxid Redox Signal* 17:1013–1040, 2012.

Ambalavanan N, Carlo WA, D'Angio CT, et al.: Cytokines associated with bronchopulmonary dysplasia or death in extremely low birth weight infants, *Pediatrics* 123:1132–1141, 2009.

Ammari A, Suri M, Milisavljevic V, et al.: Variables associated with the early failure of nasal CPAP in very low birth weight infants, *J Pediatr* 147:341–347, 2005.

Anderson PJ, Doyle LW: Neurodevelopmental outcome of bronchopulmonary dysplasia, *Semin Perinatol* 30:227–232, 2006.

Andrews WW, Goldenberg RL, Faye-Petersen O, Cliver S, Goepfert AR, Hauth JC: The Alabama Preterm Birth study: polymorphonuclear and mononuclear cell placental infiltrations, other markers of inflammation, and outcomes in 23- to 32-week preterm newborn infants, *Am J Obstet Gynecol* 195(3):803–808, 2006.

Auten RL, White C: Oxidative and nitrosative stress and bronchopulmonary dysplasia. In Abman SH, editor: *Bronchopulmonary Dysplasia*, vol 240. New York, 2009, Informa Healthcare, pp 105–117.

Bancalari E, Abdenour GE, Feller R, Gannon J, et al.: Bronchopulmonary dysplasia: clinical presentation, *J Pediatr* 95:819–823, 1979.

Bancalari E, Claure N, Gonzalez A: Patent ductus arteriosus and respiratory outcome in premature infants, *Biol Neonate* 88:192–201, 2005.

Baraldi E, Filippone M: Chronic lung disease after premature birth, *N Engl J Med* 357:1946–1955, 2007.

Beeton ML, Maxwell NC, Davies PL, et al.: Role of pulmonary infection in the development of chronic lung disease of prematurity, *Eur Respir J* 37:1424–1430, 2011.

Bell EF, Acarregui MJ: Restricted versus liberal water intake for preventing morbidity and mortality in preterm infants, *Cochrane Database Syst Rev* (1):CD000503, 2008.

Berkelhamer SK, Mestan KK, Steinhorn RH: Pulmonary hypertension in bronchopulmonary dysplasia, *Semin Perinatol* 37:124–131, 2013.

Bhandari A, Panitch HB: Pulmonary outcomes in bronchopulmonary dysplasia, *Semin Perinatol* 30:219–226, 2006.

Bhandari V, Gruen JR: The genetics of bronchopulmonary dysplasia, *Semin Perinatol* 30:185–191, 2006.

Brion LP, Primhak RA: Intravenous or enteral loop diuretics for preterm infants with (or developing) chronic lung disease, *Cochrane Database Syst Rev* (4):CD001453, 2000.

Brion LP, Primhak RA, Ambrosio-Perez I: Diuretics acting on the distal renal tubule for preterm infants with (or developing) chronic lung disease, *Cochrane Database Syst Rev* (1):CD001817, 2002.

Broström EB, Thunqvist P, Adenfelt G, et al.: Obstructive lung disease in children with mild to severe BPD, *Respir Med* 104:362–370, 2010.

Chang LY, Crapo JD: Inhibition of airway inflammation and hyperreactivity by a catalytic antioxidant, *Chest* 123(Suppl 3):446S, 2003.

Chorne N, Leonard C, Piecuch R, et al.: Patent ductus arteriosus and its treatment as risk factors for neonatal and neurodevelopmental morbidity, *Pediatrics* 119:1165–1174, 2007.

Clark RH, Kueser TJ, Walker MW, et al.: Low-dose nitric oxide therapy for persistent pulmonary hypertension of the newborn. Clinical Inhaled Nitric Oxide Research Group, *N Engl J Med* 342:469–474, 2000.

Cole FS, Alleyne C, Barks JD, et al.: NIH Consensus Development Conference statement: inhaled nitric-oxide therapy for premature infants, *Pediatrics* 127:363–369, 2011.

Cools F, Henderson-Smart DJ, Offringa M, Askie LM, et al.: Elective high frequency oscillatory ventilation versus conventional ventilation for acute pulmonary dysfunction in preterm infants, *Cochrane Database Syst Rev* (3):CD000104, 2009.

Crowley P: Prophylactic corticosteroids for preterm birth, *Cochrane Database Syst Rev* (2):CD000065, 2000.

Cummings JJ, D'Eugenio DB, Gross SJ: A controlled trial of dexamethasone in preterm infants at high risk for bronchopulmonary dysplasia, *N Engl J Med* 320:1505–1510, 1989.

Cutz E, Chiasson D: Chronic lung disease after premature birth, *N Engl J Med* 743–746, 2008.

Darlow BA, Graham PJ: Vitamin A supplementation to prevent mortality and short- and long-term morbidity in very low birthweight infants, *Cochrane Database Syst Rev* (10):CD000501, 2011.

Davis JM, Parad RB, Michele T, Allred E, et al.: Pulmonary outcome at 1 year corrected age in premature infants treated at birth with recombinant human CuZn superoxide dismutase, *Pediatrics* 111(3):469–476, 2003.

Dodd JM, Flenady V, Cincotta R, et al.: Prenatal administration of progesterone for preventing preterm birth, *Cochrane Database Syst Rev* (1):CD004947, 2006.

Doyle LW, Halliday HL, Ehrenkranz RA, et al.: Impact of postnatal systemic corticosteroids on mortality and cerebral palsy in preterm infants: effect modification by risk for chronic lung disease, *Pediatrics* 115:655–661, 2005.

Ehrenkranz RA, Walsh MC, Vohr BR, et al.: Validation of the National Institutes of Health consensus definition of bronchopulmonary dysplasia, *Pediatrics* 116:1353–1360, 2005.

Ellsbury DL, Acarregui MJ, McGuinness GA, et al.: Variability in the use of supplemental oxygen for bronchopulmonary dysplasia, *J Pediatr* 140:247–249, 2002.

Fawke J, Lum S, Kirkby J, et al.: Lung function and respiratory symptoms at 11 years in children born extremely preterm: the EPICure study, *Am J Respir Crit Care Med* 182:237–245, 2010.

Finer NN, Carlo WA, Walsh MC, et al.: Early CPAP versus surfactant in extremely preterm infants, *N Engl J Med* 362(21):1970–1979, 2010.

Fox E, Post M: Growth factors and cell-cell interactions during lung development. In Abman SH, editor: *Bronchopulmonary dysplasia*, New York, 2009, Informa Healthcare, pp 40–55.

Frank L, Sosenko IR: Failure of premature rabbits to increase antioxidant enzymes during hyperoxic exposure: increased susceptibility to pulmonary oxygen toxicity compared with term rabbits, *Pediatr Res* 29:292–296, 1991.

Gitto E, Reiter RJ, Karbownik M, et al.: Causes of oxidative stress in the pre- and perinatal period, *Biol Neonate* 81:146–157, 2002.

Goldenberg Rl, Andrews WW, Goepfert AR, et al.: The Alabama Preterm Birth Study: umbilical cord blood Ureaplasma urealyticum and Mycoplasma hominis cultures in very preterm newborn infants, *Am J Obstet Gynecol* 198(1):43.e1–e5, 2007.

Guimaraes H, Guedes MB, Rocha G, et al.: Vitamin A in prevention of bronchopulmonary dysplasia, *Curr Pharm Des* 18(1):3101–3113, 2012.

Halliday HL, Ehrenkranz RA, Doyle LW: Delayed (>3 weeks) postnatal corticosteroids for chronic lung disease in preterm infants, *Cochrane Database Syst Rev* (1):CD001145, 2003.

Halliday HL, Ehrenkranz RA, Doyle LW: Moderately early (7-14 days) postnatal corticosteroids for preventing chronic lung disease in preterm infants, *Cochrane Database Syst Rev* (1):CD001144, 2003.

Halliday HL, O'Neill C: What is the evidence for drug therapy in the prevention and management of bronchopulmonary dysplasia? In Polin RA, Bancalari E, editors: *The newborn lung*, ed 2, Philadelphia, PA, 2008, Saunders, pp 208–232.

Henderson-Smart DJ, De Paoli AG, Clark RH, Bhuta T: High frequency oscillatory ventilation versus conventional ventilation for infants with severe pulmonary dysfunction born at or near term, *Cochrane Database Syst Rev* (3):CD002974, 2009.

Hjalmarson O, Sandberg K: Abnormal lung function in healthy preterm infants, *Am J Respir Cell Mol Biol* 165(1):83–87, 2002.

Kotecha SJ, Edwards MO, Watkins WJ, et al.: Effect of preterm birth on later FEV1: a systematic review and meta-analysis, *Thorax* 68(8):760–766, 2013.

Jobe AH: Effects of chorioamnionitis on the fetal lung, *Clin Perinatol* 39:441–457, 2012.

Jobe AH, Bancalari E: Bronchopulmonary dysplasia, *Am J Respir Crit Care Med* 163:1723–1729, 2001.

Jobe AJ: The new BPD: an arrest of lung development, *Pediatr Res* 46(6):641–643, 1999.

Johnson BH, Yi M, Masood A, et al.: A critical role for the IL-1 receptor in lung injury induced in neonatal rats by 60% O₂, *Pediatr Res* 66:260–265, 2009.

Kabra NS, Schmidt B, Roberts RS, et al.: Neurosensory impairment after surgical closure of patent ductus arteriosus in extremely low birth weight infants: results from the Trial of Indomethacin Prophylaxis in Preterms, *J Pediatr* 150(3):229–234, 2007.

Kaplan HC, Tabangin ME, McClendon D, et al.: Understanding variation in vitamin A supplementation among NICUs, *Pediatrics* 126(2):e367–e373, 2010.

Kuypers E, Collins JJ, Kramer BW, et al.: Intra-amniotic LPS and antenatal betamethasone: inflammation and maturation in preterm lamb lungs, *Am J Physiol Lung Cell Mol Physiol* 302(4):L380–L389, 2012.

Lahra MM, Beeby PJ, Jeffery HE: Intrauterine inflammation, neonatal sepsis, and chronic lung disease: a 13-year hospital cohort study, *Pediatrics* 123:1314–1319, 2009.

Lavoie PM, Dube MP: Genetics of bronchopulmonary dysplasia in the age of genomics, *Curr Opin Pediatr* 22:134–138, 2010.

Liggins GC, Howie RN: A controlled trial of antepartum glucocorticoid treatment for prevention of the respiratory distress syndrome in premature infants, *Pediatrics* 50(4):515–525, 1972.

Lockwood CJ, Kuczynski E: Risk stratification and pathological mechanisms in preterm delivery, *Paediatr Perinat Epidemiol* 15(Suppl 2):78–89, 2001.

Mahut B, De Blic J, Emond S, et al.: Chest computed tomography findings in bronchopulmonary dysplasia and correlation with lung function, *Arch Dis Child Neonatal Ed* 92(6):F459–F464, 2007.

Mammel MC, Green TP, Johnson DE, et al.: Controlled trial of dexamethasone therapy in infants with bronchopulmonary dysplasia, *Cochrane Database Syst Rev* (4):CD002311, 2012.

Mirea L, Sankaran K, Seshia M, et al.: Treatment of patent ductus arteriosus and neonatal mortality/morbidities: adjustment for treatment selection bias, *J Pediatr* 161:689–694, 2012. e1.

Morley CJ, Davis PG, Doyle LW, et al.: Nasal CPAP or intubation at birth for very preterm infants, *N Engl J Med* 358(7):700–708, 2008.

Mosca F, Colnaghi M, Fumagalli MBPD: old and new problems, *J Matern Fetal Neonatal Med* 24(Suppl 1):80–82, 2011.

Mourani PM, Abman SH: Pulmonary vascular disease in bronchopulmonary dysplasia: pulmonary hypertension and beyond. *Curr Opin Pediatr* 25:329–337, 2013. http://dx.doi.org/10.1097/MOP.0b013e328360a3f6.

Moya MP, Bisset III GS, Auten Jr RL, et al.: Reliability of CXR for the diagnosis of bronchopulmonary dysplasia, *Pediatr Radiol* 31(5):339–342, 2001.

Natarajan G, Pappas A, Shankaran S, et al.: Outcomes of extremely low birth weight infants with bronchopulmonary dysplasia: impact of the physiologic definition, *Early Hum Dev* 88:509–515, 2012.

Northway Jr WH, Rosan RC, Porter DY: Pulmonary disease following respirator therapy of hyaline-membrane disease. Bronchopulmonary dysplasia, *N Engl J Med* 276(7):357–368, 1967.

Ogden BE, Murphy S, Saunders GC, et al.: Lung lavage of newborns with respiratory distress syndrome. Prolonged neutrophil influx is associated with bronchopulmonary dysplasia, *Chest* 83:31S–33S, 1983.

Onland W, Offringa M, De Jaegere AP, et al.: Finding the optimal postnatal dexamethasone regimen for preterm infants at risk of bronchopulmonary dysplasia: a systematic review of placebo-controlled trials, *Pediatrics* 123(1):367–377, 2009.

Paananen R, Husa AK, Vuolteenaho R, et al.: Blood cytokines during the perinatal period in very preterm infants: relationship of inflammatory response and bronchopulmonary dysplasia, *J Pediatr* 154:39–43, e3, 2009.

Rojas MA, Gonzalez A, Bancalari E, et al.: Changing trends in the epidemiology and pathogenesis of neonatal chronic lung disease, *J Pediatr* 126:605–610, 1995.

Romero R, Espinoza J, Kusanovic JP, et al.: The preterm parturition syndrome, *BJOG* 113(Suppl 3):17–42, 2006.

Schmidt B, Anderson PJ, Doyle LW, et al.: Survival without disability to age 5 years after neonatal caffeine therapy for apnea of prematurity, *JAMA* 307(3):275–282, 2012.

Schmidt B, Davis P, Moddemann D, et al.: Long-term effects of indomethacin prophylaxis in extremely-low-birth-weight infants, *N Engl J Med* 344:1966–1972, 2001.

Schmidt B, Roberts RS, Davis P, et al.: Caffeine for Apnea of Prematurity Trial Group. Caffeine therapy for apnea of prematurity, *N Engl J Med* 354(20):2112–2121, 2006.

Shah PS, Sankaran K, Aziz K, et al.: Outcomes of preterm infants <29 weeks gestation over 10-year period in Canada: a cause for concern? *J Perinatol* 32(2):132–138, 2012.

Shah SS, Ohlsson A: Ibuprofen for the prevention of patent ductus arteriosus in preterm and/or low birth weight infants, *Cochrane Database Syst Rev* (1):CD004213, 2006.

Shenai JP: Vitamin A supplementation in very low birth weight neonates: rationale and evidence, *Pediatrics* 104(6):1369–1374, 1999.

Shennan AT, Dunn MS, Ohlsson A, et al.: Abnormal pulmonary outcomes in premature infants: prediction from oxygen requirement in the neonatal period, *Pediatrics* 82:527–532, 1988.

Shepherd EG, Knupp AM, Welty SE, et al.: An interdisciplinary bronchopulmonary dysplasia program is associated with improved neurodevelopmental outcomes and fewer rehospitalizations, *J Perinatol* 32:33–38, 2012.

Smith VC, Zupancic JA, McCormick MC, et al.: Rehospitalization in the first year of life among infants with bronchopulmonary dysplasia, *J Pediatr* 144(6):799–803, 2004.

Soll RF: Inhaled nitric oxide for respiratory failure in preterm infants, *Neonatology* 102:251–253, 2012.

Somaschini M, Castiglioni E, Volonteri C, et al.: Genetic predisposing factors to bronchopulmonary dysplasia: preliminary data from a multicentre study, *J Matern Fetal Neonatal Med* 25(Suppl 4):127–130, 2012.

Soraisham AS, Singhal N, McMillan DD, Sauve RS, Lee SK: Canadian Neonatal Network. A multicenter study on the clinical outcome of chorioamnionitis in preterm infants, *Am J Obstet Gynecol* 200(4):372, e1-6, 2009.

Sosenko IRS, Bancalari E: New developments in the pathogenesis and prevention of bronchopulmonary dysplasia. In Bancalari E, Polin RA, editors: *The newborn lung: neonatology questions and controversies*, ed 2, Philadelphia, PA, 2012, Saunders, pp 217–233.

Stoll BJ, Hansen NI, Bell EF, et al.: Neonatal outcomes of extremely preterm infants from the NICHD Neonatal Research Network, *Pediatrics* 126(3):443–456, 2010.

Stroustrup A, Trasande L: Epidemiological characteristics and resource use in neonates with bronchopulmonary dysplasia: 1993-2006, *Pediatrics* 126(2):291–297, 2010.

Suresh GK, Davis JM, Soll RF: Superoxide dismutase for preventing chronic lung disease in mechanically ventilated preterm infants, *Cochrane Database Syst Rev* (1):CD001968, 2001.

Tanswell AK, Jankov RP: Bronchopulmonary dysplasia: one disease or two? *Am J Respir Crit Care Med* 167:1–2, 2003.

Thebaud B, Abman SH: Bronchopulmonary dysplasia: where have all the vessels gone? Roles of angiogenic growth factors in chronic lung disease, *Am J Respir Crit Care Med* 175:978–985, 2007.

Thomas W, Speer CP: Chorioamnionitis: important risk factor or innocent bystander for neonatal outcome? *Neonatology* 99:177–187, 2011.

Thome UH, Ambalavanan N: Permissive hypercapnia to decrease lung injury in ventilated preterm neonates, *Semin Fetal Neonatal Med* 14:21–27, 2009.

Van Marter LJ, Dammann O, Allred EN, et al.: Chorioamnionitis, mechanical ventilation, and postnatal sepsis as modulators of chronic lung disease in preterm infants, *J Pediatr* 140(2):171–176, 2002.

Walsh MC, Wilson-Costello D, Zadell A, et al.: Safety, reliability, and validity of a physiologic definition of bronchopulmonary dysplasia, *J Perinatol* 23:451–456, 2003.

Walsh MC, Yao Q, Gettner P, et al.: Impact of a physiologic definition on bronchopulmonary dysplasia rates, *Pediatrics* 114:1305–1311, 2004.

Watterberg KL, Demers LM, Scott SM, et al.: Chorioamnionitis and early lung inflammation in infants in whom bronchopulmonary dysplasia develops, *Pediatrics* 97:210–215, 1996.

Wilson AC: What does imaging the chest tell us about bronchopulmonary dysplasia? *Paediatr Respir Rev* 11:158–161, 2010.

Wong PM, Lees AN, Louw J, et al.: Emphysema in young adult survivors of moderate-to-severe bronchopulmonary dysplasia, *Eur Respir J* 32:321–328, 2008.

CHAPTER 12

NEONATAL APNEA

Ana Paula D. Ribeiro, MD • Elie G. Abu Jawdeh, MD • Richard J. Martin, MD

Apnea of prematurity is one of the most common conditions in the neonatal intensive care unit (NICU). In the last three decades, our understanding of respiratory control in premature infants and its underlying neuroanatomical pathways and physiologic mechanisms has greatly improved. Some management aspects of apnea in premature infants remain debatable with variation across centers and neonatologists. Through clinical cases, this chapter reviews the physiologic mechanisms causing neonatal apnea and the different management options while caring for patients with apnea of prematurity.

CASE STUDY 1

The patient is a male infant born at 26 weeks' gestation, 680 grams. He required initial intubation for surfactant when FiO$_2$ reached 0.5. Now at day 4 of nasal continuous positive air pressure (CPAP) (4 cm H$_2$O); in FiO$_2$ of 0.3, there is a spontaneous respiratory rate of 60 breaths per minute with minimal retractions and no observed apnea.

EXERCISE 1

QUESTIONS

1. What physiologic mechanisms make this infant at risk for apnea of prematurity?

2. Is CPAP likely to prevent/benefit his apnea?

3. Is this infant a candidate for xanthine therapy?

ANSWERS

1. Apnea of prematurity is mostly defined as a cessation of breathing for more than 20 seconds or a short pause in breathing accompanied by desaturation (SpO$_2$ <80%) and/or bradycardia (heart rate ≤80 beats/min) in babies less than 37 weeks' gestation (Zhao et al., 2011). It is considered a developmental disorder because it is the consequence of physiologic immaturity of respiratory control, and inversely proportional to gestational age. There are two important physiologic mechanisms implicated in apnea of prematurity: impaired respiratory drive owing

to immature respiratory control and failure to maintain airway patency.

The immaturity of respiratory control is manifested by impaired ventilatory responses to hypoxia and hypercapnia, and an exaggerated inhibitory response to stimulation of airway receptors. Hypercapnia is the major chemical stimulant of breathing and sensed primarily centrally in the brainstem. Preterm infants—especially those with apnea—exhibit decreased ventilatory responses to CO$_2$.

Chemosensitivity to hypoxia is sensed peripherally and both enhanced and reduced peripheral chemoreceptor function of the carotid bodies may predispose to apnea, bradycardia, and desaturations in the preterm infant. The O$_2$ sensitivity of the carotid body chemoreceptors *in utero* is adapted to a low PaO$_2$ of approximately 25 mmHg; after birth there is a fourfold increase in PaO$_2$, which silences or dampens these peripheral chemoreceptors. This is followed by a gradual increase in hypoxic chemosensitivity. Exaggerated peripheral chemoreceptor stimulation may be caused by repeated hypoxic episodes. Such enhanced peripheral chemosensitivity may destabilize breathing and result in respiratory pauses secondary to hypocapnia seen after hyperventilation. Thus diminished peripheral chemosensitivity may prolong apnea while increased peripheral sensitivity may precipitate apnea (Figure 12-1).

Activation of the laryngeal mucosa in premature infants can lead to apnea, bradycardia, and hypotension, by stimulation of inhibitory airway receptors. An example of this is when deep suctioning is attempted during resuscitation, which can lead to bradycardia and consequently apnea. This laryngeal chemoreflex is viewed as protective to inhibit respiration and will develop into cough and swallowing in more mature infants.

Failure to maintain airway patency is an important factor that contributes to obstructive and mixed apnea. The determinants of airway stability include anatomical structure, neuromuscular activation of airway dilators, ventilatory control, and the arousal threshold from sleep.

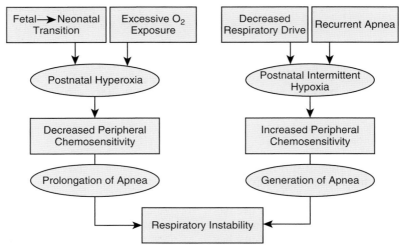

FIGURE 12-1 ■ **Proposed model illustrating the effects of hyperoxia and intermittent hypoxia on carotid chemoreceptor activities and subsequent effects on respiratory instability.** The fetal–neonatal transition combined with excessive O_2 exposure decreases peripheral chemosensitivity, which could prolong termination of an apneic event, leading to respiratory instability. On the other hand, decreased respiratory drive and recurrent apnea result in oscillations in hypoxia during development, which may lead to a long-lasting increase in peripheral chemosensory activity (sensitization). The result could be a hyperventilation and eventual apnea. (From MacFarlane PM, Ribeiro AP, Martin RJ: Carotid chemoreceptor development and neonatal apnea, *Respir Physiol Neurobiol* 185:170-176, 2013.)

Apnea is divided into three categories based on the presence or absence of upper airway obstruction. Central apnea is total cessation of inspiratory effort with a patent airway. In obstructive apnea there is inspiratory effort and also chest wall motion, although there is no nasal flow due to an obstructed airway. Mixed apnea consists of respiratory efforts against an obstructed upper airway preceded or followed by central apnea; about 50% of clinically significant cases of apnea of prematurity are due to mixed apneas.

The hypopharynx is a common site of upper airway obstruction owing to its poor muscle tone resulting in airway collapse, especially if the infant's neck is flexed. The larynx and trachea are more rigid structures and less common sites of airway obstruction, although this can be seen if there is vocal cord dysfunction, laryngeal edema or stenosis, or laryngo- or tracheomalacia.

The newborn trachea and larynx are relatively superiorly positioned, resulting in a close proximity between the epiglottis and soft palate. This configuration facilitates partitioning of the pharynx to facilitate suckling. However, this anatomy also confers a strong preference toward nasal breathing in infants. Therefore any nasal swelling can cause obstruction of the upper airway; swelling may result from constant nasal suctioning, prolonged use of a nasogastric tube, or prolonged use of nasal prongs with continuous positive pressure (NCPAP) or nasal intermittent positive pressure ventilation (NIPPV).

2. CPAP may benefit this patient's apneic episodes, because most of the longer apneas observed at <28 weeks of age are mixed apneas and continuous positive airway pressure (CPAP) acts to splint the upper airway with positive pressure and decrease the risk of upper airway closure or obstruction. CPAP also increases functional residual capacity (FRC) and improves oxygenation.

Data from healthy premature infants (32 to 36 weeks' postconceptional age) showed that supraglottic resistance was decreased with increasing CPAP pressures and this contributed to 60% of the total change observed in pulmonary resistance. By mechanically dilating the supraglottic airway and lowering resistance in both inspiration and expiration, CPAP may prevent pharyngeal collapse (Miller et al., 1990). Furthermore, CPAP improves thoracoabdominal synchrony, increases tidal volume (V_T), reduces the labored breathing index, and increases end expiratory lung volume level. These effects not only help to prevent apnea of prematurity, but also may decrease the need for intubation.

NIPPV and high flow nasal cannula (HFNC) increasingly are being used to treat apnea of prematurity. Potential benefits of the of HFNC for CPAP delivery include ease of administration, possible reduction in nasal damage, and increased ability for parents to hold and bond with their infants. These benefits must be weighed against the uncertainty of how much pressure is being delivered via the cannula, however.

In two studies comparing NIPPV and NCPAP for the management of apnea of prematurity, one showed a reduction in apnea frequency with NIPPV and the other showed a trend favoring NIPPV (Lin et al., 1998; Ryan et al., 1989). A RCT done in 2009 by Pantalitschka and colleagues on VLBW infants comparing four modes of nasal respiratory support (two modes of NIPPV and two modes of NCPAP) showed superiority of NCPAP in prevention of apnea (Pantalitschka et al., 2009). At this time there is no consensus regarding the potential benefits of NIPPV over NCPAP. Our unit at Rainbow Babies and Children's Hospital utilizes NCPAP with pressures between 3 to 6 cm H_2O for prevention of apnea of prematurity with great success. NIPPV is used mostly postextubation and HFNC is used with caution in older infants who have a continued need for oxygen.

3. Methylxanthine therapy has been used for treatment of apnea since the mid to late 1970s. Methylxanthines competitively inhibit adenosine receptors, resulting in stimulation of respiratory neural output. Although the basis of its beneficial effects is not completely understood, methylxanthine therapy reverses central hypoxic depression of breathing, increases minute ventilation, improves CO_2 sensitivity, enhances diaphragmatic activity, improves pharyngeal tone, and decreases periodic breathing.

Schmidt and colleagues published the largest randomized controlled trial of caffeine therapy for apnea of prematurity (CAP) demonstrating both respiratory and neurodevelopmental benefits for caffeine- versus placebo-treated infants (Schmidt et al., 2006; Schmidt et al., 2007). The risk of BPD was significantly reduced in the caffeine group (OR 0.63, 95% CI 0.52 to 0.76). In addition, the need for both medical (0.67, 95% CI 0.55 to 0.81) and surgical (0.32, 95% CI 0.22 to 0.45) PDA closure was reduced in the caffeine group. At 18 to 21 months follow up, caffeine-treated infants had less cognitive impairment (0.81, 95% CI 0.66 to 0.99) and decreased incidence of cerebral palsy (0.58, 95% CI 0.39 to 0.87). However, the 5-year follow up suggested attenuation of these cognitive and motor benefits (Schmidt et al., 2007).

Currently the main indications for methylxanthine therapy initiation are: (1) treatment of apnea, (2) facilitation of extubation, and (3) prophylactic use for infants at risk for apnea. Effectiveness of methylxanthine therapy in the treatment of recurrent apnea is well established. A recent Cochrane review demonstrated a decrease in both apneic episodes (RR 0.44, 95% CI 0.32 to 0.60) and the need for intermittent positive pressure ventilation (RR 0.34, 95% CI 0.12 to 0.97) with methylxanthine therapy (Henderson-Smart et al., 2010:CD000140). When caffeine is used as an apnea treatment strategy it is widely employed for infants with increased frequency and severity of apnea, especially those requiring tactile stimulation and bag-mask ventilation. Furthermore, there is evidence that methylxanthine reduces the reintubation risk in preterm infants (RR 0.48, 95%, CI 0.32 to 0.71) (Henderson-Smart et al., 2010:CD000139).

Because of increasing efforts to avoid intubation and mechanical ventilation, there is an overall shift from selective therapeutic toward widespread prophylactic use of methylxanthine therapy for apnea of prematurity. The infant in this case would be a candidate for this therapy; however, data to support the practice of prophylactic methylxanthine use in preterm infants is limited. In addition, Davis and colleagues—in a post-hoc analysis of the caffeine for apnea of prematurity (CAP) trial comparing prophylactic caffeine use and placebo—did not demonstrate significant differences in clinical outcomes except for a decrease in the risk of PDA ligation in the prophylactic caffeine group.

The two commonly used methylxanthines are caffeine and theophylline. Caffeine is favored over theophylline because of its safety profile and therapeutic advantages. Adverse effects of methylxanthines may include feeding intolerance and gastroesophageal reflux (GER), tachycardia and cardiac dysrhythmias, and (rarely) seizures. These adverse effects occur less frequently with caffeine therapy. In contrast to theophylline, caffeine has better enteral absorption, a wider therapeutic index, and is administered once daily due to a longer half life, ranging from 65 to 100 hours. Another advantage of caffeine over theophylline is absence of a need to measure serum levels, except in cases where toxicity is suspected or no clinical effects are seen.

CASE STUDY 2

The patient, a 30-week-gestation female infant, is now 3 weeks old, on full enteral feeds, and weighs 1.25 kg. The infant develops several new episodes of apnea accompanied by desaturation and bradycardia, and requires bag-mask ventilation after failure of tactile stimulation. Sepsis workup is performed and antibiotic therapy begun. Lab values are normal apart from a hematocrit of 24%.

EXERCISE 2

QUESTIONS

1. What are the mechanisms whereby sepsis produces apnea?

2. Would this infant's episodes benefit from red blood cell transfusion?

ANSWERS

1. Perinatal inflammation and infection is a major source of morbidity and mortality in premature infants. In a national cohort of ~400,000 infants, rates of early-onset sepsis were 0.98 cases per 1000 live births, revealing a continuing burden of disease with morbidity and mortality (Stoll et al., 2011). Sepsis frequently manifests as changes in breathing pattern and apneic episodes in this vulnerable population. Both viral and bacterial sepsis may result in apnea.

   In a study published in 1999 evaluating respiratory control during upper airway infection, it was observed that respiratory syncytial virus (RSV)-related apnea was more common in infants <3 months suggesting that this viral infection interferes with some respiratory control mechanisms in the process of maturation. A local release of inflammatory mediators was suggested as a mechanism of apnea related to RSV infection, implicating IL-1β (interleukin 1 beta) as positively correlated with the severity of disease (Lindgren, 1999). In 2005, new data showed that early-life RSV infection in rats is associated with significant prolongation of the apnea triggered by sensorineural stimulation. Although the mechanism is still unclear, it is widely accepted that RSV-associated apnea is caused by central inhibition of ventilatory drive, with complete absence of respiratory effort and without evidence of airway obstruction.

   Even though many studies have shown an association between proinflammatory cytokine upregulation caused by inflammation and autonomic control in the brainstem, its interaction is still poorly understood. In 2007 Hofstetter and colleagues suggested that IL-1β adversely affects respiratory control via the PGE_2 (prostaglandin E_2) pathway (Hofstetter et al., 2007). During systemic inflammation, the proinflammatory cytokine IL-1β is released into the circulation. Because it may not readily cross the blood–brain barrier (BBB), it binds to its receptor (IL-1R) located on endothelial cells of the BBB. The activation of this receptor induces the synthesis of PGH_2 (prostaglandin H_2) via COX-2 and subsequently the synthesis of PGE_2. The prostaglandin E_2 is then released into the brain and binds to its receptor (EP3R), located in respiratory control regions of the brainstem, such as the *nucleus tractus solitarius* (nTS) and the rostroventral lateral medulla (RVLM). It results in depression of central respiration-related neurons and breathing (Figure 12-2). In human neonates, C-reactive protein (CRP) is associated with elevated PGE_2 in the cerebrospinal fluid, and elevated central PGE_2 is associated with an increased apnea frequency. Therefore endogenously released prostaglandin may contribute to sepsis-induced apnea of prematurity.

   In 2011 Balan and colleagues showed that injection of lipopolysaccharide (LPS) in the airway of rat pups creates an inflammatory response measured by increased expression of mRNA for IL-1β in the brainstem, and this is associated with a decreased respiratory response to hypoxia (Balan et al., 2011). Changes in inspiratory drive are also known to occur at the level of the brainstem very soon after upper airway exposure to endotoxin or local microinjection of inflammatory cytokine in the *nucleus tractus solitarius*. This suggests that cytokine-mediated mechanisms at the brainstem initiated by systemic sepsis may be implicated in apnea of prematurity and other forms of respiratory dysregulation. Recent observations suggest that abnormalities in heart rate patterns may serve as a precursor and predictor of ensuing sepsis in neonates. If confirmed in subsequent studies careful monitoring of cardiorespiratory patterns could be a useful contributor to determining the need for sepsis workup.

2. In premature infants the hematocrit level for which a transfusion is indicated is controversial. Factors contributing to transfusion decision-making in premature infants include but are not limited to postnatal age, degree of respiratory support, and the amount of supplemental oxygen. In randomized trials both Kirpalani and colleagues and Bell and colleagues compared maintaining a high hematocrit level (liberal) versus lower (restrictive) hematocrit in premature infants (Bell et al., 2005; Kirpalani et al., 2006). Neither of these studies demonstrated a consistent benefit to maintaining a given hematocrit level and the results of the trials were contradictory.

   Premature infants have increased risk for apnea with lower hematocrit levels. Zagol and colleagues showed that the higher the hematocrit level, the less the likelihood of future apnea associated with bradycardia and oxygen desaturation (Zagol et al., 2012). Two proposed mechanisms may explain the relationship between anemia and clinically significant apneic episodes. The first suggests that anemia decreases oxygen delivery to respiratory control centers leading to hypoxic ventilatory depression. Hence

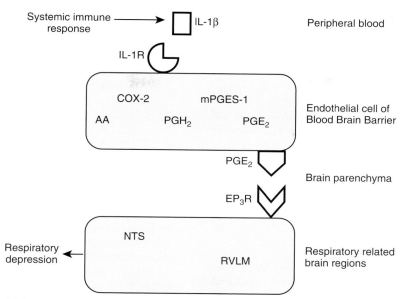

FIGURE 12-2 ■ **Model for IL-1-induced respiratory depression via a prostaglandin E2 (PGE2) mediated pathway.** During a systemic immune response, interleukin 1 (IL-1) is released into the peripheral blood stream. It binds to its receptor (IL-1R) located on endothelial cells of the blood–brain barrier. Activation of IL-1R induces the synthesis of prostaglandin H2 (PGH2) from arachidonic acid (AA) via COX-2 and the synthesis of PGE2 from PGH2 via the rate-limiting enzyme microsomal prostaglandin synthase-1 (mPGES-1). PGE2 is released into the brain parenchyma and binds to its EP3R located in respiratory control regions of the brainstem, resulting in depression of central respiration-related neurons and breathing. (Adapted from Hofstetter AO, Saha S, Siljehav V, Jakobsson PJ, Herlenius E: The induced prostaglandin E2 pathway is a key regulator of the respiratory response to infection and hypoxia in neonates, *Proc Natl Acad Sci USA* 104:9894-9899, 2007.)

RBC transfusions may decrease apnea because of improved oxygen delivery to the premature brain. The second underlying mechanism is that RBC transfusions increase oxygen stores resulting in greater stability of oxygenation in the presence of apnea, leading to less clinically significant apneic events associated with oxygen desaturation. This is consistent with a recent model analysis showing that the rate of arterial oxygen desaturation during apnea decreased with higher hemoglobin levels. In this context, will RBC transfusions improve apnea of prematurity and associated bradycardia and oxygen desaturation events? Although the literature is controversial, there is evidence that RBC transfusions decrease apnea frequency and the associated bradycardia and oxygen desaturation saturation episodes. Therefore, red blood cell transfusion should be strongly considered in infants with hematocrit levels less than 25% who have frequent apneic episodes and/or severe apnea.

The beneficial effect of red blood cell transfusion on apnea should be weighed against potential risks such as transmitted infections, and possible transfusion-related adverse reactions. Additional studies suggest a possible association between early transfusions and intraventricular hemorrhage, as well as late transfusions and necrotizing enterocolitis. Future randomized trials are needed to clarify these potential transfusion-associated risks.

CASE STUDY 3

The patient, an infant born at 24 weeks' gestation, is now 42 weeks' postmenstrual age (PMA), weighs 3.2 kg, and is taking all feeds by mouth. Supplemental oxygen and caffeine therapy were recently discontinued. Baseline oxygen saturation ranges from 94% to 100% in room air. His cardiorespiratory monitor demonstrates daily bradycardia alarms (into the 70s that self-resolve).

EXERCISE 3

QUESTIONS

1. What is the mechanism underlying these bradycardias?

2. How should discharge planning proceed?

ANSWERS

1. Several studies suggest that the majority of infants are apnea and bradycardia free by 37 to 40 weeks PMA, although extremely preterm infants may not achieve it until 43 weeks PMA.

It is very common for preterm infants such as the one described in this case to have daily and asymptomatic bradycardias. These are typically caused by short respiratory pauses, which will not be of sufficient duration to trigger an apnea alarm. Such preterm babies often have residual lung disease resulting in borderline low oxygen saturation levels in room air. When they have short respiratory pauses, their low oxygen reserve results in a brief episode of desaturation and subsequent bradycardia even if averaged SaO_2 monitors do not alarm (Figure 12-3). In these instances, the bradycardia is the result of increased vagal tone associated with hypoxia. Pharyngeal stimulation, gastric distension, upper airway obstructive crying, or straining may aggravate the problem.

2. The Collaborative Home Infant Monitoring Evaluation (CHIME) study demonstrated that apnea and bradycardia events occurred in both premature and term infants beyond discharge. Premature infants were at increased risk for extreme episodes defined as apnea lasting at least 30 seconds and heart rate (HR) <60 beats per minute (bpm) up to a PMA of 44 weeks and HR <50 bpm for PMA >44 weeks (Ramanathan et al., 2001). Home cardiorespiratory monitoring is an option for premature infants with persistent apnea, bradycardia, and hypoxemia events who are otherwise ready for hospital discharge. Because apnea and bradycardia events resolve with advancing PMA, the need for home cardiorespiratory monitoring should be reevaluated around 43 to 44 weeks PMA. At that time home monitoring can almost always be discontinued. Cardiorespiratory monitoring is not needed for premature infants who are ready for discharge and remain free of any apnea, bradycardia, and oxygen desaturation episodes.

The majority of neonatologists require a 5- to 7-day event-free period as a margin of safety before discharging home an otherwise healthy premature infant. Because of caffeine's long half life, a 7-day event-free period is recommended when caffeine has been recently discontinued. Although very uncommon, some infants continue to need caffeine therapy at hospital discharge; the use of home cardiorespiratory monitoring in this situation is controversial and there is no consensus among neonatologists. In a recent survey of an international cohort of neonatologists, discharging infants on methylxanthines was considered an indication for home monitoring for 57% of all responders (43% always and 14% sometimes) (Abu Jawdeh et al., 2013).

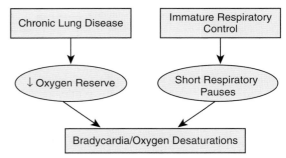

FIGURE 12-3 ■ Mechanism for (asymptomatic) bradycardia and desaturation in preterm infants.

The potential advantages and disadvantages of home monitoring should be discussed with the parents. Infants discharged home on cardiorespiratory monitors should be monitored at all times unless being directly observed by an adult. The use of home cardiorespiratory monitors equipped with an event recorder is recommended. Parents or primary care providers must demonstrate proficiency in managing the monitor, providing stimulation, and performing cardiorespiratory resuscitation. The recommended home monitor alarm settings at our center are 20 seconds for apnea and <85% for oxygen desaturation. The bradycardia alarm is set at <70 bpm for infants <44 weeks PMA, and 60 bpm when older. Home monitoring is maintained until the infant is event free for 2 to 4 weeks or has reached 43 weeks PMA and is free of events. Infants whose monitors continue to alarm beyond 44 weeks PMA may be further evaluated for other causes of apnea such as airway obstruction or seizures.

CASE STUDY 4

- *Former 35 weeks' gestation male infant now 42 weeks' PMA is at home*
- *Found 1 hour after feed coughing and choking with formula in nose and mouth; face turned blue and reported apneic*
- *Mother picked him up, blew in his face, rubbed his back, gave rescue breaths, and called emergency medical services (EMS)*
- *When EMS arrived he appeared well*
- *Admitted for 24-hour hospitalization*

EXERCISE 4

QUESTIONS

1. Did GER precipitate this episode?

2. How should this infant be evaluated?

3. What are the therapeutic options?

ANSWERS

1. This late-preterm infant presents a common dilemma that typically requires a short stay readmission. The approach to his management may cross multiple subspecialty disciplines, notably neonatology, pediatric pulmonology, and gastroenterology. From the infant's history, it is usually impossible to determine whether apnea or reflux/regurgitation was the precipitating event. Their interrelationships are summarized in Figure 12-4.

   The most important mechanism resulting in GER in preterm infants is transient relaxation of the lower esophageal sphincter (LES). The LES is composed of intrinsic smooth muscle of the esophagus and skeletal muscle of the crural diaphragm. Transient LES relaxation is defined as an abrupt decrease in LES pressure below the intragastric pressure. Refluxate may be acidic or nonacidic, the latter is more likely soon after a feed. The laryngopharyngeal region is exquisitely sensitive to afferent stimuli, which precipitate a protective response for the airway of preterm infants, comprising laryngospasm, apnea, and bradycardia. Therefore, if refluxate reaches as high as this region an apneic response might result. Recent data suggest that nonacid—rather than acid—reflux is more likely to precipitate apnea. Although this is theoretically possible, our data indicate that only about 3% of cardiorespiratory events (comprising apnea, bradycardia, and desaturation) are preceded by GER.

   Another possibility (Figure 12-4) is that apnea may be the initiating event and predispose to GER. Data from animal models and human infants have demonstrated that inhibition of respiratory neural output may be followed by a decrease in lower esophageal sphincter tone (Kiatchoosakun et al., 2002; Omari, 2009). Therefore, in the clinical scenario presented above, it is possible that spontaneous apnea was the initiating event and a subsequent regurgitation and choking aggravated the situation.

2. Infants such as this are typically hospitalized at least overnight to allay anxiety and perform a minimal diagnostic evaluation. Infants who have a history of multiple apparent life threatening events (ALTE) or are younger than 30 days of age are most likely to benefit from hospitalization. Unfortunately, our ability to identify a specific etiology for an ALTE like this is limited and there is no clear consensus on whether such an infant should receive an extensive workup. In addition to a careful history, which focuses on the possibility of a seizure disorder or feeding disturbance, we perform a simultaneous bedside evaluation for reflux and apnea.

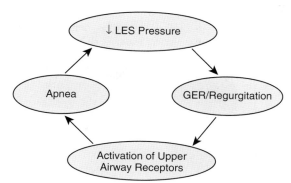

FIGURE 12-4 ■ **Potential perpetuating cycle of apnea and GER.**

The diagnostic evaluation for reflux requires a probe that measures both esophageal pH and acidic and nonacidic boluses. Esophageal pH measurement to detect reflux of acidic gastric contents in the distal esophagus is the most widely employed diagnostic test for GER in preterm infants. The test is performed by the transnasal passage of a microelectrode containing a pH sensor into the lower third of the esophagus. Various scoring techniques have been used to interpret the results of pH probe studies, and generally include the number of acid reflux episodes, average duration of the episodes, and overall proportion of time with a pH less than 4. The reflux index (RI), which consists of the sum of the periods in which pH is less than 4 as a percent of recording time, is a widely used scoring system. It is important to note that acid may not be detected postprandially in infants because milk can buffer acid contained in the refluxate, leading to underestimation of GER.

Multiple intraluminal impedance (MII) monitoring uses an esophageal catheter designed to measure impedance from multiple intraluminal recording sensors. The method permits detection of GER based on changes in electrical resistance to electrical current flow between two electrodes when a liquid and/or gas bolus moves between them and can differentiate antegrade swallows from retrograde GER. The obvious advantage of MII is the ability to assess postprandial reflux, which may be masked by milk neutralizing the acid content of the refluxate when only a pH probe is used. One reservation associated with the use of MII in preterm infants remains: namely the lack of validated normative standards in neonates.

Concurrently we assess the frequency of cardiorespiratory events and attempt to relate them temporally to evidence of GER. Given the likelihood of mixed or obstructive apnea events, respiratory inductance plethysmography (RIP) provides

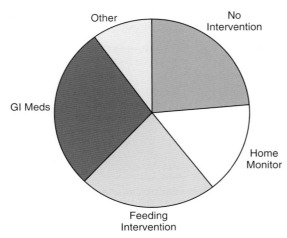

FIGURE 12-5 ■ **Discharge disposition for a cohort of 100 Rainbow Babies and Children's Hospital admissions (2008-2010) with ALTE.**

a useful alternative to standard impedance monitoring. RIP combines a band over the rib cage and abdomen and, after appropriate calibration, provides a semiquantitative measure of air flow and tidal volume. In combination with heart rate and oxygen saturation, this provides a noninvasive assessment of cardiorespiratory events. During such an overnight study it is possible to clearly characterize any events, although in the case of ALTE admissions a recurrence is unlikely.

3. After excluding any specific precipitating event by clinical history, the focus at discharge is on minimizing the risk of recurrence and protecting the infant from a future episode. In our experience at Rainbow Babies and Children's Hospital, approximately 25% of these infants will be discharged without any therapeutic intervention, whereas approximately 20% will be discharged with a cardiorespiratory monitor for a short period of time (Figure 12-5). In the absence of clear diagnostic and therapeutic guidelines for these infants, these data will vary widely between centers.

As seen in Figure 12-5, a feeding intervention, such as modifying the content or pacing of feeds, occurred in 23% of our ALTE infants, and another 28% were discharged on medications for GER. A recent study reported that 47% of ALTE admissions were discharged with a diagnosis of gastroesophageal reflux disease (GERD) (Doshi et al., 2012). There is wide variation among pediatric specialists regarding beliefs about GERD in premature infants, with pulmonologists more likely than neonatologists to report respiratory symptoms (e.g., apnea) as caused by GERD. If GER is suspected, nonpharmacologic approaches such as dietary change

(smaller frequent or thickened feeds) should be encouraged. Pharmacologic therapy that has been used in preterm infants includes histamine H-2 receptor antagonists, proton pump inhibitors, and prokinetic agents. These have not been definitively shown to be effective in improving symptoms and may be associated with adverse sequelae. Therefore, they should be used sparingly and only continued in the face of documented clinical benefit.

SUGGESTED READINGS

Abu Jawdeh EG, O'Riordan MA, Limrungsikul A, Bandyopadhyay A, Argus BM, Nakad PE, et al.: Prevalence of prophylactic caffeine use among an international cohort of neonatologists, *J Neonatal Perinatal Med* 6(3):251–256, 2013.

Abu-Shaweesh JM, Martin RJ: Neonatal apnea: what's new? *Pediatr Pulmonol* 43:937–944, 2008.

Aranda JV, Cook CE, Gorman W, Collinge JM, Loughnan PM, Outerbridge EW, et al.: Pharmacokinetic profile of caffeine in the premature newborn infant with apnea, *J Pediatr* 94:663–668, 1979.

Aranda JV, Gorman W, Bergsteinsson H, Gunn T: Efficacy of caffeine in treatment of apnea in the low-birth-weight infant, *J Pediatr* 90:467–472, 1977.

Baer VL, Lambert DK, Henry E, Snow GL, Butler A, Christensen RD: Among very-low-birth-weight neonates is red blood cell transfusion an independent risk factor for subsequently developing a severe intraventricular hemorrhage? *Transfusion* 51:1170–1178, 2011.

Balan KV, Kc P, Hoxha Z, Mayer CA, Wilson CG, Martin RJ: Vagal afferents modulate cytokine-mediated respiratory control at the neonatal medulla oblongata, *Respir Physiol Neurobiol* 178:458–464, 2011.

Bell EF, Strauss RG, Widness JA, Mahoney LT, Mock DM, Seward VJ, et al.: Randomized trial of liberal versus restrictive guidelines for red blood cell transfusion in preterm infants, *Pediatrics* 115:1685–1691, 2005.

Christensen RD: Associations between "early" red blood cell transfusion and severe intraventricular hemorrhage, and between "late" red blood cell transfusion and necrotizing enterocolitis, *Semin Perinatol* 36(4):283–289, 2012.

Christensen RD, Ilstrup S: Recent advances toward defining the benefits and risks of erythrocyte transfusions in neonates, *Arch Dis Child Fetal Neonatal Ed* 98:F365–F372, 2013.

Claudius I, Keens T: Do all infants with apparent life-threatening events need to be admitted? *Pediatrics* 119:679–683, 2007.

Committee on Fetus and Newborn: Apnea, sudden infant death syndrome, and home monitoring, *Pediatrics* 111:914–917, 2003.

Corvaglia L, Zama D, Spizzichino M, Aceti A, Mariani E, Capretti MG, et al.: The frequency of apneas in very preterm infants is increased after non-acid gastro-esophageal reflux, *Neurogastroenterol Motil* 23, 2011. 303–307,e152.

Cross KW, Oppe TE: The effect of inhalation of high and low concentrations of oxygen on the respiration of the premature infant, *J Physiol* 117:38–55, 1952.

Crowley M, Kirpalani H: A rational approach to red blood cell transfusion in the neonatal ICU, *Curr Opin Pediatr* 22:151–157, 2010.

Darnall RA: The role of CO(2) and central chemoreception in the control of breathing in the fetus and the neonate, *Respir Physiol Neurobiol* 173:201–212, 2010.

Davis PG, Schmidt B, Roberts RS, Doyle LW, Asztalos E, Haslam R, et al.: Caffeine for Apnea of Prematurity trial: benefits may vary in subgroups, *J Pediatr* 156:382–387, 2010.

DeMaio JG, Harris MC, Deuber C, Spitzer AR: Effect of blood transfusion on apnea frequency in growing premature infants, *J Pediatr* 114:1039–1041, 1989.

Di Fiore J, Arko M, Herynk B, Martin R, Hibbs AM: Characterization of cardiorespiratory events following gastroesophageal reflux in preterm infants, *J Perinatol* 30:683–687, 2010.

Di Fiore JM, Arko MK, Miller MJ, Krauss A, Betkerur A, Zadell A, et al.: Cardiorespiratory events in preterm infants referred for apnea monitoring studies, *Pediatrics* 108:1304–1308, 2001.

Doshi A, Bernard-Stover L, Kuelbs C, Castillo E, Stucky E: Apparent life-threatening event admissions and gastroesophageal reflux disease: the value of hospitalization, *Pediatr Emerg Care* 28:17–21, 2012.

Elgellab A, Riou Y, Abbazine A, Truffert P, Matran R, Lequien P, et al.: Effects of nasal continuous positive airway pressure (NCPAP) on breathing pattern in spontaneously breathing premature newborn infants, *Intensive Care Med* 27:1782–1787, 2001.

Golski CA, Rome ES, Martin RJ, Frank SH, Worley S, Sun Z, et al.: Pediatric specialists' beliefs about gastroesophageal reflux disease in premature infants, *Pediatrics* 125:96–104, 2010.

Gresham K, Boyer B, Mayer C, Foglyano R, Martin R, Wilson CG: Airway inflammation and central respiratory control: results from in vivo and in vitro neonatal rat, *Respir Physiol Neurobiol* 178:414–421, 2011.

Henderson-Smart DJ, Davis PG: Prophylactic methylxanthines for endotracheal extubation in preterm infants, *Cochrane Database Syst Rev* CD000139, 2010.

Henderson-Smart DJ, De Paoli AG: Methylxanthine treatment for apnoea in preterm infants, *Cochrane Database Syst Rev* CD000140, 2010.

Henderson-Smart DJ, De Paoli AG: Prophylactic methylxanthine for prevention of apnoea in preterm infants, *Cochrane Database Syst Rev* CD000432, 2010.

Hofstetter AO, Saha S, Siljehav V, Jakobsson PJ, Herlenius E: The induced prostaglandin E2 pathway is a key regulator of the respiratory response to infection and hypoxia in neonates, *Proc Natl Acad Sci U S A* 104:9894–9899, 2007.

Joshi A, Gerhardt T, Shandloff P, Bancalari E: Blood transfusion effect on the respiratory pattern of preterm infants, *Pediatrics* 80:79–84, 1987.

Katz ES, Mitchell RB, D'Ambrosio CM: Obstructive sleep apnea in infants, *Am J Respir Crit Care Med* 185:805–816, 2012.

Khan A, Qurashi M, Kwiatkowski K, Cates D, Rigatto H: Measurement of the CO2 apneic threshold in newborn infants: possible relevance for periodic breathing and apnea, *J Appl Physiol* 98:1171–1176, 2005.

Kiatchoosakun P, Dreshaj IA, Abu-Shaweesh JM, Haxhiu MA, Martin RJ: Effects of hypoxia on respiratory neural output and lower esophageal sphincter pressure in piglets, *Pediatr Res* 52:50–55, 2002.

Kirpalani H, Whyte RK, Andersen C, Asztalos EV, Heddle N, Blajchman MA, et al.: The Premature Infants in Need of Transfusion (PINT) study: a randomized, controlled trial of a restrictive (low) versus liberal (high) transfusion threshold for extremely low birth weight infants, *J Pediatr* 149:301–307, 2006.

Kirpalani H, Zupancic JA: Do transfusions cause necrotizing enterocolitis? The complementary role of randomized trials and observational studies, *Semin Perinatol* 36:269–276, 2012.

Lin CH, Wang ST, Lin YJ, Yeh TF: Efficacy of nasal intermittent positive pressure ventilation in treating apnea of prematurity, *Pediatr Pulmonol* 26:349–353, 1998.

Lindgren C: Respiratory control during upper airway infection mechanism for prolonged reflex apnoea and sudden infant death with special reference to infant sleep position, *FEMS Immunol Med Microbiol* 25:97–102, 1999.

Lorch SA, Srinivasan L, Escobar GJ: Epidemiology of apnea and bradycardia resolution in premature infants, *Pediatrics* 128:e366–e373, 2011.

MacFarlane PM, Ribeiro AP, Martin RJ: Carotid chemoreceptor development and neonatal apnea, *Respir Physiol Neurobiol* 185:170–176, 2013.

Martin RJ: *Management of apnea of prematurity*, Waltham, MA, 2013, UpToDate.

Martin RJ, Fanaroff AA, Walsh MC: *Fanaroff and Martin's neonatal-perinatal medicine: diseases of the fetus and infant*, 9th ed., St. Louis, MO, 2011, Mosby/Elsevier.

Martin RJ, Hibbs AM: *Gastroesophageal reflux in premature infants*, Waltham, MA, 2013, UpToDate.

Miller MJ, DiFiore JM, Strohl KP, Martin RJ: Effects of nasal CPAP on supraglottic and total pulmonary resistance in preterm infants, *J Appl Physiol* 68:141–146, 1990.

Moorman JR, Carlo WA, Kattwinkel J, Schelonka RL, Porcelli PJ, Navarrete CT, et al.: Mortality reduction by heart rate characteristic monitoring in very low birth weight neonates: a randomized trial, *J Pediatr* 159:900–906, 2011. e901.

Natarajan G, Botica ML, Thomas R, Aranda JV: Therapeutic drug monitoring for caffeine in preterm neonates: an unnecessary exercise? *Pediatrics* 119:936–940, 2007.

Omari TI: Apnea-associated reduction in lower esophageal sphincter tone in premature infants, *J Pediatr* 154:374–378, 2009.

Pantalitschka T, Sievers J, Urschitz MS, Herberts T, Reher C, Poets CF: Randomised crossover trial of four nasal respiratory support systems for apnoea of prematurity in very low birthweight infants, *Arch Dis Child Fetal Neonatal Ed* 94:F245–F248, 2009.

Pesce AJ, Rashkin M, Kotagal U: Standards of laboratory practice: theophylline and caffeine monitoring. National Academy of Clinical Biochemistry, *Clin Chem.* 44:1124–1128, 1998.

Ramanathan R, Corwin MJ, Hunt CE, Lister G, Tinsley LR, Baird T, et al.: Cardiorespiratory events recorded on home monitors: Comparison of healthy infants with those at increased risk for SIDS, *JAMA* 285:2199–2207, 2001.

Ryan CA, Finer NN, Peters KL: Nasal intermittent positive-pressure ventilation offers no advantages over nasal continuous positive airway pressure in apnea of prematurity, *Am J Dis Child* 143:1196–1198, 1989.

Sabogal C, Auais A, Napchan G, Mager E, Zhou BG, Suguihara C, et al.: Effect of respiratory syncytial virus on apnea in weanling rats, *Pediatr Res* 57:819–825, 2005.

Sanchez R, Toy P: Transfusion related acute lung injury: a pediatric perspective, *Pediatr Blood Cancer* 45:248–255, 2005.

Sands SA, Edwards BA, Kelly VJ, Davidson MR, Wilkinson MH, Berger PJ: A model analysis of arterial oxygen desaturation during apnea in preterm infants, *PLoS Comput Biol* 5:e1000588, 2009.

Sasidharan P, Heimler R: Transfusion-induced changes in the breathing pattern of healthy preterm anemic infants, *Pediatr Pulmonol* 12:170–173, 1992.

Schmidt B, Anderson PJ, Doyle LW, Dewey D, Grunau RE, Asztalos EV, et al.: Survival without disability to age 5 years after neonatal caffeine therapy for apnea of prematurity, *JAMA* 307:275–282, 2012.

Schmidt B, Roberts RS, Davis P, Doyle LW, Barrington KJ, Ohlsson A, et al.: Caffeine therapy for apnea of prematurity, *N Engl J Med* 354:2112–2121, 2006.

Schmidt B, Roberts RS, Davis P, Doyle LW, Barrington KJ, Ohlsson A, et al.: Long-term effects of caffeine therapy for apnea of prematurity, *N Engl J Med* 357:1893–1902, 2007.

Seidel D, Blaser A, Gebauer C, Pulzer F, Thome U, Knupfer M: Changes in regional tissue oxygenation saturation and desaturations after red blood cell transfusion in preterm infants, *J Perinatol* 33(4):282–287, 2013.

Slocum C, Arko M, Di Fiore J, Martin RJ, Hibbs AM: Apnea, bradycardia and desaturation in preterm infants before and after feeding, *J Perinatol* 29:209–212, 2009.

Stokowski LA: A primer on apnea of prematurity, *Adv Neonatal Care* 5:155–170, 2005. quiz 171–154.

Stoll BJ, Hansen NI, Sanchez PJ, Faix RG, Poindexter BB, Van Meurs KP, et al.: Early onset neonatal sepsis: the burden of group B Streptococcal and *E. coli* disease continues, *Pediatrics* 127:817–826, 2011.

Uauy R, Shapiro DL, Smith B, Warshaw JB: Treatment of severe apnea in prematures with orally administered theophylline, *Pediatrics* 55:595–598, 1975.

Zagol K, Lake DE, Vergales B, Moorman ME, Paget-Brown A, Lee H, et al.: Anemia, apnea of prematurity, and blood transfusions, *J Pediatr* 161:417–421, 2012. e411.

Zhao J, Gonzalez F, Mu D: Apnea of prematurity: from cause to treatment, *Eur J Pediatr* 170:1097–1105, 2011.

CHAPTER 13

NEONATAL SEPSIS

Karen M. Puopolo, MD, PhD • Gabriel J. Escobar, MD

Bacterial sepsis continues to be a major cause of morbidity and mortality among term and low birth weight, preterm newborns. Improvements in the obstetric management of women with risk factors for perinatal infections as well as advancements in neonatal intensive care have decreased the incidence, morbidity, and mortality from neonatal early-onset sepsis (EOS). Implementation of bundled approaches to infection has also improved the outlook for very low birth weight (VLBW) infants at risk for late-onset, nosocomial (hospital-acquired) sepsis (LOS). However, when neonatal infection does occur the consequences can be severe. Neurologic sequelae may result from central nervous system (CNS) infection and inflammation, as well as from secondary hypoxemia resulting from septic shock, pulmonary hypertension, and parenchymal lung disease. Accurate evaluation of sepsis risk and prompt and appropriate initiation of antibiotics are critical components of neonatal care.

This chapter is divided into two sections, discussing EOS and LOS separately. In each section, we begin by reviewing the pathogenesis, epidemiology, and microbiology of EOS and LOS. We will then present cases in each section that illustrate key issues with regard to clinical risk factors associated with each type of infection, laboratory tests that can be used to further assess for the presence of infection, and appropriate choices for empiric antibiotic therapy. The cases discussed here all occurred in the authors' centers. The EOS cases will include both term and preterm infants, whereas the LOS cases will focus on infection that occurs among continuously hospitalized, primarily VLBW infants.

PATHOGENESIS OF EOS

EOS has long been recognized as infection originating during the intrapartum period, via the amniotic cavity to the fetus, originally termed the "amniotic infection syndrome" (Benirschke, 1960; Blanc, 1961). This pathogenesis distinguishes bacterial and fungal EOS from neonatal congenital viral infections such as congenital rubella or enteroviral infection, which are acquired *in utero* via maternal viremia, placental invasion, and fetal infection. Benirschke in 1959 used placental histology and fetal and neonatal autopsies to demonstrate correlations between bacteria isolated from the maternal vagina and those found in infected neonatal lungs. He also correlated the extent of inflammatory change within the placenta and umbilical cord with characteristics of labor, and with neonatal infection, demonstrating that both were associated with premature birth, length of labor, and duration of rupture of membranes (ROM). Blanc in 1961 argued that, "Objective criteria of intrauterine exposure to infection may be derived from our knowledge of the pathogenesis of prenatal infection and might help to screen 'high risk' babies." He further suggested that "objective criteria" should include significant maternal fever, premature and/or prolonged labor, prolonged ROM, and persistent fetal tachycardia. Although intrapartum characteristics may provide opportunity for the development of EOS, the immune characteristics of the newborn also contribute to the vulnerability of newborns to invasive infection. Neonatal defense against infection immediately after birth requires effective innate immune responses. Activation of pattern-recognition receptors such as the toll-like receptor family (TLRs) and subsequent release of cytokines can be skewed in all newborn infants. A predominance of Th2-type, antiinflammatory cytokines instead of Th1-type inflammatory molecules such as interferons and tumor necrosis factor-alpha are typical for neonates. Genetic variation in TLRs may increase the risk of EOS. Newborns are also hampered by reduced phagocytic and bactericidal function of both antigen-presenting cells and neutrophils, relative to adults, with ready depletion of mature and immature neutrophils caused by defects in neutrophil recruitment and aggregation (Wynn & Levy, 2010). Finally, most pathogens causing EOS require complement, opsonic antibody, and neutrophil-based defenses for optimal defense against invasive infection. Not only do all newborns have

TABLE 13-1   Incidence of EOS

Category	Sites	Years	Cases	Incidence (per 1000)	Reference
All live births	CDC multistate surveillance	1998-2000	408	1.6	(7)
All live births	CDC multistate surveillance	2005-2008	658	0.77	(6)
≥37 weeks	14 birth hospitals	1993-2007	301	0.53	(8)
≥37 weeks	CDC multistate	2005-2008	369	0.49	(6)
34-36 weeks	248 affiliated NICUs	1996-2007	527	6.4	(9)
<1500 g	NICHD NRN 16 NICUs	2002-2003	102	17.0	(10)
<1500 g	NICHD NRN 16 NICUs	2006-2009	147	11.0	(11)

decreased levels of complement compared to adults, an individual newborn's immunoglobulin profile is derived from the mother via transplacental transfer of IgG from mother to fetus in the second half of pregnancy. The risk of EOS caused by the gram-positive bacterium Group B *Streptococcus* (*Streptococcus agalactiae*, GBS) in the newborn is inversely related to the maternal levels of serotype-specific antibody directed against the surface polysaccharide capsule of GBS (Baker & Kasper, 1976). Generally, all of the immune deficits of the newborn are relatively worse in the premature infant, contributing to the increased risk of EOS among preterm births.

In summary, the pathogenesis of EOS is that of ascending colonization of the maternal genital tract with maternal gastrointestinal and genitourinary flora; subsequent colonization of the placenta, umbilical cord, and fetus; and transition from colonization to invasive infection. Increased time for the progression of these pathologic events provided by prolonged labor and duration of ROM, and the relatively poor innate and acquired immune defenses of the fetus and newborn, provide further opportunity for development of EOS.

EPIDEMIOLOGY OF EOS

The overall incidence of EOS has decreased significantly since the first Centers for Disease Control and Prevention (CDC) recommendations for intrapartum antibiotic prophylaxis (IAP) against GBS were published in 1996. Approximately 30% of women are now treated with intrapartum antibiotics for the combined purposes of GBS IAP and secondary prevention of EOS when there is concern for maternal

chorioamnionitis (Verani, McGee, & Schrag, 2010). Recent United States CDC surveillance studies demonstrate the overall incidence of EOS to be ~1 to 2 cases per 1000 live births (Weston, Pondo, & Lewis, 2011). The incidence is lower among term infants, higher among moderately premature infants, and highest among VLBW (<1500 g) infants (Table 13-1). EOS-attributable mortality is inversely proportional to gestational age (GA) at birth; whereas only 1% to 2% among infected infants born ≥37 weeks' gestation die of EOS, approximately ¼ of EOS-affected infants born at 22 to 36 weeks' gestation die of the infection (Stoll et al., 2011; Weston, Pondo, & Lewis, 2011). Among VLBW infants, 35% of EOS-infected infants die, compared to 11% of those without culture-confirmed EOS (Stoll, Hansen, & Higgins, 2005).

MICROBIOLOGY OF EOS

The bacterial species responsible for EOS vary by geographic region and time period and reflect resident maternal gastrointestinal and genitourinary tract species. In the United States, GBS emerged in the 1970s to become the primary bacterial cause of neonatal EOS (Franciosi, Knostman, & Zimmerman, 1973; McCracken, 1973). Despite widespread implementation of IAP to prevent neonatal GBS disease, GBS remains the single most frequent cause of EOS among term infants, although *E. coli* is now the most frequent EOS pathogen in VLBW infants (Figure 13-1) (Bizarro et al., 2005; Phares et al., 1999-2005; Stoll, Hansen, & Higgins, 2005; Stoll, Hansen, & Higgins, 2010). Other enteric bacilli causing EOS include *Klebsiella*, *Hemophilus*, and *Enterobacter* species and the anaerobe *B. fragilis*. Less

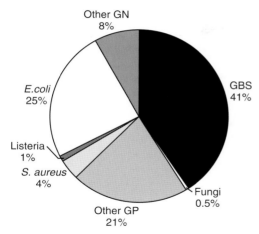

Other GN
8%

E.coli
25%

GBS
41%

Listeria
1%

S. aureus
4%

Fungi
0.5%

Other GP
21%

FIGURE 13-1 ■ **Microbiology of early-onset sepsis.**

common organisms that can cause serious early-onset disease include *Listeria monocytogenes* and *Citrobacter diversus*. Staphylococci and enterococci can be recovered from infants with EOS, but are more commonly causes of late-onset, hospital-acquired sepsis. Fungal species account for 2% to 3% of EOS infections, primarily in VLBW infants (Hornik et al., 2012; Puopolo & Eichenwald, 2010; Stoll, Hansen, & Higgins, 2005).

CASE STUDY 1

The pediatric delivery room team is called to the vaginal delivery of a 38⁶⁄₇-week infant born to a 30-year-old G2P1→2 mother because of meconium-stained fluid. The prenatal history is unremarkable; the mother received standard prenatal care and her GBS screening culture from 35 weeks' gestation was negative. The labor was spontaneous, with ROM 10 hours prior to delivery. Just prior to delivery, the mother developed a fever to 102.7° F; however, there was not sufficient time to administer intrapartum antibiotics. The infant emerged vigorous with spontaneous cry and good tone; the assigned Apgar scores were 9 at both 1 and 5 minutes of life. The birth weight was 3880 grams. The obstetric team plans to administer antibiotics to the mother postpartum until she becomes afebrile, because of a concern for chorioamnionitis.

EXERCISE 1

QUESTION

1. How should this infant be managed?
   a. Because the infant appears entirely well, no further intervention is necessary and the infant may "room-in" with the mother.

   b. Because the mother had intrapartum fever and there is concern for chorioamnionitis, the infant should be transferred to the special care nursery or NICU for a "rule out sepsis" evaluation. Once a blood culture has been obtained, the infant should be transferred to the well baby nursery and "room-in" with the mother.
   c. The infant should be transferred to the special care nursery or NICU to evaluate the infant for possible EOS. Once a blood culture has been obtained, the infant should receive empiric antibiotic therapy until the blood culture results are negative.

ANSWER

1. **c.** This case illustrates one of the most difficult issues in the management of neonatal EOS. Most infants with EOS become ill in the first day of life, but only ~50% of infected infants are symptomatic in the delivery room; ~90% are clinically symptomatic by 24 hours of life and the remainder by age 72 hours (Verani, McGee, & Schrag, 2010). Among infants who are ill-appearing at birth, evaluation for EOS and institution of empiric antibiotic therapy directed to the most common causes of EOS are standard neonatal care. Among infants who appear well at birth, an assessment of the magnitude of risk of EOS should be made to decide on the best course of care.

   Multiple studies have assessed the role of specific maternal and neonatal characteristics in predicting risk of neonatal EOS. Because GBS has been the single most common bacterial cause of EOS in the United States over the past 40 years, many studies focus on the risk of GBS-specific EOS. A summary of risk factors for EOS is shown in Table 13-2. Although many of the factors listed are interactive (e.g., very long duration of ROM is associated with preterm birth), the most significant risk factor for EOS is gestational age (GA). The incidence of EOS is ~0.5 cases/1000 among those born at ≥37 weeks, compared to ~3.0 cases/1000 live births at <37 weeks' gestation (Weston et al., 2011) (Figure 13-2, A). Much of the risk disparity among preterm infants is attributable to the 10-fold higher incidence among premature, VLBW infants (Table 13-1). Post-dates delivery also presents an increased risk of EOS, with an incidence of EOS roughly 1.5-fold higher among births occurring ≥41 weeks compared to 37 to 40 weeks (Puopolo et al., 2011). Although the reason for an increasing incidence of EOS among post-date pregnancies is not entirely known, it has been attributed to decreased integrity of amniotic membranes and partial cervical dilatation.

TABLE 13-2 **Risk Factors for EOS**

Maternal or Neonatal	Risk Factor	Risk Categories	Reference
Maternal	Age or race	• <20 vs. ≥20 years • Black vs. non-black	5, 6, 16-20
Maternal	GBS status	Positive, negative or unknown	4, 5, 21-25
Maternal	Intrapartum fever	• >37.5° C • ≥38.0° C • ≥102° F	5, 19, 26-31
Maternal	Duration of ROM	• 12 hours • ≥18 hours • >24 hours	2, 19, 29-33
Maternal	Intrapartum antibiotics	• GBS-specific • Any antibiotic • Administration time relative to delivery	8, 18, 25
Maternal	Obstetrical interventions	• # of vaginal exams • Internal fetal monitor • Membrane stripping	5, 17
Neonatal	Gestational age and or birth weight	• <37 weeks • ≥28 weeks • <1500 grams • <2500 grams	6, 8, 21, 29, 34
Neonatal	Clinical condition	Well-appearing vs. symptomatic	29, 36, 37

Another very strong predictor of EOS is the infant's clinical status. One study of infants born ≥37 weeks found bacteremia among 0.5% of evaluated, asymptomatic infants versus 3.2% of evaluated, symptomatic infants (Johnson et al., 1997). Another study of infants born ≥35 weeks found bacteremia among 0.4% of evaluated, symptomatic infants versus 0.04% of all asymptomatic infants born in that GA range (Mukhopadhyay, Eichenwald, & Puopolo, 2011). We found an adjusted odds ratio for EOS of 0.26 (95% confidence interval, 0.11 to 0.63) among asymptomatic infants when compared to symptomatic infants evaluated for EOS (Escobar et al., 2000). However, in each of these studies, EOS did occur among asymptomatic infants (with risk factors for sepsis) at a rate that was 2 to 3 times than that of the entire birth cohort.

Thus for the infant in Case Study 1, term birth and asymptomatic status reduce the odds that the infant will suffer EOS, and may suggest that the best of course of action is that in choice "a." Before leaving the infant in the delivery room, a few other factors listed in Table 13-2 should be considered. Intrapartum characteristics are also significant predictors of EOS. Many of the studies identifying these factors were conducted prior to the widespread use of intrapartum antibiotics to prevent GBS-specific EOS. We recently conducted a study of risk factors for EOS among infants born ≥34 weeks' gestation in the era of GBS IAP and quantified the risk associated with many of the factors listed in Table 13-2, using both bivariate analyses and multivariate logistic regression models (Puopolo et al., 2011). Graphical representation of risk associated with intrapartum maternal temperature and duration of ROM is shown in Figure 13-2, *B* and 13-2, *C*. Maternal intrapartum fever may signal the development of infection of the uterine compartment, and the relationship shown in Figure 13-2, *A* suggests that the height of fever correlates with risk of EOS in the newborn. In other words, the magnitude of the febrile response may be more important than the mere presence of an elevated temperature. Although prior studies of EOS considered different cut-off values for duration of ROM—12, 18, or 24 hours—as particularly risky, in fact the relationship of ROM with risk of EOS increases in a monotonic fashion.

Final issues for consideration in Case Study 1 are maternal GBS colonization and maternal intrapartum antibiotic administration. Multiple studies demonstrate that women are variably colonized with GBS in their gastrointestinal and genitourinary tracts; point-prevalence studies of pregnant

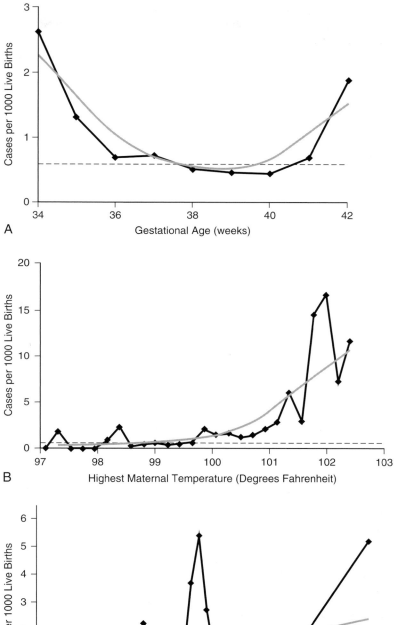

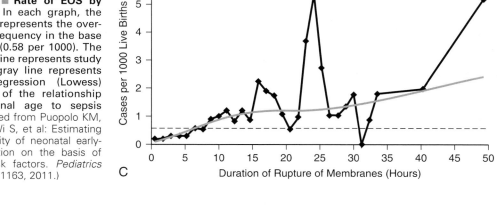

FIGURE 13-2 ■ Rate of EOS by risk factor. In each graph, the dotted line represents the overall sepsis frequency in the base population (0.58 per 1000). The black solid line represents study data. The gray line represents a local regression (Lowess) smoothing of the relationship of gestational age to sepsis rate. (Adapted from Puopolo KM, Draper D, Wi S, et al: Estimating the probability of neonatal early-onset infection on the basis of maternal risk factors. *Pediatrics* 128:e1155-e1163, 2011.)

women report colonization rates of 10% to 30% (Verani, McGee, & Schrag, 2010) although one longitudinal study of 1248 nonpregnant, sexually active women found that nearly 60% were colonized at least once over the course of a year (Meyn et al., 2002). Because maternal GBS colonization is not universal, multivariate analyses of risk factors for GBS-specific EOS demonstrate that maternal GBS status is the overwhelming predictor of risk, with odds ratio >200 (Benitz,

Gould, & Druzin, 1999). As noted above, the CDC recommends IAP to decrease the risk of infant GBS colonization and invasive infection. The current recommendations for GBS IAP and the impact of these recommendations are shown in Box 13-1 and Figure 13-3. GBS IAP has been effective in decreasing the national incidence of GBS-specific EOS. However, the

---

<table>
<tr><td>**BOX 13-1**</td><td>**Indications for GBS Intrapartum Antibiotic Prophylaxis**</td></tr>
</table>

- Previous infant with invasive GBS disease
- GBS bacteriuria during any trimester of the current pregnancy
- Positive GBS vaginal–rectal screening culture at 35 to 37 weeks' gestation during current pregnancy
- Unknown GBS status at the onset of labor (culture not done, incomplete, or results unknown) and any of the following:
  - Delivery at <37 weeks' gestation
  - Amniotic membrane rupture ≥18 hours
  - Intrapartum temperature ≥100.4° F (≥38.0° C)
  - Intrapartum nucleic acid amplification test positive for GBS

Note that GBS IAP is not indicated if cesarean delivery is performed before onset of labor on a woman with intact amniotic membranes, regardless of GBS colonization status or gestational age.

Adapted from: Verani JR, McGee L, Schrag SJ, et al: Prevention of perinatal group B streptococcal disease—revised guidelines from CDC, 2010, MMWR Recomm Rep 59:1-36, 2010.

---

results of prenatal GBS screening at 35 to 37 weeks' gestation can be discordant with true maternal colonization at the time of delivery ~4% to 5% of the time (Yancey et al., 1996). Most GBS-specific EOS among term infants now occurs in those born to mothers who have screened GBS negative (Puopolo, Madoff, & Eichenwald, 2005; Van Dyke et al., 2009).

So what is the best choice for our infant in Case Study 1? The 2010 revised CDC guidelines for prevention of perinatal GBS disease contain guidelines for secondary prevention of all bacterial-cause EOS (Figure 13-4). The American Academy of Pediatrics Committee on the Fetus and Newborn (COFN) has endorsed these guidelines, with minor modifications contained in the footnote to Figure 13-4 (Brady & Polin, 2013). CDC and COFN standards would advise choice "c". Although the infant is born at term to a GBS-negative mother, and duration of ROM is less than 18 hours, the obstetric concern for chorioamnionitis suggests that the most prudent course of action is to obtain a neonatal blood culture and begin empiric antibiotic therapy pending the blood culture results and the infant's clinical course. We recently developed a multivariate risk model for EOS that integrates GA, maternal intrapartum fever, duration of ROM, maternal GBS status, and intrapartum antibiotic use to estimate the risk of EOS (available at *http://www. dor.kaiser.org/external/DORExternal/research/ InfectionProbabilityCalculator.aspx* or *http://www. newbornsepsiscalculator.org*). Use of this calculator would estimate a probability of culture-confirmed infection of 5.7/1000 live births, roughly 10 times higher than the baseline risk

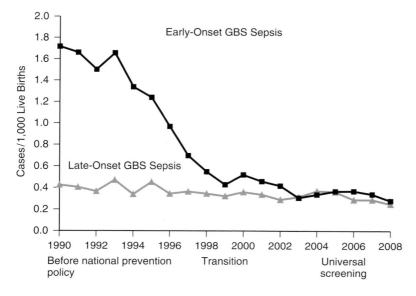

FIGURE 13-3 ■ Impact of GBS prophylaxis on incidence of GBS-specific EOS. (Adapted from National Center for Immunization and Respiratory Diseases, Division of Bacterial Diseases: Early-onset group B streptococcal disease prevention: for clinicians, 2010. Accessed February 17, 2014 at http:// www.cdc.gov/groupbstrep/ clinicians/neonatal-providers.html #slidesets.)

among infants born at 38 to 40 weeks' gestation, and high enough to support choice "c." In reality, this was the course taken. The infant's blood culture grew GBS within 12 hours of incubation, but a repeat blood culture was negative, lumbar puncture for cerebrospinal fluid (CSF) evaluation after antibiotic therapy was reassuring, and the infant remained clinically well.

CASE STUDY 2

The pediatric delivery room team is called to the vaginal delivery of a 39⅝-week infant born to a 32-year-old G1P0→1 mother because of a prenatal history notable for insulin-dependent gestational diabetes. The mother received standard prenatal care and her GBS screening culture at 36 weeks' gestation was negative. Labor was induced and membranes ruptured 9.5 hours prior to delivery.

The mother developed a fever to 100.8° F late in her labor course. The obstetric team did not administer intrapartum antibiotics because they were not concerned about developing chorioamnionitis, attributing the intrapartum fever to the lengthy induction and use of epidural analgesia. The infant emerged vigorous with spontaneous cry and good tone; the assigned Apgar scores were 7 at 1 minute and 8 at 5 minutes of life. The birth weight was 3520 grams. The infant did not require supplemental oxygen, but retractions and tachypnea were present at 15 minutes of life, and so the infant was taken to the NICU for observation. Because of the respiratory distress and intrapartum fever, a complete blood cell (CBC) and blood culture were obtained in the first hour of life. However, by 2 hours of life the respiratory rate and oxygen saturations were normal, and the retractions have resolved.

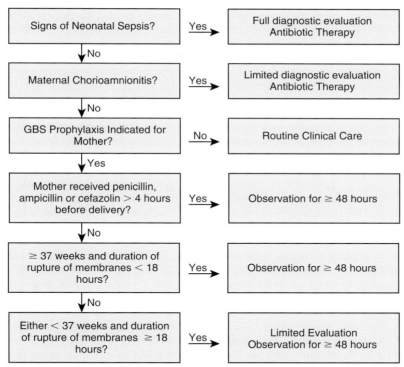

FIGURE 13-4 ■ **Algorithm for secondary prevention of GBS EOS.** Limited evaluation consists of blood culture and CBC with differential ± CRP at birth or at 6 to 12 hours of life. Full diagnostic evaluation consists of these items as well as chest radiograph and lumbar puncture if appropriate. The American Academy of Pediatrics Committee on Fetus and Newborn endorses these guidelines with the following exceptions: (a) Well-appearing infants born at 35 to 36 weeks' gestation in the setting of inadequate indicated GBS prophylaxis may be treated with observation for ≥48 hours if ROM <18 hours. (b) Well-appearing infants born ≥37 weeks in the setting of inadequate indicated GBS prophylaxis may be treated with observation for ≥48 hours if ROM ≥18 hours or with limited evaluation if close observation is not possible. (c) Well-appearing infants born <37 weeks' gestation in the setting of inadequate indicated GBS prophylaxis may have CBC with differential ± CRP at 6 to 12 hours of life, with blood culture only obtained if laboratory data is abnormal. COFN recommends that the duration of antimicrobial therapy for healthy-appearing infants without evidence of bacterial infection be no more than 48 hours. In small preterm infants, some may continue antibiotics for up to 72 hours while awaiting bacterial culture results. (From Verani JR, McGee L, Schrag SJ, et al: Prevention of perinatal group B streptococcal disease—revised guidelines from CDC, 2010, *MMWR Recomm Rep* 59:1-36, 2010.)

EXERCISE 2

QUESTION

1. How should this infant be managed?
   a. Because the infant now appears entirely well, nothing more is needed and the infant should be transferred back to the mother.
   b. Because the mother had intrapartum fever and the infant had some respiratory distress, you should be concerned about EOS. Await the results of the CBC and C-reactive protein and begin empiric antibiotic therapy (following a blood culture) if the results are abnormal.
   c. Begin empiric antibiotic therapy regardless of the laboratory results, and treat until the blood culture results are reported as negative.

ANSWER

1. **b.** This case presents several difficulties in EOS risk assessment. Using what we learned in Case Study 1, we summarize: term infant, well-appearing by 2 hours of age, mother GBS negative, with intrapartum maternal fever but no obstetric concern for chorioamnionitis. The CDC 2010 guidelines for secondary prevention of EOS would not advocate for evaluation of this infant because of concern for chorioamnionitis, but the initial symptoms of respiratory distress can justify concern for infection in a symptomatic infant. Using this Sepsis Risk Score multivariate approach, the predicted probability of culture-confirmed infection is 1.04/1000, or roughly twice the baseline risk in the term population. As the clinician, you are reassured by the resolution of the initial respiratory distress, but a bit uncomfortable with the history of the maternal fever. When there is uncertainty about the need for blood culture and/or initiation of antibiotics, neonatal clinicians have relied on two common laboratory tests to aid their risk assessment for EOS: the total white blood cell (WBC) and neutrophil indices, and the C-reactive protein (CRP).

The total WBC and neutrophil indices (absolute neutrophil count [ANC]), absolute band count, and the ratio of immature to total neutrophils (I:T ratio) are readily available and commonly used to evaluate both symptomatic and asymptomatic infants at risk for sepsis. Interpretation of these values has been compromised by the relatively small size of studies used to determine normal values, and the array of conditions that may affect these values. Maternal fever, neonatal asphyxia, meconium aspiration syndrome, pneumothorax, and hemolytic disease have all been associated with neutrophilia; maternal pregnancy-induced hypertension and preeclampsia are associated with neonatal neutropenia and thrombocytopenia. Interpretation of neonatal WBC values has relied on dichotomizing values as "normal" or "abnormal" based on small studies, such as the 1979 study by Manroe and colleagues. The development of electronic medical records has permitted larger analyses. A 2008 study of 30,354 WBC values from the Intermountain Healthcare system stratified neutrophil values by time after birth and by GA; infants with blood culture–proven EOS, chromosomal abnormalities, extremely low or high WBC results, and those born to mothers with preeclampsia were excluded (Schmutz et al., 2008). This study found a higher upper limit of ANC than the Manroe study, although neutropenia was defined similarly (ANC <2500/mm^3 for term infants, and <1000/mm^3 for preterm infants.)

One challenge to using the WBC in newborns is the "roller coaster" shape of the WBC, ANC, and I:T curves in the first 72 hours of life, suggesting that optimal interpretation of WBC data to predict EOS should account for the natural rise and fall in WBC during this period. One study of 856 near-term and term newborn infants born to mothers with suspected chorioamnionitis evaluated the use of serial WBC components obtained at <1 hour, 12 hours, and 24 hours of life to predict clinical and culture-proven EOS (Jackson et al., 2004). The authors noted multiple abnormal values in all study infants compared to the Manroe standard curves and concluded that single or serial neutrophil values have no utility in prediction of clinical or culture-proven EOS. Two recent studies used very large datasets to evaluate the use of WBC and its components in predicting EOS. In a study that included 67,623 CBC and blood culture pairs obtained in the first 72 hours of life from infants ≥34 weeks' gestation (including 245 cases of blood culture–proven infection) (Newman et al., 2010), the best combination of sensitivity and specificity occurred when specimens were tested beyond 4 hours of life (Figure 13-5). Both the WBC and the ANC were most predictive of infection when they were low (WBC <5,000/mm^3; ANC <1,000/mm^3). Elevated WBC (>20,000/mm^3) and low platelet counts (<150 × 10^3/µl) were largely non-informative in the study newborns. The I:T ratio was the most informative of the three metrics if measured beyond 4 hours of life; low values (<0.15) were reassuring, whereas elevated values (>0.30) were associated with EOS. Adjusting for factors such as birth weight, maternal preeclampsia, gender, and mode of delivery did not improve the overall predictive value of the

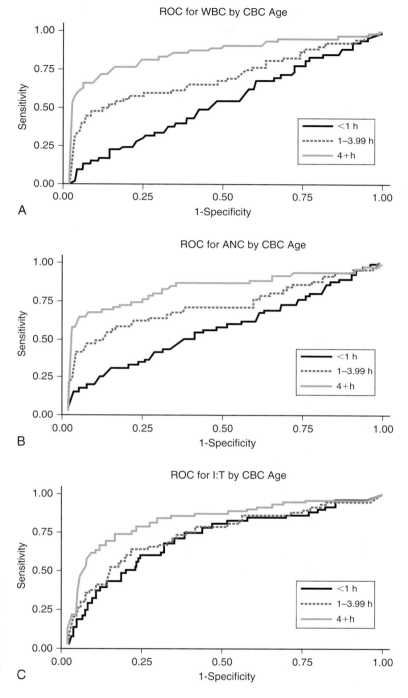

FIGURE 13-5 ■ **Receiver-operator curves for WBC and differential in prediction of EOS according to age at the time of the CBC.** (Adapted from Newman T, Puopolo K, Wi S, et al: Interpreting complete blood counts soon after birth in newborns at risk for sepsis. *Pediatrics* 126:903-909, 2010.)

WBC and its components. This study supports the use of CBC only after the first few hours of life, when placed in the proper clinical context (e.g., when used as part of an algorithm to evaluate infants for sepsis risk).

The second large study used an administrative database and a cohort of 166,092 infants of all GA to analyze CBC and blood cultures obtained in the first 72 hours of life (Hornik et al., 2012a). This study calculated mean values for WBC, ANC, I:T ratio and platelets for each of the first 3 days of life, but did not account for age in hours after birth. This study also found that a low total WBC count (<5000/mm³), low ANC (<1500/mm³), and elevated I:T (>0.5) had the highest odd ratios for EOS, whereas elevated total WBC >20,000/mm^3 and low platelet counts were of no use in predicting EOS among study infants with GA >36 weeks.

CRP is a nonspecific marker of inflammation or tissue necrosis that is produced by the liver in response to interleukin-6 release from activated inflammatory and endothelial cells. Many of the same noninfectious conditions that can affect the WBC in newborns—maternal fever, neonatal asphyxia, meconium aspiration syndrome, pneumothorax, or hemolysis—have been associated with elevated CRP. Although elevations in CRP (>1 mg/dL) are found in the course of culture-confirmed infection, a single determination of CRP at birth lacks sensitivity for EOS (Benitz et al., 1998; Benitz, 2010). CRP determinations are most useful for their negative predictive accuracy (i.e., they are helpful for identifying infants with a low probability of infection). Excluding a value obtained at birth, the negative predictive accuracy of serial CRP determinations is >98%; however, single CRP determinations are not useful for identifying infants with positive blood cultures (Benitz, 2010). The predictive ability of an elevated CRP level at 6 to 12 hours of life is not much different from that of having an I:T ratio >0.3 after 4 hours of life.

Therefore in Case Study 2, the results of a CBC with differential or CRP obtained in the first hour of life is unlikely to provide information that will inform the risk of EOS and help with the decision to begin antibiotics in this infant. The rapid resolution of symptoms, relatively low predicted probability of EOS by multivariate analysis and guidance provided by the CDC and COFN guidelines would all support clinical observation. Laboratory testing at 6 to 12 hours of life may be more helpful in determining the risk of EOS, and would be another reasonable management option, with institution of empiric antibiotic therapy if that testing was not reassuring. In reality, this infant was managed by choice "b." The CBC results were WBC 20,900/mm^3, I:T ratio 0.13, ANC 16,500/mm^3 and platelet count 302 × 10^3/ul, and although these were obtained at 1 hour of life, they were interpreted by the caregivers as normal. CRP was not obtained and antibiotics were not given. The infant was returned to the nursery for close observation, remained well, and the blood culture was negative.

CASE STUDY 3

The pediatric delivery team is called to the delivery of a male premature infant at 27⁶/₇ weeks' gestation. The prenatal history is notable for cerclage placement at 14 weeks' gestation. The mother *presented at 26²/₇ weeks with premature ROM (PROM) but she was not in preterm labor. She received a course of betamethasone and was treated with penicillin G for 48 hours until a GBS screen sent on admission was negative. Because she was afebrile without evidence of preterm labor, she was admitted to the high-risk obstetric service for expectant management. Per local obstetric policy, she was given erythromycin for 7 days to increase latency. On the day of delivery, the mother developed a fever to 101.4° F with onset of contractions; she was taken for a cesarean section delivery owing to fetal breech position. The infant emerged with minimal respiratory effort and was intubated in the delivery room; Apgar scores were 5 at 1 minute, 5 at 5 minutes, and 8 at 10 minutes. The birth weight was 1200 grams. In the first 6 hours of life, the infant developed increasing respiratory failure despite the administration of exogenous surfactant, but improved on high-frequency ventilation. He remained hemodynamically stable. You are concerned about EOS and obtain a blood culture and CBC with differential. The total WBC is 21,760/mm³, with an I:T ratio 0.14 and ANC 11,098/mm³. The platelet count is 190 × 10³/ul. You do not perform a lumbar puncture due to the infant's respiratory instability.*

EXERCISE 3

QUESTION

1. How should this infant be managed?
   a. Begin ampicillin and gentamicin pending blood culture results because most bacteria causing EOS are still sensitive to these antibiotics.
   b. Begin cefotaxime and gentamicin pending blood culture results because this baby is at risk for an ampicillin-resistant infection.
   c. Begin ampicillin and cefotaxime pending blood cultures results because this baby is at risk for an ampicillin-resistant infection and some organisms causing EOS are inherently resistant to cephalosporins.
   d. Administer intravenous immunoglobulin (IVIG) and broad-spectrum antibiotics since this baby is likely deficient in maternally acquired antibody.

ANSWER

1. **c.** This case illustrates many of the concerns raised in the EOS assessment of preterm infants. Using what we learned in Case Studies 1 and 2, we can summarize: preterm, VLBW infant, born to a woman with 10 days of PROM who developed fever and preterm labor. The infant is critically ill from birth; the total WBC, neutrophil

indices, and platelet values obtained within the first hour of life are within normal ranges. In contrast to the EOS assessment of term infants, the assessment of preterm, VLBW infants presents several unique challenges. First, we know that the baseline risk of EOS in the VLBW population is relatively high (~1% to 2%)—at least 20 times higher than term infants, making the choice to rule out infection the default position of most clinicians. Second, VLBW birth is frequently associated with recognized risk factors for EOS, as in this case. The presence of prolonged PROM and the obstetric diagnosis of chorioamnionitis raise the estimated risk considerably above baseline risk (Dutta et al., 2010; Jackson et al., 2012). Combined with the presence of critical illness, both the CDC and COFN recommendations—and common sense—support the initiation of antibiotics in this infant.

Antibiotic choice for empiric treatment of EOS should include broad coverage based on the known microbiology of infection, and usually includes a β-lactam antibiotic and an aminoglycoside (commonly ampicillin and gentamicin). As shown in Figure 13-1, the microbiology of EOS among all live births is dominated by gram-positive organisms GBS (and other streptococci) and *E. coli*. Ampicillin and gentamicin remain a good choice for empiric treatment of EOS in term and late-preterm infants because GBS, most other streptococci, and many *E. coli* are sensitive to ampicillin, and *E. coli* remain sensitive to gentamicin and other aminoglycosides (Stoll et al., 2011). However, in VLBW infants, *E. coli* and other gram-negative organisms predominate and ampicillin and gentamicin alone may not be sufficient, especially when there is a significant risk of infection. The reported incidence of ampicillin resistance in *E. coli* EOS isolates ranges from 40% to 85% (Puopolo & Eichenwald, 2010; Stoll et al., 2005; Stoll, Hansen, & Sanchez, 2011). Other gram-negative enteric isolates causing EOS such as *Klebsiella* species are also resistant to ampicillin. Addition of a third-generation cephalosporin (such as cefotaxime) to empiric EOS therapy will insure adequate coverage for such organisms.

Specific factors associated with ampicillin-resistant infections include preterm birth and prior prolonged maternal antepartum and intrapartum antibiotic treatment (Bizzarro et al., 2008; Puopolo & Eichenwald, 2010; Schrag et al., 2006; Stoll et al., 2002a). With the implementation of IAP against GBS, a practice that primarily prevents beta-lactam sensitive infections, an increasing *proportion* of EOS cases are caused by gram-negative organisms (Clark et al.,

2006; Puopolo & Eichenwald, 2010). Whether intrapartum prophylaxis policies are contributing to an absolute increase in the *incidence* of EOS caused by ampicillin-resistant gram-negative organisms is a matter of ongoing controversy. CDC surveillance and reviews of published data conclude that there is no evidence of an increase in non-GBS or ampicillin-resistant EOS among term infants (Clark et al., 2006). However, increases in non-GBS EOS and ampicillin-resistant EOS are reported in VLBW infants (Bizzarro et al., 2008; Stoll et al., 2002a). Trends in the microbiology of EOS likely vary to some extent by institution, and may be influenced by local obstetric practices as well as by local variation in indigenous bacterial flora. Ultimately, decisions about empiric antibiotic therapy for EOS or LOS are best informed by an understanding of both national and local data. However, in the absence of local data suggesting otherwise, the best course of action in Case Study 3 is choice "c" due to the high risk of any EOS as well as ampicillin-resistant EOS in this case. Choice "c" is better than choice "b" primarily because use of a cephalosporin and gentamicin will not provide coverage for the less common EOS organisms *Enterococci* and *Listeria*, both of which are inherently resistant to cephalosporins. The decision to use ampicillin and cefotaxime is best made with the understanding that the antibiotic choice should be simplified to the narrowest combination (or discontinued altogether) when blood culture results are known at 48 to 72 hours of incubation.

Some clinicians might consider using IVIG in the treatment of VLBW infants with suspected EOS, because of the importance of opsonic antibody in immune defense against polysaccharide-encapsulated organisms such as GBS and *E. coli* and the relatively inadequate immunoglobulin reserves among premature infants. Metaanalyses of relatively small, randomized trials of the use of IVIG in the acute treatment of suspected or proven neonatal sepsis conducted before 2011 showed a decrease in mortality of borderline significance (Ohlsson & Lacy, 2010). However, a recent multicenter, randomized, placebo-controlled trial of IVIG for adjunctive therapy in suspect EOS involving nearly 3500 primarily VLBW infants showed no effect on the outcomes of suspected or culture-confirmed EOS (NIS Collaborative Group et al., 2011). In light of this study, choice "d" would not be generally recommended. Other immunomodulatory agents such as the recombinant white cell growth factors G-CSF and GM-CSF, activated protein C, and pentoxifylline have been trialed in small numbers of infants or in adults with sepsis

(Cohen-Wolkowicz, Benjamin, & Capparelli, 2009). None of these therapies can currently be recommended for use in neonates.

Early-onset meningitis complicates 4% to 10% of EOS cases (Bizzarro et al., 2008; Stoll et al., 2011). Data on early-onset meningitis may underestimate the total burden of this complication since many clinicians do not perform lumbar punctures before initiating antibiotic therapy, especially among unstable VLBW infants like that described in Case Study 3. If lumbar puncture is not performed prior to starting antibiotics, it is reasonable to dose empiric antibiotics using meningitic dosing until blood culture results are known and/or lumbar puncture is performed. In Case Study 3, ampicillin-resistant *E. coli* grew from the blood cultures; later CSF analyses did not indicate the presence of meningitis.

A final issue to consider that may be unique to VLBW infants is the potential risk of antibiotic therapy itself. The relatively high risk of EOS, the frequent presence of specific risk factors for EOS, including critical illness, and concerns about the modifying effects of intrapartum antibiotic administration lead many clinicians to treat VLBW infants with prolonged antibiotic courses for presumed culture-negative EOS. Although clinicians make this choice to optimize infant outcomes, recent studies have called into question the safety of this approach. Several reports have noted an association with prolonged antibiotic exposures in the first week of life and a subsequent increased risk of late-onset infection, necrotizing enterocolitis (NEC), and death, even when controlled for initial severity of illness (Cotton et al., 2006; Cotten et al., 2009; Kuppala et al., 2011; Vanaja et al., 2011). One study was able to demonstrate a linear increase in risk of NEC with total duration of antibiotic exposure, in the absence of blood culture–confirmed infection (Vanaja et al., 2011). Ultimately, the clinician must make an informed judgment about extended antibiotic treatment in the absence of culture-confirmed infection based on the likelihood of infection for an individual infant, the presence of intrapartum risk factors, infant condition, and the perceived risk/benefit ratio of antibiotic therapy.

PATHOGENESIS OF LATE-ONSET SEPSIS (LOS)

This section will focus on LOS that occurs among premature, VLBW infants. Most cases of late-onset sepsis are now classified as healthcare-associated infections because they occur while the infants are receiving treatment for other conditions in an ICU setting. The most common healthcare infections are central line–associated bloodstream infections (CLABSI) and ventilator associated pneumonia (VAP). Preterm newborn infants hospitalized in a NICU have multiple risk factors for healthcare-associated infections, including host defense impairments associated with premature birth, acquisition of pathogenic bacteria and fungi from the NICU environment, and need for invasive monitoring and procedures (central venous lines, urinary catheters, endotracheal tubes, and chest tubes). Furthermore, even less invasive procedures—such as peripheral IVs and CPAP prongs—may be associated with superficial abrasions that can lead to transient bacteremias or soft tissue infections that can lead to LOS.

The relative immune deficiencies of the newborn reviewed above in the section "Pathogenesis of EOS" also contribute to the pathogenesis of LOS, including alterations in TLR responses, reduced neutrophil function, and relative deficiencies in complement and immunoglobulin. The lack of maternally derived opsonic antibody is especially problematic for very low gestation infants (those born ≤28 weeks) and likely contributes to the vulnerability of VLBW infants to infections with relatively nonvirulent species such as coagulase-negative *Staphylococci* (CONS). VLBW infants are also more likely than term infants to be born to women with complications of pregnancy such as preeclampsia and placental dysfunction. These conditions can lead to fetal growth restriction and neonatal bone marrow dysfunction, with prolonged periods of leukopenia and neutropenia that also contribute to the pathogenesis of healthcare-associated infections. It is important to remember that many of these same issues are also applicable to term and near-term infants, particularly those with congenital anomalies that require prolonged NICU care and the presence of central venous lines (CVLs).

EPIDEMIOLOGY OF LOS

The incidence of LOS is inversely related to both GA and birth weight and varies by center. Among VLBW infants born ≤28 weeks' gestation in NICHD Neonatal Research Network (NRN) centers from 2003 to 2007, 36% had at least one episode of culture-confirmed LOS, with rates ranging from 18% to 51% among the 20 individual centers (Stoll et al., 2010). Figure 13-6 shows data on LOS evaluation and confirmed infection among infants born at our

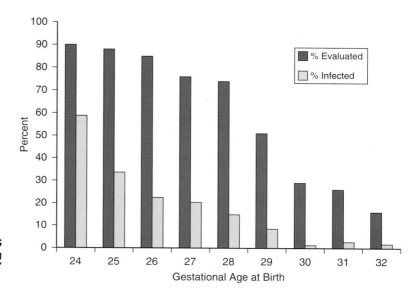

FIGURE 13-6 ■ **Frequency of LOS evaluation and infection among infants born at ≤32 weeks' gestation.**

centers from 2008 to 2010. Concern for the presence of LOS contributes to a very high rate of LOS evaluation at our centers; a mean of 2.4 evaluations per infant were performed among infants born ≤28 weeks' gestation, and 26% suffered at least one episode of LOS. Meningitis complicates LOS in ~5% of infants for whom a lumbar puncture is performed and can occur in the absence of bacteremia (Stoll et al., 2004). LOS-attributable mortality is inversely proportional to GA at birth, but overall LOS increases mortality among VLBW infants by ~10% (Stoll et al., 2002b). LOS-attributable mortality is significantly associated with the infecting organism. Gram-positive organisms such as CONS rarely contribute to mortality, but infection-attributable mortality is significant for gram-negative (19% to 36%) and *Candida* infections (22% to 32%) (Downey, Smith, & Benjamin, 2010). The underlying cause of LOS is related to the presence of CVLs in ~60% of cases; NEC, urinary tract infections, and soft tissue infections may also lead to bacteremia.

MICROBIOLOGY OF LOS

The microbial species responsible for LOS vary by center, likely reflecting difference in the local population as well as specific hospital flora. The predominant isolate in most reports is CONS, but there is site-specific variation observed in the relative proportion of infections due to methicillin-sensitive and methicillin-resistant *Staphylococcus aureus* (MSSA and MRSA), gram-negative species, and to *Candida* species. Aggregate data from the NICHD NRN, Pediatrix, and our centers

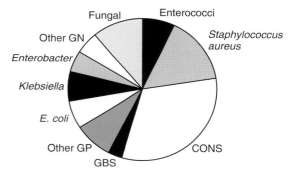

FIGURE 13-7 ■ **Microbiology of LOS.**

is shown in Figure 13-7 (Hornik et al., 2012; Stoll et al, 2002b; and unpublished data). Most (~90%) of LOS among VLBW infants is due to ampicillin-resistant species. Highly resistant species such as MRSA, vancomycin-resistant enterococci (VRE), extended-spectrum beta-lactamase (ESBL)–producing *E. coli* and *Klebsiella* species, and *Enterobacter* species that contain chromosomally encoded, inducible β-lactamases (AmpC-encoded cephalosporinases) are all reported with increasing frequency among NICU populations (Benenson et al., 2013; Cantey et al., 2013; Lessa et al., 2009). Fungal species account for 6% to 18% of LOS infections and primarily occur among infants with birth weight <1000 grams (Downey, Smith, & Benjamin, 2010; Feja et al., 2005; Stoll et al., 2002b).

CASE STUDY 4

An infant was born at 28⁵⁄₇ weeks gestation with a birth weight 910 grams, by cesarean section owing *to severe maternal preeclampsia. The mother was treated with betamethasone, magnesium sulfate, and antihypertensive medications prior to delivery. The infant's course was complicated by respiratory distress syndrome (RDS) requiring intubation and surfactant therapy, hypotension treated with dopamine, and a patent ductus arteriosus (PDA) treated with indomethacin. Umbilical venous and arterial catheters (UVC and UAC) were placed at birth and the UAC removed on the eighth day of life. On the eleventh day of life, the infant was tolerating 10 mL/kg/day feedings but became increasingly tachycardic. Ventilatory support was increased because of CO_2 retention and increasing oxygen requirements. Feedings were stopped and a blood culture was obtained. The CBC had the following values: WBC 8800/mm³, ANC 6090, I:T 0.26, platelet count 30 × 10³/ul. Of note, at birth the infant's WBC was 4900/mm³, with I:T 0.0, ANC 1420/mm³ and platelet count 220 × 10³/ul; over the following 10 days, the WBC had ranged from 6000 to 10,000/mm³, the platelet count >150 × 10³/ul, I:T <0.1, and ANC >2000/mm³.*

EXERCISE 4

QUESTION

1. What is the next most appropriate step?
   a. Begin antibiotics because of the infant's clinical instability and multiple risk factors for LOS.
   b. Do not begin antibiotics because the total WBC count and differential counts are reassuring and the infant's respiratory deterioration is unrelated to infection.
   c. Begin antibiotics because of the clinical instability and multiple risk factors for LOS but perform lumbar puncture before giving antibiotics.

ANSWER

1. **a** or **c.** The assessment of LOS risk among VLBW infants is complicated because the NICU course of these infants is often marked by physiologic instability owing to global organ-system immaturity. In addition, the relatively high risk of infection among the lowest GA infants often leads to the default position of evaluating the infant for LOS and beginning empiric antibiotic therapy with any sign of instability. Such an approach leads to high cumulative exposures to antibiotics, despite recent evidence that antibiotic exposures themselves may increase the subsequent risk of LOS, NEC, fungal sepsis, and death among the most premature babies (Cotton et al., 2006; Cotten et al., 2009; Kuppala et al., 2011; Vanaja et al., 2011). A real-time assessment of risk that goes beyond GA and

birth weight is the optimal approach. Table 13-3 provides a list of the major clinical characteristics associated with increased risk of LOS. In Case Study 4, multiple risk factors are present: low GA, low birth weight, use of an umbilical venous catheter, mechanical ventilation since birth, and total parenteral nutrition (TPN) administration. This combination of risk factors with acute clinical instability justifies a LOS evaluation and empiric treatment. Choices "a" and "c" are both reasonable. A lumbar puncture should only be done in an infant who is clinically stable.

Given the difficulties in assessing LOS risk within a population of infants with a relatively high baseline incidence of infection, clinicians turn to the same tests—CBC and CRP—as discussed above for EOS. Optimal interpretation of these tests in the hospitalized preterm infant

TABLE 13-3 Risk Factors for LOS Among VLBW Infants

Category	Factor Associated with Increased Risk	References
Gestational age	Risk inversely proportional to both gestational age and to birth weight	34, 61
Postnatal age	Risk peaks ~8-14 days of life Most LOS occurs before 28 days of age	62
Feeding		
NPO	Later postnatal age at initiation of feeding	61
MM vs formula	Formula feeding increases risk compared to mother's own milk feeding	68, 69
Technicalities of Care		
Central venous lines	Odds ratio of LOS increases 1.5-fold with 8-14 days of CVL use	61
Mechanical ventilation	Odds ratio of LOS increases 4-fold after 8-14 days on ventilator	61
TPN	Odds ratio of LOS increases 20-fold after 3 weeks of TPN administration	61
Medications		
H2 blockers	Increased risk with antacid therapy	70
Early antibiotic exposures	>5 days of empiric antibiotics	58
Medical complications	RDS, PDA, NEC all increase risk	61, 62

is difficult because of the effects of maternal diseases on neonatal bone marrow responses, as well as the multitude of noninfectious issues that can result in an inflammatory response. Several small studies have examined the ability of components of the CBC to predict late-onset sepsis, only two of which focused on VLBW infants (Fanaroff et al., 1998; Sarkar et al., 2006). A large study using the administrative data set of the Pediatrix medical group assessed the relationship between CBC and LOS (Hornik et al., 2012). In this study, 69,854 cultures were obtained from 37,826 infants. 13.8 % of the cultures were positive. Those data were matched with results from CBC counts obtained near the time of the sepsis evaluations. Although there was an association of sepsis with abnormal total WBC counts, neutrophil indices and low platelet counts, none of them possessed adequate sensitivity to reliably rule out sepsis. This study had several limitations including a CBC/culture matching algorithm that did not include time of day, leading to potential inclusion of CBCs that may have been drawn as much as 2 days before the blood culture or as late as a day after. In addition, the study could not distinguish primary cultures from "test of cure" cultures after identification of a bacteremic infant.

A single determination of CRP at time of LOS evaluation lacks sensitivity for culture-confirmed infection and should not be used to guide the decision to initiate empiric antibiotics (Benitz, 2010; Benitz et al., 1998). The performance of serial CRP determinations at time of evaluation, at 8 to 24 hours, and again at 48 hours for culture-confirmed LOS is better, although ~25% of culture-confirmed cases of LOS did not have even one abnormal CRP value among three serial values obtained (Benitz, 2010).

The blood culture from Case Study 4 grew MSSA within 12 hours of incubation. It should be noted that the CBC obtained at the time of LOS evaluation prompted clinical concern because of the acute differences in the values obtained compared to all other values obtained since birth. Because the isolate was a recognized pathogen, a CVL was in place at the time of infection, and there was no other identified cause of the infection, this episode was considered a central line–associated bloodstream infection (CLABSI) per National Healthcare Safety Network criteria (CDC, 2012).

CASE STUDY 5

A female infant was born at 24⁶/₇ weeks with a birth weight 600 grams, by vaginal delivery following preterm labor. The mother received a full course of

betamethasone prior to delivery. ROM occurred at delivery and the mother was afebrile. The infant's course was complicated by RDS requiring intubation and surfactant therapy; hypotension treated briefly with dopamine; and a PDA treated with indomethacin. UVC and peripheral arterial lines were placed at birth. The infant was given antibiotics to rule out EOS and these were discontinued when the blood culture from birth was sterile at 48 hours of incubation. On the seventh day of life, the infant's respiratory status is stable on low conventional ventilatory settings in 21% oxygen, but she develops acute abdominal distention and bilious aspirates while receiving 5 mL/kg/day of mother's milk feeding. An abdominal radiograph shows a largely gasless abdomen. The feedings are stopped and a blood culture is obtained. The CBC shows a WBC 3380/mm³, ANC 1622/mm³, I:T 0.51, platelet count 51 × 10³/ul. In the prior 6 days of life, the infant had five CBCs, each with normal values.

EXERCISE 5

QUESTION

1. What is the next most appropriate step?
   a. Because the infant has multiple risk factors for LOS, including the presence of a central venous line, begin vancomycin to treat for the possibility of coagulase negative staphylococcal sepsis.
   b. Because you are concerned about the infant's abdominal status, begin ampicillin and gentamicin and initiate a workup to rule out NEC.
   c. Because you are concerned about the infant's abdominal status, her increased risk of CLABSI, and her abnormal WBC and differential, begin vancomycin and gentamicin to cover almost all bacterial causes of infection.
   d. Same as (c), but begin antifungal agents as well since the baby was born at 24 weeks' gestation.

ANSWER

1. **c** or **d.** Empiric antibiotic choice for LOS should consider the risk factors present; the possible source of infection; the severity of illness at presentation; and the known microbiology of infection within a center. Choices for suspected CLABSI should include coverage for the most common gram-positive organisms (CONS, MSSA) as well as gram-negative organisms. Many centers use vancomycin and an aminoglycoside (gentamicin or tobramycin). For centers with a known low incidence of MRSA (and/or ongoing screening policies for MRSA carriage),

nafcillin or oxacillin and an aminoglycoside can be used safely to minimize total empiric use of vancomycin and reserve the use of this antibiotic for situations in which culture results mandate its use (Chiu et al., 2011). Centers with known high rates of gentamicin or cephalosporin-resistant gram-negative colonization and infection may opt to use a 4th generation cephalosporin (such as cefepime) or a carbapenem such as meropenem in combination with a penicillinase-resistant penicillin (oxacillin or nafcillin) or vancomycin. When there is concern for NEC with perforation, the addition of anaerobic coverage (clindamycin and metronidazole are common choices) to a standard regimen or the use of piperacillin/tazobactam for both broad-spectrum gram-negative and anaerobic coverage should be considered. Empiric antifungal treatment is often reserved for infants who, in addition to the predictors listed in Table 13-3, have specific risk factors for fungal LOS (GA <26 weeks, birth weight <750 grams, broad-spectrum antibiotic treatment in the week prior to LOS evaluation) (Benjamin et al., 2010). Centers with known high rates of fungal infection (>10% of all LOS) may have lower thresholds for the use of empiric antifungal therapy.

Overall, the clinician must make a judgment both about the likelihood of LOS and the severity of the present illness. In this case, given the abrupt change in CBC values, combined with concern for CLABSI and NEC, either choice "c" or choice "d" would also be justified. The infant in Case Study 5 developed increasing abdominal distention and discoloration over several hours, with severe respiratory decompensation eventual bowel perforation. The blood culture drawn at the time of presentation grew *Klebsiella pneumoniae* at 12 hours of incubation. The isolate was ampicillin-resistant, but sensitive to cephalosporins and gentamicin. Unfortunately, the infant in Case Study 5 died despite maximal intensive care that included emergent surgical decompression of the abdomen. Because the likely cause of the bacteremia was the compromised bowel, this was not considered a case of CLABSI.

CASE STUDY 6

An infant was born at 30 weeks with birth weight 1300 grams suffers a CLABSI with blood culture growing MSSA. This is the fourth CLABSI that has occurred in your 50-bed NICU in the past 3 months; the other infants had birth weight <1200 grams and had either a percutaneously inserted central catheter (PICC) or UVC in place at the time of infection. The other organisms isolated included CONS and Candida albicans. Your hospital infection

control officer publicly states that your NICU has a terrible rate of infection compared to other NICUs and places you in charge of creating an approach to CLABSI prevention.

EXERCISE 6

QUESTION

1. How should you proceed?
   a. Convene a committee of neonatologists to develop criteria to remove central lines sooner.
   b. Meet with the NICU nursing director to review daily CVL care, because the nurses perform all daily CVL care, including line and dressing changes.
   c. Do (a) and (b) but also work with the infection control officer to determine the baseline rates of infection in your NICU and benchmark those to national standards.
   d. Do (a), (b), and (c), but within a multidisciplinary committee you convene to review all aspects of CVL care. Review literature on best practices to prevent CLABSI and implement multiple reforms for CVL insertion, daily care, and removal.

ANSWER

1. **d.** In addition to the impact of LOS on VLBW mortality, these infections also result in increased short-term severity of illness, increased duration of NICU hospitalization, and increased risk of long-term neurodevelopmental impairment (Schlapbach et al., 2011; Stoll et al., 2004). The observed variation in LOS rates among centers, even when controlled for infant severity of illness, has prompted efforts to identify best practices to prevent LOS. If you are placed in charge of LOS-reduction efforts in the 21st century, there is significant literature to guide your approach to infection reduction, including specific practice recommendations from quality consortiums such as Vermont-Oxford Network (Kilbride, Powers, & Wirtshafter, 2003a and b), the California Perinatal Quality Care Collaborative (Bowles et al., 2008), from national organizations such as CDC (O'Grady, Alexander, & Burns, 2011) and IDSA (Beekmann et al., 2012), and from individual center experiences (Bizzarro et al., 2010). All of these organizations emphasize the importance of multidisciplinary approaches to infection reduction that both recognize the multiple clinical inputs into best practices, and the importance of multidisciplinary cooperation to mediate practice change. The basic tenets of NICU infection reduction are shown in Table 13-4, all of which support choice "d."

TABLE 13-4 Basic Components of NICU Infection Reduction

Category	Actions
General	Optimize hand hygiene practices
	Monitor compliance with all practice recommendations
Feeding practices	Guidelines for the initiation and advancement of enteral feeding of VLBW infants
	Support breast milk feeding for VLBW infants
Infusion practices	CDC-recommended practices for duration of TPN, intravenous fluid and medication infusions
Central line management	CVL insertion and daily line care checklists
	Guidelines for CVL necessity and removal
	Dedicated PICC placement teams
Disinfection and blood culture practices	Sterile skin preparation for blood culture, blood drawing, and peripheral IV placement
	Adequate volume of blood in culture bloods (minimum 1 mL in pediatric bottles)
Antibiotic stewardship	Guidelines for antibiotic initiation, choice and discontinuation
	Surveillance for colonization with antibiotic-resistant organisms
	Isolation and precautions for patients colonized or infected with antibiotic-resistant organisms
	Fluconazole prophylaxis targeted to high-risk infants
Infection accounting	Real-time data collection for central line days, culture results and antibiotic resistance patterns
	Communication with staff regarding CLABSI and overall LOS incidence
	Root cause analysis at time of LOS event

Preventative therapeutic approaches to VLBW infection have also been investigated. Multiple studies have been conducted using prophylactic administration of IVIG to prevent VLBW LOS. A metaanalysis of 19 trials revealed that although the use of IVIG to prevent LOS resulted in a 3% to 4% decrease in LOS, IVIG was not associated with a decrease in mortality or other serious outcomes and is generally not recommended (Ohlsson & Lacy, 2004). Recent trials of probiotic therapies and lactoferrin show promise in preventing both NEC and LOS, but neither are currently commercially available in the United States (Manzoni et al., 2009; Saiman, 2006). Administration of fluconazole prophylaxis to prevent *Candida* colonization and subsequent infection of high-risk infants is effective in reducing fungal LOS, with recent data supporting the safety of this practice (Healy, Campbell, Zaccaria, & Baker, 2008; Kaufman et al., 2001; Kaufman et al., 2011). However, fluconazole prophylaxis should only be considered in infants weighing <750 grams in a NICU with a high rate of fungal infections.

SUGGESTED READINGS

Alexander JM, Gilstrap LC, Cox SM, et al: Clinical chorioamnionitis and the prognosis for very low birth weight infants, *Obstet Gynecol* 91:725–729, 1998.

Alexander JM, McIntire DM, Leveno KJ: Chorioamnionitis and the prognosis for term infants, *Obstet Gynecol* 94:274–278, 1999.

Baker CJ, Barrett FF: Transmission of group B streptococci among parturient women and their neonates, *J Pediatr* 83:919–925, 1973.

Baker CJ, Kasper DL: Correlation of maternal antibody deficiency with susceptibility to neonatal group B streptococcal infection, *N Engl J Med* 294:753–756, 1976.

Beekmann SE, Diekema DJ, Huskins WC, et al: Infectious Diseases Society of America Emerging Infections Network. Diagnosing and reporting of central line-associated bloodstream infections, *Infect Control Hosp Epidemiol* 33(9):875–882, 2012.

Benenson S, Levin PD, Block C, et al: Continuous surveillance to reduce extended-spectrum β-lactamase *Klebsiella pneumoniae* colonization in the neonatal intensive care unit, *Neonatology* 103(2):155–160, 2013.

Benirschke K: Routes and types of infection in the fetus and the newborn, *Am J Dis Child* 99:714–721, 1960.

Benitz WE: Adjunct laboratory tests in the diagnosis of early-onset neonatal sepsis, *Clin Perinatol* 37:421–438, 2010.

Benitz WE, Gould JB, Druzin ML: Risk factors for early-onset group B streptococcal sepsis: Estimation of odds ratios by critical literature review, *Pediatrics* 103:e77, 1999.

Benitz WE, Han MY, Madan A, et al: Serial serum C-reactive protein levels in the diagnosis of neonatal infection, *Pediatrics* 102(4):e41, 1998.

Benjamin Jr DK, Stoll BJ, Gantz MG, et al: Neonatal candidiasis: epidemiology, risk factors, and clinical judgment, *Pediatrics* 126(4):e865–e873, 2010.

Bizzarro MJ, Dembry LM, Baltimore RS, et al: Changing patterns in neonatal *Escherichia coli* sepsis and ampicillin resistance in the era of intrapartum antibiotic prophylaxis, *Pediatrics* 121(4):689–696, 2008.

Bizzarro MJ, Raskind C, Baltimore RS, et al: Seventy-five years of neonatal sepsis at Yale: 1928-2003, *Pediatrics* 116:595–602, 2005.

Bizzarro MJ, Sabo B, Noonan M, et al: A quality improvement initiative to reduce central line-associated bloodstream infections in a neonatal intensive care unit, *Infect Control Hosp Epidemiol* 31(3):241–248, 2010.

Blanc WA: Pathways of fetal and early neonatal infection. Viral placentitis, bacterial and fungal chorioamnionitis, *J Pediatr* 59:473–496, 1961.

Bowles S, Pettit J, Mickas N, et al for the California Perinatal Quality Collaborative. Neonatal hospital-acquired infection prevention. Accessed June 20, 2013 at http://www.cpqcc.org/quality_improvement/qi_toolkits/hospital_acquired_infection_prevention_rev_march_2008.

Boyer KM, Gadzala CA, Burd LI, et al: Selective intrapartum chemoprophylaxis of neonatal group B streptococcal early-onset disease. I. epidemiologic rationale, *J Infect Dis* 148:795–801, 1983.

Boyer KM, Gadzala CA, Kelly PD, et al: Selective intrapartum chemoprophylaxis of neonatal Group B Streptococcal early-onset disease. III. Interruption of mother-to-infant transmission, *J Infect Dis* 148:810–816, 1983.

Boyer KM, Gotoff SP: Prevention of early-onset neonatal group B streptococcal disease with selective intrapartum chemoprophylaxis, *N Engl J Med* 314:1665–1669, 1986.

Brady MT, Polin RA: Prevention and management of infants with suspected or proven neonatal sepsis, *Pediatrics* 132(1):166–168, 2013.

Cantey JB, Sreeramoju P, Jaleel M, et al: Prompt control of an outbreak caused by extended-spectrum β-lactamase-producing *Klebsiella pneumoniae* in a neonatal intensive care unit, *J Pediatr* 163:672–679, 2013.

Centers for Disease Control and Prevention (CDC): *National healthcare safety newtwork device associated module: Central line–associated bloodstream infection (CLABSI) event,* 2012. Accessed July 15, 2013 at http://www.cdc.gov/nhsn/PDFs/pscManual/4PSC_CLABScurrent.pdf.

Centers for Disease Control and Prevention (CDC): Perinatal group B streptococcal disease after universal screening recommendations–United States, 2003-2005, *MMWR Morb Mortal Wkly Rep* 56:701–705, 2007.

Chiu CH, Michelow IC, Cronin J, Ringer SA, Ferris TG, Puopolo KM: Effectiveness of a guideline to reduce vancomycin use in the neonatal intensive care unit, *Pediatr Infect Dis J* 30(4):273–278, 2011.

Clark RH, Bloom BT, Spitzer AR, et al: Empiric use of ampicillin and cefotaxime, compared with ampicillin and gentamicin, for neonates at risk for sepsis is associated with an increased risk of neonatal death, *Pediatrics* 117:67–74, 2006.

Cohen-Wolkowiez M, Benjamin Jr DK, Capparelli E: Immunotherapy in neonatal sepsis: advances in treatment and prophylaxis, *Curr Opin Pediatr* 21(2):177–181, 2009.

Cohen-Wolkowiez M, Moran C, Benjamin DK, et al: Early and late onset sepsis in late preterm infants, *Pediatr Infect Dis J* 28:1052–1056, 2009.

Cotten CM, McDonald S, Stoll B, et al: The association of third-generation cephalosporin use and invasive candidiasis in extremely low birth-weight infants, *Pediatrics* 118:717–722, 2006.

Cotten CM, Taylor S, Stoll B, et al: Prolonged duration of initial empirical antibiotic treatment is associated with increased rates of necrotizing enterocolitis and death for extremely low birth weight infants, *Pediatrics* 123:58–66, 2009.

Downey LC, Smith PB, Benjamin Jr DK: Risk factors and prevention of late-onset sepsis in premature babies, *Early Hum Dev* 86(suppl 1):7–12, 2010.

Dutta S, Reddy R, Sheikh S, et al: Intrapartum antibiotics and risk factors for early onset sepsis, *Arch Dis Child Fetal Neonatal Ed* 95:F99–F103, 2010.

Escobar GJ, Li DK, Armstrong MA, et al: Neonatal sepsis workups in infants ≥2000 grams at birth: a population-based study, *Pediatrics* 106:256–263, 2000.

Fanaroff AA, Korones SB, Wright LL, et al: Incidence, presenting features, risk factors and significance of late-onset septicemia in very-low-birth-weight infants. The National Institute of Child Health and Human Development Neonatal Research Network, *Pediatr Infect Dis J* 17:593–598, 1998.

Feja KN, Wu F, Roberts K, et al: Risk factors for candidemia in critically ill infants: a matched case–control study, *J Pediatr* 147:156–161, 2005.

Fishman SG, Gelber SE: Evidence for the clinical management of chorioamnionitis, *Semin Fetal Neonatal Med* 17:46–50, 2012.

Franciosi RA, Knostman JD, Zimmerman RA: Group B streptococcal neonatal and infant infections, *J Pediatr* 82:707–718, 1973.

Graham III PL, Begg MD, Larson E, et al: Risk factors for late onset gram-negative sepsis in low birth weight infants hospitalized in the neonatal intensive care unit, *Pediatr Infect Dis J* 25(2):113–117, 2006.

Healy CM, Campbell JR, Zaccaria E, Baker CJ: Fluconazole prophylaxis in extremely low birth weight neonates reduces invasive candidiasis mortality rates without emergence of fluconazole-resistant *Candida* species, *Pediatrics* 121(4):703–710, 2008.

Hornik CP, Benjamin DK, Becker KC, et al: Use of the complete blood cell count in early-onset neonatal sepsis, *Pediatr Infect Dis J* 31(8):799–802, 2012.

Hornik CP, Benjamin DK, Becker KC, et al: Use of the complete blood cell count in late-onset neonatal sepsis, *Pediatr Infect Dis J* 31:803–807, 2012.

Hornik CP, Fort P, Clark RH, et al: Early and late onset sepsis in very-low-birth-weight infants from a large group of neonatal intensive care units, *Early Hum Dev* 88(suppl 2):S69–S74, 2012.

Hyde TB, Hilger TM, Reingold A, et al: Trends in incidence and antimicrobial resistance of early-onset sepsis: population-based surveillance in San Francisco and Atlanta, *Pediatrics* 110:690–695, 2002.

Hylander MA, Strobino DM, Dhanireddy R: Human milk feedings and infection among very low birth weight infants, *Pediatrics* 102(3):E38, 1998.

Jackson GL, Engle WD, Sendelbach DM, et al: Are complete blood cell counts useful in the evaluation of asymptomatic neonates exposed to suspected chorioamnionitis? *Pediatrics* 113:1173–1180, 2004.

Jackson GL, Rawiki P, Sendelbach D, et al: Hospital course and short-term outcomes of term and late preterm neonates following exposure to prolonged rupture of membranes and/or chorioamnionitis, *Pediatr Infect Dis J* 31(1):89–90, 2012.

Johnson CE, Whitwell JK, Pethe K, et al: Term newborns who are at risk for sepsis: are lumbar punctures necessary? *Pediatrics.* 99:e10–e14, 1997.

Kaufman D, Boyle R, Hazen KC, et al: Fluconazole prophylaxis against fungal colonization and infection in preterm infants, *N Engl J Med* 345(23):1660–1666, 2001.

Kaufman DA, Cuff AL, Wamstad JB, et al: Fluconazole prophylaxis in extremely low birth weight infants and neurodevelopmental outcomes and quality of life at 8 to 10 years of age, *J Pediatr* 158(5):759–765, 2011.

Kilbride HW, Powers R, Wirtschafter DD, et al: Evaluation and development of potentially better practices to prevent neonatal nosocomial bacteremia, *Pediatrics* 111(4 Pt 2):e504–e518, 2003.

Kilbride HW, Wirtschafter DD, Powers RJ, et al: Implementation of evidence-based potentially better practices to decrease nosocomial infections, *Pediatrics* 111(4 Pt 2):e519–e533, 2003.

Kuppala VS, Meinzen-Der J, Morrow AL, et al: Prolonged initial empirical antibiotic treatment is associated with adverse outcomes in premature infants, *J Pediatr* 159:720–725, 2011.

Lessa FC, Edwards JR, Fridkin SK, et al: Trends in incidence of late-onset methicillin-resistant Staphylococcus aureus infection in neonatal intensive care units: data from the National Nosocomial Infections Surveillance System, 1995-2004, *Pediatr Infect Dis J* 28(7):577–581, 2009.

Manroe BL, Weinberg AG, Rosenfeld CR, et al: The neonatal blood count in health and disease. I. Reference values for neutrophilic cells, *J Pediatr* 95:89–98, 1979.

Manzoni P, Decembrino L, Stolfi I, et al: Lactoferrin and prevention of late-onset sepsis in the pre-term neonates, *Early Hum Dev* 86(suppl 1):59–61, 2010.

Manzoni P, Rinaldi M, Cattani S, et al: Bovine lactoferrin supplementation for prevention of late-onset sepsis in very low-birth-weight neonates: a randomized trial, *JAMA* 302(13):1421–1428, 2009.

McCracken Jr GH: Group B streptococci: the new challenge in neonatal infections, *J Pediatr* 82:703–706, 1973.

Meyn LA, Moore DM, Hillier SL, et al: Association of sexual activity with colonization and vaginal acquisition of group B *Streptococcus* in nonpregnant women, *Am J Epidemiol* 155:949–957, 2002.

Moore MR, Schrag SJ, Schuchat A: Effects of intrapartum antimicrobial prophylaxis for prevention of group-B-streptococcal disease on the incidence and ecology of early-onset neonatal sepsis, *Lancet Infect Dis* 3(4):201–213, 2003.

Mukhopadhyay S, Eichenwald EC, Puopolo KM: Impact of neonatal sepsis evaluation on asymptomatic infants born at ≥35 weeks gestation, *J Perinatol* 33(3):198–205, 2011.

Newman TB, Puopolo KM, Wi S, et al: Interpreting complete blood counts soon after birth in newborns at risk for sepsis, *Pediatrics* 126:903–909, 2010.

NIS Collaborative Group, Brocklehurst P, Farrell B, King A, Juszczak E, Darlow B, et al: Treatment of neonatal sepsis with intravenous immune globulin, *N Engl J Med* 365(13):1201–1211, 2011.

O'Grady NP, Alexander M, Burns LA, et al: *Guidelines for the prevention of intravascular catheter-related infections,* 2011. Accessed July 15, 2013 at http://www.cdc.gov/hicpac/pdf/guidelines/bsi-guidelines-2011.pdf.

Ohlsson A, Lacy J: Intravenous immunoglobulin for suspected or subsequently proven infection in neonates, *Cochrane Database Syst Rev* (3):CD001239, 2010.

Ohlsson A, Lacy JB: Intravenous immunoglobulin for preventing infection in preterm and/or low-birth-weight infants, *Cochrane Database Syst Rev* (1):CD000361, 2004.

Phares CR, Lynfield R, Farley MM, et al: Epidemiology of invasive group B streptococcal disease in the United States, 1999-2005, *JAMA* 299:2056–2065, 2008.

Puopolo KM, Draper D, Wi S, et al: Estimating the probability of neonatal early-onset infection on the basis of maternal risk factors, *Pediatrics* 128:e1155–e1163, 2011.

Puopolo KM, Eichenwald EC: No change in the incidence of ampicillin-resistant, neonatal, early-onset sepsis over 18 years, *Pediatrics* 125:e1031–e1038, 2010.

Puopolo KM, Madoff LC, Eichenwald EC: Early-onset group B streptococcal disease in the era of maternal screening, *Pediatrics* 115:1240–1246, 2005.

Saiman L: Strategies for prevention of nosocomial sepsis in the neonatal intensive care unit, *Curr Opin Pediatr* 18(2):101–106, 2006.

Sarkar S, Bhagat I, Hieber S, et al: Can neutrophil responses in very-low-birth-weight infants predict the organisms responsible for late-onset bacterial or fungal sepsis? *J Perinatol* 26:501–505, 2006.

Schlapbach LJ, Aebischer M, Adams M, et al: Impact of sepsis on neurodevelopmental outcome in a Swiss National Cohort of extremely premature babies, *Pediatrics* 128:e348–e357, 2011.

Schmutz N, Henry E, Jopling J, et al: Expected ranges for blood neutrophil concentrations of neonates: the Manroe and Mouzinho charts revisited, *J Perinatol* 28:275–281, 2008.

Schrag S, Gorwitz R, Fultz-Butts K, Schuchat A: Prevention of perinatal group B streptococcal disease. Revised guidelines from CDC, *MMWR Recomm Rep* 51(RR-11):1–22, 2002.

Schrag SJ, Hadler JL, Arnold KE, et al: Risk factors for invasive, early-onset *Escherichia coli* infections in the era of widespread intrapartum antibiotic use, *Pediatrics* 118:570–576, 2006.

Schuchat A, Oxtoby M, Cochi S, et al: Population-based risk factors for neonatal group B streptococcal disease: results of a cohort study in metropolitan Atlanta, *J Infect Dis* 162:672–677, 1990.

Schuchat A, Zywicki SS, Dinsmoor MJ, et al: Risk factors and opportunities for prevention of early-onset neonatal sepsis: a multicenter case-control study, *Pediatrics* 105:21–26, 2000.

Stoll BJ, Hansen N, Fanaroff AA, et al: Changes in pathogens causing early-onset sepsis in very-low-birth-weight infants, *N Engl J Med* 347:240–247, 2002.

Stoll BJ, Hansen N, Fanaroff AA, et al: Late-onset sepsis in very low birth weight neonates: the experience of the NICHD Neonatal Research Network, *Pediatrics* 110:285–291, 2002.

Stoll BJ, Hansen N, Fanaroff AA, et al: To tap or not to tap: high likelihood of meningitis without sepsis among very low birth weight infants, *Pediatrics* 113(5):1181–1186, 2004.

Stoll BJ, Hansen NI, Adams-Chapman I, et al: Neurodevelopmental and growth impairment among extremely low-birth-weight babies with neonatal infection, *JAMA* 292:2357–2365, 2004.

Stoll BJ, Hansen NI, Bell EF, et al: Neonatal outcomes of extremely preterm infants from the NICHD Neonatal Research Network, *Pediatrics* 126:443–456, 2010.

Stoll BJ, Hansen NI, Higgins RD, et al: Very low birth weight preterm infants with early onset neonatal sepsis: the predominance of gram-negative infections continues in the National Institute of Child Health and Human Development Neonatal Research Network, 2002-2003, *Pediatr Infect Dis J* 24:635–639, 2005.

Stoll BJ, Hansen NI, Sánchez PJ, et al: Early onset neonatal sepsis: the burden of Group B streptococcal and *E. coli* continues, *Pediatrics* 127:817–826, 2011.

Van Dyke MK, Phares CR, Lynfield R, et al: Evaluation of universal antenatal screening for group B, *Streptococcus. N Engl J Med* 360:2626–2636, 2009.

Vanaja N, Alexander VN, Northrup V, et al: Antibiotic exposure in the newborn intensive care unit and the risk of necrotizing enterocolitis, *J Pediatr* 159:392–397, 2011.

Verani JR, McGee L, Schrag SJ: Division of Bacterial Diseases, National Center for Immunization and Respiratory Diseases, Centers for Disease Control and Prevention. Prevention of perinatal group B streptococcal disease—revised guidelines from CDC, *MMWR Recomm Rep* 2010(59):1–36, 2010.

Weston EY, Pondo T, Lewis MM, et al: The burden of invasive early-onset neonatal sepsis in the United States, 2005-2008, *Pediatr Infect Dis J* 30:937–941, 2011.

Wynn JL, Levy O: Role of innate host defenses in susceptibility to early onset neonatal sepsis, *Clin Perinatol* 37:307–377, 2010.

Yancey MK, Schuchat A, Brown LK, et al: The accuracy of late antenatal screening cultures in predicting genital group B streptococcal colonization at delivery, *Obstet Gynecol* 88:811–815, 1996.

CHAPTER 14

PATENT DUCTUS ARTERIOSUS

William E. Benitz, MD

While the fetus remains *in utero*, the ductus arteriosus is an essential component of the circulation, permitting blood to flow right-to-left from the pulmonary artery to the descending aorta, bypassing the fluid-filled lungs and returning to the placenta for gas exchange. At birth, the low resistance placental circulation is removed and pulmonary vascular resistance rapidly decreases, coincident with aeration of the lungs, resulting in reversal of ductal flow, which quickly becomes predominantly left-to-right, from the descending aorta into the pulmonary artery and onward to the lungs. Pulmonary blood flow therefore exceeds net systemic cardiac output until after the ductus closes. In term babies, the ductus normally constricts and becomes functionally occluded by the fourth postnatal day. If the ductus does not close, hemodynamic effects of a persistent left-to-right ductal shunt may become pathologic, potentially requiring active management. Persistent ductal patency for more than a few days in a term infant is usually associated with another significant underlying pathology, such as a syndromic condition or congenital heart disease, and will almost always require medical intervention. In preterm infants, however, closure of the ductus is often substantially delayed and in some instances may not occur at all. Preterm infants with prolonged ductal patency have an increased risk for numerous adverse outcomes, but the best strategies for evaluation and treatment may not be known. Consequently, these infants often present very difficult management dilemmas. The case studies presented in this chapter will present some of these challenges and suggest strategies for addressing them.

EPIDEMIOLOGY

CASE STUDY 1

An 840-gram infant was delivered vaginally at 27 weeks' gestation following spontaneous onset of preterm labor at 25 weeks. Her mother had been treated with indomethacin for tocolysis and

magnesium sulfate for fetal neuroprotection. She had received two doses of betamethasone more than 24 hours prior to delivery. The baby was vigorous at birth and responded well to support with continuous positive airway pressure by nasal mask and supplemental oxygen at an FiO$_2$ of 0.35.

EXERCISE 1

QUESTIONS

1. Which of the following most accurately reflects the probability that this infant will have a patent ductus arteriosus (PDA) at 7 days of age, in the absence of interventions intended to close the ductus?
   a. 10%
   b. 20%
   c. 33%
   d. 67%
   e. 90%

2. Which of the following features of this baby's perinatal history are associated with an increased risk of prolonged ductal patency?
   a. Estimated gestational age (EGA) <28 weeks
   b. Birth weight <1000 grams
   c. Prenatal exposure to indomethacin
   d. Prenatal exposure to magnesium sulfate
   e. Treatment with antenatal steroids

ANSWERS

1. **d.**

2. **All except e.**
   In normal infants born after 36 weeks' gestation, the ductus constricts and becomes functionally closed in most by 72 hours and in all by 96 hours of age (Figure 14-1) (Gentile, 1981). Even within this group of late-preterm and term infants, the timing of ductal closure is related to maturity, with all infants >40 weeks' gestation but only 50% and 80% of those born at 36 to 38 or 38 to 40 weeks, respectively, achieving closure by 40 hours of age. Among preterm infants, rates of ductal patency and the length of the delay in achieving ductal closure progressively increase with decreasing birth

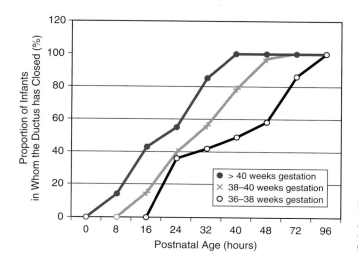

FIGURE 14-1 ■ Timing of ductal closure in late preterm and term infants. (From Gentile R, Stevenson G, Dooley T, et al: Pulsed Doppler echocardiographic determination of time of ductal closure in normal newborn infants, *J Pediatr* 98:443-448, 1981.)

TABLE 14-1   **Timing of Spontaneous Closure of the Ductus Arteriosus**

Patient Group	Percentage of Infants with Closed Ductus		
	By Day 4	By Day 7	By Discharge
EGA >38 weeks	100	100	100
EGA 30-37 weeks	90	98	98
EGA 27-28 weeks	22	36	NA
EGA 25-26 weeks	20	32	NA
EGA 24 weeks	8	13	NA
BW 1000-1500 g	35	67	94
BW <1000 g	21	34	NA

BW, Birth weight; *EGA*, estimated gestational age.
Adapted from Clyman RI, Couto J, Murphy GM: Patent ductus arteriosus: are current neonatal treatment options better or worse than no treatment at all? Semin Perinatol 36:123-129, 2012.

weight or maturity (Table 14-1). Because two out of three infants born at <1000 grams still have a PDA on Day 7 (Table 14-1), the correct answer to question 1 is "d" (67%).

Early observations suggested that spontaneous ductal closure could nearly always be expected given sufficient time, but this sometimes took several months (Perloff, 1971). However, changes in practice—including widespread use of treatments to close the ductus, antenatal steroids to induce lung maturity, exogenous surfactant to ameliorate respiratory distress syndrome (RDS), better strategies for respiratory support, and shifting demographics with greatly increased survival rates among very low birth weight (VLBW) and extremely low birth weight (ELBW) infants—have made application of those observations to current practice untenable. Recent data show that

the ductus usually closes without treatment in preterm infants who are >28 weeks' gestation (73%) (Koch, 2006), >1000 grams at birth (94%) (Nemerofsky, 2008), or do not have RDS (97%) (Reller, 1993). Case series reporting outcomes for less mature, smaller infants with RDS are nearly impossible to interpret because of nearly universal use of therapies to achieve ductal closure. In a cohort of infants <31 weeks' gestation who were in the placebo arm of a randomized clinical trial, ductal closure occurred in 60% of infants by 3 days of age (Van Overmeire, 2004) and in a cohort of infants 26 to 31 weeks' gestation who required assisted ventilation and had echocardiographic confirmation of PDA on Day 3 of life, ductal closure occurred by 9 days of age in 78% of infants (Van Overmeire, 2001). Half of the 500- to 999-gram infants assigned to the placebo arm of the Trial of Indomethacin Prophylaxis in Preterms (TIPP) never developed signs of a hemodynamically significant PDA (Schmidt, 2001). Observational data from preterm infants <1000 grams with a persistent PDA at hospital discharge suggest that the PDA will close in about 75% of those (Jhaveri, 2010) by the end of the first year. Although the evidence is fragmentary, these data are sufficient to demonstrate that spontaneous closure of the ductus should be expected in many, if not most, preterm infants.

A number of perinatal factors, in addition to prematurity and low birth weight, influence the risk of prolonged ductal patency. PDA is more common among infants who are small for gestational age, exposed to indomethacin for tocolysis before delivery, or given magnesium sulfate for neuroprotection (Katayama, 2011), and less frequent after antenatal administration of glucocorticoids. The correct answer to Question 2 is therefore "All except e,"

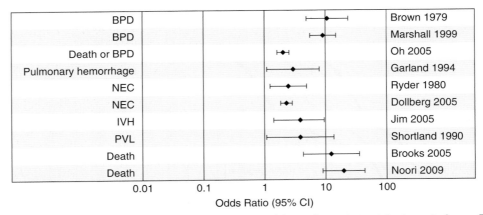

FIGURE 14-2 ■ **Odds ratios for adverse outcomes associated with persistent patent ductus arteriosus.** Black diamonds represent the point estimates for each odds ratio and the error bars represent the 95% confidence interval for those estimates. None of these confidence intervals include 1, so all outcomes are statistically more likely to occur in preterm infants with persistent PDA ($P < 0.05$). Values for each odds ratio point estimate are provided in the text. (Data from suggested readings: Brooks, 2005; Brown, 1979; Dollberg, 2005; Garland, 1994; Jim, 2005; Marshall, 1999; Noori, 2012; Oh, 2005; Ryder, 1980; and Shortland, 1990.)

because that item (antenatal steroid exposure) is associated with a *lower* risk of PDA. A strong relationship between PDA and RDS has been recognized for many years. Although the causal nature of this association remains uncertain, PDA is consequently more common among infants who require ventilatory assistance or exogenous surfactant. This infant's requirement for support with positive airway pressure and supplemental oxygen, presumably owing to RDS, are an additional risk factor for PDA. The spontaneous onset of preterm labor and failure of tocolytic therapy may be signs of an intrauterine bacterial infection, another factor that would predispose to persistent PDA (Dessardo, 2012).

EXERCISE 2

QUESTION

1. At 7 days of age, a large PDA is documented by echocardiography. Which of the following conditions are associated with persistent patency of the ductus arteriosus at age 7 days?
   a. Pulmonary hemorrhage
   b. Bronchopulmonary dysplasia
   c. Necrotizing enterocolitis
   d. Prolonged requirement for respiratory support
   e. Intraventricular hemorrhage
   f. Death

ANSWER

1. **All except a.**
   Delayed closure of the ductus arteriosus was first recognized more than 50 years ago as

a common correlate of more severe respiratory distress in premature infants. It has subsequently been linked to numerous adverse outcomes, including prolonged ventilation, bronchopulmonary dysplasia (BPD), necrotizing enterocolitis (NEC), impaired renal function, intraventricular hemorrhage (IVH), periventricular leukomalacia (PVL), cerebral palsy, and death (Benitz, 2010). These complications are often attributed to a large left-to-right ductal shunt, resulting in excessive pulmonary perfusion and systemic organ ischemia, but the causal nature of these associations remains to be determined. Early, severe pulmonary hemorrhage is associated with ductal patency at 12 to 18 hours of age (Garland, 1994), but later pulmonary hemorrhage (after the first week) is not related to persistent ductal patency.

The strength of associations between PDA and adverse outcomes are quite impressive (Figure 14-2). One study of infants seen at two Boston hospitals in 1978 demonstrated that PDA increased the odds of BPD more than 10-fold (OR 10.7) (Brown, 1979). A population-based study of preterm infants in North Carolina in 1994 found an odds ratio for BPD of 9.0 (Marshall, 1999), and a multicenter trial conducted between 1999 and 2001 reported an odds ratio for death or BPD of 2.0 (Oh, 2005). Data collected at two Boston hospitals from 1989 to 1992 revealed that ductal patency at 12 to 18 hours of age was associated with an odds ratio for early, severe pulmonary hemorrhage of 3.0 (Garland, 1994). A multicenter study of NEC from the late 1970s demonstrated an odds ratio of 2.5 (Ryder, 1980), and an Israeli national analysis of NEC cases from the late 1990s found an odds ratio of 2.3 (Dollberg, 2005). The odds ratios for IVH (Jim, 2005) and that for periventricular leukomalacia (Shortland, 1990) have both been estimated to be 3.9. Infants in whom the ductus remains open despite treatment with indomethacin are much more likely to die before hospital discharge than those whose ductus closes without treatment. In data from a single center in Western Australia, persistent PDA after treatment was associated with an odds ratio for neonatal death of 12.3 (versus infants with spontaneous closure); after adjustment for gestational age and Clinical Risk Index for Babies (CRIB) score, the adjusted odds ratio was still 4.0 (95% CI 1.1 to 14.5) (Brooks, 2005). A similar analysis from Oklahoma found an unadjusted odds ratio of 19.3; adjustment for perinatal factors, level of maturity, disease severity, and morbid pathologies resulted in an adjusted odds ratio of 16.8 (95% CI 6.1 to 46.6) (Noori, 2009). Confidence intervals for these odds ratios are shown in Figure 14-2; all are statistically significant. Despite the magnitude of these associations, they do not prove a causal role for persistent ductal patency in production of those adverse outcomes. Nonetheless, these results (and others like them) have provided great impetus for the hypothesis that elimination of ductal patency might substantially improve long-term outcomes for preterm infants.

CLINICAL PRESENTATION AND DIAGNOSTIC EVALUATION

CASE STUDY 1 (continued)

EXERCISE 3

QUESTIONS

1. Which of the following physical findings on the seventh day after birth might suggest the diagnosis of persistent ductal patency?
   a. Bounding radial arterial pulses
   b. Palpable pulses in the palms of the hands
   c. Pulsus paradoxus
   d. Hyperdynamic precordium
   e. Systolic murmur
   f. To-and-fro murmur in systole and diastole
   g. Bilateral rales
   h. Hepatomegaly
   i. Cool extremities
   j. Intermittent cyanotic episodes
   k. Absent bowel sounds

2. Which of the following radiographic findings on the seventh day after birth might suggest the presence of a PDA?
   a. Cortical hyperostosis of long bones
   b. Cardiomegaly
   c. Increased lung lucency
   d. Prominent pulmonary vascular markings
   e. Pulmonary edema with a small heart
   f. Elevation of the left hemidiaphragm

3. Which of the following clinical conditions during the second week after birth might suggest the presence of a PDA?
   a. Oliguria with increasing blood urea nitrogen (BUN) levels
   b. Feeding intolerance
   c. Central apnea episodes
   d. Persistent jaundice
   e. Inability to wean respiratory support

ANSWERS

1. **a**, **b**, **d**, **e**, **g**, and **h**.

2. **b** and **d**.

3. **a** and **e**.

Persistent ductal patency in a preterm infant may become evident through findings on physical examination or because of signs of circulatory or respiratory impairment. A persistent PDA may first become apparent from development of the characteristic coarse systolic murmur heard best along the left sternal border. However, many infants with a large PDA may have no audible murmur, despite having a large left-to-right shunt and substantial pulmonary overcirculation. The murmur may become audible or increase in intensity only as the ductus constricts, resulting in higher velocity and more turbulent shunt flow. The increased left ventricular stroke volume imposed by a large left-to-right shunt may produce a prominent precordial impulse or hyperactive precordium. Arterial pulses often are prominent, bounding, or palpable where they normally are not (e.g., in the palms). Reduced systemic diastolic pressures with widened pulse pressures are common in preterm infants >1000 grams, but lower systolic, diastolic, and mean arterial pressures without an increased pulse pressure are more typical in those <1000 grams. Congestive heart failure may be evident as rales, hepatomegaly, or peripheral edema. These findings are nonspecific, insensitive, and do not reliably predict echocardiography results (Skelton, 1994). Similar physical findings may be present in infants with other circulatory disorders, such as aortopulmonary window, hemitruncus, or arteriovenous malformations, or in hyperdynamic conditions, such as anemia, fever, or sepsis. Choices "a," "b," "d," "e," "g," and "h" are correct answers to Question 1.

Pulsus paradoxus, or phasic decreases in systolic blood pressure in synchrony with respiration, should not accompany PDA. If that finding is observed in an infant with a large heart and signs of congestive heart failure, pericardial effusion and tamponade should be considered. The continuous "machinery" or "to-and-fro" murmur typical of PDA in older children is rarely found in neonates. The "runoff" effect of left-to-right ductal shunting into the pulmonary circulation is very rarely sufficient to result in overt signs of compromised systemic perfusion, such as cool extremities or lactic acidemia; such findings should suggest other causes of compromised systemic cardiac output, such as hypovolemia or sepsis. Cyanotic episodes associated with a PDA would imply periods of right-to-left shunting, which should not occur unless there is pulmonary edema or another pathology, such as pulmonary hypertension or right ventricular outflow tract obstruction. Bowel ischemia is a potential adverse effect of the "ductal steal," but experience has shown that feedings can be continued despite ductal patency (Jhaveri, 2010), so loss of bowel sounds would not be expected as a sign of PDA. Choices "c," "f," "i," "j," and "k" are therefore not correct answers to Question 1.

PDA is frequently suspected only because excessive pulmonary blood flow leads to pulmonary edema, which results in increasing oxygen requirement, decreasing lung compliance, or inability to wean the infant from supplemental oxygen, distending airway pressure, or positive pressure ventilation. Systemic hemodynamic effects include hepatomegaly and peripheral edema, as well as signs of suboptimal organ perfusion. In particular, a large ductal shunt may compromise renal blood flow, resulting in oliguria and chemical signs of prerenal renal failure (rising BUN without a proportionate increase in serum creatinine). Because of these effects, "b" and "d" are correct answers to Question 2 and "a" and "e" are correct answers to Question 3.

Cortical hyperostosis may result from prolonged administration of prostaglandin E_1 (alprostadil) to maintain ductal patency of the ductus in infants with ductus-dependent congenital heart disease, but does not result from ductal patency itself. Excessive pulmonary blood flow may lead to decreased, but not increased, radiolucency of the lungs. A small heart in an infant with pulmonary edema should suggest capillary leak or pulmonary venous or lymphatic obstruction; PDA is unlikely to be the cause of the lung findings. Paralysis of the left hemidiaphragm may follow surgical ligation of the ductus, but is rarely associated with a PDA alone. Although feeding intolerance has been proposed as a criterion for assessment of the hemodynamic significance of PDA (Noori, 2012), a moderate PDA does not cause feeding intolerance or require discontinuation of feeding, as noted above. Feeding intolerance in an infant with PDA suggests a severe ductal steal resulting in either significant bowel ischemia or severe congestive heart failure with bowel edema; in either case, other clinical signs would be prominent. A PDA does not affect central nervous system or hepatic function, so central apnea or prolonged jaundice would not be expected associations. Items "a," "c," "e," and "f" are therefore not correct answers to Question 2, and "b", "c", and "d" are not correct answers to Question 3.

CASE STUDY 2

Between 7 and 10 days of age, the infant described in Case Study 1 continues to require support with nasal continuous positive airway pressure (NCPAP) and has a gradually increasing oxygen requirement. Her heart rate is 175 beats per minute and blood pressure is 35/18 (mean 26). She has a soft systolic murmur, full pulses, and her liver edge is palpable 2 cm below the right costal margin.

EXERCISE 4

QUESTIONS

1. Which of the following diagnostic studies will be most useful in determining whether the clinical findings in this infant are associated with presence of a PDA?
   a. Chest radiograph
   b. Color Doppler echocardiography
   c. Serum level of B-type natriuretic peptide (BNP)
   d. Serum level of troponin T
   e. Magnetic resonance angiography

2. Which of the above diagnostic studies might be useful in assessment of the severity of the hemodynamic derangements resulting from a large left-to-right PDA shunt?

ANSWERS

1. **b.**

2. **All except e.**

The definitive diagnostic test for PDA is color Doppler echocardiography, which permits direct visualization of ductal anatomy, as shown in Figure 14-3, measurement of the ductal diameter, and assessment of the direction of ductal blood flow throughout the cardiac cycle. The correct answer to Question 1 is clearly "b." If the ductus is found to be patent, echocardiography may also provide useful information about its hemodynamic effects. Large shunts are associated with a ratio of left atrial to aortic root dimensions (LA:Ao ratio) >2:1; ductal diameter >3.0 mm; dilation of the left ventricle; and reduced or reversed diastolic flow in the descending aorta or in the cerebral, renal, or mesenteric arteries. Left ventricular dysfunction may be associated with a high velocity mitral regurgitant jet (>2.0 m/s), an increased ratio of early passive to late atrial filling (E/A >1.5), or shortening of the left ventricular isovolumic relaxation time (IVRT <40 ms). Such measurements may have utility as indicators of hemodynamic significance of a PDA (McNamara, 2007), particularly as components of a composite scoring system, but no individual measurement appears to be highly reliable. High composite scores incorporating nine echocardiographic measurements acquired prior to treatment of PDA appear to be predictive of chronic lung disease (Sehgal, 2013). The relationship of these measurements, or scores based on them, to other adverse outcomes potentially attributable to ductal shunting remains to be established. Nonetheless, extension of echocardiography to hemodynamic

assessment—rather than only diagnosis—of PDA promises to provide better constructs for selection of subjects for clinical trials, and eventually more rational criteria for treatment to close a problematic ductus.

Serum biomarkers may also be useful in assessment of hemodynamic significance, guiding treatment, or prediction of sequelae of PDA. Levels of B-type natriuretic peptide (BNP) or NT-pro-BNP (an inactive byproduct of BNP synthesis) are elevated in the plasma of infants with PDA (Choi, 2005; Flynn, 2005), decrease after PDA closure (El-Khuffash, 2007; Sanjeev, 2005), and correlate with echocardiographic findings (El-Khuffash, 2007; Flynn, 2005; Sanjeev, 2005). Discontinuation of indomethacin as soon as BNP levels decreased in response to treatment reduced the number of doses given, but did not change other outcomes, suggesting a role in assessment of the response to or guiding duration of treatment (Attridge, 2009). Both severe IVH (grade III or IV) and worse neurodevelopmental outcomes are more frequent in preterm infants (<32 weeks' gestation) with PDA who had elevated levels of NT-pro-BNP at 48 hours of age (El-Khuffash, 2007; El-Khuffash, 2011). Elevated plasma troponin T levels at 48 hours of age correlate with echocardiographic findings (presence of PDA and shunt estimates) (El-Khuffash, 2008b), death or grade II-IV IVH (El-Khuffash, 2008a), and increased risk for poor neurodevelopmental outcome at 2 years of age (El-Khuffash, 2011). Although these observations suggest that selection of infants based on these biomarkers may lead to improved outcomes, that hypothesis has not been tested. Therefore, these analytes are correct answers to Question 2, but not Question 1.

PDA may be associated with cardiomegaly, increased pulmonary vascular markings, or signs of pulmonary edema on chest radiographs. These signs are nonspecific and insensitive (Davis, 1995). While conventional radiographs may suggest the presence of PDA, they cannot substitute for echocardiography for confirmation of the diagnosis. Heart size and the severity of pulmonary edema may help in assessment of hemodynamic significance. Choice "a" is therefore not correct for Question 1, but is correct for Question 2. Magnetic resonance angiography can provide excellent images of the ductus, but does not provide simultaneous functional information. Although it could be used to confirm the diagnosis, bedside echocardiography remains the preferred method. Choice "e" is not a correct answer for either Question 1 or 2.

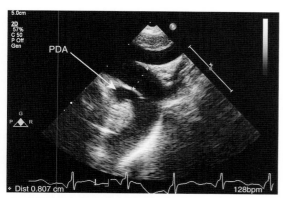

FIGURE 14-3 ■ Echocardiographic image patent ductus arteriosus *(arrow)* entering the descending aorta, just distal to the aortic arch (indicated by measurement markers) and the left subclavian artery takeoff. (From Emani SM: Patent ductus arteriosus, coarctation of the aorta, and vascular rings. In Sellke FW, Del Nido PJ, Swanson SJ, editors: *Sabiston and Spencer surgery of the chest*, ed 8, Philadelphia, PA, 2010, Saunders, pp 1781-1795.)

PROPHYLAXIS

CASE STUDY 3

A 980-gram baby was born at 31 weeks' gestation after a pregnancy complicated by chronic hypertension and rapidly worsening preeclampsia. His mother received magnesium sulfate for her preeclampsia, but had to be delivered urgently less than 12 hours after a single dose of betamethasone. He was hypotonic with poor respiratory effort, and required intubation and initiation of positive pressure ventilation in the delivery room. After the initial dose of surfactant, he stabilized on moderate ventilator settings (PIP of 16 cm H_2O, PEEP of 5 cm H_2O, rate 36 breaths per minute, and FiO_2 of 0.45) with the following blood gases: pH of 7.21, PaO_2 of 63 mmHg, $PaCO_2$ of 57 mmHg, HCO_3 of 22 mEq/L. A chest radiograph demonstrated bilateral diffuse granular lung densities and air bronchograms. A serum magnesium level was 4.5 mEq/L. Other blood chemistries and hematologic findings were unremarkable.

EXERCISE 5

QUESTIONS

1. Which of the following clinical outcomes would be *less* likely to occur after ligation of the ductus arteriosus on the day of birth?
   a. Early, severe pulmonary hemorrhage
   b. Severe IVH
   c. NEC
   d. BPD
   e. Neurodevelopmental impairment at age 18 to 22 months
   f. Ductal ligation
   g. Death

2. Which of the same clinical outcomes would be *less* likely to occur after treatment of this infant with indomethacin, beginning within 6 hours after birth?

3. Which of the same clinical outcomes would be *less* likely to occur after treatment of this infant with ibuprofen beginning within 6 hours after birth?

ANSWERS

1. **c, f.**

2. **a, b, f.**

3. **f.**

If persistent ductal patency is so common and the associated morbidities so severe, as

described, it seems logical that intervening to close the ductus as soon as possible might be beneficial. This hypothesis has been tested extensively. In a single, small (84 subjects) trial of prophylactic ligation, infants who weighed <1000 grams at birth were randomized to either surgical ligation on the first day after birth or expectant management (Cassady, 1989). Not surprisingly, fewer babies in the early ligation group required subsequent surgical ligation, but there were no effects on rates of mortality, chronic lung disease (as defined at that time), IVH, severe (> grade 2) IVH, or retinopathy of prematurity (ROP). Significantly fewer infants in the early ligation group developed NEC (OR 0.20, 95% CI 0.06 to 0.68), possibly because initiation of feedings was significantly delayed in the surgical group. Unfortunately, that result has not been replicated in studies of ductal closure by other methods. Effects on other listed outcomes were not reported. A more recent reanalysis of data from that trial found an increased risk of BPD, defined as a need for supplemental oxygen at 36 weeks' postmenstrual age, in the early ductal ligation group (OR 3.8, 95% CI 1.1 to 12.5) (Clyman, 2009). The answers to Question 1, above, are therefore "c" and, of course, "f" (although it remains uncertain whether a reduction in the risk of NEC, answer "c", is a direct effect of ductal closure or is even reproducible).

Prophylaxis with indomethacin is the most extensively studied approach to accelerating closure of the ductus. In this strategy, treatment with indomethacin is initiated in all qualifying preterm infants soon after birth without waiting for confirmation of prolonged ductal patency. Two small trials of enterally administered indomethacin demonstrated efficacy in ductal closure, but no effects on mortality, chronic lung disease, IVH, or ROP. Twenty randomized controlled trials of intravenous indomethacin enrolled nearly 3000 subjects who were randomized to either early treatment with intravenous indomethacin or placebo, typically beginning within the first 6 to 12 hours after birth. Although rate and/or severity of IVH—not PDA—was the primary outcome for about half of these trials, all reported rates of persistent PDA, as well as several other outcomes. The results of these trials are summarized in Figure 14-4. Although indomethacin prophylaxis is associated with a substantial reduction in the rate of persistent PDA (OR 0.27, 95% CI 0.23 to 0.32), there was no improvement in other outcomes, with the exception of lower rates of IVH, IVH > grade 2, and PVL. Despite lower rates of these neurosonographic findings, long-term neurodevelopmental

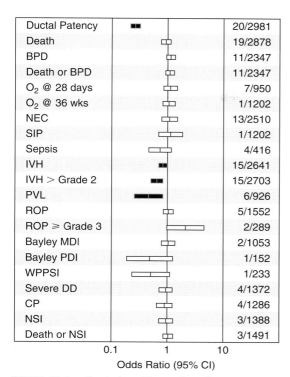

Ductal Patency		20/2981
Death		19/2878
BPD		11/2347
Death or BPD		11/2347
O$_2$ @ 28 days		7/950
O$_2$ @ 36 wks		1/1202
NEC		13/2510
SIP		1/1202
Sepsis		4/416
IVH		15/2641
IVH > Grade 2		15/2703
PVL		6/926
ROP		5/1552
ROP ⩾ Grade 3		2/289
Bayley MDI		2/1053
Bayley PDI		1/152
WPPSI		1/233
Severe DD		4/1372
CP		4/1286
NSI		3/1388
Death or NSI		3/1491

0.1   1   10

Odds Ratio (95% CI)

FIGURE 14-4 ■ **Pooled odds ratios for outcomes observed in randomized controlled trials of indomethacin prophylaxis.** Bars represent the 95% confidence intervals for each outcome; the line at the midpoint of each bar denotes the odds ratio (OR) point estimate. OR significantly different from 1 are indicated by black bars (two-tailed P < 0.05). The number of trials (N) and total included subjects (n) for each outcome are shown on the right (N/n). *BPD,* Bronchopulmonary dysplasia; *CLD,* chronic lung disease; *NEC,* necrotizing enterocolitis; *SIP,* spontaneous intestinal perforation; *IVH,* intraventricular hemorrhage; *PVL,* periventricular leukomalacia; *ROP,* retinopathy of prematurity; *MDI,* Mental Development Index; *PDI,* Psychomotor Development Index; *CP,* cerebral palsy. (Adapted from Benitz WE. Treatment of persistent patent ductus arteriosus in preterm infants: time to accept the null hypothesis? *J Perinatol* 30:241-252, 2010.)

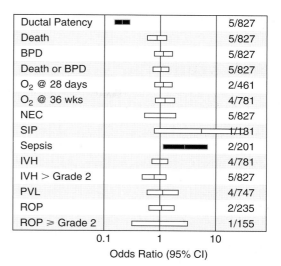

Ductal Patency		5/827
Death		5/827
BPD		5/827
Death or BPD		5/827
O$_2$ @ 28 days		2/461
O$_2$ @ 36 wks		4/781
NEC		5/827
SIP		1/181
Sepsis		2/201
IVH		4/781
IVH > Grade 2		5/827
PVL		4/747
ROP		2/235
ROP ⩾ Grade 2		1/155

0.1   1   10

Odds Ratio (95% CI)

FIGURE 14-5 ■ **Pooled odds ratios for outcomes observed in randomized controlled trials of ibuprofen prophylaxis.** Symbols and abbreviations are as indicated for Figure 14-4. (Adapted from Benitz WE: Treatment of persistent patent ductus arteriosus in preterm infants: time to accept the null hypothesis? *J Perinatol* 30:241-252, 2010.)

outcomes were not improved. The confidence intervals for effects on the most important long-term outcomes (death, BPD, NEC, ROP, severe developmental delay, CP, and neurosensory impairment) are narrow and were not statistically different from "no effect." Data regarding effects on pulmonary hemorrhage are not included in Figure 14-4, because the criteria for that diagnosis do not appear to be consistent among the five trials for which that outcome is reported (Alfaleh, 2008; Bada, 1989; Bandstra, 1988; Couser, 1996; Domanico, 1994). Collectively, these trials did not identify a significant effect on rates of pulmonary hemorrhage over the hospital course, but a detailed analysis

(Alfaleh, 2008) demonstrated reduction in the frequency of early, severe pulmonary hemorrhage after indomethacin prophylaxis. That effect was not associated with a reduction in bronchopulmonary dysplasia or other long-term morbidities. The correct answers to Question 2 are therefore "a," "b," and "f."

There are fewer trials of ibuprofen prophylaxis, and none report long-term follow up data. The effects of prophylaxis with early initiation of ibuprofen are summarized in Figure 14-5. Ibuprofen is effective in reducing the rate of persistent ductal patency (OR 0.24, 95% CI 0.17 to 0.33), but there were no significant effects on other reported outcomes. Importantly, the reduction in rates of IVH observed with indomethacin was not achieved with ibuprofen. The only correct answer to Question 3 is therefore "f".

Prophylactic intervention to accelerate ductal closure in at-risk preterm infants therefore appears to be justified only by the expectation of reduction in severe IVH or severe early pulmonary hemorrhage with indomethacin prophylaxis or (possibly) in NEC with prophylactic ligation. Use of prophylaxis may be appropriate in settings where rates of these complications are high, but otherwise, these potential benefits do not appear to outweigh potential hazards (see below). Routine prophylactic treatment of all ELBW or VLBW neonates cannot be recommended (Hamrick, 2010).

TREATMENT

CASE STUDY 4

A 690-gram baby was born at 27 weeks' gestation. The pregnancy had been uncomplicated until his mother presented with bulging membranes and then quickly progressed to delivery, affording no opportunity for antenatal treatments. The baby was vigorous at birth and was assigned Apgar scores of 5 and 7 at 1 and 5 minutes of age, respectively. He was initially stabilized on NCPAP with an FiO_2 of 0.40, but steadily worsening respiratory distress required intubation and administration of two doses of surfactant in the first 24 hours after birth. On the third day after birth, he continued to require positive pressure ventilation with an FiO_2 of 0.52. Vital signs included a heart rate of 165 beats per minute and transduced blood pressure of 40/24 (mean 29) mmHg. A coarse systolic murmur was audible and he had normal pulses and peripheral perfusion. A chest radiograph demonstrated bilateral pulmonary parenchymal densities with indistinct diaphragmatic and cardiothymic silhouettes. Echocardiography demonstrated a PDA 1.5 mm in diameter, with bidirectional but predominantly left-to-right shunting.

EXERCISE 6

QUESTION

1. For which of the following treatment strategies is there evidence supporting an expectation of an improvement in long-term outcomes for this infant?
   a. Treatment with indomethacin 0.2 mg/kg/dose IV every 12 hours for three doses
   b. Treatment with ibuprofen 10 mg/kg/dose once, then 5 mg/kg/dose daily for 2 days
   c. Surgical ligation within the next 48 hours
   d. None of the above

ANSWER

1. **d.**

   Despite the apparent lack of benefit from universal intervention to induce early ductal closure, it is not unreasonable to hypothesize that selective intervention if the ductus remains open beyond the age at which closure normally occurs in term infants (Figure 14-1) might be advantageous. There is surprisingly little empiric data that addresses this hypothesis, but it is not entirely untested. Four randomized trials—three using indomethacin (Hammerman, 1986;

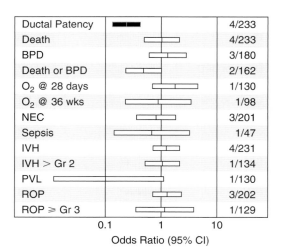

Ductal Patency		4/233
Death		4/233
BPD		3/180
Death or BPD		2/162
O_2 @ 28 days		1/130
O_2 @ 36 wks		1/98
NEC		3/201
Sepsis		1/47
IVH		4/231
IVH > Gr 2		1/134
PVL		1/130
ROP		3/202
ROP ≥ Gr 3		1/129

0.1   1   10
Odds Ratio (95% CI)

FIGURE 14-6 ■ **Pooled odds ratios for outcomes observed in randomized controlled trials of ibuprofen or indomethacin treatment of asymptomatic preterm infants.** Symbols and abbreviations are as indicated for Figure 14-4.

Mahony, 1982; Weesner, 1987) and one using ibuprofen (Aranda, 2009)—have examined the effects of treatment of infants in whom the ductus remains patent, as confirmed by echocardiography, on the third or fourth postnatal day, but who do not have overt clinical signs of hemodynamic compromise (e.g., two or more of the following: bounding pulses, hyperdynamic precordium, pulmonary edema, increased heart size by chest radiograph, systolic murmur). Like prophylactic treatment, indomethacin and ibuprofen are both effective for inducing ductal closure when initiated at a few days of age (OR for persistent patency 0.23, 95% CI 0.12 to 0.41), but no other beneficial effects were found (Figure 14-6). Unlike immediate prophylactic therapy, treatment delayed for even a few days, until after the period of greatest risk for IVH, does not appear to have a favorable effect on IVH or severe IVH. There have been no published trials of surgical ligation of the ductus in infants without clinical signs of significant hemodynamic effects. Because these data provide no evidence of benefit from treatment to induce ductal closure in asymptomatic infants, it is not possible to proceed with any of the listed treatment strategies with confidence that it represents the optimal course, so the correct answer to Question 1 is "d".

In a similar vein, selection of infants for intervention only when clinical signs of significant hemodynamic consequences of the PDA become evident may identify a cohort for whom treatment might be beneficial. The next exercise will explore that hypothesis.

CASE STUDY 5

Echocardiography performed at 10 days of age in the infant described in Case Studies 1 and 2 confirmed the presence of a patent ductus, 2.2 mm in diameter, with continuous left-to-right flow throughout both systole and diastole. The next day, examination revealed bilateral rales, a coarse systolic murmur, and bounding radial pulses, as well as the previously noted hepatomegaly.

EXERCISE 7

QUESTION

1. For which of the following treatment strategies is there evidence supporting an expectation of improvement in the long-term outcome for this infant?
   a. Treatment with indomethacin 0.2 mg/kg/ dose IV every 12 hours for three doses
   b. Treatment with ibuprofen 10 mg/kg/dose once, then 5 mg/kg/dose daily for 2 days
   c. Surgical ligation within the next 48 hours
   d. None of the above

ANSWER

1. **d.**

   Waiting for the effects of ductal patency to produce clinical signs does not appear to increase the likelihood that treatment will lead to measureable benefits. There is a shocking paucity of empiric data on this matter (Benitz, 2010). Two early studies of surgical ligation enrolled and randomized a total of 56 subjects, but demonstrated no benefit other than ductal closure itself. Eight randomized trials of enteral indomethacin that followed up on the seminal observations that this treatment induces ductal constriction (Friedman, 1976; Heymann, 1976) were published in the early 1980s, confirming induction of ductal closure (OR 0.14, 95% CI 0.07 to 0.25) and suggesting a reduction in mortality (OR 0.33, 95% CI 0.15 to 0.74). Only one of these reported other outcomes (NEC, BPD, or death), with no evident benefit. The results of six trials of intravenous indomethacin for symptomatic PDA are summarized in Figure 14-7. Although effective in promoting ductal closure (OR 0.17, 95% CI 0.10 to 0.28), no other benefits are apparent. The strength of this conclusion is limited, however, because most of these trials did not report outcomes other than ductal closure, BPD, and death. That reservation notwithstanding, the fact that beneficial effects of ductal closure have not been demonstrated with

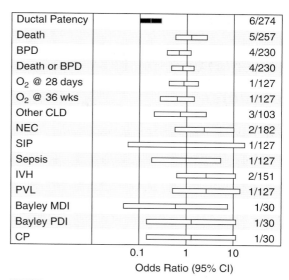

FIGURE 14-7 ■ Pooled odds ratios for outcomes observed in randomized controlled trials of intravenous indomethacin treatment of symptomatic preterm infants. Symbols and abbreviations are as indicated for Figure 14-4. (Adapted from Benitz WE: Treatment of persistent patent ductus arteriosus in preterm infants: time to accept the null hypothesis? *J Perinatol* 30:241-252, 2010.)

any treatment or prophylaxis strategy leaves little doubt that early, routine treatment to close the PDA in preterm infants is not beneficial and therefore is not indicated (Benitz, 2010). As was the case for asymptomatic babies, the correct answer to Question 1 is "d."

The lack of long-term benefit from treatment to close a PDA may not imply that there are no short-term advantages. It is commonly believed, for example, that closing the ductus with a cyclooxygenase inhibitor or ligation reliably leads to a reduction in requirements for oxygen supplementation or mechanical support of ventilation. The next exercise will examine these possibilities.

CASE STUDY 6

An 1140-gram infant was born at 31 weeks' gestation to a mother with newly recognized preeclampsia, by urgent cesarean section because of a type 3 fetal heart tracing and suspected placental abruption. He was flaccid at birth, responded poorly to stimulation and bag-mask ventilation, and required intubation and positive pressure ventilation before 3 minutes of age. He was given Apgar scores of 1 (HR <100), 3 (HR >100, body pink), and 5 (HR >100, body pink, some flexion, grimace) at 1, 5 and 10 minutes, respectively. Cord blood gases (arterial) were pH of 6.75, PaO$_2$ of 12 mmHg, PaCO$_2$ of 106 mmHg, HCO$_3$ of 14.0 mEq/L, and base excess of −18.7 mEq/L. Because of concern about the perceived high risk of IVH, he was started on a course of indomethacin prophylaxis (0.1 mg/kg/dose daily for 3 days) soon after arrival in the NICU.

EXERCISE 8

QUESTIONS

1. Which of the following short-term effects can be expected to result from this use of indomethacin in infants similar to the one described in this case study?
   a. Earlier closure of the ductus arteriosus
   b. More use of indomethacin to close a PDA
   c. Fewer surgical PDA ligations
   d. Lower oxygen requirements from days 3 through 7
   e. Decreased requirements for mechanical respiratory support
   f. Reduced urine output
   g. Lower rates of grade III or IV intraventricular hemorrhage

2. Which of those short-term effects could be expected to result from early treatment with ibuprofen in such infants?

ANSWERS

1. **a**, **c**, **f**, and **g.**

2. **a** and **c.**

   Early administration of indomethacin as prophylaxis for IVH or for treatment of PDA reliably results in earlier ductal closure, and, consequently, less frequent need for subsequent treatment with indomethacin or surgical ligation. Therefore, answers "a" and "c" are correct and "b" is not. However, such treatments fail to result in less severe respiratory disease or to reduce the requirements for supplemental oxygen or other respiratory therapies, as many had expected. On the contrary, infants treated with prophylactic or early indomethacin require more surfactant doses (Yaseen, 1997) as well as more oxygen (Schmidt, 2006; Van Overmeire, 2001; Yaseen, 1997) and higher airway pressures (Van Overmeire, 2001) over the first 7 to 10 days after birth. Data demonstrating the latter effects are presented in Figure 14-8. Answers "d" and "e" are therefore not correct.

   Blood flow in cerebral (Austin, 1992), mesenteric (Coombs, 1990; Pezzati, 1999), and renal (Pezzati, 1999) arteries is reduced after treatment with indomethacin, resulting in lower cerebral oxygen saturations, decreased glomerular

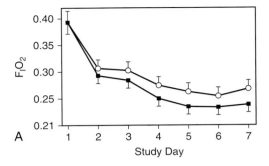

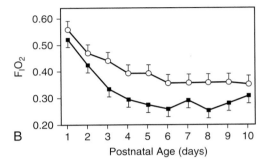

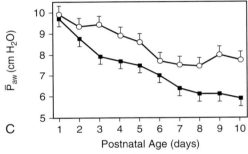

FIGURE 14-8 ■ **Effects of early indomethacin on requirements for respiratory support. A,** The daily mean FiO_2 for ELBW (<1000 g) infants randomized to prophylactic indomethacin (n = 496) or placebo (n = 503) soon after birth. **B** and **C,** Supplemental oxygen requirement **(B)** and mean airway pressure **(C)** in infants <28 weeks' gestation treated with early (day 3; n = 23) or late (day 7; n = 21) indomethacin. Data points represent mean ± standard error. All differences are significant (p <0.05) for day 3 and after. Open symbols and dashed lines represent the early indomethacin groups; filled symbols and solid lines represent placebo **(A)** or late indomethacin **(B** and **C)** groups. (Data in **A** from Schmidt B, Davis P, Moddemann D, et al: Long-term effects of indomethacin prophylaxis in extremely-low-birth-weight infants. *N Engl J Med* 344:1966-1972, 2001. **B** and **C** adapted from Benitz WE: Treatment of persistent patent ductus arteriosus in preterm infants: time to accept the null hypothesis? *J Perinatol* 30:241-252, 2010.)

filtration, and decreased urine production. Choice "f" is therefore a correct answer. Fortunately, these hemodynamic changes apparently do not lead to more frequent complications, including BPD, NEC, bowel perforation, ROP, or neurodevelopmental impairment, or to increased mortality rates (Benitz, 2010). There is an increased risk of spontaneous intestinal perforation if indomethacin is given to preterm infants who are also receiving hydrocortisone, however (Watterberg, 2004). As noted previously, indomethacin prophylaxis reduces the rates of IVH and grade III or IV IVH, although the mechanism of this effect and its relationship to these local effects on cerebral blood flow remain uncertain. Choice "g" therefore is also a correct answer.

Ibuprofen is equally effective with indomethacin for achieving ductal closure, and its use is associated with less frequent requirements for additional treatment with indomethacin or surgical ligation. Choices "a" and "c," but not "b," are correct for this drug too. No placebo-controlled studies have examined the effects of ibuprofen treatment on requirements for respiratory support. In direct comparisons to indomethacin, ibuprofen-treated infants required slightly fewer days of ventilator support or supplemental oxygen; early effects on mean airway pressure and F_IO_2, if any, have not been reported, so there is no evidence that "d" and "e" are correct. In comparison to those associated with indomethacin, the effects of ibuprofen on cerebral, renal, and mesenteric blood flow are minimal or small. Ibuprofen may produce measureable effects on renal function, such as a slight increase in serum creatinine, but usually does not cause significant oliguria. Although neither indomethacin nor ibuprofen has been associated with substantially increased or decreased rates of NEC in placebo-controlled trials, head-to-head comparisons suggest that NEC is less frequent in preterm infants treated with ibuprofen than in those who receive indomethacin (Ohlsson, 2013). Ibuprofen does not appear to have neuroprotective effects similar to those of indomethacin, as no reduction in IVH rates has been reported from ibuprofen trials. The possibility of an increase in the risk of neurologic injury with ibuprofen has been raised by *in vitro* experiments demonstrating bilirubin displacement from albumin by ibuprofen (Ahlfors, 2004), but the practical significance of those observations remains uncertain.

CASE STUDY 7

A 550-gram baby was born at 24 weeks' gestation, 2 weeks after his mother was found to have cervical dilation and bulging membranes by regularly scheduled ultrasonography. Labor was suppressed with indomethacin, and a course of antenatal corticosteroids was completed the day before delivery. Vaginal birth followed recurrence of labor, despite *tocolytic treatment with magnesium sulfate. The baby required intubation in the delivery room because of a persistent lack of respiratory effort. He continued to require positive pressure ventilation, with slowly increasing requirements for ventilation and oxygen supplementation. By Day 15 after birth, he required support with high-frequency oscillatory ventilation with an FiO_2 of 0.72, and was being treated for hypotension with hydrocortisone (3 mg/kg/day) and dopamine (18 µg/kg/min). On examination, he had a heart rate of 190 beats per minute, blood pressure of 31/17 (mean 23), a loud systolic murmur, bounding pulses, and an enlarged liver. His chest radiograph showed a large heart, shunt vascularity, and perihilar pulmonary edema. Echocardiography confirmed persistent ductal patency, with a 2.5 mm transductal diameter, LA:Ao ratio of 2.1, left ventricular distension, continuous left-to-right shunting, and reversal of diastolic low in the descending aorta.*

EXERCISE 9

QUESTION

1. Which of the following are *potential* short-term (within 3 to 4 days) consequences of immediate surgical ligation of the ductus in this infant?
   a. Resolution of hypotension
   b. Circulatory collapse
   c. Marked respiratory improvement
   d. Left diaphragm paresis
   e. Worsening pulmonary edema

ANSWER

1. **All of the above.**

   Surgical ligation is a safe, expeditious, and reliable way to eliminate the effects of a large left-to-right ductal shunt. The immediate effects of this surgery are difficult to predict, however. Elimination of the low resistance shunt into the pulmonary circulation should increase the blood pressure, and observation for that effect often provides intraoperative assurance to the anesthesiologist and surgeon that the correct vessel has been ligated. However, as many as one-third of preterm infants develop severe left ventricular dysfunction within hours of the surgery, resulting in circulatory and respiratory collapse requiring major escalations in cardiotonic and ventilatory support (Teixeira, 2008). This complication occurs less frequently with increasing postnatal age, so it may be preferable to defer surgery until after one month of age (if feasible). Some infants have substantial respiratory improvement following surgery, but this is not always the case. In the best case, elimination of excessive pulmonary blood flow leads to resolution of pulmonary edema and marked respiratory improvement. Ventricular dysfunction may produce the opposite effect, however. Paresis of the left hemidiaphragm resulting from left phrenic nerve injury is not uncommon, and may greatly delay weaning from assisted ventilation. Left vocal cord paralysis, which may occur in as many as two-thirds of ELBW infants who undergo ductal ligation (Benjamin, 2010; Clement, 2008), prolongs assisted ventilation, oxygen supplementation, and hospitalization, and increases the likelihood of BPD, feeding difficulties, tube feeding, and permanent voice impairment (Roksund, 2010). Other early complications include chylothorax, pneumothorax, and phrenic or recurrent laryngeal nerve injury (Benitz, 2011), and long-term sequelae include increased risks of BPD (Chorne, 2007; Clyman, 2009) and neurodevelopmental impairment (Kabra, 2007). Some adverse outcomes may result from the circumstances creating the need for surgery rather than the surgery itself, so it is not certain that they could be averted by avoidance of surgery. Because of these unpredictable and widely variable responses to surgical ductal ligation, all of the options are correct answers to Question 1.

Nearly all of the trials that provide evidence that early, routine ductal closure in preterm infants does not produce better outcomes were conducted in the first week or two after birth, and interventions to close the PDA if it persisted into the third or fourth week were common, even for subjects assigned to the placebo arms. Those data therefore do not allow the conclusion that intervention to close the ductus is not beneficial at any age in preterm infants. In fact, the consequences of large left-to-right shunts in the second half of the first postnatal month and beyond in ELBW infants are unknown, as are the possible indications for, potential benefits from, optimal timing of, and best method for achieving later ductal closure. If there is a benefit from later intervention, it is not apparent whether optimal management might consist of immediate ligation or a trial of cyclooxygenase inhibitor prior to ligation. Similarly, the possibility remains that some infants may benefit from early ductal closure, either because they were not well represented in prior clinical trials or by virtue of selection using echocardiographic or biomarker criteria as discussed above. It does seem likely that there are some infants, perhaps including the baby described in Case Study 7, for whom treatment benefits eventually will be demonstrated

in well-designed clinical trials. Until those trials produce the evidence needed to guide care, it will be necessary to base management on individualized clinical judgment.

ALTERNATIVES TO DUCTAL CLOSURE

CASE STUDY 8

At 1 week of age, the baby described in Case Study 4 remained intubated and on positive pressure ventilation, but he had stabilized on low ventilator settings (PIP 15, PEEP 4, rate 24) with an FiO_2 of 0.28. Blood gases were pH of 7.21, PaO_2 of 95 mmHg, $PaCO_2$ of 42 mmHg, HCO_3 of 27.4 mEq/L, base excess -3.3 mEq/L. He was receiving trophic feedings of maternal milk (2 mL every 3 hours) and parenteral nutrition with a total fluid intake at 150 mL/kg/day. His blood pressure was 44/19, his murmur persisted, and his arterial pulses were prominent. A chest radiograph showed mild cardiomegaly and pulmonary congestion. Laboratory studies were significant for the following values: creatinine 0.9 mg/dL, urea nitrogen 43 mg/dL, albumin 1.6 g/dL, hemoglobin 7.8 g/dL, hematocrit 24.

EXERCISE 10

QUESTIONS

1. Which of the following summarizes the best strategy for managing the presumed PDA in this infant?
   a. Ignore it.
   b. Monitor for signs of decompensation without interventions.
   c. Implement measures to mitigate PDA effects.
   d. Begin a course of ibuprofen.
   e. Request ligation.

2. If no intervention is offered to close this infant's PDA, which of the following measures might be appropriate steps to ameliorate the potential adverse effects of the presumed PDA?
   a. Reduce the ventilator rate and/or PIP.
   b. Increase PEEP to 6 cm H_2O.
   c. Increase FiO_2 to 0.34.
   d. Restrict fluid intake to 120 mL/kg/day.
   e. Increase acetate content in parenteral nutrition fluid.
   f. Reduce amino acid content in parenteral nutrition fluid.
   g. Add albumin to parenteral nutrition fluid.
   h. Transfuse red blood cells.

ANSWERS

1. **c.**

2. **a**, **b**, and **h.**

There is little evidence to guide correct answers to these questions. Given the lack of evidence for benefit from medical or surgical closure of the ductus and the modest apparent impact that PDA is having in this infant, the correct answer to Question 1 is probably "c." The potential effects of PDA may be important, so it should not simply be ignored, and measures to prevent complications probably are preferable to treatment of complications after they develop, so monitoring alone may not be the best choice. Several reports provide reassurance that adoption of less aggressive management strategies is consistent with favorable outcomes. Management of VLBW infants with symptomatic PDA using fluid restriction to 130 to 150 mL/kg/day, diuretics, and captopril (to reduce systemic vascular resistance) decreased the need for either indomethacin or ligation (in only 1.6% and 3.6% of infants, respectively), yet produced outcomes that compared favorably with Vermont Oxford Network benchmarks (Pietz, 2007). Outcomes comparable to or better than those reported to multicenter collaboratives were also achieved in ventilated infants ≤30 weeks gestation who had a PDA demonstrated by echocardiography, using "conservative management" consisting of fluid restriction to 130 mL/kg/day, reduction of the inspiratory time to 0.35 seconds (from 0.4 to 0.45 seconds), and an increased end expiratory pressure (to 4.5 cm H_2O), (Vanhaesebrouck, 2007). The PDA closed without treatment in more than 95% of those infants. At another center, adoption of a strategy of selective rather than universal PDA ligation for infants whose ductus remained open after indomethacin prophylaxis decreased the rate of surgery in that high-risk cohort from 100% to 72% (Jhaveri, 2010). Therefore, 28% of the babies in the latter era avoided surgery. In those infants, the ductus closed spontaneously before hospital discharge in one-third, after discharge but before 6 months of age in one-third, and remained patent or was closed by transcatheter coiling in the remaining one-third. It is worth noting, however, that ligation was considered in the latter era only for infants who developed signs of circulatory compromise. Therefore, surgeries were performed at a later age, resulting in significantly more days of exposure to ductal shunting in infants who had surgery. However, prolonged exposure to the effects of PDA was not associated with any increase in adverse outcomes (BPD, sepsis, ROP, IVH ≥grade III, neurologic injury, or death), and the risk of NEC was actually substantially lower (adjusted OR 0.25, 95% CI 0.07 to 0.95). This favorable change in the incidence of NEC is all the more remarkable because it was also associated with continuation of feedings despite presence of a PDA, in contrast to the earlier practice of interrupting enteric nutrition under those circumstances. Another study compared outcomes of infants requiring respiratory support with moderate to large PDAs before and after adoption of selective rather than liberal criteria for treatment with indomethacin or ligation. The revised approach relied primarily on modest fluid restriction (to approximately 130 to 140 mL/kg/day); indomethacin or ligation was reserved for infants who could not be weaned from positive pressure ventilation or could not maintain adequate oxygenation and ventilation on NCPAP (Kaempf, 2012). Despite less use of indomethacin or ligation in the second era (in 26% vs. 79% and 33% vs. 45% of infants, respectively), neither the requirements for respiratory support nor rates of multiple morbidities (BPD, IVH, PVL, NEC, etc.) were affected. However, the rate of death or BPD as a combined outcome was greater (54% vs. 40%) in the second era. In the infants discharged home with PDA, the ductus closed spontaneously in 70% within 1 year. These reports do not provide strong evidence that any of these approaches constitutes a "best practice" for PDA management, but they do indicate that more tolerant approaches to preterm babies with PDA do not lead to worse outcomes. In concert with the previously described evidence that early, routine intervention to close the ductus does not improve outcomes, these observations suggest that the correct answer to Question 1 should be "c." Which measures to use—those chosen in these observational studies or others not yet tested—remains to be determined in trials targeted to evaluate their efficacy.

Until evidence to guide management is available, judgment will have to rely on considerations of the pathophysiology of ductal shunting. The consequences of such shunting can be categorized as follows: excessive pulmonary blood flow, compromised perfusion of other organs, and congestive heart failure. Even large left-to-right shunts may not result in pulmonary edema unless pulmonary fluid fluxes are additionally disturbed by factors such as surfactant deficiency, low serum oncotic forces, or capillary leak syndrome. When pulmonary edema develops, the alveolar-arterial oxygen gradient increases and lung compliance decreases. Systemic cardiac output and perfusion of vital organs may be compromised by the "ductal steal" of a large left-to-right shunt. Doppler ultrasound may demonstrate decreased, absent, or reversal of diastolic flow in the descending aorta and in the middle cerebral, superior mesenteric, and renal arteries (Groves, 2008). Early changes in cerebral blood flow velocities associated with PDA have been correlated with later development of periventricular leukomalacia (although the causal relationship is uncertain) (Pladys, 2001). Reduced renal blood flow correlates with impaired renal function (Vanpee, 1993), and changes in mesenteric artery flow may be related to development of NEC (Dollberg, 2005). In term infants with congenital heart disease requiring surgical correction, retrograde flow in the descending aorta during diastole is associated with an increased risk of NEC (Carlo, 2007). The implications of diastolic flow reversal in preterm infants with PDA have not been formally evaluated, however. These ischemic effects of large ductal shunt may be compounded by myocardial dysfunction resulting from a greatly increased volume workload on the left heart, leading to atrial and ventricular distension, echocardiographic signs of ventricular dysfunction, ST segment depression (Way, 1979), or elevated serum troponin levels (El-Khuffash, 2008b).

This disturbed pathophysiology can be addressed at each of those levels (Benitz, 2011). Excessive pulmonary blood flow may be mitigated by measures that increase pulmonary vascular resistance, including permissive hypercapnia, increased distending airway pressure, transfusion to increase the hematocrit, and avoidance of alkalosis, excessive supplemental oxygen, and pulmonary vasodilator agents such as nitric oxide. These measures also augment systemic cardiac output and organ perfusion. Systemic afterload reduction (e.g., captopril) and avoidance or very judicious use of systemic vasopressor drugs will reduce the driving force behind the left-to-right ductal shunt. Careful attention to support of total cardiac output through ensuring adequacy of preload and provision of inotropic support may also be helpful. When adrenal insufficiency is suspected, supplemental hydrocortisone may increase blood pressure. Standard methods for management of congestive heart failure—preload reduction through fluid restriction and diuretics, inotropic support, and afterload reduction—should be effective. Published data suggest that modest fluid restriction, to approximately 140 mL/kg/day, is sufficient in this setting.

In addition to consideration of these hemodynamic factors, management should address other factors that may directly contribute to organ compromise, prolong ductal patency, or independently influence outcomes through mechanisms not related to the PDA. Conditions that may augment development of pulmonary edema, such as hypoproteinemia or capillary leak, should be prevented or treated. Optimal nutrition is the key to prevention of hypoproteinemia, but is not always sufficient. Hypoproteinemia may be most quickly corrected by administration of albumin (along with diuresis to remove the concomitant salt load); however, the administration of albumin is controversial because of safety concerns. Capillary leak should be avoided by prevention of bacterial infection using meticulous infection control methods. Similarly, circumstances that may increase the risk of injury to the brain (infection, anemia, hypoglycemia), kidneys (hypovolemia, nephrotoxic drugs), or bowel must be minimized. Closure of the ductus may be delayed by excessive fluid administration (especially above 180 mL/kg/day), hospital-acquired bacterial infection (particularly coagulase-negative *Staphylococcus*), and possibly by diuretic therapy. Although furosemide does not appear to interfere with ductal closure in response to indomethacin (Lee, 2010), it may delay closure in infants who are not treated with cyclooxygenase inhibitors (Green, 1983). None of these strategies have been evaluated in clinical trials, and the net effect of each may depend on the balance between conflicting actions. For example, aggressive use of furosemide may help in management of pulmonary edema and congestive heart failure, but may have adverse effects if it results in hypovolemia, metabolic alkalosis, or prolonged ductal patency.

These considerations suggest the following answers to Question 2. Answers "a" and "b" are correct, because allowing an increase in $Paco_2$ should induce pulmonary arteriolar constriction, and an increase in PEEP might increase pulmonary vascular resistance and decrease the transpulmonary arteriovenous pressure gradient. Increasing the Fio_2 ("c") would not be helpful, as that might reduce pulmonary vascular resistance and increase pulmonary blood flow. Since the Pao_2 is already high, a reduction in Fio_2 would be a better response. Fluid restriction ("d") would be appropriate, but it is important to make sure the nutritional intake is adequate to support normal growth. Increasing the acetate content in parenteral fluids ("e") would exacerbate the existing mild metabolic alkalosis, potentially increasing pulmonary blood flow. Reducing the amino acid content of the nutritional fluids ("f") might help reduce the BUN level; however, this might perpetuate the hypoalbuminemia.

Adding albumin to the parenteral nutrition fluid ("g") might help increase the serum albumin level and favor mobilization of third space fluid from the lungs and elsewhere, but that practice has safety concerns and is usually discouraged. Transfusion with red blood cells ("h"), with a goal hematocrit in the upper 40s or greater, may help limit excessive pulmonary blood flow (because of differential effects on systemic and pulmonary vascular rheology) and will reduce the total cardiac output required to meet metabolic demand; however, the role of this strategy in infants with PDA has not been established.

Managing patent ductus in preterm infants remains one of the most challenging tasks in neonatal medicine. Beyond the knowledge that induced early closure of the ductus does not improve long-term results, there is little empiric evidence to guide the treatment of this condition. Acceptance of ductal patency while attending to its hemodynamic consequences is increasingly accepted as the best initial approach to management, particularly in infants >1000 grams, in whom the ductus will nearly always close without intervention. Smaller infants, particularly those with RDS, may require treatment to address ductal patency, but the indications for intervention, optimal timing, and best treatment(s) are unknown. While we seek answers to these questions, management of the preterm infant with patent ductus should be approached with humility, circumspection, and patience.

SUGGESTED READINGS

Ahlfors CE: Effect of ibuprofen on bilirubin-albumin binding, *J Pediatr* 144:386–388, 2004.

Alfaleh K, Smyth JA, Roberts RS, et al: Prevention and 18-month outcomes of serious pulmonary hemorrhage in extremely low birth weight infants: results from the trial of indomethacin prophylaxis in preterms, *Pediatrics* 121:e233–238, 2008.

Aranda JV, Clyman R, Cox B, et al: A randomized, double-blind, placebo-controlled trial on intravenous ibuprofen L-lysine for the early closure of nonsymptomatic patent ductus arteriosus within 72 hours of birth in extremely low-birth-weight infants, *Am J Perinatol* 26:235–245, 2009.

Attridge JT, Kaufman DA, Lim DS: B-type natriuretic peptide concentrations to guide treatment of patent ductus arteriosus, *Arch Dis Child Fetal Neonatal Ed* 94:F178–F182, 2009.

Austin NC, Pairaudeau PW, Hames TK, et al: Regional cerebral blood flow velocity changes after indomethacin infusion in preterm infants, *Arch Dis Child* 67:851–854, 1992.

Bada HS, Green RS, Pourcyrous M, et al: Indomethacin reduces the risks of severe intraventricular hemorrhage, *J Pediatr* 115:631–637, 1989.

Bandstra ES, Montalvo BM, Goldberg RN, et al: Prophylactic indomethacin for prevention of intraventricular hemorrhage in premature infants, *Pediatrics* 82:533–542, 1988.

Benitz WE: Learning to live with patency of the ductus arteriosus in preterm infants, *J Perinatol* 31(suppl 1): S42–S48, 2011.

Benitz WE: Treatment of persistent patent ductus arteriosus in preterm infants: time to accept the null hypothesis? *J Perinatol* 30:241–252, 2010.

Benjamin JR, Smith PB, Cotten CM, et al: Long-term morbidities associated with vocal cord paralysis after surgical closure of a patent ductus arteriosus in extremely low birth weight infants, *J Perinatol* 30:408–413, 2010.

Brooks JM, Travadi JN, Patole SK, et al: Is surgical ligation of patent ductus arteriosus necessary? The Western Australian experience of conservative management, *Arch Dis Child Fetal Neonatal Ed* 90:F235–F239, 2005.

Brown ER: Increased risk of bronchopulmonary dysplasia in infants with patent ductus arteriosus, *J Pediatr* 95:865–866, 1979.

Carlo WF, Kimball TR, Michelfelder EC, et al: Persistent diastolic flow reversal in abdominal aortic Doppler-flow profiles is associated with an increased risk of necrotizing enterocolitis in term infants with congenital heart disease, *Pediatrics* 119:330–335, 2007.

Cassady G, Crouse DT, Kirklin JW, et al: A randomized, controlled trial of very early prophylactic ligation of the ductus arteriosus in babies who weighed 1000 g or less at birth, *N Engl J Med* 320:1511–1516, 1989.

Choi BM, Lee KH, Eun BL, et al: Utility of rapid B-type natriuretic peptide assay for diagnosis of symptomatic patent ductus arteriosus in preterm infants, *Pediatrics* 115:e255–261, 2005.

Chorne N, Leonard C, Piecuch R, et al: Patent ductus arteriosus and its treatment as risk factors for neonatal and neurodevelopmental morbidity, *Pediatrics* 119:1165–1174, 2007.

Clement WA, El-Hakim H, Phillipos EZ, et al: Unilateral vocal cord paralysis following patent ductus arteriosus ligation in extremely low-birth-weight infants, *Arch Otolaryngol Head Neck Surg* 134:28–33, 2008.

Clyman R, Cassady G, Kirklin JK, et al: The role of patent ductus arteriosus ligation in bronchopulmonary dysplasia: reexamining a randomized controlled trial, *J Pediatr* 154:873–876, 2009.

Clyman RI, Couto J, Murphy GM: Patent ductus arteriosus: are current neonatal treatment options better or worse than no treatment at all? *Semin Perinatol* 36:123–129, 2012.

Coombs RC, Morgan ME, Durbin GM, et al: Gut blood flow velocities in the newborn: effects of patent ductus arteriosus and parenteral indomethacin, *Arch Dis Child* 65:1067–1071, 1990.

Couser RJ, Ferrara TB, Wright GB, et al: Prophylactic indomethacin therapy in the first twenty-four hours of life for the prevention of patent ductus arteriosus in preterm infants treated prophylactically with surfactant in the delivery room, *J Pediatr* 128:631–637, 1996.

Davis P, Turner-Gomes S, Cunningham K, et al: Precision and accuracy of clinical and radiological signs in premature infants at risk of patent ductus arteriosus, *Arch Pediatr Adolesc Med* 149:1136–1141, 1995.

Dessardo NS, Mustac E, Dessardo S, et al: Chorioamnionitis and chronic lung disease of prematurity: a path analysis of causality, *Am J Perinatol* 29:133–140, 2012.

Dollberg S, Lusky A, Reichman B: Patent ductus arteriosus, indomethacin and necrotizing enterocolitis in very low birth weight infants: a population-based study, *J Pediatr Gastroenterol Nutr* 40:184–188, 2005.

Domanico RS, Waldman JD, Lester LA, et al: Prophylactic indomethacin reduces the incidence of pulmonary hemorrhage and patent ductus arteriosus in surfactant-treaed infants <1250 g, *Pediatr Res* 35:331A, 1994.

El-Khuffash A, Barry D, Walsh K, et al: Biochemical markers may identify preterm infants with a patent ductus arteriosus at high risk of death or severe intraventricular haemorrhage, *Arch Dis Child Fetal Neonatal Ed* 93:F407–F412, 2008a.

El-Khuffash AF, Amoruso M, Culliton M, et al: N-terminal pro-B-type natriuretic peptide as a marker of ductal haemodynamic significance in preterm infants: a prospective observational study, *Arch Dis Child Fetal Neonatal Ed* 92:F421–F422, 2007.

El-Khuffash AF, Molloy EJ: Influence of a patent ductus arteriosus on cardiac troponin T levels in preterm infants, *J Pediatr* 153:350–353, 2008b.

El-Khuffash AF, Slevin M, McNamara PJ, et al: Troponin T, N-terminal pro natriuretic peptide and a patent ductus arteriosus scoring system predict death before discharge or neurodevelopmental outcome at 2 years in preterm infants, *Arch Dis Child Fetal Neonatal Ed* 96:F133–F137, 2011.

Flynn PA, da Graca RL, Auld PA, et al: The use of a bedside assay for plasma B-type natriuretic peptide as a biomarker in the management of patent ductus arteriosus in premature neonates, *J Pediatr* 147:38–42, 2005.

Friedman WF, Hirschklau MJ, Printz MP, et al: Pharmacologic closure of patent ductus arteriosus in the premature infant, *N Engl J Med* 295:526–529, 1976.

Garland J, Buck R, Weinberg M: Pulmonary hemorrhage risk in infants with a clinically diagnosed patent ductus arteriosus: a retrospective cohort study, *Pediatrics* 94:719–723, 1994.

Gentile R, Stevenson G, Dooley T, et al: Pulsed Doppler echocardiographic determination of time of ductal closure in normal newborn infants, *J Pediatr* 98:443–448, 1981.

Green TP, Thompson TR, Johnson DE, et al: Furosemide promotes patent ductus arteriosus in premature infants with the respiratory-distress syndrome, *N Engl J Med* 308:743–748, 1983.

Groves AM, Kuschel CA, Knight DB, et al: Does retrograde diastolic flow in the descending aorta signify impaired systemic perfusion in preterm infants? *Pediatr Res* 63:89–94, 2008.

Hammerman C, Strates E, Valaitis S: The silent ductus: its precursors and its aftermath, *Pediatr Cardiol* 7:121–127, 1986.

Hamrick SE, Hansmann G: Patent ductus arteriosus of the preterm infant, *Pediatrics* 125:1020–1030, 2010.

Heymann MA, Rudolph AM, Silverman NH: Closure of the ductus arteriosus in premature infants by inhibition of prostaglandin synthesis, *N Engl J Med* 295:530–533, 1976.

Jhaveri N, Moon-Grady A, Clyman RI: Early surgical ligation versus a conservative approach for management of patent ductus arteriosus that fails to close after indomethacin treatment, *J Pediatr* 157:381–387, 2010.

Jim WT, Chiu NC, Chen MR, et al: Cerebral hemodynamic change and intraventricular hemorrhage in very low birth weight infants with patent ductus arteriosus, *Ultrasound Med Biol* 31:197–202, 2005.

Kabra NS, Schmidt B, Roberts RS, et al: Neurosensory impairment after surgical closure of patent ductus arteriosus in extremely low birth weight infants: results from the Trial of Indomethacin Prophylaxis in Preterms, *J Pediatr* 150:229–234, 2007.

Kaempf JW, Wu YX, Kaempf AJ, et al: What happens when the patent ductus arteriosus is treated less aggressively in very low birth weight infants? *J Perinatol* 32:344–348, 2012.

Katayama Y, Minami H, Enomoto M, et al: Antenatal magnesium sulfate and the postnatal response of the ductus arteriosus to indomethacin in extremely preterm neonates, *J Perinatol* 31:21–24, 2011.

Koch J, Hensley G, Roy L, et al: Prevalence of spontaneous closure of the ductus arteriosus in neonates at a birth weight of 1000 grams or less, *Pediatrics* 117:1113–1121, 2006.

Lee BS, Byun SY, Chung ML, et al: Effect of furosemide on ductal closure and renal function in indomethacin-treated preterm infants during the early neonatal period, *Neonatology* 98:191–199, 2010.

Mahony L, Carnero V, Brett C, et al: Prophylactic indomethacin therapy for patent ductus arteriosus in very-low-birth-weight infants, *N Engl J Med* 306:506–510, 1982.

Marshall DD, Kotelchuck M, Young TE, et al: Risk factors for chronic lung disease in the surfactant era: a North Carolina population-based study of very low birth weight infants, *Pediatrics* 104:1345–1350, 1999.

McNamara PJ, Sehgal A: Towards rational management of the patent ductus arteriosus: the need for disease staging, *Arch Dis Child Fetal Neonatal Ed* 92:F424–F427, 2007.

Nemerofsky SL, Parravicini E, Bateman D, et al: The ductus arteriosus rarely requires treatment in infants >1000 grams, *Am J Perinatol* 25:661–666, 2008.

Noori S: Pros and cons of patent ductus arteriosus ligation: hemodynamic changes and other morbidities after patent ductus arteriosus ligation, *Semin Perinatol* 36:139–145, 2012.

Noori S, McCoy M, Friedlich P, et al: Failure of ductus arteriosus closure is associated with increased mortality in preterm infants, *Pediatrics* 123:e138–e144, 2009.

Oh W, Poindexter BB, Perritt R, et al: Association between fluid intake and weight loss during the first ten days of life and risk of bronchopulmonary dysplasia in extremely low birth weight infants, *J Pediatr* 147:786–790, 2005.

Ohlsson A, Walia R, Shah SS: Ibuprofen for the treatment of patent ductus arteriosus in preterm and/or low birth weight infants, *Cochrane Database Syst Rev* 4:CD003481, 2013.

Perloff JK: Therapeutics of nature—the invisible sutures of "spontaneous closure," *Am Heart J* 82:581–585, 1971.

Pezzati M, Vangi V, Biagiotti R, et al: Effects of indomethacin and ibuprofen on mesenteric and renal blood flow in preterm infants with patent ductus arteriosus, *J Pediatr* 135:733–738, 1999.

Pietz J, Achanti B, Lilien L, et al: Prevention of necrotizing enterocolitis in preterm infants: a 20-year experience, *Pediatrics* 119:e164–e170, 2007.

Pladys P, Beuchee A, Wodey E, et al: Patent ductus arteriosus and cystic periventricular leucomalacia in preterm infants, *Acta Paediatr.* 90:309–315, 2001.

Reller MD, Rice MJ, McDonald RW: Review of studies evaluating ductal patency in the premature infant, *J Pediatr* 122:S59–S62, 1993.

Roksund OD, Clemm H, Heimdal JH, et al: Left vocal cord paralysis after extreme preterm birth, a new clinical scenario in adults, *Pediatrics* 126:e1569–1577, 2010.

Ryder RW, Shelton JD, Guinan ME: Necrotizing enterocolitis: a prospective multicenter investigation, *Am J Epidemiol* 112:113–123, 1980.

Sanjeev S, Pettersen M, Lua J, et al: Role of plasma B-type natriuretic peptide in screening for hemodynamically significant patent ductus arteriosus in preterm neonates, *J Perinatol* 25:709–713, 2005.

Schmidt B, Davis P, Moddemann D, et al: Long-term effects of indomethacin prophylaxis in extremely-low-birth-weight infants, *N Engl J Med* 344:1966–1972, 2001.

Schmidt B, Roberts RS, Fanaroff A, et al: Indomethacin prophylaxis, patent ductus arteriosus, and the risk of bronchopulmonary dysplasia: further analyses from the Trial of Indomethacin Prophylaxis in Preterms (TIPP), *J Pediatr* 148:730–734, 2006.

Sehgal A, Paul E, Menahem S: Functional echocardiography in staging for ductal disease severity: role in predicting outcomes, *Eur J Pediatr* 172:179–184, 2013.

Shortland DB, Gibson NA, Levene MI, et al: Patent ductus arteriosus and cerebral circulation in preterm infants, *Dev Med Child Neurol* 32:386–393, 1990.

Skelton R, Evans N, Smythe J: A blinded comparison of clinical and echocardiographic evaluation of the preterm infant for patent ductus arteriosus, *J Paediatr Child Health* 30:406–411, 1994.

Teixeira LS, Shivananda SP, Stephens D, et al: Postoperative cardiorespiratory instability following ligation of the preterm ductus arteriosus is related to early need for intervention, *J Perinatol* 28:803–810, 2008.

Vanhaesebrouck S, Zonnenberg I, Vandervoort P, et al: Conservative treatment for patent ductus arteriosus in the preterm, *Arch Dis Child Fetal Neonatal Ed* 92:F244–F247, 2007.

Van Overmeire B, Allegaert K, Casaer A, et al: Prophylactic ibuprofen in premature infants: a multicentre, randomised, double-blind, placebo-controlled trial, *Lancet* 364:1945–1949, 2004.

Van Overmeire B, Van de Broek H, Van Laer P, et al: Early versus late indomethacin treatment for patent ductus arteriosus in premature infants with respiratory distress syndrome, *J Pediatr* 138:205–211, 2001.

Vanpee M, Ergander U, Herin P, et al: Renal function in sick, very low-birth-weight infants, *Acta Paediatr* 82:714–718, 1993.

Watterberg KL, Gerdes JS, Cole CH, et al: Prophylaxis of early adrenal insufficiency to prevent bronchopulmonary dysplasia: a multicenter trial, *Pediatrics* 114:1649–1657, 2004.

Way GL, Pierce JR, Wolfe RR, et al: ST depression suggesting subendocardial ischemia in neonates with respiratory distress syndrome and patent ductus arteriosus, *J Pediatr* 95:609–611, 1979.

Weesner KM, Dillard RG, Boyle RJ, et al: Prophylactic treatment of asymptomatic patent ductus arteriosus in premature infants with respiratory distress syndrome, *South Med J* 80:706–708, 1987.

Yaseen H, al Umran K, Ali H, et al: Effects of early indomethacin administration on oxygenation and surfactant requirement in low birth weight infants, *J Trop Pediatr* 43:42–46, 1997.

CHAPTER 15

NEONATAL HYPOTENSION

Tai-Wei Wu, MD • Shahab Noori, MD • Istvan Seri, MD, PhD

Hypotension of the premature newborn is a condition commonly encountered in the neonatal intensive care setting. Although no definite cut-off values exist in considering a given newborn to be "hypotensive," certain blood pressure ranges will cause significant anxiety among caregivers. The goal of this chapter is to illustrate the complexity involved in the diagnosis and management of neonatal hypotension and guide the clinician in decision-making using available evidence and a physiology-based individualized approach when caring for patients with neonatal circulatory compromise. We present a real case with a type of cardiovascular compromise frequently seen in the neonatal intensive care unit (NICU) and ask the reader to make clinical decisions. Along with the description of the course of the patient, we also present current evidence for and the pitfalls of the definition, diagnosis, and management of neonatal hypotension and provide some data on clinically relevant outcome measures. Last, supplanting the case with additional information, we hope the reader arrives at a logical, reasonable, and pathophysiology-focused treatment plan.

CASE STUDY 1

An 805-gram male preterm infant was born at 24½ weeks' gestation via vaginal delivery. The pregnancy was complicated by preterm, prolonged rupture of membranes (PPROM), without clinical signs of chorioamnionitis or excessive vaginal bleeding. The infant emerged apneic and limp with a heart rate less than 60 beats per minute. Positive pressure ventilation was begun immediately and the patient received chest compressions for about 1 minute. After stabilization in the delivery room, the patient was transferred to the NICU for further management with diagnoses of extreme prematurity, suspected perinatal depression, and respiratory distress syndrome.

In the NICU, initial arterial blood gas (ABG) values were determined as follows: pH of 7.05, $PaCO_2$ of 92 mmHg, PaO_2 of 102 mmHg, bicarbonate of 25 mEq/L, and base deficit of 5 mEq/L.

The patient was initially ventilated with a conventional ventilator on relatively high settings with a fractional inspired oxygen concentration (FiO_2) of 0.35. The chest x-ray was consistent with respiratory distress syndrome and a dose of surfactant was administered. Because of a persistent respiratory acidosis, the infant was then placed on high-frequency oscillatory ventilation (HFOV) with subsequent normalization of blood gases. Umbilical arterial and venous catheters were successfully inserted. Maintenance fluid administration with 10% dextrose-water and amino acids was started at a rate of 120 mL/kg/day. At 12 hours of age, the ABG showed a pH of 7.35, $PaCO_2$ of 37 mmHg, PaO_2 of 47 mmHg, bicarbonate of 20 mEq/L, and base deficit of 6 mEq/L. Systolic, diastolic, and mean blood pressures were 31, 25, and 28 mmHg, respectively, and the capillary refill time (CRT) was less than 2 seconds. The infant's hematocrit was 47%.

EXERCISE 1

QUESTION

1. What is the most appropriate course of action to improve this infant's hemodynamic status?
   a. No intervention and continue to monitor closely.
   b. Give a 10 to 20 mL/kg normal saline bolus.
   c. Start dobutamine drip at 5 mcg/kg/min and titrate.
   d. Start dopamine drip at 2 mcg/kg/min and titrate.
   e. Start epinephrine drip at 0.025 mcg/kg/min and titrate.

ANSWER

1. From our experience, many physicians would continue to monitor the patient closely perhaps because of the reassuring mean blood pressure reading and CRT. However, before we commit to an option, let us examine what determines systemic blood pressure and explore how "normal" blood pressure is commonly defined.

DETERMINANTS OF BLOOD PRESSURE

In fundamental fluid mechanics, pressure within a tube is described by Ohm's law:

$$\text{Pressure Gradient} = \text{Flow} \times \text{Resistance}$$

Applying this equation to the cardiovascular system, the equation becomes:

$$\text{Mean Blood Pressure} - \text{Right Atrial Pressure} =$$
$$\text{Cardiac Output} \times \text{Systemic Vascular Resistance}$$

Thus, blood pressure (the dependent variable) is the product of two independent variables: cardiac output and systemic vascular resistance (SVR). The heart pumps a certain volume of blood per minute (cardiac output = stroke volume × heart rate) into the arterial bed, where it meets a given resistance. Stroke volume is determined by preload, contractility, and afterload and the heart rate is affected by a number of factors including but not restricted to autonomic sympathetic-parasympathetic balance, catecholamine production and release, and temperature. Adequate circulating blood volume and ventricular compliance are necessary for appropriate filling of the heart chambers during diastole resulting in the generation of necessary sarcomere stretch prior to ventricular contraction. The Frank-Starling law describes sarcomere length-dependent changes of cardiac contractility, where increased preload, up to a certain point, improves myocardial contractility (Figure 15-1). During systole, SVR contributes to afterload as the heart has to generate a pressure to overcome the resistance and produce forward flow. In addition to the blood pressure generated, afterload is directly determined by the diameter and is inversely related to the thickness of the left ventricle. An increase in afterload shifts the Frank-Starling curve and decreases stroke volume (Figure 15-2, *A* and *B*).

A number of etiologic factors have been suggested to cause hypotension and circulatory compromise in preterm neonates during the first 24 hours ("early postnatal transitional period") (Noori, Stavroudis, & Seri, 2012). These factors include abnormal regulation of vascular tone, relative adrenal insufficiency, and the inability of the immature myocardium to adapt to the sudden increase in SVR, especially when the cord is clamped immediately after delivery. In addition, in patients with immediate cord clamping, the lack of transfusion of additional blood from the placenta also results in a suboptimal intravascular volume status, further compromising cardiovascular transition in this vulnerable patient

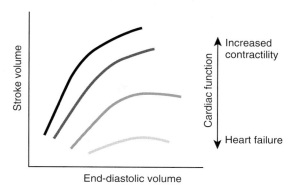

FIGURE 15-1 ■ **Frank-Starling curves of the heart represented as the relationship between end-diastolic volume and stroke volume.** In a normal heart stroke volume increases with increases in end-diastolic volume (sarcomere stretch). However, in a heart with depressed function, the Frank-Starling curve shifts downward and to the right and increases in end-diastolic volume only minimally augment stroke volume. (From Hanft LM, Korte FS, McDonald KS: Cardiac function and modulation of sarcomeric function by length, *Cardiovasc Res* 77[4]:627-636, 2008.)

population (Garofalo & Abenhaim, 2012; Rabe et al., 2012).

From the equation based on Ohm's law, we can appreciate that when cardiac output changes, the infant can still maintain blood pressure in the normal range by adjusting the SVR in the opposite direction. Accordingly, and based on the compensatory capacity of the immature cardiovascular system to maintain blood pressure in the given patient, we can classify the hemodynamic status of a newborn into four major categories:

1. Cardiac dysfunction *with* compensatory increase in vasomotor tone
2. Cardiac dysfunction *without* adequate compensation in vasomotor tone
3. Vasomotor dysregulation leading to vasodilation *with* compensation in cardiac output
4. Vasomotor dysregulation leading to vasodilation *without* adequate compensation in cardiac output (Figure 15-3)

Please note that we did not include the absolute volume status of the patient in the classification and that hypotension only manifests if cardiac output or vasomotor tone does not adequately adjust in compensation. In addition, we must emphasize that in a number of patients, the compensatory increase in vasomotor tone might result in compromised systemic blood flow despite "normal" blood pressure values. On the other hand, in patients with vasomotor dysregulation, the compensatory increase in cardiac

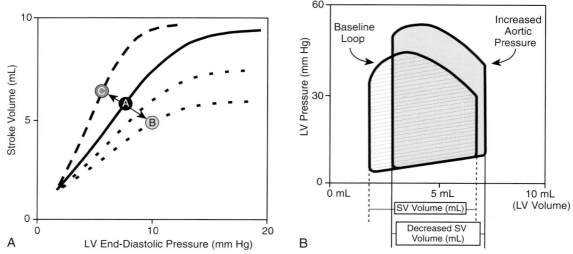

FIGURE 15-2 ■ Depiction of the effect of increasing afterload (represented by aortic pressure) on the left ventricle end-diastolic pressure–stroke volume relationship (Frank-Starling curves; **A**) and the left ventricle volume–pressure relationship (volume-pressure loop; **B**) adjusted for the neonatal heart with heart rate, inotropy, and left ventricle wall thickness held constant. A shift in the stroke volume–LV end-diastolic pressure relationship from A to B and A to C occurs with increased and decreased afterload, respectively (**A**). In **B**, the baseline (control) volume pressure loop is depicted by the stripes and the shift in and change of the pressure-volume loop in response to the change in afterload is shown in gray. The decrease in stroke volume and the increase in end-diastolic and end-systolic left ventricle pressure in response to the increased afterload are represented by the right and upward shift and narrowing of the pressure volume loop (**B**). (Modified from Klabunde RA: Effects of preload, afterload, and inotropy on ventricular pressure-volume loops. In Klabunde RA, editors: *Cardiovascular physiology concepts.* ed 2, Philadelphia, PA, 2011, Lippincott Williams & Wilkins. http://www.cvphysiology.com/Cardiac%20Function/CF025.htm.)

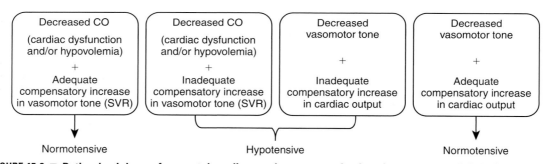

FIGURE 15-3 ■ **Pathophysiology of neonatal cardiovascular compromise in primary myocardial dysfunction and primary abnormal vascular tone regulation with or without compensation by the unaffected other variable.** This figure illustrates why blood pressure can remain in the "normal" range when there is appropriate compensatory increase in either vasomotor tone or cardiac output. In the hypotensive scenarios, there is inadequate compensatory increase in these variables. *CO,* Cardiac output.

output might result in adequate organ blood flow despite blood pressure values in the perceived "hypotensive" range.

NORMATIVE BLOOD PRESSURE DATA

A number of investigators have reported population-based normal ranges of blood pressure values based on gestational age, postnatal age, or birth weight. The majority of the data support the notion that larger and more mature infants

have higher blood pressures. In addition, blood pressure increases with postnatal age (Table 15-1) (Watkins, West, & Cooke, 1989). One common clinical practice is to consider the minimum acceptable mean blood pressure value to equal the gestational age of the infant. This rather simplistic but practical approach is based on the 1992 recommendations from the Joint Working Group of the British Association of Perinatal Medicine ("Development of audit measures and guidelines...", 1992). However, there is no evidence to support the validity and/or clinical relevance of this practice. Others will advocate the

TABLE 15-1 Average Mean Blood Pressure (MBP) and the 10th Percentile MBP for 131 Very Low Birth Weight Infants Throughout the First 3 Days of Postnatal Life (MBP/10th Percentile of MBP)

Birth Weight (g)	Time (h) Postnatal Age								
	3	12	24	36	48	60	72	84	96
500	35/23	36/24	37/25	38/26	39/28	41/29	42/30	43/31	44/33
600	35/24	36/25	37/26	39/27	40/28	41/29	42/31	44/32	45/33
700	36/24	37/25	38/26	39/28	42/29	42/30	43/31	44/32	45/34
800	36/25	37/26	39/27	40/28	41/29	42/31	44/32	45/33	46/34
900	37/25	38/26	39/27	40/29	42/30	43/31	44/32	45/34	47/35
1000	38/26	39/27	40/28	41/29	42/31	43/32	45/33	46/34	47/35
1100	38/27	39/37	40/29	42/30	43/31	44/32	45/34	46/35	48/36
1200	39/27	40/28	41/29	42/30	43/32	45/33	46/34	47/35	48/37
1300	39/28	40/29	41/30	43/31	44/32	45/33	46/35	48/36	49/37
1400	40/28	42/29	42/30	43/32	44/33	46/34	47/35	48/36	49/38
1500	40/29	42/30	43/31	44/32	45/33	46/35	48/36	49/37	50/38

Numbers refer to average MBP/tenth percentile for MBP.
From Watkins AMC, West CR, Cooke RWI: Blood pressure and cerebral haemorrhage and ischaemia in very low birthweight infants, Early Hum Develop *19:103-110,1989.*

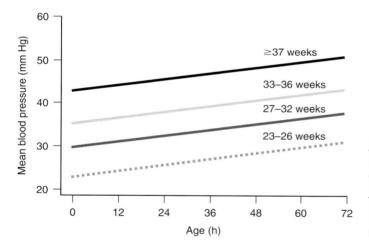

FIGURE 15-4 ■ **Mean blood pressure (two-tail, 80% confidence interval) in 103 infants born at gestational ages of 23 to 43 weeks during the first 72 postnatal hours; the higher the gestational and postnatal age, the higher the mean blood pressure.** (From Nuntnarumit P, Yang W, Bada-Ellzey HS: Blood pressure measurements in the newborn, *Clin Perinatol* 26:981, 1999.)

use of population-based norms as the accepted blood pressure range (Figure 15-4) (Nuntnarumit, Yang, & Bada-Ellzey, 1999). Finally, based on the presumptive lower elbow of the cerebral blood flow autoregulatory range, others have proposed the use of 28 to 30 mmHg as the critical lower limit of acceptable blood pressure in preterm infants during the immediate transitional period. Furthermore, it has been suggested that at mean arterial pressure below 28 to 30 mmHg, the compromised and pressure passive cerebral blood flow contributes to the occurrence of intraventricular hemorrhage and periventricular leukomalacia. However, a high level of evidence supporting this notion is lacking.

From these differing approaches, one can easily see why it has become extremely difficult to appropriately define neonatal hypotension and

to reach a general consensus on blood pressure management in the preterm neonate. The main reason for the confusion in defining neonatal hypotension is the simple fact that aside from heart rate, blood pressure is the only continuously and routinely monitored hemodynamic variable. As blood pressure is the dependent variable in the equation determining systemic blood flow (CO = BP / SVR), a clinically relevant definition of hypotension and its treatment cannot be solely based on the blood pressure value. Indeed, evidence from randomized control studies is lacking on clinically relevant outcome measures of treatment of preterm infants with mean arterial pressures below gestational and postgestational age-dependent norms. Even more concerning are the findings of a recent study indicating that conducting such a randomized control trial might not be feasible in the United States primarily because of the difficulties in obtaining parental consent in a timely manner and because of the significant bias among neonatologists for how to manage preterm neonates with hypotension (Batton et al., 2012). On the other hand, a number of studies have found an association between early hypotension and subsequent peri/intraventricular hemorrhage (P/IVH) and poor neurodevelopmental outcome in premature infants. Of note, although the association between early postnatal hypotension and subsequent brain injury has been established, causation remains to be proven.

In summary, ensuring that the patient's blood pressure is in the "normal range" may be falsely reassuring, as blood pressure might be in the normal range while systemic and especially end-organ perfusion is compromised. This notion brings us to the discussion of monitoring and treating low blood pressure versus low systemic/organ blood flow. Which approach is a more impactful predictor of outcome and how do they correlate with each other?

BLOOD PRESSURE VERSUS BLOOD FLOW: WHICH ONE IS A BETTER PREDICTOR FOR OUTCOME?

As discussed earlier, blood pressure has traditionally been the conventional determinant of initiating clinical intervention in the newborn with cardiovascular compromise. It is readily obtainable and frequently monitored invasively in the critical care setting. Blood pressure obtained through the umbilical arterial catheter and peripheral arterial line strongly correlate with one another with values approaching of 0.98 for systolic pressure and 0.97 for diastolic pressure (Butt & Whyte, 1984). The correlation between noninvasive oscillometric measurements and invasive blood pressure measurements is also acceptable provided that appropriate cuff size is being used (0.45 to 0.55 cuff width-to-arm ratio), adequate pain control is provided, and there is an absence of movements or procedures (Dannevig et al., 2005; Emery & Greenough, 1993) during the measurements.

As stated earlier, a common pitfall among clinicians is the assumption that normal blood pressure translates to normal flow to the organs. Yet, blood pressure in the perceived normal range does not always imply normal systemic or organ blood flow. In the first 12 hours after delivery, very preterm infants are likely to be in the "compensated phase" of shock, where neuroendocrine compensatory mechanisms maintain normal blood flow to the vital organs (brain, heart, and adrenal glands) while nonvital organ blood flow and overall systemic blood flow are decreased. Of the very low birth weight (VLBW) infants who present initially with normal blood pressure and low systemic blood flow, up to 80% will eventually fail to compensate and go on to develop low blood pressures considered by many as hypotension. Indeed, Kluckow and Evans found a poor correlation between mean blood pressure and left ventricular output (LVO) in preterm infants, even with a closed ductus arteriosus during the first 24 hours after delivery (r = 0.38) (Figure 15-5) (Kluckow & Evans, 1996). Thus, relying on blood pressure alone may result in unnecessary treatment in certain situations or a delay in initiating treatment in a timely manner in others.

As for the correlation between systemic blood flow during the immediate postnatal period and morbidity and long-term outcomes, data are mostly available from studies where superior vena cava (SVC) flow was used as a surrogate of systemic blood flow. Although assessment of SVC flow has its technical limitations and thus requires a large number of patients to be included in a given study, its use as a surrogate of systemic blood flow is an intuitively reasonable approach in patients with the fetal channels open. Indeed, a significant association between low SVC flow and P/IVH and abnormal neurodevelopment at 3 years of age has been found. The same group of researchers also found no effect of treatment of low SVC flow with dopamine or dobutamine on death and neurodevelopmental disability compared to group of preterm neonates with normal SVC flow (Osborn et al., 2007). However, because the study did not include a nontreated control group with low SVC flow, used fixed doses of inotropes without titration to an optimum hemodynamic effect, and utilized SVC flow as a surrogate of systemic blood flow, the findings must be viewed with caution.

Now we will turn our attention to the currently available clinical tools to directly or indirectly evaluate systemic and end-organ perfusion along with the limitations of these approaches.

INDIRECT MEASURES OF ORGAN PERFUSION

Clinical findings of hypotension and compromised organ blood flow can manifest as decreased capillary refill time (CRT), development of lactic acidosis, and/or decreased/absent urine output. These are often incorporated into routine physical exams by the astute physician in the assessment of the hemodynamic status of the newborn.

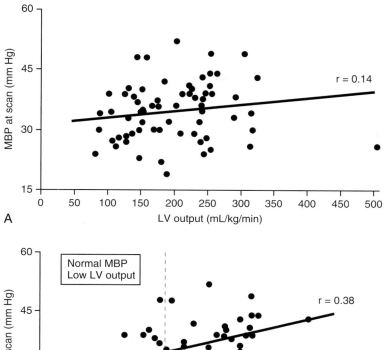

FIGURE 15-5 ■ Scatterplots illustrating the poor correlation between mean blood pressure (*MBP*) and left ventricular output (*LVO*) in 67 preterm infants requiring ventilation **(A)** and in 45 preterm infants with closed ductus arteriosus **(B)**. (From Kluckow M, Evans N: Relationship between blood pressure and cardiac output in preterm infants requiring mechanical ventilation, *J Pediatr* 129[4]:506-512, 1996.)

Capillary Refill Time

CRT (seconds) is assessed by pressing the skin for 3 to 5 seconds and then measuring the time it takes for the capillary bed to refill and for the skin to return to its baseline color. The forehead and sternum are considered the most appropriate and reliable sites for measurement of CRT and a value of >3 seconds is generally considered as abnormal. CRT in the newborn does not correlate with blood pressure and has poor sensitivity and specificity in the detection of decreased systemic blood flow. Thus, in our case, the normal CRT might be reassuring, but does not necessarily mean that systemic flow was indeed normal. Various factors are at play, including the site of assessment, duration of digital pressure, skin maturity, skin and ambient temperature, interobserver variability, presence of compensated shock, and medications. In a study of 128 infants less than 30 weeks' gestation a CRT of 3 seconds only had a 55% sensitivity and 81% specificity in detecting low SVC blood flow (<41 mL/kg/min). The sensitivity improved to 78% when a CRT of <3 seconds was combined with a mean blood pressure of <30 mmHg (Osborn, Evans, & Kluckow, 2004).

Lactic Acidosis

When organ blood flow has decreased to a critical level, tissue hypoxia occurs and anaerobic metabolism ensues, resulting in increased production of lactic acid. The finding of lactic acidosis (>2.5 mmol/L) is thus a relatively late finding in neonatal circulatory compromise, and the associated decrease in pH must be differentiated from metabolic acidosis secondary to renal or, less frequently, enteral bicarbonate wasting of the preterm neonate. In severe circulatory collapse, lactic acid may accumulate primarily in the severely underperfused tissue bed and not be evident in the centralized systemic circulation. In that situation, the severity of acidosis initially might not be fully appreciated by the clinician. Thus, following the resuscitation of these patients, lactic acidosis might first increase despite signs of improved tissue oxygen delivery. In addition, one needs to be aware that when epinephrine is administered to manage neonatal cardiovascular compromise, lactic acid production will increase independent of the circulatory status and the patient's response to the treatment. This occurs because epinephrine enhances hepatic glycogenolysis and glycolysis, via its selective beta-2 adrenoreceptor-mediated effects. Therefore, in the setting of hypotension treated by continuous infusion of epinephrine, lactic acid levels may become elevated and thus repeated assessment of lactic acidosis can no longer serve as an initial reliable surrogate measure of tissue hypoperfusion (Valverde et al., 2006).

Oliguria/Anuria

Similar to the development of lactic acidosis, decreased urine output is a relatively late and indirect sign of neonatal shock. As a filtering organ, the kidney receives around 20% of the cardiac output but it only requires approximately 5% to maintain cellular integrity and function. Thus, in the early, compensated phase of shock the kidney is among the nonvital organs with the most significant decrease in tissue perfusion. Unfortunately, as urine output significantly decreases following delivery in every neonate, changes in urine output are difficult to use as early indirect evidence of compensated shock in the preterm neonate during the first postnatal day(s). On the other hand, as the immature renal tubules are unable to reabsorb solutes and water appropriately, the developmentally regulated glomerulotubular imbalance might result in relatively higher urine output even in the face of decreased glomerular filtration rate. Therefore, as with lactic acid measurements, it requires repeated assessment of urine output and serum creatinine values along with a thorough understanding of developmental renal physiology to fully understand the renal response to cardiovascular compromise in the preterm neonate during the first postnatal days.

DIRECT MEASURES OF ORGAN PERFUSION BY BEDSIDE EQUIPMENT

Assessment of systemic blood flow and organ blood flow distribution is a complex and difficult undertaking especially because cardiovascular changes are dynamic in nature. Many factors can alter systemic and organ blood flow in seconds, including changes in tissue oxygen delivery and metabolic demand for oxygen, developmentally regulated changes in vital organ assignment, medications, volume and type of fluid administration, and so forth. Therefore, it is not sufficient to obtain single measurements periodically. Rather, the cardiovascular status needs to be continuously evaluated if possible or, at least, with multiple data points over time. In addition the physician must take into account the clinical context and the changes in the patient's condition.

CASE SUMMARY AND ADDITIONAL HEMODYNAMIC INFORMATION

Case Summary

- 24½-week gestation, 805-grams very preterm neonate born after PPROM without evidence of chorioamnionitis or bleeding
- Emerged depressed and required resuscitation including chest compressions
- Received surfactant and during the first postnatal hours was transitioned from conventional mechanical ventilation to HFOV due to respiratory compromise
- At 12 hours of age patient had mild metabolic acidosis on ABG (pH of 7.35, $PaCO_2$ of 37 mmHg, PaO_2 of 47 mmHg, bicarbonate of 20 mEq/L, and base deficit of 6 mEq/L) and his systolic, diastolic, and mean blood pressures were 31, 25, and 28 mmHg, respectively. His CRT was less than 2 seconds and his hematocrit was 47%.

Additional Hemodynamic Information

To more objectively and directly assess the infant's cardiovascular status (Lemson, Nusmeier, & van der Hoeven, 2011; Soleymani et al., 2012), an echocardiogram (Figure 15-6) was performed at bedside. The study revealed poor myocardial contractility, minimal septal and posterior left ventricular wall movement, and a shortening fraction of 20% (normal 28% to 44%). In addition, right ventricular output (RVO) was diminished at 49 mL/kg/min (normal 150 to 300 mL/kg/min). Let us interpret the echocardiography findings first.

Shortening fraction (SF) is a measure of left ventricular (LV) systolic function and is calculated as follows:

$$SF\,(\%) = \frac{\left(\begin{array}{l} LV\ end\ diastolic\ diameter - \\ LV\ end\ systolic\ diameter \end{array}\right)}{LV\ end\ diastolic\ diameter} \times 100$$

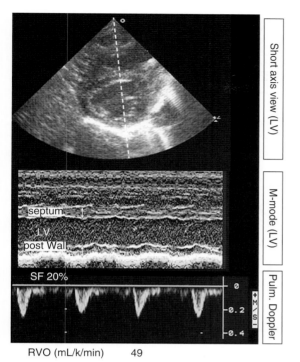

Short axis view (LV)

M-mode (LV)

Pulm. Doppler

septum

LV
post Wall

SF 20%

RVO (mL/k/min)   49

FIGURE 15-6 ■ Bedside echocardiography of case patient on the first postnatal day. There was minimal septal and left ventricular posterior wall movement. Shortening fraction (SF = 20%) and right cardiac output (RVO = 49 mL/kg/min) were depressed. Normal SF = 28% to 44% and RVO = 150 to 300 mL/kg/min.

Normal SF ranges between 28% and 44%, but in extremely preterm infants, especially in early postnatal period, a value in low 20s may be normal. However, this measure is affected by both preload and afterload and thus values below the normal range may indicate intrinsic myocardial dysfunction and/or changes in the loading condition of the heart.

RVO may first appear to the reader as a measurement of blood flow to the pulmonary circulation. However, it is also a measure of the blood flow returning to the right side of the heart from the rest of the body. Therefore, in the absence of a significant atrial shunting, RVO also represents systemic blood flow. In the newborn, especially the preterm infant during the transitional period, LVO is not a reliable measure of systemic blood flow due to the presence of shunting through the patent ductus arteriosus (PDA) and/or the foramen ovale. In the presence of left-to-right shunting through the PDA, LVO will overestimate true systemic blood flow, as a portion of the LVO is shunted through the ductus to the pulmonary circulation. Thus, in the presence of a left-to-right shunting at the PDA, LVO becomes a measure for both systemic and

pulmonary blood flow. In patients with left-to-right shunting across the PDA, assessment of RVO or SVC flow is believed to be a better measure of systemic blood flow. However, both techniques have their significant technical and pathophysiology-related limitations. For instance, significant left-to-right shunting through the foramen ovale renders RVO a less appropriate measure of systemic flow. The reader can better appreciate the complexity of the concept described here by looking at the schematic diagram in Figure 15-7.

In summary, based on the principles of cardiovascular physiology and assessment of the available data we conclude that relying on blood pressure *or* blood flow *alone* cannot provide the necessary information for the clinician on which the diagnosis and treatment of neonatal cardiovascular compromise can be based. Rather, using *both* blood pressure *and* the available direct and indirect measures of systemic and organ blood flow holds the promise to facilitate the timely diagnosis and initiation of appropriate, pathophysiology-driven treatment of neonatal shock. However, it must be emphasized that efficacy of any intervention must be assessed by *both* its short-term hemodynamic benefits *and* its impact on long-term neurodevelopmental outcome.

DISCUSSION OF ANSWERS

Let us now see how the additional information affects the reader's clinical decision-making process:

Choice a. "No intervention, continue close monitoring."

This choice may appear appropriate after the initial case presentation with the reassuring routinely monitored hemodynamic variables such as blood pressure, CRT, and urine output. However, even without the availability of echocardiography, careful analysis of the history should raise suspicion for possible myocardial dysfunction. During resuscitation, the need for chest compressions places the patient at a high risk for myocardial dysfunction secondary to ischemic injury. In addition, the narrow pulse pressure (31–25 = 6 mmHg) should have raised significant concerns, as it can be a sign of low stroke volume. The changes in arterial blood pressure throughout the cardiac cycle are primarily determined by the stroke volume and the compliance of the aorta. In simplified terms, the diastolic arterial pressure of the newborn is closely related to SVR, while the systolic arterial pressure is related to the stroke volume because the compliance of aorta only changes minimally.

Assessment of Systemic Blood Flow during
Transition (1-24 hours)

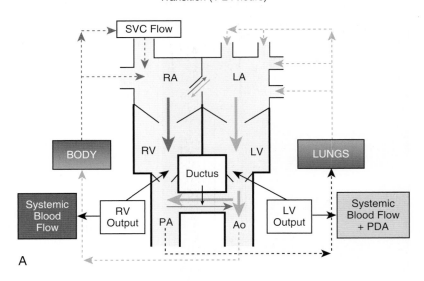

A

Assessment of Systemic Blood Flow during
Transition (24-72 postnatal hours)

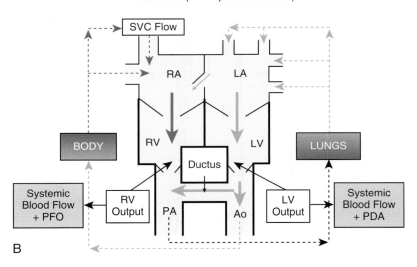

B

FIGURE 15-7 ■ Blood flow diagrams during 1 to 24 hours (**A**) and 24 to 72 hours (**B**) after delivery. Please note that in the presence of a patent ductus arteriosus (*PDA*) and absence of significant atrial shunting, right ventricular (*RV*) output represents systemic blood flow and left ventricular (*LV*) output represents blood flow returning through the left atrium to the left ventricle and distributed between the pulmonary (via the left-to-right PDA flow) and systemic circulation.

If now we add the findings of the echocardiography study to our analytical process, it becomes even more evident that the patient might benefit from receiving inotropic support. The poor myocardial contractility and decreased RVO (i.e., the surrogate measure of systemic blood flow) indicate that it is prudent to intervene before systemic hypoperfusion leads to ischemic cellular injury. In this case, the treating physician chose to continue to monitor the patient clinically. Cardiac function spontaneously improved by 72 hours after birth (Figure 15-8); however, a bilateral grade four P/IVH was detected at this time. Although clearly we do not have the evidence that early

initiation and careful titration of inotropic support with dobutamine (Martinez, Padbury, & Thio, 1992; Robel-Tillig et al., 2007) would have necessarily altered the course, it is reasonable to assume that this patient was at a very high risk for developing P/IVH because of his extreme prematurity, the perinatal depression, and the resultant myocardial dysfunction. The initial tissue ischemia caused by the myocardial dysfunction was then followed by improvement in systemic perfusion upon recovery of the cardiovascular status, resulting in reperfusion of the organs including the brain. The hypoperfusion-reperfusion cycle may be important in the pathogenesis of P/IVH.

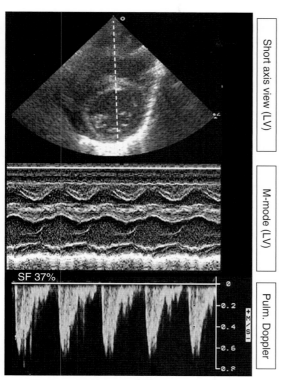

Short axis view (LV)

M-mode (LV)

Pulm. Doppler

SF 37%

RVO (mL/k/min)   228

FIGURE 15-8 ■ **Bedside echocardiography of case patient at 72 hours of postnatal life**. Although the patient did not received inotropic support, both shortening fraction (SF = 37%) and right ventricular output both normalized (RVO = 228 mL/kg/min) by the third postnatal day.

Choice b. "Give a 10 TO 20 mL/kg normal saline bolus."

Although absolute hypovolemia is the most common cause of hypotension in the pediatric patient population, decreased circulating blood volume does not appear to be the primary cause of early hypotension in most preterm neonates. This assumption is supported by the lack of a significant correlation between blood volume (measured by indocyanine green dye dilution method) and mean arterial blood pressure in preterm neonates during the first postnatal day (Wright & Goodall, 1994). Dopamine administration has also been found to be more effective than volume administration in the treatment of early hypotension in the preterm newborn (Lundstrøm, Pryds, & Greisen, 2000). Thus, these findings suggest that hypovolemia is unlikely to be a main cause of hypotension in the early transitional period, especially in the absence of acute blood loss or increased urine output. However, as discussed earlier, delayed cord clamping improves cardiovascular adaptation in preterm infants in part by increasing circulating blood volume. Therefore,

hypovolemia might yet be one of the *contributing factors* to the pathogenesis of early hypotension in many preterm neonates. It is unclear whether, in the absence of delayed cord clamping, early and careful use of blood transfusions can mimic the beneficial hemodynamic effects of delayed cord clamping. However, there are a number of proposed additional benefits of delayed cord clamping, such as transfusion of the patient's own blood rich in stem cells, which clearly cannot be achieved using the postnatal transfusion approach. Finally, it is important to note that excessive volume administration can negatively impact myocardial contractility, increase edema formation, and decrease ventilation and oxygenation.

Choices c, d, and e. Start dobutamine (c), dopamine (d) and epinephrine (e) and titrate as appropriate.

Before selecting your drug of choice, it will be worthwhile to review the mechanisms of actions of each medication (Table 15-2) (Noori & Seri, 2012).

Dobutamine is a synthetic catecholamine and is classified as an inotrope because of its predominant β-adrenergic cardiac effects with less prominent β-adrenergic vascular and minimal α_1-adrenergic effects. Thus, dobutamine significantly increases myocardial contractility and also provides some afterload relief. However, it should be noted that especially at higher doses, dobutamine might impair diastolic function. *Dopamine* is a naturally occurring catecholamine classified as a vasopressor-inotrope. Dopamine exerts complex dose-dependent vascular, myocardial, renal, and endocrine effects and, owing to developmentally regulated differences in cardiovascular adrenergic receptor expression, its dose-response curve differs in neonates from that seen in adults. At low doses, dopamine stimulates dopamine receptors (≥0.5 μg/kg/min) to induce primarily renal and mesenteric vasodilatation, direct renal tubular epithelial actions, and complex endocrine effects. At low-medium doses of dopamine (≥2 to 4 μg/kg/min), cardiovascular effects of vascular α-1 adrenoreceptor stimulation become apparent via increases in SVR and mild increase in myocardial contractility. Finally, at somewhat higher doses (4 to 8 μg/kg/min), the drug-induced stimulation of the β-1 and β-2 adrenoreceptors results in increased myocardial contractility and heart rate; thus cardiac output increases. At even higher doses of dopamine, the α-1 adrenoreceptor stimulation-induced peripheral vasoconstriction predominates. This can result in significant peripheral vasoconstriction, an increase in afterload and blood pressure, with variable and sometimes negative effects on

TABLE 15-2   **Estimated Relative Cardiovascular Receptor Stimulatory Effects of Inotropes, Lusitropes, and Vasopressors**

| | Adrenergic, Dopaminergic, and Vasopressin Receptors | | | | | |
| | α_1/α_2 | β_2 | α_1 | β_1/β_2 | DA_1/DA_2 | V_{1a} |
	VASCULAR	VASCULAR	CARDIAC	CARDIAC	VASCULAR/CARDIAC	VASCULAR
Phenylephrine	++++	0	+	0	0	0
Norepinephrine	++++	+/0	++	++++	0	0
Epinephrine	++++	++++	++	++++	0	0
Dopamine*	++++	++	++	+++	++++	0
Dobutamine[†]	+/0	++	++	++++	0	0
Isoprenaline	0	+++	0	++++	0	0
Vasopressin	0	0	0	0	0	++++
PDE-III inhibitors	0	0	0	0	0	0
PDE-V inhibitors	0	0	0	0	0	0

From Noori S, Seri I: Neonatal blood pressure support: the use of inotropes, lusitropes, and other vasopressor agents, Clin Perinatol 39(1):221-238, 2012.

$\alpha_1/\alpha_2/\beta_1/\beta_2$, Subtypes of α- and β-adrenoreceptors; DA, dopamine; DOB, dobutamine; PDE, phosphodiesterase enzymes; PDE-III inhibitors used in neonates, amrinone, milrinone; PDE-V inhibitors used in neonates, sildenafil; V_{1a}, vasopressin reception expressed in the vasculature.
*Dopamine also has serotoninergic actions.
[†]Efficacy of dobutamine is independent of its affinity for adrenoreceptors.

systemic blood flow. Keep in mind that the above dosing effects may not necessarily hold true in the critically ill premature infant, owing to the immature cardiovascular system, the developmentally regulated differences in cardiovascular adrenoreceptor expression, and relative adrenocortical insufficiency (Noori & Seri, 2012; Seri, 1995). Epinephrine is a vasopressor-inotrope that has direct β-adrenergic myocardial and vascular effects at lower doses (0.01 to 0.1 µg/kg/min) and strong α-adrenergic effects at medium to high doses (>0.1 µg/kg/min). Thus, epinephrine administration results in significant increases in myocardial contractility and cardiac output and peripheral vascular resistance and blood pressure. However, one must keep in mind that inappropriately high doses of vasopressor inotropes (dopamine, epinephrine, and norepinephrine) might induce an overwhelming increase in systemic vascular resistance, potentially resulting in decreased systemic blood flow. On the other hand, by decreasing myocardial compliance, high doses of dobutamine might decrease ventricular filling and thus cardiac output.

In our case, there was evidence of significant myocardial dysfunction on echocardiogram with an adequate compensatory increase in vascular resistance to maintain mean blood pressure in the "normal" range resulting, however, in a severely compromised systemic blood flow. Because dobutamine is a pure inotrope with mild peripheral vasodilatory effects, it has the best hemodynamic profile to enhance myocardial contractility

without increasing afterload. Thus dobutamine should effectively increase cardiac output and organ blood flow in this infant and *is the most appropriate medication to provide hemodynamic support*. However, it remains to be proven whether the use of a dobutamine infusion in a "normotensive" very preterm neonate with myocardial dysfunction and resultant systemic hypoperfusion will decrease the incidence of brain injury.

Dopamine and epinephrine both can be helpful in improving cardiac output in patients with shock caused primarily by excessive vasodilation with or without myocardial dysfunction. However, the vasoconstrictive effects of these medications, especially at higher doses, can be counterproductive by increasing left ventricular afterload and decreasing systemic perfusion.

Although milrinone was not included as a choice among the answers, it might be a drug to be considered in the case described in this chapter. Milrinone is a lusitrope with documented positive inotropic effects in infants, children, and adults. However, because milrinone might not have a significant positive inotropic effect in preterm or term neonates during the first postnatal days and it has been found ineffective in very preterm neonates with compromised systemic blood flow during the first postnatal day, its routine use in the clinical practice in preterm neonates in the immediate postnatal period cannot be recommended at present.

Finally, a number of studies have found that in preterm infants with cardiovascular compromise not responding to conventional doses of vasopressor-inotropes, administration of low doses of steroids is followed by increases in blood pressure (Helbock, Insoft, & Conte, 1993; Ng et al., 2006; Seri, Tan, & Evans, 2001) and improvement in systemic and organ blood flow (Noori et al., 2006). The genomic and nongenomic effects of gluco- and mineralocorticoids (Biniwale, Sardesai, & Seri, 2013; Seri, Tan, & Evans, 2001) and the documented high incidence of relative adrenal insufficiency of preterm infants are thought to explain these findings (Ng et al., 2004). As exposure of the preterm neonate to even low doses of dexamethasone during the postnatal first days and weeks is associated with long-term neurodevelopmental sequelae, low-dose hydrocortisone, thought to be devoid of such effects, has been used and perhaps overused to treat hypotension and cardiovascular compromise in very preterm neonates during the transitional period. However, low-dose hydrocortisone is not devoid of side effects. Most concerning is the significant increase in spontaneous ileal perforations, especially when hydrocortisone is coadministered with indomethacin or ibuprofen (Attrdige et al., 2006; Watterberg et al., 2004). In the present case, where myocardial dysfunction was the primary underlying etiology of the cardiovascular compromise, exposure to low-dose hydrocortisone only would have been considered if myocardial function had not improved following dobutamine administration.

CONCLUSION

As discussed in this chapter, treatment of hypotension and circulatory compromise in the premature newborn is complicated and the clinician should not focus solely on blood pressure findings to guide management. First, the gestational- and postnatal-age–dependent normal range of blood pressure is not well defined in preterm infants during the first postnatal days. In addition, there is no evidence that treatment of neonatal "hypotension" affects clinically relevant long-term outcome measures. Blood pressure in the perceived normal range can also be falsely reassuring because the infant may be in the early, "compensated" phase of shock. On the other hand, low blood pressure does not always imply poor organ perfusion because myocardial compensation may provide for appropriate organ blood flow even at relatively lower perfusion pressures. Thus it is no wonder that no consensus exists on the diagnosis and treatment of early hypotension in the preterm infant.

Based on the available evidence and the principles of cardiovascular physiology briefly presented in this chapter, the authors advocate that both blood pressure and indirect and/or direct measures of systemic and organ blood flow be taken into consideration when decision about the initiation of treatment of suspected shock in preterm neonates is being considered. Accordingly, in routine clinical care blood pressure should be used as one of the screening tools for cardiovascular compromise and the indirect clinical and laboratory signs of systemic and organ blood flow such as CRT, urine output, and lactic acidosis should be incorporated in assessment of cardiovascular function. Unfortunately, as our case demonstrated, clinical assessment of cardiovascular function is not always reliable and additional tools such as functional echocardiography are necessary in many cases to complement the physical examination. Finally, we urge the physician to have a high index of suspicion for myocardial dysfunction in neonates born with a perinatal insult such as described in the case. On the other hand, in neonates with perinatal infection, a high index of suspicion for poor vascular tone regulation should be considered and these patients might respond to carefully titrated dopamine or epinephrine treatment. A bedside echocardiogram may help to assess the suspected underlying myocardial dysfunction, abnormal vasomotor tone regulation, or both and provide more objective information on the status of systemic and organ blood flow.

SUGGESTED READINGS

Attridge JT, Clark R, Walker MW, Gordon PV: New insights into spontaneous intestinal perforation using a national data set: (2) two populations of patients with perforations, *J Perinatol* 26(3):185–188, 2006.

Bada HS, Korones SB, Perry EH, Arheart KL, Ray JD, Pourcyrous M, et al.: Mean arterial blood pressure changes in premature infants and those at risk for intraventricular hemorrhage, *J Pediatr* 117(4):607–614, 1990.

Batton B, Batton D, Riggs T: Blood pressure during the first 7 days in premature infants born at postmenstrual age 23 to 25 weeks, *Am J Perinatol* 24(2):107–115, 2007.

Batton BJ, Li L, Newman NS, Das A, Watterberg KL, Yoder BA, et al.: Feasibility study of early blood pressure management in extremely preterm infants, *J Pediatr* 161(1):65–69, 2012. e1.

Biniwale M, Sardesai S, Seri I: Steroids and vasopressor-resistant hypotension, *Current Pediatric Reviews* 9:75–83, 2013.

Butt WW, Whyte H: Blood pressure monitoring in neonates: comparison of umbilical and peripheral artery catheter measurements, *J Pediatr* 105(4):630–632, 1984.

Cunningham S, Symon AG, Elton RA, Zhu C, McIntosh N: Intra-arterial blood pressure reference ranges, death and morbidity in very low birthweight infants during the first seven days of life, *Early Hum Dev* 56(2-3):151–165, 1999.

Dannevig I, Dale HC, Liestøl K, Lindemann R: Blood pressure in the neonate: three non-invasive oscillometric pressure monitors compared with invasively measured blood pressure, *Acta Paediatr* 94(2):191–196, 2005.

Dempsey EM, Barrington KJ: Evaluation and treatment of hypotension in the preterm infant, *Clin Perinatol* 36(1):75–85, 2009.

Development of audit measures and guidelines for good practice in the management of neonatal respiratory distress syndrome: Report of a Joint Working Group of the British Association of Perinatal Medicine and the Research Unit of the Royal College of Physicians, *Arch Dis Child* 67(10 Spec No):1221–1227, 1992.

Doyle L, Davis P: Postnatal corticosteroids in preterm infants: systematic review of effects on mortality and motor function, *J Paediatr Child Health* 36:101–107, 2000.

Eidem B, O'Leary P: Basic techniques. In Eidem B, Cetta F, O'Leary P, editors: *Echocardiography in pediatric and adult congenital heart disease*, Philadelphia, PA, 2010, Lippincott Williams & Wilkins, pp 29–47.

Emery EF, Greenough A: Assessment of non-invasive techniques for measuring blood pressure in preterm infants of birthweight less than or equal to 750 grams, *Early Hum Dev* 33(3):217–222, 1993.

Fanaroff JM, Wilson-Costello DE, Newman NS, Montpetite MM, Fanaroff AA: Treated hypotension is associated with neonatal morbidity and hearing loss in extremely low birth weight infants, *Pediatrics* 117(4):1131–1135, 2006.

Garofalo M, Abenhaim HA: Early versus delayed cord clamping in term and preterm births: a review, *J Obstet Gynaecol Can* 34(6):525–531, 2012.

Goldstein RF, Thompson RJ, Oehler JM, Brazy JE: Influence of acidosis, hypoxemia, and hypotension on neurodevelopmental outcome in very low birth weight infants, *Pediatrics* 95(2):238–243, 1995.

Greisen G: Autoregulation of vital and nonvital organ blood flow in the preterm and term neonate. In Kleinman C, Seri I, editors: *Neonatology questions and controversies: hemodynamics and cardiology*, 2nd ed, Philadelphia, PA, 2012, Saunders/Elsevier, pp 29–47.

Hanft LM, Korte FS, McDonald KS: Cardiac function and modulation of sarcomeric function by length, *Cardiovasc Res* 77(4):627–636, 2008.

Helbock HJ, Insoft RM, Conte FA: Glucocorticoid-responsive hypotension in extremely low birth weight newborns, *Pediatrics* 92:715–717, 1993.

Hunt RW, Evans N, Rieger I, Kluckow M: Low superior vena cava flow and neurodevelopment at 3 years in very preterm infants, *J Pediatr* 145(5):588–592, 2004.

Kanik E, Ozer EA, Bakiler AR, Aydinlioglu H, Dorak C, Dogrusoz B, et al.: Assessment of myocardial dysfunction in neonates with hypoxic-ischemic encephalopathy: is it a significant predictor of mortality? *J Matern Fetal Neonatal Med* 22(3):239–242, 2009.

Kluckow M, Evans N: Low superior vena cava flow and intraventricular haemorrhage in preterm infants, *Arch Dis Child Fetal Neonatal Ed* 82(3):F188–F194, 2000. a.

Kluckow M, Evans N: Relationship between blood pressure and cardiac output in preterm infants requiring mechanical ventilation, *J Pediatr* 129(4):506–512, 1996.

Kluckow M, Evans N: Superior vena cava flow in newborn infants: a novel marker of systemic blood flow, *Arch Dis Child Fetal Neonatal Ed* 82(3):F182–F187, 2000. b.

Kluckow M, Seri I: Clinical presentations of neonatal shock: the very low birth weight neonate during the first postnatal day. In Kleinman C, Seri I, editors: *Neonatology questions and controversies: hemodynamics and cardiology*, 2nd ed, Philadelphia, PA, 2012, Saunders/Elsevier, pp 237–267.

Lemson J, Nusmeier A, van der Hoeven JG: Advanced hemodynamic monitoring in critically ill children, *Pediatrics* 128(3):560–571, 2011.

Limperopoulos C, Bassan H, Kalish LA, Ringer SA, Eichenwald EC, Walter G, et al.: Current definitions of hypotension do not predict abnormal cranial ultrasound findings in preterm infants, *Pediatrics* 120(5):966–977, 2007.

Lundstrøm K, Pryds O, Greisen G: The haemodynamic effects of dopamine and volume expansion in sick preterm infants, *Early Hum Dev* 57(2):157–163, 2000.

Martens SE, Rijken M, Stoelhorst GM, van Zwieten PH, Zwinderman AH, Wit JM, et al.: Is hypotension a major risk factor for neurological morbidity at term age in very preterm infants? *Early Hum Dev* 75(1-2):79–89, 2003.

Martinez AM, Padbury JF, Thio S: Dobutamine pharmacokinetics and cardiovascular responses in critically ill neonates, *Pediatrics* 89(1):47–51, 1992.

McLean C, Noori S, Cayabab R, Seri I: Cerebral circulation and hypotension in the premature infant—diagnosis and treatment. In Perlman J, editor: *Neonatology questions and controversies: neurology*, 2nd ed, Philadelphia, PA, 2012, Saunders/Elsevier.

Munro MJ, Walker AM, Barfield CP: Hypotensive extremely low birth weight infants have reduced cerebral blood flow, *Pediatrics* 114(6):1591–1596, 2004.

Ng PC, Lee CH, Bnur FL, Chan IH, Lee AW, Wong E, et al.: A double-blind, randomized, controlled study of a "stress dose" of hydrocortisone for rescue treatment of refractory hypotension in preterm infants, *Pediatrics* 117:367–375, 2006.

Ng PC, Lee CH, Lam CW, et al.: Transient adrenocortical insufficiency of prematurity and systemic hypotension in very low birthweight infants, *Arch Dis Child Fetal Neonatal Ed* 89:F119–126, 2004.

Noori S, Friedlich P, Wong P, Ebrahimi M, Siassi B, Seri I: Hemodynamic changes after low-dosage hydrocortisone administration in vasopressor-treated preterm and term neonates, *Pediatrics* 118:1456–1466, 2006.

Noori S, McCoy M, Anderson M, Ramji F, Seri I: Temporal relationships of the changes in cardiac function and cerebral blood flow to intra/periventricular hemorrhage in extremely preterm infants, *Journal of Pediatrics*, 2013. resubmitted.

Noori S, Seri I: Neonatal blood pressure support: the use of inotropes, lusitropes, and other vasopressor agents, *Clin Perinatol* 39(1):221–238, 2012.

Noori S, Wu TW, Seri I: pH effects on cardiac function and systemic vascular resistance in preterm infants, *J Pediatr* 162(5):958–963, 2013. e1.

Nuntnarumit P, Yang W, Bada-Ellzey HS: Blood pressure measurements in the newborn, *Clin Perinatol* 26(4):981–996, 1999. x.

Osborn DA, Evans N, Kluckow M: Clinical detection of low upper body blood flow in very premature infants using blood pressure, capillary refill time, and central-peripheral temperature difference, *Arch Dis Child Fetal Neonatal Ed* 89(2):F168–173, 2004.

Osborn DA, Evans N, Kluckow M, Bowen JR, Rieger I: Low superior vena cava flow and effect of inotropes on neurodevelopment to 3 years in preterm infants, *Pediatrics* 120(2):372–380, 2007.

Paradisis M, Evans N, Kluckow M, Osborn D: Randomized trial of milrinone versus placebo for prevention of low systemic blood flow in very preterm infants, *J Pediatr* 154(2):189–195, 2009.

Pellicer A, Bravo MC, Madero R, Salas S, Quero J, Cabañas F: Early systemic hypotension and vasopressor support in low birth weight infants: impact on neurodevelopment, *Pediatrics* 123(5):1369–1376, 2009.

Rabe H, Diaz-Rossello JL, Duley L, Dowswell T: Effect of timing of umbilical cord clamping and other strategies to influence placental transfusion at preterm birth on maternal and infant outcomes, *Cochrane Database Syst Rev* 8:CD003248, 2012.

Rademaker KJ, Uiterwaal CS, Groenendaal F, Venema MM, van Bel F, Beekv FJ, et al.: Neonatal hydrocortisone treatment: neurodevelopmental outcome and MRI at school age in preterm-born children, *J Pediatr* 150:351–357, 2007.

Robel-Tillig E, Knüpfer M, Pulzer F, Vogtmann C: Cardiovascular impact of dobutamine in neonates with myocardial dysfunction, *Early Hum Dev* 83(5):307–312, 2007.

Seri I: Cardiovascular, renal, and endocrine actions of dopamine in neonates and children, *J Pediatr* 126(3):333–344, 1995.

Seri I, Tan R, Evans J: Cardiovascular effects of hydrocortisone in preterm infants with pressor-resistant hypotension, *Pediatrics* 107:1070–1074, 2001.

Shinwell ES, Karplus M, Reich D, et al.: Early postnatal dexamethasone treatment and increased incidence of cerebral palsy, *Arch Dis Child Fetal Neonatal Ed* 83:F177–181, 2000.

Soleymani S, Borzage M, Noori S, Seri I: Neonatal hemodynamics: monitoring, data acquisition and analysis, *Expert Rev Med Devices* 9(5):501–511, 2012.

Strozik KS, Pieper CH, Cools F: Capillary refilling time in newborns–optimal pressing time, sites of testing and normal values, *Acta Paediatr* 87(3):310–312, 1998.

Valverde E, Pellicer A, Madero R, Elorza D, Quero J, Cabañas F: Dopamine versus epinephrine for cardiovascular support in low birth weight infants: analysis of systemic effects and neonatal clinical outcomes, *Pediatrics* 117(6):e1213–1222, 2006.

Watkins AM, West CR, Cooke RW: Blood pressure and cerebral haemorrhage and ischaemia in very low birth-weight infants, *Early Hum Dev* 19(2):103–110, 1989.

Watterberg KL, Gerdes JS, Cole CH, Aucott SW, Thilo EH, Mammel MC, et al.: Prophylaxis of early adrenal insufficiency to prevent bronchopulmonary dysplasia: a multicenter trial, *Pediatrics* 114:1649–1657, 2004.

Watterberg KL, Shaffer ML, Mishefske MJ, et al.: Growth and neurodevelopmental outcomes after early low-dose hydrocortisone treatment in extremely low birth weight infants, *Pediatrics* 120(1):40–48, 2007.

Weindling M, Paize F: Peripheral haemodynamics in newborns: best practice guidelines, *Early Hum Dev* 86(3): 159–165, 2010.

Wright IM, Goodall SR: Blood pressure and blood volume in preterm infants, *Arch Dis Child Fetal Neonatal Ed* 70(3):F230–F231, 1994.

CHAPTER 16

CONGENITAL HEART DISEASE IN THE NEWBORN PERIOD

Ganga Krishnamurthy, MBBS • Veniamin Ratner, MD •
Stéphanie Levasseur, MD, FRCPC • S. David Rubenstein, MD

Children with congenital heart disease (CHD) have structural defects of the heart and/or great vessels that are present before birth. Defects range from relatively simple lesions, which neither induce clinical signs nor require therapy, to complex life-threatening lesions, which require surgery in the neonatal period.

CHD is the most common birth defect. Recent prevalence estimates for CHD range from 6 to 10 per 1000 live births. Approximately 40,000 infants are born with a congenital heart defect each year in the United States.

One of every four infants with CHD has *critical CHD* (i.e., a defect that requires either a surgical or a transcatheter procedure within the first year of life for survival). Ductal dependent heart defects, which require the ductus arteriosus to remain patent after birth, are examples of critical lesions.

FETAL CIRCULATION

Prior to the time of birth, the fetus is dependent on the uteroplacental unit for survival. The relatively oxygen-rich blood from the placenta enters the inferior vena cava via the umbilical vein and ductus venosus. Preferential streaming of blood occurs in the right atrium between the blood returning via the superior vena cava (relatively oxygen poor) and that returning from the inferior vena cava (Rudolph, 2009). The more highly saturated blood from the inferior vena cava crosses the foramen ovale to the left side of the heart, facilitating delivery of blood with relatively high oxygen content to the fetal myocardium and brain (Edelstone et al., 1979). Deoxygenated fetal blood returning from the superior vena cava travels through the right ventricle, across the ductus arteriosus, and down the descending aorta to the placenta, where oxygen and carbon dioxide transfer occurs via simple diffusion. Both the fetal right and left ventricles are responsible for blood flow to the systemic circuit and placenta. Because the resistance in the fetal pulmonary vasculature is high, less than 15% of right ventricular output is delivered to the lungs (Rudolph, 2009). Thus, the parallel fetal circulatory system promotes efficient oxygen delivery in a relatively hypoxic environment (Figure 16-1, *A*).

The fetal circulation is forgiving to neonates with even the most severe forms of CHD. Intra- and extracardiac shunts allow fetal circulatory adaptations to abnormal heart anatomy. For example, if there is severe obstruction to either ventricular outflow tract, diversion of flow into the other ventricle and great vessel occurs across the foramen ovale and the ductus arteriosus.

CASE STUDY 1

A 3.2 kg infant is born via a cesarean section at 36 weeks' gestation to a primigravida woman with an unremarkable history. The infant is mildly tachypneic, but there is no grunting. There are no risk factors for infection. At 5 minutes of life, the preductal saturation value on FiO_2 of 0.21% is 92% and the post ductal value is 84%.

EXERCISE 1

QUESTION

1. What is the best course of action for this infant?
   a. Continued observation
   b. Consultation with pediatric cardiology
   c. Stat echocardiogram
   d. Four extremity blood pressures
   e. Arterial blood gas determination from the left radial artery.

ANSWER

1. **a.**

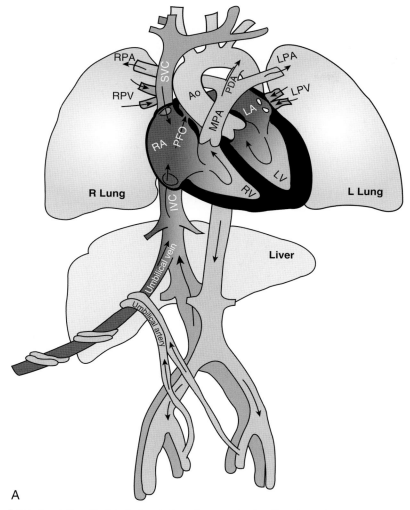

FIGURE 16-1 ■ A, Fetal circulation **B,** Adult circulation. Arrows depict direction of blood flow. *SVC,* Superior vena cava; *IVC,* inferior vena cava; *RA,* right atrium; *LA,* left atrium; *RV,* right ventricle; *LV,* left ventricle; *PFO,* patent foramen ovale; *MPA,* main pulmonary artery; *RPA,* right pulmonary artery; *LPA,* left pulmonary artery; *PDA,* patent ductus arteriosus; *RPV,* right pulmonary veins; *LPV,* left pulmonary veins; *Ao,* aorta; *R Lung,* right lung; *L Lung,* Left lung.

Transitional Circulation

Most of the circulatory changes that happen in the transition from intra- to extrauterine life occur in the first few moments after birth, with additional circulatory adjustments occurring over a period of several weeks. The primary events that trigger the alteration in blood flow patterns are removal of the low resistance placental circuit and the establishment of alveolar ventilation (Rudolph, 2009). With establishment of alveolar gas volume, there is a substantial decline in pulmonary vascular resistance and a several-fold increase in pulmonary blood flow. A rise in left atrial pressure results from an increase in pulmonary venous return and allows closure of the foramen ovale, abolishing the atrial level

shunt. The higher oxygen tension in the blood initiates the postnatal closure of the ductus arteriosus, establishes complete separation of pulmonary and systemic blood flows, and leads to a circulation in series (Figure 16-1, *B*). In full-term infants, functional closure of the ductus arteriosus is initiated within the first hours and days following birth; anatomic closure follows quickly thereafter.

Postnatal closure of fetal shunts can be life threatening in babies with ductal dependent CHD. Closure of the ductus arteriosus can lead to severe hypoxemia when there is obstruction to pulmonary blood flow and decreased perfusion to vital organs when there is obstruction to systemic blood flow. Postnatal closure of the foramen ovale can cause severe hypoxemia in

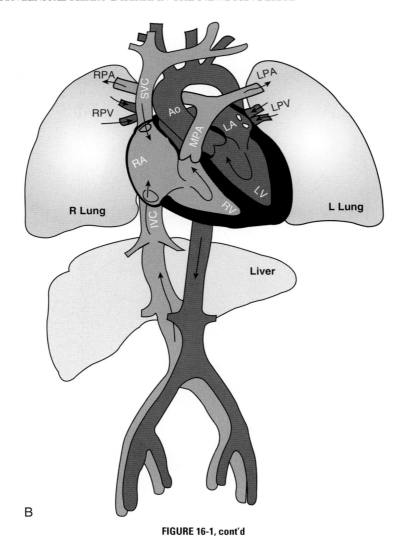

FIGURE 16-1, cont'd

babies with d-Transposition of the great arteries and intact ventricular septum. In this lesion, the aorta arises from the right ventricle and the pulmonary artery arises from the left ventricle. After birth, the circulation remains in parallel and severe hypoxemia may result if the shunt at the atrial level is abolished. Only adequate mixing at the atrial level will permit a stable transition. Transition to extrauterine life may also be difficult in babies with hypoplastic left heart syndrome with mitral atresia and an intact or restrictive atrial septum. Because of restricted egress of pulmonary venous return, pulmonary edema quickly ensues, and hence these babies are severely hypoxemic from birth with signs of inadequate cardiac output. However, with the few exceptions described previously, most babies with CHD should transition normally from the fetal circulation.

SCREENING METHODS FOR CHD

Although antenatal diagnosis of CHD is increasing, a significant proportion of babies with CHD are not diagnosed before birth. Postnatal diagnosis of CHD in the delivery room or the newborn nursery is possible only if signs of CHD manifest during the hospital stay or if there is a universal screening protocol utilizing pulse oximetry. In a recently published review of 20-year trends in the diagnosis of life-threatening cardiovascular malformations, 62% of babies with such lesions presented prior to discharge from the hospital, 25% of babies with critical CHD were diagnosed after discharge from the nursery, and 5% were diagnosed at autopsy (Figure 16-2) (Wren et al., 2008). Babies with left sided obstructive lesions such as coarctation of the aorta were more likely to be diagnosed after discharge from the nursery

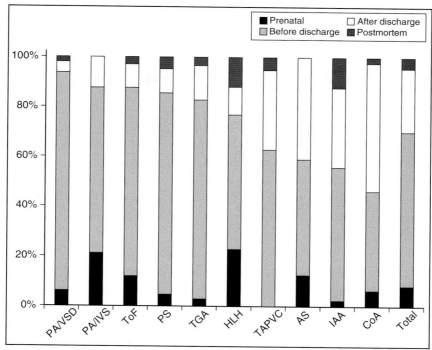

FIGURE 16-2 ■ Congenital heart disease and timing of diagnosis. *PA/VSD*, Pulmonary atresia, ventricular septal defect; *PA/IVS*, pulmonary atresia, intact ventricular septum; *ToF*, tetralogy of Fallot; *PS*, pulmonary stenosis; *TGA*, transposition of the great arteries; *HLH*, hypoplastic left heart syndrome; *TAPVC*, totally anomalous pulmonary venous connection; *AS*, aortic stenosis; *IAA*, interrupted aortic arch; *CoA*, coarctation of the aorta. (Adapted from Wren C, et al: Twenty-year trends in diagnosis of life-threatening neonatal cardiovascular malformations, *Arch Dis Child Fetal Neonatal Ed* 93[1]:F33-F35, 2008, with permission from BMJ Publishing Group Ltd.)

(Figure 16-2), whereas those who had cyanotic CHD were more likely to be identified while still in the nursery.

Critical CHD is difficult to uncover in asymptomatic newborn infants because many congenital heart defects do not produce visible central cyanosis despite severe hypoxemia. Screening by pulse oximetry provides an opportunity to detect clinically silent hypoxemia in critical CHD. In September 2011, the U.S. Department of Health and Human Services recommended that all newborns be screened for critical CHD prior to discharge from the newborn nursery, using pulse oximetry. This recommendation has been endorsed by several national organizations including the American Academy of Pediatrics. Pulse oximetry has now been included in the Recommended Uniform Screening Panel for newborns across several states, but implementation is far from universal. The proposed newborn screening strategy is described in Figure 16-3.

Screening by pulse oximetry is highly specific for detection of critical CHD (99.9%) and has moderate sensitivity (70%). The false positive rate is very low (0.035%) when screening occurs after 24 hours of age (Mahle et al., 2009, 2012). It is important to note that although pulse oximetry is generally a reliable screening tool, it can miss lesions, particularly those that involve obstruction to systemic blood flow.

Neonates with critical CHD may escape detection at all three stages of screening, i.e., antenatal ultrasound, routine neonatal examination in the nursery, and pulse oximetry. A high index of suspicion, along with prompt and timely recognition of babies with critical CHD, improves prognosis.

EVALUATION OF NEONATES FOR CHD

History

As mentioned previously, most babies with critical CHD follow an ordinary transition to extrauterine life, and the perinatal history is often unremarkable. The *absence* of important clinical information that would foster the consideration of an alternative diagnosis is a notable feature of CHD. For example, babies with severely obstructed totally anomalous pulmonary venous connection commonly present with respiratory distress and cyanosis within the first 24 hours of

Pulse oximetry screening algorithm

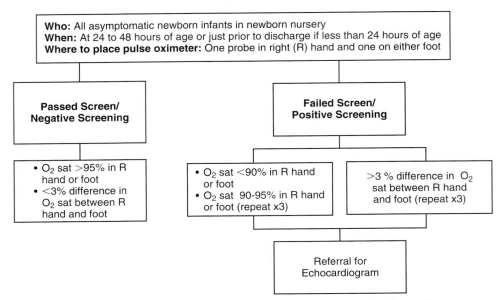

FIGURE 16-3 ■ **Algorithm for pulse oximetry screening for congenital heart disease.**

life. However, respiratory distress is a common symptom in neonates and has several etiologies. Fortunately, in most of these other disorders, the etiology is apparent from the history. Respiratory distress owing to surfactant deficiency is seen in preterm or late-preterm infants and is rarely encountered in infants born at term. Respiratory distress caused by an invasive bacterial infection is likely if there is a maternal history of prolonged rupture of membranes, a history of chorioamnionitis or maternal vaginal carriage of Group B streptococcus. In the presence of such historical data, a diagnosis of the usual etiologies of respiratory distress (e.g., sepsis or surfactant deficiency) is easily made. It is the *absence* of such relevant historical information that makes a diagnosis of CHD more likely.

Babies with cyanotic CHD usually present with cyanosis or cyanotic "spells." Lesions, which cause obstruction to pulmonary blood flow or poor mixing, often present during the initial hospital stay in the nursery. In these patients, cyanosis is not noticed at birth because the ductus arteriosus is still patent. Parents or medical caretakers may initially note transient cyanosis during crying or feeding. As the ductus arteriosus begins to close, cyanosis becomes more apparent and persistent. Most importantly, despite the cyanosis, a history of respiratory distress with dyspnea is usually not elicited.

Parents of babies with left sided obstructive lesions may report an increase in the rate of breathing, irritability, and progressive difficulty in feeding. These symptoms emerge as systemic blood flow becomes compromised with closure of the ductus arteriosus. Infants usually present after nursery discharge, typically within the first 2 weeks of life. As circulatory failure ensues, patients may present to the emergency room in extremis.

Babies with large left-to-right shunts manifest symptoms of heart failure (e.g., rapid respirations, diaphoresis, feeding difficulties). These symptoms are subtle at first, usually appear by 4 to 6 weeks of age, and worsen over time.

PHYSICAL EXAMINATION

General Physical Examination

Anthropometric measurements: Weight, height, and head circumference should be measured. A small head circumference is noted in some babies with CHD, e.g., hypoplastic left heart syndrome. In babies with congestive cardiac failure who are several weeks old, comparison of current weight to birth weight may uncover inadequate interim growth.

Vital signs: Tachycardia (normal heart rate 120 to 160 beats/minute) in babies with CHD may be reflective of depressed ventricular function. An increased respiratory rate (normal 40 to 60 breaths/minute) may be caused by pulmonary edema, excessive pulmonary blood flow, or metabolic acidosis. Blood pressure should be measured in all four extremities. Normally, the measured blood pressure in the lower extremities is a little higher than that measured in the upper extremities. A blood pressure gradient of greater than 10 to 20 mmHg between the right arm and lower extremities may indicate coarctation of the aorta or interruption of the aortic arch. Systemic hemoglobin oxygen saturation should be measured using pulse oximetry. Ideally, both preductal (right hand) and postductal (any foot) hemoglobin oxygen saturation values should be recorded simultaneously. Normally, both pre-ductal and postductal saturations are above 95% with minimal difference in measurements. Low (<95%) preductal or postductal saturation may be suggestive of cyanotic CHD.

General exam: CHD often has an underlying genetic etiology with recognizable patterns indicative of a chromosomal abnormality or syndrome. Underlying hypoxemia with central cyanosis is best recognized in the buccal mucosa, lips, and tongue. Cool extremities, feeble pulses, mottled skin, and prolonged capillary refill time indicate poor cardiac output and systemic perfusion. Peripheral pulses are globally diminished when ventricular function is depressed. Disparity in both pulses and blood pressure between the upper and lower extremities suggests juxta-ductal coarctation of the aorta or interruption of the aortic arch distal to the origin of the left subclavian artery.

Cardiovascular exam: The site of precordial activity should be noted. Dextrocardia should be suspected if the precordial impulse or activity is noted in the right hemithorax rather than the left. Parasternal impulse rather than an apical impulse is normal in neonates and signifies right ventricular dominance. A prominent parasternal impulse is noted with right ventricular pressure overload (right ventricular outflow tract obstructive lesions, pulmonary hypertension and d-Transposition of the great arteries). A diminished parasternal impulse is noted in right ventricular inflow obstruction (e.g., tricuspid atresia or tricuspid stenosis with hypoplasia of the right ventricle). Left ventricular volume overload in infants with left-to-right shunts (large ventricular septal defect, large patent ductus arteriosus) causes a prominent and hyperdynamic apical impulse.

Abnormalities of the first heart sound are rarely appreciated in newborns. Split S_1 may be seen in infants with Ebstein anomaly. Soon after birth, when the pulmonary vascular resistance is still elevated, closure of both aortic and pulmonary valves occurs almost simultaneously. Hence, a single S_2 is commonly heard. As the pulmonary vascular resistance falls, the pulmonary valve closes after the aortic valve and a split S_2 becomes apparent. A rapid heart rate makes it difficult to appreciate physiologic splitting of the second heart sound in newborn infants. Fixed splitting of the second heart sound in newborns is heard when pulmonary blood flow is excessive, as in unobstructed total or partial anomalous pulmonary venous connection. Wide, fixed splitting of the second heart sound occurs in atrial septal defects but is not typically heard in the newborn period. A split second heart sound is also appreciated when there is right ventricular obstruction or conduction delay. A single second heart sound is appreciated when there is only one semilunar valve, as in pulmonary or aortic atresia or truncus arteriosus. A loud pulmonic component is heard in pulmonary hypertension, whereas a soft P_2 may suggest pulmonary stenosis. Stenosis of semilunar valves, a bicuspid aortic valve or a dysplastic truncal valve (truncus arteriosus) may produce additional sounds or ejection clicks. A midsystolic click is sometimes appreciated in Ebstein anomaly or with mitral valve prolapse.

Murmurs are often associated with structural abnormalities of the heart. Quite often, the murmurs are innocent and bear little clinical significance. It may be difficult for the inexperienced practitioner to distinguish innocent from pathologic murmurs. A systematic approach to evaluation may assist in identifying an underlying anatomic malformation causing the cardiac murmur. The intensity, quality, location, radiation, duration, and timing of the murmur should be assessed. Murmurs can occur during systole, diastole, or continuously during the entire cardiac cycle. Timing and duration of murmurs during the different phases of systole or diastole should be noted. A harsh murmur of at least grade 3 intensity, best heard in the left lower sternal border and occupying the whole duration of systole, is likely to be secondary to a ventricular septal defect. A harsh 3- to 4-grade intensity murmur with a crescendo-decrescendo configuration, best heard in the upper right sternal border and radiating to the carotids, may suggest stenosis of the aortic valve. A murmur heard continuously across systole and diastole and best appreciated in the left upper sternal border is probably due to a widely patent ductus arteriosus. Innocent murmurs are common in the newborn period. Innocent murmurs are softer, occur in systole, and have accompanying symptoms. It is extremely important to note that the absence of murmur does *not* rule out CHD.

Pulmonary exam: Respiratory rate, effort, quality of breath sounds, and the presence of adventitious sounds should be assessed. Babies with significant left-to-right shunts and increased pulmonary blood flow are tachypneic and show an increased respiratory effort. Most babies with cyanotic CHD exhibit normal respiratory activity despite low oxygen saturation. A *normal* respiratory exam in the presence of cyanosis *strongly* suggests CHD.

Abdominal exam: Location and size of the liver should be assessed. A left sided liver is present in situs inversus and a midline liver is often noted in heterotaxy syndromes. Hepatomegaly suggests hepatic congestion and right ventricular dysfunction or volume overload. Neonates with hepatic arteriovenous malformation and high output cardiac failure may have a bruit over the liver.

Evaluation

Chest radiograph: Characteristic chest radiographs may be useful in the diagnosis of some CHD. However, in most cases of CHD, chest radiographs are rarely diagnostic.

Electrocardiogram: A 12-lead electrocardiogram (ECG) often reveals typical ECG findings in some types of CHD. However, a normal ECG should *not* rule out the presence of a serious underlying CHD.

Hyperoxia test: Hyperoxia test is helpful in differentiating hypoxemia caused by structural heart disease from that caused by lung disease. Arterial blood gas is obtained at baseline and after exposure to 100% oxygen under an oxyhood for at least 15 minutes. Babies with structural heart disease do not show a significant increase in PaO_2 (remains less than 150 mmHg) after exposure to 100% oxygen.

Echocardiogram: An immediate cardiology consultation should be requested when CHD is suspected. Echocardiogram is often the only definitive procedure required to confirm a diagnosis of structural heart disease.

Blood tests: Baseline blood work includes complete blood count to help rule out infection, serum chemistry to assess for electrolyte and renal function abnormalities, and an arterial blood gas with lactate level to assess gas exchange and the presence or absence of lactic acidosis.

Early Management and Stabilization

Airway, breathing, and circulation must be assessed in patients with signs consistent with pulmonary or cardiac disease. In patients presenting with severe hypoxia and increased respiratory effort, intubation and mechanical ventilation may assist in improving gas exchange. Circulation cannot be reestablished without a patent ductus arteriosus in ductal

dependent lesions. Prostaglandin E1 (PGE-1) infusion can reopen a closing ductus arteriosus and must be initiated as soon as ductal dependent CHD is suspected. It is not necessary to wait for an echocardiogram for confirmatory evidence prior to initiating a PGE-1 infusion except in cases of totally anomalous pulmonary venous connection where an infusion of PGE-1 has the potential to increase pulmonary edema, thereby worsening oxygenation. Reopening the ductus arteriosus will improve oxygen saturation in patients with ductal dependent pulmonary circulation and systemic perfusion will improve in patients with ductal dependent systemic circulation after initiating a PGE-1 infusion. Correction of hypovolemia and initiation of cardiotonic drugs to enhance inotropy may be required in patients presenting in cardiogenic shock. Metabolic derangements including hypoglycemia and hypocalcemia should be corrected. Early transfer to a cardiac center is important.

The three **major** presenting features of CHD in the newborn period are *central cyanosis, decreased perfusion to the body, and tachypnea.* The predominant clinical manifestation depends upon the type of CHD. The following case studies provide examples of typical presentations of CHD.

EVALUATION OF THE CYANOTIC NEWBORN

CASE STUDY 2

You are asked to attend an elective cesarean section delivery at 39 weeks of a 32-year-old gravida 2, para 1 woman. Routine prenatal laboratory tests are unremarkable. Normal fetal anatomy was noted on an 18-week screening ultrasound.

A term male infant with a vigorous cry is handed to you. APGAR scores of 8 and 8 at 1 and 5 minutes respectively are assigned. You provide free flow oxygen at 1 minute of life for cyanosis. There is minimal improvement in skin color. At 20 minutes of life, you note that the baby's face, oral mucosa, and tongue continue to have a bluish hue but the abdomen and both legs appear pinker. The baby is breathing comfortably (respiratory rate is 50 breaths/minute) with neither grunting nor subcostal retractions, i.e., without dyspnea. The lungs are clear to auscultation with equal air entry. The precordium is quiet, the heart rate and rhythm are normal, and there are no murmurs heard. The second heart sound appears loud. Peripheral pulses are normal. There is no hepatomegaly. Chest radiograph shows well-aerated lung fields with no focal pathology, a normal heart size, and a left aortic arch.

EXERCISE 2

QUESTIONS

1. Indicate whether the following statements are true (T) or false (F):
   a. Both central and peripheral cyanosis signal underlying arterial hypoxemia.
   b. Clinical recognition of central cyanosis is easier in neonates with anemia than in those with a normal hemoglobin concentration.
   c. This infant's cyanosis is most likely related to extrapulmonary right-to-left shunting of blood.

2. What etiologies might be responsible for the central cyanosis in this newborn infant?

3. What test might be used to distinguish cardiac disease from pulmonary disease?

ANSWERS

1. **a**: F; **b**: F; **c**:T.

2. See Figure 16-4.

3. Hyperoxia test.

Because the normal systemic arterial oxygen saturation in fetal life is around 60% to 65%, generalized cyanosis at birth is a normal finding but transient. In most babies who are born at term, skin color improves rapidly as alveolar ventilation is established. Persistent cyanosis is abnormal. Cyanosis signals the presence of elevated levels of deoxyhemoglobin in the underlying capillaries. At least 3 to 5 grams/dL of deoxyhemoglobin should be present in the microcirculation for cyanosis to be apparent.

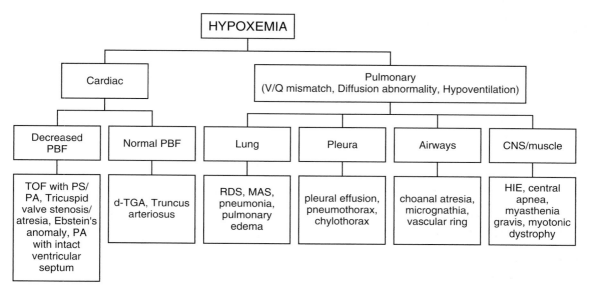

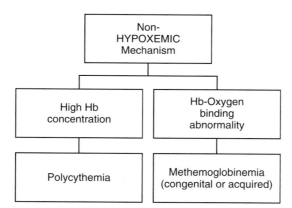

FIGURE 16-4 ■ **Pathophysiologic mechanisms of and examples of conditions that can cause central cyanosis.** *PBF,* Pulmonary blood flow; *CNS,* central nervous system; *TOF,* tetralogy of Fallot; *PS,* pulmonary stenosis; *PA,* pulmonary atresia; *d-TGA,* d-Transposition of the great arteries; *RDS,* respiratory distress syndrome; *MAS,* meconium aspiration syndrome; *HIE,* hypoxic ischemic encephalopathy; *Hb,* hemoglobin.

Cyanosis may not be recognized if deoxyhemoglobin levels are less than this critical amount. For example, let us assume that this infant has a total hemoglobin concentration of 18 grams/dL and an oxygen saturation of 83%. The calculated oxyhemoglobin concentration for this infant would be 15 grams/dL (0.83 × 18 grams/dL) and the calculated deoxyhemoglobin level would be 3 grams/dL (18 to 15 grams/dL). At this absolute concentration of deoxyhemoglobin, cyanosis is likely to be apparent. In the same example, if the absolute concentration of deoxyhemoglobin were 2 grams/dL, this infant would *not* appear cyanotic despite an abnormal hemoglobin oxygen saturation of 89% (oxyhemoglobin concentration = 16/18 grams/dL or 89%).

It is important to note that hemoglobin concentration determines the saturation level at which cyanosis is visible and detected (Figure 16-5). Cyanosis may not be appreciated in newborn infants with normal hemoglobin levels unless oxygen saturation falls below 85%. Cyanosis is identified at a higher level of hemoglobin saturation in newborns with polycythemia. For example, if the hemoglobin concentration were 22 grams/dL, cyanosis would be detected at a saturation of 86% (22–3 grams/dL= 19 grams/dL, 19/22 = 86%). Cyanosis is more difficult to detect in patients with anemia. In anemic infants, the hemoglobin saturation has to fall profoundly before cyanosis is visible. For example, if the hemoglobin concentration is 6 grams/dL, cyanosis would be noticeable only if the hemoglobin saturation fell below 50% (6–3 grams/dL = 3 grams/dL, 3/6 = 50%). Other factors that affect detection of cyanosis include skin pigmentation, fetal hemoglobin concentration, and conditions that influence the position of the hemoglobin-oxygen dissociation curve.

Cyanosis that is restricted to the periphery (e.g., nail beds, hands, and feet), is called peripheral cyanosis. Sluggish peripheral circulation associated with hypothermia, vasomotor instability, or polycythemia causes increased oxygen extraction by the tissues and elevated levels of deoxyhemoglobin in the microcirculation. However, in peripheral cyanosis, oxygen tension and saturation of hemoglobin in the systemic circulation are normal. Peripheral cyanosis is a common condition in newborn infants. It is usually innocuous unless it is associated with low cardiac output states.

Central cyanosis is more ominous and never a normal finding. It is caused by elevated levels of deoxyhemoglobin and reduced levels of oxyhemoglobin in the *circulation*. Unlike peripheral cyanosis, central cyanosis is most often indicative of underlying *hypoxemia*. Hypoxemia results from two underlying pathophysiologic mechanisms: (1) reduced oxygen tension in pulmonary venous blood (and thereby in the aorta); or (2) extrapulmonary right-to-left shunting of systemic venous blood with low PaO_2 into the systemic arterial circuit.

Conditions that lead to V/Q mismatch and intrapulmonary right-to-left shunting or those that result in impairment of oxygen diffusion across the alveolar epithelium lead to decreased oxygen tension in pulmonary venous blood. Etiologies for low oxygen tension in pulmonary veins include but are not limited to: pulmonary (respiratory distress syndrome, meconium aspiration, pneumonia), airway abnormalities (choanal atresia), neurologic, neuromuscular or muscular (myotonic dystrophy), and skeletal anomalies (severe scoliosis, thoracic dystrophies). Extrapulmonary right-to-left shunting occurs in the setting of cyanotic CHD or persistent pulmonary

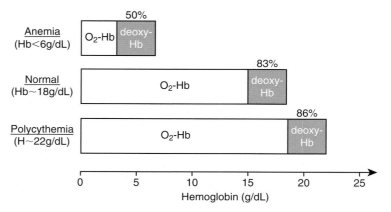

Cyanosis and Hb concentration

FIGURE 16-5 ■ **Effect of hemoglobin concentration and cyanosis.** *Hb,* Hemoglobin; *O₂-Hb,* oxyhemoglobin.

hypertension. Other pathophysiologic mechanisms that may cause central cyanosis but that are not associated with hypoxemia include polycythemia (excessive hemoglobin concentration and high levels of circulating deoxyhemoglobin) and abnormalities of hemoglobin-oxygen binding (congenital or acquired methemoglobinemia). Figure 16-4 lists conditions that cause central cyanosis in newborn infants.

It is possible to distinguish cyanosis caused by CHD from other conditions that cause hypoxemia and systemic arterial desaturation. Diseases involving the lung parenchyma (e.g., pneumonia, meconium aspiration) or involving the pleural space (e.g., effusion or pneumothorax) commonly affect gas exchange and oxygenation. In these conditions, other clinical features suggestive of respiratory disease (e.g., nasal flaring, grunting, dyspnea) accompany cyanosis, as does hypercarbia. Infants born with congenital neurologic, muscular, or neuromuscular conditions may present with cyanosis and hypercarbia owing to decreased respiratory effort from hypotonia. In neonates with cyanotic CHD, cyanosis is often the *sole* clinical feature. The *absence* of respiratory distress and hypercarbia in a cyanotic infant should raise a strong suspicion of CHD.

Hypoxemia caused by extrapulmonary right-to-left shunting in CHD can be distinguished from that caused by pulmonary venous desaturation by employing the hyperoxia test.

The primary determinant of hemoglobin-oxygen association is the partial pressure of oxygen in the blood (Figure 16-6). Oxygen

binds readily to hemoglobin in the lungs where the partial pressure of oxygen is high and dissociates from hemoglobin in tissues where the partial pressure is much lower. Because of the sigmoidal properties of the hemoglobin-oxygen dissociation curve, increasing partial pressure of oxygen beyond 100 mmHg does not produce significantly greater binding of oxygen to hemoglobin; hence, there is negligible increase in hemoglobin oxygen saturation and oxygen content when alveolar partial pressure of oxygen is increased beyond 100 mmHg. The hyperoxia test utilizes the sigmoidal properties of the hemoglobin-oxygen dissociation curve to differentiate hypoxemia caused by intrinsic lung disease from that caused by cyanotic CHD. The PaO_2 from an arterial blood gas is measured at baseline and after administering 100% oxygen for at least 10 to 15 minutes. The partial pressure of oxygen in the alveolus, pulmonary vein, and aorta is reduced in babies with parenchymal lung disease. An increase in inspired oxygen concentration to 100% increases alveolar partial pressure of oxygen, which in turn results in a higher pulmonary vein oxygen tension and a higher oxygen tension and saturation in the aorta. Typically, in babies with intrinsic lung disease, the PaO_2 increases to greater than 150 mmHg after exposure to 100% oxygen for 10 to 15 minutes.

Babies with cyanotic CHD are hypoxemic primarily due to right-to-left shunting of systemic venous blood into the systemic arterial circuit. The systemic arterial circuit therefore has an admixture of pulmonary venous blood (with PaO_2 of 100 mmHg and oxygen saturation of 100%) and systemic venous blood (with PaO_2 of approximately 40 mmHg and oxygen saturation of approximately 70%). Administering 100% oxygen to patients with cyanotic CHD and no lung disease will increase alveolar and pulmonary venous partial pressure of oxygen (to above 600 mmHg), but will not increase the oxygen saturation of pulmonary venous blood. As mentioned previously, due to the sigmoidal properties of the hemoglobin-oxygen dissociation curve, increasing alveolar partial pressure of oxygen beyond 100 mmHg does not cause a significantly greater binding of oxygen to hemoglobin. As noted in Figure 16-6, neither the oxygen saturation nor the oxygen content at PaO_2 of 100 mmHg and at 600 mmHg is remarkably different. Hence, as administering 100% oxygen does not significantly alter the oxygen saturation and content of the pulmonary venous blood, the net oxygen saturation and PaO_2 in the arterial circuit in babies with cyanotic CHD is not changed significantly. Typically, the PaO_2 in babies with cyanotic

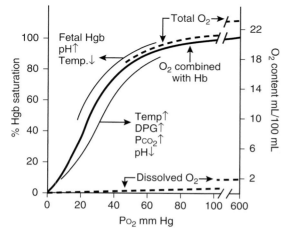

Hemoglobin-oxygen Dissociation Curves

FIGURE 16-6 ■ Oxyhemoglobin-dissociation curve demonstrating the sigmoid relationship between PaO_2 of the blood and hemoglobin saturation and the linear relationship between dissolved oxygen and PaO_2.

CHD remains below 100 mmHg despite exposure to 100% oxygen. The one exception to the rule is persistent fetal circulation where PaO_2 may remain below 100 mmHg despite a normal intracardiac anatomy.

Examples of congenital heart lesions likely to present with central cyanosis include those that involve restriction of blood flow to the lungs, e.g., severe pulmonary valve stenosis or atresia, and tetralogy of Fallot with severe valvar and/or subvalvar pulmonary stenosis. In these lesions, a combination of right-to-left shunting of desaturated blood across a patent foramen ovale into the left side of the heart and into the aorta, and decreased blood flow into the lungs causes arterial hypoxemia and central cyanosis. Typically, these defects are diagnosed when constriction of the ductus arteriosus causes further decrease in pulmonary blood flow. Defects without restriction to pulmonary blood flow but characterized by the admixture of desaturated blood in the aorta may also present with central cyanosis. These include d-Transposition of the great arteries, where the aorta arises from the right ventricle and the pulmonary artery arises from the left ventricle; and truncus arteriosus, where there is a single arterial trunk and tricuspid atresia. Table 16-1 lists congenital heart lesions likely to present with central cyanosis.

EXERCISE 3

QUESTION

1. What is the next step in the evaluation of the infant in Case Study 2?

ANSWER

1. Place two pulse oximetry sensors: one on the right hand, the other on a foot. Preductal and postductal hemoglobin oxygen saturation measurements are critical in the evaluation of a neonate for CHD. A pulse oximetry sensor placed on the right hand in an infant with a presumed left aortic arch and a normal branching pattern of the head vessels measures preductal hemoglobin oxygen saturation; a sensor on either leg measures postductal saturation. A pulse oximetry sensor on the left hand is not an accurate reflection of preductal oxygen saturation because the origin of the left subclavian artery is close to the region where the ductus arteriosus connects to the aorta. By 60 minutes of life, babies with a structurally normal heart and good transition to extrauterine life have similar values for pre- and postductal hemoglobin saturation (>95%).

EXERCISE 4

QUESTION

1. In which conditions would you expect the preductal saturation to be higher than the postductal saturation value and in which congenital heart lesion would you expect the reverse to be true?

ANSWER

1. Preductal saturation > postductal saturation: persistent pulmonary hypertension of the newborn and left heart obstructive lesions such as critical coarctation or interrupted aortic arch.

TABLE 16-1 Congenital Heart Lesions Likely to Present with Central Cyanosis

A. Right ventricular inflow/outflow abnormality	Defect
Tricuspid valve stenosis/atresia	Stenosis/atresia of tricuspid valve
Ebstein anomaly	Inferior displacement of tricuspid valve
Pulmonary atresia with intact ventricular septum	Atresia of pulmonary valve
Pulmonary stenosis	Subvalvar, valvar, or supravalvar obstruction to pulmonary blood flow
Tetralogy of Fallot with pulmonary stenosis or atresia	Anterior malalignment of the conal septum leading to variable degree of obstruction to pulmonary blood flow, overriding aorta, ventricular septal defect, and right ventricular hypertrophy
B. Without right ventricular inflow/outflow abnormality	**Defect**
Transposition of the great arteries	Ventriculoarterial discordance: aorta arises from the right ventricle, pulmonary artery arises from the left ventricle
Truncus arteriosus	Single arterial trunk arises from the ventricles with variable origins of the pulmonary arteries from the trunk
Totally anomalous pulmonary venous connection with obstruction	Abnormal connection of all the pulmonary veins to the systemic venous system

Postductal saturation > preductal saturation: d-Transposition of the great arteries with pulmonary hypertension or with coarctation of the aorta.

Postductal oxygen saturation may be lower than the preductal oxygen saturation (differential cyanosis) in babies whose pulmonary vascular resistance is elevated and shunting across the patent ductus arteriosus is predominantly right (desaturated blood) to left. Differential cyanosis is also noted in neonates with critical coarctation of aorta or interrupted aortic arch where the right ventricle provides flow into the descending aorta via the ductus arteriosus. Reverse differential cyanosis occurs when the postductal saturation is *higher* than the preductal saturation. In this scenario, the descending aorta has an admixture of blood with higher oxygen tension and saturation than seen in the right subclavian artery. Causes of reverse differential cyanosis include d-Transposition of the great arteries with pulmonary hypertension, or d-Transposition of the great arteries with coarctation of the aorta. In simple d-Transposition of the great arteries, blood with "high" oxygen tension enters the pulmonary artery from the left ventricle and is shunted into the descending aorta in the face of elevated pulmonary vascular resistance or in the presence of either coarctation or interruption of the aorta.

CASE STUDY 2 (continued)

Pulse oximetry readings from the right hand and left foot are 60% and 80% respectively. The baby continues to breathe comfortably with unchanged skin color despite oxygen administration by nasal cannula at 1.5 L/minute and FiO$_2$ of 1.0. Peripheral pulses are normal. A baseline arterial blood gas obtained from the right radial artery: pH of 7.32, PCO$_2$ of 40 mmHg, PaO$_2$ of 34 mmHg, base deficit of −2, and bicarbonate of 21 mEq/L. The PaO$_2$ after a hyperoxia test was 40 mmHg.

EXERCISE 5

QUESTION

1. What is the most likely diagnosis in Case Study 2?

ANSWER

1. d-Transposition of the great arteries. A centrally cyanotic infant without respiratory distress and a positive hyperoxia test suggests an underlying cyanotic CHD. Reverse differential cyanosis, absent murmur but loud S$_2$ (anterior aortic valve in d-transposed great vessels), and a normal sized heart without oligemic lung fields, makes

the diagnosis of d-Transposition of the great arteries most likely.

CASE STUDY 2 (continued)

The pediatric cardiologist confirms the diagnosis of d-Transposition of the great arteries. The interventricular septum is intact and concern about a restrictive foramen ovale is confirmed. The pediatric cardiologist suggests starting a PGE-1 infusion at 0.01 micrograms/kg/minute and to make arrangements for transfer to a cardiac care center where a balloon atrial septostomy may be performed to improve mixing.

In babies with d-Transposition of the great arteries, the aorta arises from the right ventricle and the pulmonary artery arises from the left ventricle (Figure 16-7; Video 16-1). After birth, the circulation remains in parallel and desaturated blood returning to the right atrium recirculates into the aorta. For survival to occur, adequately oxygenated blood from the left side of the heart must enter the systemic circulation through septal defects at the atrial or ventricular level or at the level of the ductus arteriosus. If the ventricular septum is intact and the foramen ovale becomes restrictive after birth, there are no other major venues for adequate mixing of oxygenated and deoxygenated blood. Babies are consequently profoundly hypoxemic and cyanotic in the first minutes to hours after birth. Survival depends upon the rapid creation of an atrial level communication through a transcatheter route. Only interventional cardiologists at cardiac centers can perform these procedures and urgent transfer to such centers is critical.

A simple d-Transposition of the great arteries without critical outflow tract obstruction is not a ductal dependent lesion because there is neither restriction to pulmonary nor systemic blood flow. However, the majority of blood flow into the lungs and into the aorta is *ineffective*. Oxygenated blood in the left ventricle is pumped back into the lungs and desaturated blood in the right ventricle is pumped into the aorta. PGE-1 is instituted to increase "effective" pulmonary and systemic blood flows (Figure 16-8). Maintaining patency of the ductus arteriosus promotes aorta to pulmonary artery shunting thereby increasing effective pulmonary blood flow (desaturated blood from aorta to pulmonary artery through the ductus arteriosus). The increased pulmonary blood flow will in turn increase left atrial pressure and increase effective systemic oxygenated blood flow (oxygenated blood shunts from left atrium to right atrium across the foramen ovale). Sometimes, the anticipated improvement in oxygenation does not occur after initiating

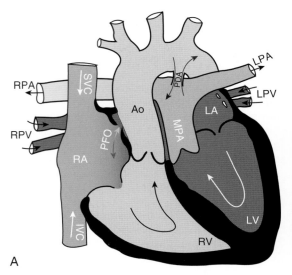

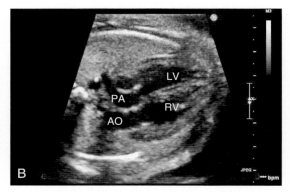

A

B

FIGURE 16-7 ■ **A,** Cartoon of d-Transposition of the great arteries. Arrows depict direction of blood flow. **B,** Outflow tract view on echocardiogram in fetus with d-Transposition of the great arteries showing the transposed relationship (LV-PA and RV-AO) of the ventricles and great vessels. **B,** Outflow tract view on echocardiogram in fetus with d-Transposition of the great arteries showing the transposed relationship (LV-PA and RV-AO) of the ventricles and great vessels. *SVC,* Superior vena cava; *IVC,* inferior vena cava; *RA,* right atrium; *LA,* left atrium; *RV,* right ventricle; *LV,* left ventricle; *PFO,* patent foramen ovale; *MPA,* main pulmonary artery; *RPA,* right pulmonary artery; *LPA,* left pulmonary artery; *PDA,* patent ductus arteriosus; *RPV,* right pulmonary veins; *LPV,* left pulmonary veins; *Ao,* aorta.

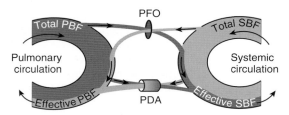

FIGURES 16-8 ■ **Cartoon depicting the relative contributions of oxygenated and desaturated blood in pulmonary and systemic circulations and areas of mixing in d-Transposition of the great arteries and intact ventricular septum.** Effective pulmonary blood flow (PBF) denotes desaturated blood directed toward the pulmonary circulation. Effective systemic blood flow (SBF) denotes oxygenated blood directed towards the systemic circulation. *PFO,* Patent foramen ovale; *PDA,* patent ductus arteriosus.

PGE-1 because the foramen ovale is restrictive. An urgent balloon atrial septostomy (a bedside procedure that enlarges the foramen ovale) is required to improve mixing (Video 16-2). Once the balloon atrial septostomy is performed, systemic oxygenation usually improves dramatically. *After a few days of observation, an elective arterial switch procedure is performed.* This procedure involves switching the great vessels so that they connect to the appropriate ventricles. In addition the coronary arteries are transferred to their new location in the neoaorta. In the current era, operative survival and long-term outcomes after the arterial switch procedure are excellent.

CYANOTIC NEWBORN WITH CARDIOMEGALY

CASE STUDY 3

You are called to the well-baby nursery to evaluate a 4-hour-old female baby who was noted to have a cyanotic spell during a crying episode. This infant was born at 39 weeks' gestation to a 24- year-old gravida 2, para 1 woman. The mother's pregnancy was unremarkable and delivery was by elective cesarean section. APGAR scores were 8 and 9 at 1 and 5 minutes respectively. The infant was apparently "well" until the nurse noticed the cyanotic spell. This infant's vital signs are as follows: temperature: 36.8° C, heart rate 160 beats/minute, respiratory rate 65 breaths/minute, blood pressure 93/45, pre- and postductal saturations are 70% and 75%, respectively. This infant appears nondysmorphic, active, and vigorous but with central cyanosis. She has mild tachypnea but appears to be breathing comfortably. Both lung fields receive equal air entry and are clear to auscultation. Her precordium is active, multiple heart sounds are heard, and a 3/6-pansystolic murmur is heard in the lower left parasternal region. The liver is palpable 2 cm below the right costal margin in the midclavicular line. Peripheral pulses and perfusion are normal. A chest radiograph is shown in Figure 16-9.

An ECG reveals tall P waves, rightward QRS axis, and right ventricular conduction delay. Arterial blood gas: pH of 7.35, PCO$_2$ of 32 mmHg,

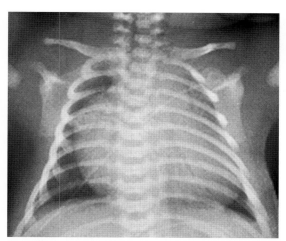

FIGURE 16-9 ■ **Chest radiograph of patient described in Case Study 3.**

1. Sepsis/pneumonia
2. Hypoglycemia
3. Hypothermia
4. Gastroesophageal reflux
5. Airway obstruction
6. Congenital heart disease
7. Persistent pulmonary hypertension
8. Intracranial hemorrhage related to birth trauma
9. Apnea, seizures
10. Effects of maternal sedation
11. Hypermagnesemia
12. Inborn errors of metabolism

PaO$_2$ of 36 mmHg, HCO$_3$ of 22 mEq/L. Complete blood count: white blood cell (WBC) 18 × 10^9/L, hemoglobin 17 grams/dL, hematocrit 49%, platelet count 224 × 10^9/L. WBC differential includes 55% neutrophils, 35% lymphocytes, and no bands. Pediatric cardiology consult has been requested.

EXERCISE 6

QUESTIONS

1. Under what conditions should cyanosis be considered a normal finding in a newborn infant?

2. What is the most likely cause of cyanosis in the case?

ANSWERS

1. Cyanotic or "blue" spells can be seen in otherwise "well" babies. By definition, benign cyanotic "spells" are transitory and brief. These spells typically occur during crying and resolve rapidly when the baby is calm and quiet. The hemoglobin oxygen saturation measurement by pulse oximetry is normal after resolution of the cyanotic episode. There are no other symptoms or signs, and these babies are well appearing and have a normal examination.

   In the absence of a benign history as described, all other cyanotic spells should be considered abnormal and an underlying cause must be sought. Several conditions can result in cyanotic spells in the newborn period (Box 16-1). Most of these conditions can be differentiated through careful historical evaluation, a thorough physical examination, and select investigative studies.

   Babies with cyanotic CHD may present with cyanotic spells in the well-baby nursery. Typically, even if cyanosis resolves, the hemoglobin oxygen saturation measurement by pulse oximetry is *not* normal and is generally below 95%. A low oxygen saturation and an abnormal precordial examination, as noted in this case study are strongly suggestive of a cyanotic CHD.

2. In this case, the most likely cause of the cyanosis in this infant is incompetence of the tricuspid valve. The early auscultation of a parasternal pansystolic murmur is most likely to be related to a tricuspid regurgitant murmur. Regurgitation across the tricuspid valve can be seen in structurally normal as well as abnormal hearts. The most common cause of tricuspid regurgitation in structurally normal hearts occurs with pulmonary hypertension for a short time after birth and is generally transient. A flail tricuspid valve caused by necrosis or rupture of papillary muscle in the setting of perinatal asphyxia may result in severe tricuspid valve regurgitation. Congenital cardiac anomalies that cause tricuspid regurgitation include Ebstein anomaly and pulmonary atresia with intact ventricular septum. Other congenital abnormalities of the tricuspid valve such as dysplasia of the tricuspid valve, abnormal chordal attachments of the tricuspid valve, unguarded tricuspid valve (where there is no valvar apparatus), or cleft tricuspid valve leaflet are quite rare. The identification of several heart sounds, including split first and second heart sounds and third and fourth sounds, makes the diagnosis of a primary abnormality of the tricuspid valve, especially Ebstein anomaly, more likely.

   In Ebstein anomaly, the tricuspid valve is abnormal (Figure 16-10; Video 16-3). The septal and posterior leaflets are displaced inferiorly and are usually tethered to the right ventricular wall.

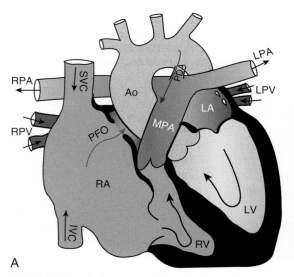
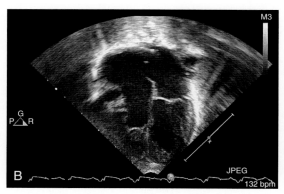

FIGURE 16-10 ■ **A,** Cartoon of Ebstein anomaly. Arrows depict direction of blood flow. **B,** Four chamber view on echocardiogram of patient with Ebstein anomaly. The displaced tricuspid valve and atrialized portion of right ventricle are clearly seen. *SVC,* Superior vena cava; *IVC,* inferior vena cava; *RA,* right atrium; *LA,* left atrium; *RV,* right ventricle; *LV,* left ventricle; *PFO,* patent foramen ovale; *MPA,* main pulmonary artery; *RPA,* right pulmonary artery; *LPA,* left pulmonary artery; *PDA,* patent ductus arteriosus; *RPV,* right pulmonary veins; *LPV,* left pulmonary veins; *Ao,* aorta.

Mobility of the tricuspid valve is further limited by abnormal chordal attachments. Varying degrees of tricuspid regurgitation occur, resulting in right atrial enlargement. A high right atrial pressure promotes right-to-left shunting across a patent foramen ovale or an atrial septal defect. The region of the right ventricle between the tricuspid valve annulus and the inferiorly displaced valve leaflets is called the atrialized portion of the right ventricle and has no role in right ventricular output. During systole, blood from the right ventricle regurgitates into the right atrium, especially in the setting of elevated pulmonary vascular resistance as seen in the newborn period. Pulmonary blood flow across the pulmonary valve may be minimal under these conditions. Therefore, pulmonary blood flow may be dependent upon the patency of the ductus arteriosus while pulmonary vascular resistance is still elevated. Hence Ebstein anomaly is often diagnosed when the ductus arteriosus begins to constrict, further decreasing blood flow into the lungs. As a result, values of hemoglobin oxygen saturation fall and cyanosis becomes apparent.

Babies with Ebstein anomaly and moderate to severe tricuspid valve regurgitation may have a hyperdynamic precordium due to volume overload of the right ventricle. The tricuspid regurgitant murmur is best heard along the lower left sternal border. S_1 is split due to increased flow across the tricuspid valve. S_2 is often split due to right ventricular conduction delay. Third and fourth heart sounds are often appreciated

and may be related to vibrations of the abnormal tricuspid valve. Multiple heart sounds and a parasternal pansystolic murmur in a cyanotic newborn are suggestive of Ebstein anomaly.

EXERCISE 7

QUESTION

1. What are the causes of a massive cardiothymic silhouette in the newborn period?

ANSWER

1. Chest radiograph and ECG are useful diagnostic tools in the evaluation of babies with CHD. The position and contour of the cardiovascular silhouette on chest radiographs is informative. Dextrocardia and presence of a right-sided stomach bubble or a midline liver may indicate complex CHD including heterotaxy syndromes. The presence or absence of a thymic shadow and sidedness of the aortic arch should be assessed. An absent thymic shadow (first day of life) may suggest 22q11.2 deletion syndrome and raises the possibility of a conotruncal malformation (congenital abnormalities of cardiac outflow tracts). Characteristic radiographic features are noted in some types of CHD (e.g., Coeur en Sabot or boot-shaped heart in tetralogy of Fallot, "egg on string" appearance in d-Transposition of the great arteries). Prominence of pulmonary vasculature indicates excessive pulmonary blood flow; relatively oligemic lung fields suggest

paucity of blood flow to the lungs. Pulmonary venous congestion and pulmonary edema are noted in totally anomalous pulmonary venous connection with obstruction.

Very few cardiac conditions cause a massive cardiothymic silhouette as seen on chest radiographs. Most neonatal cases of enlarged cardiac shadow on x-rays are caused by an enlarged right atrium (Ebstein anomaly, pulmonary atresia with intact ventricular septum). Other causes include cardiomegaly owing to increase in myocardial mass or length (hypertrophic or dilated cardiomyopathy), enormous increase in right ventricular volume and pressure overload (large arteriovenous malformations), cardiac or mediastinal tumors, and pericardial effusions. The two most common causes of massive cardiomegaly in a *cyanotic* newborn are Ebstein anomaly and pulmonary atresia with intact ventricular septum. In both these conditions, massive right atrial enlargement results from tricuspid regurgitation.

The ECG is a useful tool that may help distinguish Ebstein anomaly from pulmonary atresia with intact ventricular septum. In both, tall P waves suggestive of right atrial enlargement are seen. In Ebstein anomaly, preexcitation suggestive of Wolff-White-Parkinson syndrome may be seen, as may a right ventricular conduction delay. A paucity of right ventricular forces is more usual in pulmonary atresia with intact ventricular septum where the right ventricle is hypoplastic.

EXERCISE 8

QUESTION

1. What intervention(s) may improve the oxygen saturation in this patient?

ANSWER

1. Increase the inspired oxygen concentration and consider starting inhaled nitric oxide. Consider using PGE-1. As mentioned previously, the atrialized portion of the right ventricle contributes minimally towards right ventricular output. In the neonatal period, when the pulmonary vascular resistance is elevated, the right ventricle may not be able to generate adequate systolic pressure to open the pulmonary valve. The pulmonary valve is hence "functionally" atretic, as blood does not flow across it (Figure 16-11). During this time, pulmonary blood flow is dependent upon the patency of the ductus arteriosus. Hypoxemia and cyanosis may worsen if the ductus arteriosus constricts or closes.

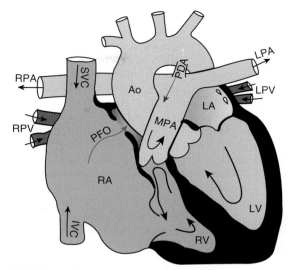

FIGURES 16-11 ■ Cartoon depicting functional pulmonary atresia in Ebstein anomaly. Arrows depict direction of blood flow. *SVC,* Superior vena cava; *IVC,* inferior vena cava; *RA,* right atrium; *LA,* left atrium; *RV,* right ventricle; *LV,* left ventricle; *PFO,* patent foramen ovale; *MPA,* main pulmonary artery; *RPA,* right pulmonary artery; *LPA,* left pulmonary artery; *PDA,* patent ductus arteriosus; *RPV,* right pulmonary veins; *LPV,* left pulmonary veins; *Ao,* aorta.

Antegrade flow across the pulmonary valve in the setting of functional pulmonary atresia may be promoted by decreasing the pulmonary vascular resistance, which may be accomplished by increasing the concentration of inspired oxygen or by providing inhaled nitric oxide. Oxygen and/or inhaled nitric oxide may be weaned over the course of several days as the pulmonary vascular resistance declines, antegrade flow across the pulmonary valve increases, and right-to-left flow across the foramen ovale or atrial septal defect diminishes. In the case of anatomic obstruction, ductal patency is of course critical until an intervention to open the pulmonary outflow tract can be performed. The differentiation of functional vs. true pulmonary outflow obstruction can be difficult and requires consultation with pediatric cardiology and investigation with echocardiography. The institution of PGE-1 until the exact physiology is determined is indicated.

CASE STUDY 3 (continued)

The pediatric cardiologist confirms the diagnosis of Ebstein anomaly with moderate to severe tricuspid regurgitation and functional pulmonary atresia. Inspired oxygen is increased to 50% by nasal cannula. Oxygen saturation improves steadily to above 90%. After 3 to 4 days, oxygen is weaned back to 21% and the patient is discharged home on the seventh day of life with a hemoglobin saturation of 85%.

Severity of Ebstein anomaly varies. Patients with mild abnormalities of the tricuspid valve and minimal regurgitation may remain asymptomatic and require no intervention. Some may present with transient cyanosis in the newborn period as the patient described in this case study. More severe cases can present with cardiac failure and/or cyanosis in infancy.

Management of the patient with Ebstein anomaly varies and is based on the clinical presentation. With severe restriction to pulmonary blood flow in the neonatal period, a palliative aortopulmonary shunt may be required to provide a stable source of pulmonary blood flow. In others, exclusion of the tricuspid valve by oversewing it may also be required. Definitive repair with tricuspid valvuloplasty or tricuspid valve replacement may be performed in patients in whom symptoms emerge later in childhood, adolescence, or adulthood.

MURMUR IN NEONATE

CASE STUDY 4

You receive a call from a pediatrician in the well-baby nursery who wishes to transfer a 12-hour-old male infant to the neonatal intensive care unit (NICU) after a murmur was discovered in the admission physical examination. The mother is a 26-year-old primigravida. The pregnancy was uneventful. This infant was born at 39 weeks' gestation by normal spontaneous vaginal delivery. APGAR scores were 9 and 9 at 1 and 5 minutes, respectively. On examination, the infant appears comfortable, pink, and not in any apparent cardiorespiratory distress. The birth weight is 3.56 kg. Vital signs are as follows: heart rate is 150 beats/minute, respiratory rate is 50 breaths/ minute, blood pressure is 68/45 mmHg (right arm), preductal and postductal hemoglobin saturations are 86%. The baby is breathing comfortably, with neither tachypnea nor chest retractions. Precordial examination is significant for a prominent parasternal impulse. A harsh 3/6 ejection systolic murmur is best heard over the left upper sternal border. Peripheral pulses and blood pressure are normal.

Chest radiograph reveals mild cardiomegaly, left aortic arch, and mildly oligemic lung fields with no focal lung pathology. ECG reveals a normal sinus rhythm, rightward QRS axis, and right ventricular hypertrophy. Pediatric cardiology consultation is awaited.

EXERCISE 9

QUESTIONS

1. On a physical examination, what features are used to differentiate an innocent murmur from a pathologic murmur?

2. Which of the following statements about murmurs is true?
   a. The most common innocent murmur in the newborn period is peripheral pulmonary artery stenosis.
   b. Absence of murmur in the newborn period rules out CHD.

ANSWERS

1. Routine newborn physical examination within 24 hours of birth and again prior to discharge offers a critical window during which presymptomatic infants with CHD may be detected. Reported prevalence of murmurs in term newborns is highly variable. In most large series, the prevalence of murmurs in the newborn period is less than 1%.

   Cardiac murmurs may be innocent and of no consequence or may be associated with structural abnormalities of the heart. In one large series, more than 54% of babies in whom a murmur was noted in the newborn period had CHD (Ainsworth et al., 1999). See below for characteristics of innocent and pathologic murmurs.

2. **a.** The most common lesions recognized from murmurs are those with left-to-right shunts, particularly ventricular septal defects. The remaining 46% in the same series (mentioned previously) (Ainsworth et al., 1999) had either a structurally normal heart or physiologic findings that accounted for the murmur, e.g., physiologic branch pulmonary artery stenosis. Common "innocent" murmurs heard in the newborn period include peripheral pulmonary artery stenosis (PPS), a closing ductus arteriosus, or Still murmur. The typical murmur of PPS is described as a low-grade, 1-2/6 mid-systolic ejection murmur best heard in the left upper sternal area and radiating to the axilla and back. PPS murmurs generally resolve in most patients by 6 months of age. This murmur is caused by turbulence created by the relative size discrepancy between the main and branch pulmonary arteries. Still murmur is generally heard in young, school-aged children but occasionally can be heard in newborn infants. Still murmur is a low-grade systolic murmur with a musical quality and is best heard in the lower left parasternal regions.

   Certain qualities may differentiate pathologic from innocent murmurs: high grade—grade 3 intensity or higher, harsh quality, murmurs extending through systole and best noted in the left upper sternal border, and those associated with an abnormal S_2 are most likely pathologic and indicative of an underlying structural heart disease.

A high baseline heart rate and a rapidly evolving transitional circulation make the task of examination of the cardiovascular system in the neonate particularly challenging. Discriminating innocent from pathologic murmurs may be a difficult task for most pediatricians, particularly those in training. It is important to note that in a significant proportion of infants who presented later with cardiac failure or died owing to cardiovascular collapse, a murmur present in the neonatal period was not recognized as pathologic (Abu-Harb et al., 1994). The decision to refer all murmurs heard in the newborn period or to selectively refer those with pathologic characteristics for evaluation by a pediatric cardiologist will ultimately depend upon the experience and skill of the primary caregiver.

Conversely, the absence of a murmur *does not* rule out CHD. Many serious congenital heart lesions do not present with a murmur at all. Some may not have yet developed the physiologic changes needed for the murmur to be detected in the newborn nursery. In the same large series described previously, 47% of infants who were eventually diagnosed with CHD later in infancy had no murmur in the neonatal period (Ainsworth et al., 1999). The infant in our case study has a prominent precordial impulse suggestive of right ventricular pressure overload. An ejection systolic murmur, best appreciated in the left upper sternal border, is likely related to an obstruction of the right ventricular outflow tract at the supravalvar, valvar, or subvalvar levels. A low hemoglobin saturation of 86% suggests right-to-left shunting. Oligemic lung fields on chest radiograph indicate reduced blood flow to the lungs.

CASE STUDY 4 (continued)

A diagnosis of critical valvar pulmonary stenosis is confirmed on echocardiogram by the pediatric cardiologist. The ductus arteriosus is restrictive. The cardiologist requests that a PGE-1 infusion be started immediately at 0.01 mcg/kg/min. The hemoglobin saturation increases to 94%. The next day, the infant undergoes a successful transcatheter balloon valvuloplasty.

One of the most common causes of obstruction to the right ventricular outflow tract is pulmonary valve stenosis (Figure 16-12; Video 16-4). The pulmonary valve may be domed without distinct separation into leaflets or the leaflets may be fused at the commissures. Sometimes, especially in patients with Noonan syndrome, the valve leaflets are thickened and dysplastic. Obstruction at the pulmonary valve causes right ventricular hypertrophy, particularly of

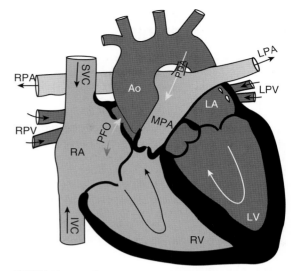

FIGURE 16-12 ■ **Cartoon depicting valvar pulmonary stenosis.** Arrows depict direction of blood flow. *SVC,* Superior vena cava; *IVC,* inferior vena cava; *RA,* right atrium; *LA,* left atrium; *RV,* right ventricle; *LV,* left ventricle; *PFO,* patent foramen ovale; *MPA,* main pulmonary artery; *RPA,* right pulmonary artery; *LPA,* left pulmonary artery; *PDA,* patent ductus arteriosus; *RPV,* right pulmonary veins; *LPV,* left pulmonary veins; *Ao,* aorta.

the infundibulum, which may contribute to the right ventricular outflow tract obstruction.

There are varying degrees of valvar pulmonary stenosis. Mild pulmonary valve stenosis rarely progresses and usually requires no treatment. Moderate or severe obstruction to the pulmonary valve is progressive and therapy is required. Severe obstruction to the right ventricular outflow tract (critical pulmonary stenosis) can cause compromise of pulmonary blood flow and requires ductal patency to provide an alternate source of pulmonary blood flow.

Transcatheter balloon valvuloplasty is curative when obstruction is restricted to the valvar level (Video 16-5). Neonatal transcatheter balloon valvuloplasty is very successful; surgical or transcatheter reinterventions are rarely required.

After balloon valvuloplasty, PGE-1 infusion is usually discontinued. Over the course of the next 48 hours, a decline in oxygen saturations is expected as the ductus arteriosus closes. Decline in oxygen saturation is due to continued right-to-left atrial shunting in the setting of diminished right ventricular compliance caused by right ventricular hypertrophy. As right ventricular hypertrophy regresses over several weeks to months, right ventricular compliance will improve, right-to-left shunting across the foramen ovale will diminish, and the hemoglobin oxygen saturation will improve.

CYANOTIC NEWBORN WITH RESPIRATORY DISTRESS

CASE STUDY 5

A full-term male neonate is born to a 23-year-old primigravida whose prenatal laboratory tests are unremarkable, including a negative cervical culture Group B Streptococcus. Membranes ruptured 4 hours prior to delivery; the amniotic fluid was clear. There is no history of maternal fever during labor. Labor was spontaneous and uncomplicated; vaginal delivery occurred at 39 weeks of gestation. APGAR scores of 9 and 9 are assigned. You are called to evaluate this infant at 12 hours of life in the newborn nursery for grunting respirations. On physical examination, you find a 3 kg nondysmorphic, centrally cyanotic male infant of term gestation with significant respiratory distress manifest by nasal flaring and subcostal and intercostal chest retractions. Air entry is equal bilaterally; diffuse rales are appreciated. On precordial examination, the second heart sound appears loud. A 2/6 systolic murmur is appreciated over the upper left sternal border. His abdomen is not distended; however, the liver is palpable 1 to 2 cm below the right costal margin. The extremities are warm and distal pulses appear fairly strong. You bring him to the NICU for further management. Vital signs: respiratory rate 85 to 90 breaths/minute, heart rate 168 beats/minute, blood pressure 76/46, hemoglobin saturation is 60% breathing room air. He is placed on nasal prong continuous positive airway pressure (CPAP), but is intubated shortly thereafter for a persistently low saturation value of 65% and continuing respiratory distress. On conventional mechanical support and inspired oxygen of 1.0, his saturation measured by pulse oximetry is 68%. Arterial blood gas: pH of 7.32, PCO_2 of 42 mmHg, PaO_2 of 35 mmHg, HCO_3 of 20 meq/L, base deficit of −2/SaO_2 65%.

A chest radiograph obtained on admission is shown in Figure 16-13. Complete blood count: WBC 15×10^9/L, hemoglobin 18 grams/dL, platelet count 245×10^9/L. Differential: 54% neutrophils, no bands, and 35% lymphocytes.

EXERCISE 10

QUESTION

1. Which of the following diagnoses is most consistent with this infant's clinical course and chest radiograph?
   a. Transient tachypnea of the newborn
   b. Respiratory distress syndrome
   c. Totally anomalous pulmonary venous connection with obstruction
   d. Large ventricular septal defect

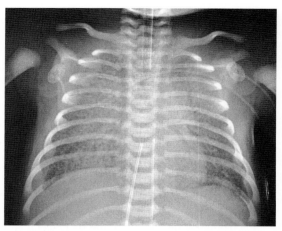

FIGURES 16-13 ■ **Chest radiograph of patient described in Case Study 5.**

ANSWER

1. **c.** It is not uncommon for newborn infants to have respiratory distress. The timing of onset of symptoms, contributory information from prenatal and delivery history, and a thorough physical examination help in establishing the correct diagnosis. Respiratory distress in the term infant may have several etiologies including transient tachypnea of the newborn (TTN), pneumonia, aspiration or air-leak syndromes, pleural effusions, or CHD.

   TTN is a common cause of respiratory distress in the term and near-term infant. The underlying pathophysiologic mechanism is attributed to delayed absorption of alveolar fluid. Signs suggestive of lung disease are noted at birth or soon thereafter. A chest radiograph typically shows hyperinflated lungs with alveolar edema and fluid in the interstitium and interlobar fissures. Respiratory distress in neonates with TTN is generally mild; a supplemental oxygen requirement exceeding 40% is unusual and signs usually resolve within 24 to 48 hours. Vertical transmission of microorganisms from infected amniotic fluid or the lower genital tract may result in pneumonia and early-onset sepsis. These neonates may exhibit signs of respiratory distress either at birth or within the first 24 hours of life. Nonspecific signs suggestive of infection may be present, including temperature instability, apnea, lethargy, glucose instability, poor feeding, or abdominal distension. The severity of clinical signs can vary from mild respiratory distress to fulminant sepsis with shock. Leukopenia, absolute or relative neutropenia, and an elevated I:T ratio reinforce the diagnosis of pneumonia and bacterial sepsis. On a chest radiograph, severe cases of pneumonia may resemble the reticulogranular pattern seen in premature infants with surfactant deficiency because they have surfactant inactivation. In less severe cases, patchy pulmonary infiltrates are seen.

Clinical signs in neonates with air-leak syndromes or pleural effusions can vary in severity depending upon the degree of air or fluid accumulation and extent of respiratory and/or hemodynamic compromise. The chest radiograph is diagnostic in both these conditions. Neonates may aspirate meconium, blood, or amniotic fluid. Obstruction of airways leads to respiratory distress. Infants may become symptomatic soon after or in the first hours following birth. The degree of respiratory distress varies and depends upon the extent of obstruction of the small airways. The chest radiograph often shows patchy areas of infiltrate and collapse along with areas of hyperinflation. Respiratory distress syndrome is usually a disease of the premature infant. Typically, this disorder is seen when delivery occurs before 34 weeks of gestation. Symptoms are present at birth and vary in severity with the most severe symptoms noted in lower gestational ages. The chest radiograph shows a typical reticulogranular pattern in lungs with low volumes.

Some forms of CHD may present with respiratory distress. Typically, respiratory distress in the setting of CHD occurs when there is:

• Too much pulmonary blood flow
• Obstruction to flow in pulmonary veins

Excessive pulmonary blood flow occurs in lesions with an abnormal communication between the pulmonary and systemic circuit either at the level of the atria, ventricles, or the great vessels. Examples of such lesions include large atrial or ventricular septal defects, atrioventricular septal defects, large patent ductus arteriosus, aortopulmonary window, truncus arteriosus, or totally abnormal pulmonary venous connection without obstruction. Typically, symptoms of increased respiratory effort manifest when there is a substantial decline in pulmonary vascular resistance and left-to-right shunt volume increases. As the pulmonary vascular resistance is still elevated after birth, the above lesions rarely exhibit symptoms of pulmonary overcirculation at birth or in the first few days of life.

Some or all four pulmonary veins may not return normally to the left atrium. Instead, the pulmonary veins may establish an abnormal communication with a systemic venous channel (Figure 16-14). If there is significant resistance to flow in the anomalous pulmonary venous pathway, pulmonary venous

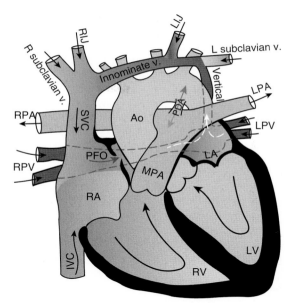

FIGURE 16-14 ■ Cartoon depicting supradiaphragmatic totally anomalous pulmonary vein connection. Arrows depict direction of blood flow. *SVC,* Superior vena cava; *IVC,* inferior vena cava; *RIJ, LIJ,* right and left jugular vein; *r, l subclavian v,* right, left subclavian vein; *vertical v,* vertical vein; *RA,* right atrium; *LA,* left atrium; *RV,* right ventricle; *LV,* left ventricle; *PFO,* patent foramen ovale; *MPA,* main pulmonary artery; *RPA,* right pulmonary artery; *LPA,* left pulmonary artery; *PDA,* patent ductus arteriosus; *RPV,* right pulmonary veins; *LPV,* left pulmonary veins; *Ao,* aorta.

hypertension ensues. When the hydrostatic pressure within the pulmonary veins exceeds oncotic pressure, pulmonary edema follows. The decrease in lung compliance results in respiratory distress and the alveolar diffusion abnormality from edema results in hypoxemia and reduced hemoglobin oxygen saturation. Timing of symptoms depends upon the number and degree of obstructed pulmonary veins. In isolated totally anomalous pulmonary venous connection with obstruction, symptoms of respiratory distress and cyanosis are seen within the first 24 hours after birth but are rarely noted at birth.

Finally, increased left atrial pressure may secondarily cause pulmonary venous hypertension and pulmonary edema and hence respiratory distress. Examples of lesions causing an increased left atrial pressure include hypoplastic left heart syndrome with mitral atresia and a restrictive or intact atrial septum, severe mitral or aortic valve stenosis or regurgitation, decreased left ventricular systolic or diastolic function secondary to cardiomyopathy, or obstruction to the left ventricular outflow tract. Infants with these lesions typically show signs of decreased perfusion in addition to respiratory distress.

Totally anomalous pulmonary venous connection must be excluded in term infants presenting with respiratory distress, especially when there are chest radiographic findings of pulmonary edema and a normal heart size (Figure 16-13). Totally anomalous pulmonary venous connection may be classified into different types based on the location of drainage of the pulmonary veins. Supracardiac, cardiac, and infracardiac types reflect the areas of connection of the pulmonary veins. Totally anomalous pulmonary venous connection may be also classified based on whether they are obstructed or not. The degree of obstruction often varies and the clinical presentation depends upon the severity of obstruction. Patients with *unobstructed* total anomalous pulmonary venous connection generally present with symptoms of pulmonary overcirculation and cardiac failure by 4 to 6 weeks of age.

CASE STUDY 5 (continued)

On an echocardiogram, the pediatric cardiologist makes the diagnosis of infracardiac totally anomalous pulmonary venous connection with obstruction. The four pulmonary veins join to form a confluence, which drains via a long vertical vein into the portal vein. Pulmonary artery pressure is elevated; right ventricular systolic function is mildly depressed; the foramen ovale is not restrictive. Flow through the patent ductus arteriosus is right-to-left in systole. He recommends urgent transfer to a cardiac surgical center.

The hemoglobin oxygen saturation as measured by pulse oximetry is no higher than 70% and he is placed on conventional mechanical ventilation with a peak inspiratory pressure of 22 mmHg, positive end expiratory pressure of 5 mmHg, and FiO$_2$ of 1.0.

EXERCISE 11

QUESTION

1. While awaiting transport, a medical student suggests adding inhaled nitric oxide to improve oxygenation. This intervention will most likely:
   a. Improve oxygenation by increasing pulmonary blood flow
   b. Worsen oxygenation by increasing pulmonary blood flow

ANSWER

1. **b.** Totally anomalous pulmonary venous connection with obstruction is a surgical emergency. Urgent transfer to a cardiac center where surgery can be performed is critical for survival. Infants with obstructed totally anomalous pulmonary venous connection exhibit hypoxemia, the severity of which varies with the degree of obstruction.

Several factors contribute to the hypoxemia: (1) pulmonary edema and the secondary diffusion abnormality lead to low oxygen tension and saturation in the pulmonary veins; (2) mixing of oxygenated and deoxygenated blood—pulmonary venous return mixes with systemic venous return; and (3) hypoxic reflex pulmonary artery vasoconstriction leads to pulmonary artery hypertension, right-to-left shunting across the ductus arteriosus, and decreased pulmonary blood flow. Pulmonary artery vasoconstriction in the setting of pulmonary venous obstruction and hypertension restricts blood flow into the lungs and protects the pulmonary bed from worsening alveolar edema. Maneuvers that decrease pulmonary vascular resistance, e.g., inhaled nitric oxide, are expected to lead to an increase in pulmonary blood flow. In the setting of fixed downstream obstruction, pulmonary edema is likely to worsen if blood flow into the pulmonary circuit is greater than that drained from it. Therefore, the use of pulmonary vasodilators in an effort to improve oxygenation may be counterproductive and may be ill advised.

Employing optimal ventilator strategies that improve oxygenation—but do not negatively impact right ventricular function—is desired. Hence, increasing inspired oxygen concentration and optimizing positive end expiratory pressure and mean airway pressure to maintain functional residual capacity of the lung may improve oxygenation. Excessive increases in positive end expiratory pressure or mean airway pressure will increase intrathoracic pressure and negatively affect right ventricular performance. The most important goal is to meet the oxygen needs of the body rather than applying arbitrary goal targets of oxygen saturation. Therefore, in the absence of metabolic acidosis, a "low" oxygen saturation may be accepted while awaiting the arrival of the transport team. In severe cases, when oxygen deficit is profound or when right ventricular function is severely depressed, extracorporeal support may be considered for stabilization prior to operative intervention.

EXERCISE 12

QUESTION

1. The same medical student asks if PGE-1 may be used in this patient. The most appropriate answer to the question posed above is:
   a. PGE-1 is absolutely contraindicated in *all* cases of obstructed totally anomalous pulmonary venous connection.
   b. PGE-1 may be used in *some* cases of obstructed totally anomalous pulmonary venous connection.

ANSWER

1. **b.** The use of PGE-1 in obstructed total anomalous pulmonary venous connection is controversial. There may be a role for its use in select cases; however, PGE-1 must always be used with caution. In obstructed total anomalous pulmonary venous connection, PGE-1 may be employed to "off-load" the failing right ventricle or when left ventricular inflow or outflow is inadequate. The latter can occur when the foramen ovale is "restrictive." In total anomalous pulmonary venous connection, left ventricular preload and hence output is dependent upon right-to-left shunting across the foramen ovale. If the foramen is small and "restrictive," left ventricular preload or filling is reduced and hence left ventricular stroke volume is reduced. A posteriorly deviated interventricular septum (in the setting of severe pulmonary hypertension and right ventricular dilatation) can lead to encroachment of left ventricular cavity and impede left ventricular filling and output.

As long as the ductus arteriosus is widely patent, right ventricular output may be diverted into the systemic circuit. However, when such a "pop-off" mechanism is unavailable, the systolic performance of the right ventricle may deteriorate in the face of increased afterload (increased pulmonary vascular resistance and a restrictive ductus arteriosus). Hence, maintaining ductal patency by administering PGE-1 infusion may help preserve right ventricular systolic function or delay its deterioration. Although adding PGE-1 infusion may worsen oxygen saturation, the net oxygen delivery will likely improve as the systemic output improves. It is important to note that the pulmonary vasodilatory properties of PGE-1 may also worsen oxygenation by mechanisms described previously. In this patient, as the ductus arteriosus is widely patent, the foramen ovale is not restrictive, and the right ventricular systolic function is preserved, the use of PGE-1 is not indicated.

NEONATE WITH DECREASED PERFUSION

CASE STUDY 6

A 10-day-old female infant born at 39 weeks of gestation arrives at the emergency room of the community hospital where you are covering. She was born by normal spontaneous vaginal delivery at the same hospital and was discharged home within 48 hours. The mother's pregnancy, labor, and delivery were unremarkable. A normal neonatal admission and discharge physical examinations were documented in the hospital records. This infant was feeding and voiding appropriately while in the hospital. By parental account, their infant became progressively "fussy." She breathed faster and required a longer time for each bottle-feeding. On the day of presentation she fed no more than 1 ounce of formula and hadn't voided since the night before.

Vital signs: Temperature 36.8, heart rate 190 beats/minute, noninvasive blood pressure from the right arm 78/50 mmHg, respiratory rate 78 breaths/minute, SaO$_2$ from the right hand is 98%. Weight is 3.3 kg (birth weight and discharge weight are 3.5 and 3.4 kg). The infant appears alert but irritable. She is in moderate respiratory distress with nasal flaring and has subcostal and intercostal retractions. Equal breath sounds are heard bilaterally and fine rales are heard at both lung bases. The precordium is hyperdynamic, pulmonary component of the second heart sound is loud, and no murmurs are appreciated on auscultation. The liver is palpable 4 cm below the right costal margin. Lower extremity pulses are difficult to palpate. Her feet are cool to touch. There are no skin lesions; the capillary refill is 5 seconds CBC: WBC 15 × 10^9/L, Hct 40%, platelet count 23 × 10^9/L. Differential count 50% neutrophils, 35% lymphocytes, and no bands. Serum chemistry panel: sodium 145 mEq/L, potassium 5 mEq/L, chloride 110 mEq/L, bicarbonate 14 mEq/L, blood urea nitrogen 40 mg/dL, creatinine 1.0 mg/dL. The chest radiograph shows pulmonary edema and cardiomegaly and a left aortic arch. Blood culture is pending. Intravenous antibiotics have been administered.

EXERCISE 13

QUESTION

1. This infant's clinical presentation is most consistent with a:
    a. Left heart obstructive lesion
    b. Right heart obstructive lesion
    c. Adrenal Insufficiency
    d. Sepsis

ANSWER

1. **a.** Newborn infants with obstruction to left ventricular output may be difficult to distinguish from those with sepsis. The clinical presentation is often similar but careful and thorough physical examination and historical evaluation may help in establishing an accurate clinical diagnosis.

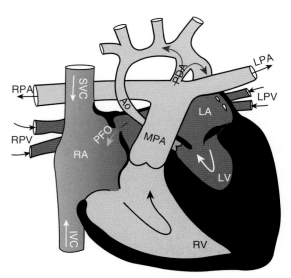

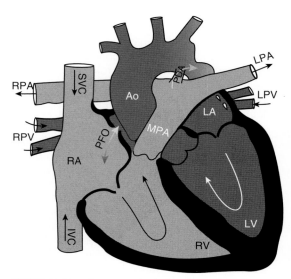

FIGURE 16-15 ■ Cartoon depicting hypoplastic left heart syndrome. Arrows depict direction of blood flow. *SVC,* Superior vena cava; *IVC,* inferior vena cava; *RA,* right atrium; *LA,* left atrium; *RV,* right ventricle; *LV,* left ventricle; *PFO,* patent foramen ovale; *MPA,* main pulmonary artery; *RPA,* right pulmonary artery; *LPA,* left pulmonary artery; *PDA,* patent ductus arteriosus; *RPV,* right pulmonary veins; *LPV,* left pulmonary veins; *Ao,* aorta.

FIGURE 16-16 ■ Cartoon depicting juxtaductal coarctation of the aorta. Arrows depict direction of blood flow. *SVC,* Superior vena cava; *IVC,* inferior vena cava; *RA,* right atrium; *LA,* left atrium; *RV,* right ventricle; *LV,* left ventricle; *PFO,* patent foramen ovale; *MPA,* main pulmonary artery; *RPA,* right pulmonary artery; *LPA,* left pulmonary artery; *PDA,* patent ductus arteriosus; *RPV,* right pulmonary veins; *LPV,* left pulmonary veins; *Ao,* aorta.

Obstruction to left ventricular outflow may occur at different levels. Examples include coarctation of the aorta, interrupted aortic arch, hypoplasia of the aortic arch, and valvar or subvalvar aortic stenosis. In extreme cases, the entire left sided structures may be exceedingly small (hypoplastic left heart syndrome). Severity of obstruction to flow from the left ventricle is variable and can range from mild (coarctation with minimal obstruction) to severe (hypoplastic left heart syndrome where the minute left ventricle is ill equipped to support the systemic circulation) (Figure 16-15).

Coarctation of the aorta refers to narrowing of the aorta, usually discrete, and in the juxtaductal region (Figure 16-16). Interrupted aortic arch may be of several types based on the level of interruption. Interruption usually occurs between the left subclavian artery and the left common carotid artery but may occur proximal or distal to this location.

The right ventricle supports flow into the aorta distal to the level of the obstruction via the ductus arteriosus, which is usually patent at 24 to 48 hours of life. Functional closure occurs by 4 days in most infants and anatomic closure follows over the next several days and weeks. Critical left sided obstructive lesions depend upon right ventricular output and ductal patency to support the systemic circulation. Once the ductus arteriosus closes, the left ventricle

has to support the entire systemic circulation. Obstruction to left ventricular output imposes an increase in afterload to the left ventricle and because the neonatal heart is unable to handle acute pressure overload, left ventricular systolic function deteriorates. An increase in left atrial pressure results in pulmonary edema, causing both an increase in respiratory work and feeding difficulties. The decrease in systemic blood flow and organ perfusion leads to a switch to anaerobic bioenergetics and metabolic acidosis. Left ventricular performance worsens with metabolic acidosis and circulatory function is further compromised.

Left sided obstructive lesions may be particularly challenging to diagnose. These patients are rarely symptomatic during their brief stay in the nursery. If the diagnosis is not made prior to discharge from the nursery, babies with critical left sided obstructive lesions may present with signs of evolving or established circulatory failure and cardiogenic shock. Patients with fulminant sepsis may present in a similar fashion, but will likely have supporting laboratory indices favoring a diagnosis of invasive bacterial infection.

CASE STUDY 6 (continued)

Femoral artery pulses are difficult to appreciate, whereas both brachial artery pulses are felt easily. You ask that noninvasive blood pressure be measured in all four extremities: right arm 78/50 mmHg, left arm 66/40 mmHg. After several failed attempts, blood pressure on the lower extremities is obtained: right leg 30/22 mmHg, left leg 34/22 mmHg. Pulse oximetry reading from sensor on the right hand is 98%; a similar sensor on the foot shows a poor tracing.

EXERCISE 14

QUESTION

1. Of the following, the most likely diagnosis is:
   a. Juxtaductal coarctation of the aorta
   b. Hypoplastic left heart syndrome
   c. Aortic valve stenosis
   d. Interrupted aortic arch

ANSWER

1. **a.** As described previously, obstruction to left ventricular outflow can occur at different levels. When such an obstruction is suspected, clinical evaluation and vital sign measurements may offer clues to the level of obstruction (Table 16-2). A good starting point is to palpate femoral pulses. It is generally difficult to feel femoral pulses easily in newborn infants unless hips are abducted. In this optimal position, one should be able to easily palpate femoral artery pulses. If there is difficulty in feeling both femoral pulses, comparison should be made with brachial artery pulses. If brachial artery pulses are very strong and femoral pulses are poor, the level of aortic obstruction is below the level of the left subclavian artery (if the arch is leftward) or below the level of the right subclavian artery (if the arch is rightward). If the right brachial pulse is easily felt, but the left brachial and both femoral pulses are equally diminished, the arch is likely to be interrupted proximal to the

origin of the left subclavian artery. Sometimes, in severe coarctation of the aorta, the adjacent subclavian artery also may be narrowed; hence the pulse on that arm may be difficult to appreciate or may be of lower amplitude than that of the contralateral arm. When both brachial and femoral pulses are diminished and the perfusion is poor, significant depression in cardiac performance is likely. The other possibility is the presence of an aberrant right subclavian artery arising distal to the obstruction. Feeling the carotid pulses may differentiate the two. When cardiac output is severely compromised, carotid pulses are also difficult to palpate. However, in coarctation of the aorta with an aberrant right subclavian artery, the carotid pulse amplitude will be very strong. Blood pressure measurement in the four extremities should show the same differences as that revealed by pulse strength. When obstruction is more proximal, e.g., aortic stenosis or hypoplastic left heart syndrome, there is no difference in pulse amplitude or blood pressure between the four extremities.

In this patient who presents with pulses and blood pressure differential between the upper and lower extremities, juxtaductal coarctation of the aorta is the most likely diagnosis.

EXERCISE 15

QUESTION

1. A pediatric cardiologist is not readily available. The emergency room physician requests your assistance in the management of this infant. The best option is:
   a. To start PGE-1 infusion right away prior to echocardiogram and arrival of pediatric cardiologist
   b. Wait for pediatric cardiologist and echocardiogram to start PGE-1 infusion

TABLE 16-2   Level of Obstruction of Aortic Arch

Femoral Pulses	Right Brachial Pulse	Left Brachial Pulse	Possible Site of Obstruction
++	++	++	No obstruction
+/−	++	+	Juxtaductal coarctation of the aorta (left brachial pulse may be diminished due to narrowing extending into the left subclavian artery)
+/−	++	+/−	Interruption of the aortic arch proximal to the left subclavian artery (left brachial and femoral pulses are similar)
+/−	+/−	+/−	• Diminished left ventricular performance • Aortic stenosis • Hypoplastic left heart syndrome • Aberrant origin of the right subclavian artery distal to the level of obstruction

++, Normal pulse; +, palpable pulse but diminished; −, absent pulse.

ANSWER

1. **a.** PGE-1 must be started right away if critical left heart obstruction is suspected. It is not necessary to wait for a confirmatory echocardiogram if one cannot be obtained readily. Other therapeutic interventions such as volume resuscitation and inotropic therapy are rarely effective unless the ductus arteriosus is reopened and systemic blood flow is reestablished. PGE-1 is administered as a continuous infusion owing to its rapid metabolism. Low doses of PGE-1 (0.01 mcg/kg/min to 0.05 mcg/kg/min) are usually adequate to maintain patency of an open ductus arteriosus. A higher dose of PGE-1 (0.1 to 0.2 mcg/kg/min) may be effective in reopening a functionally closed ductus arteriosus. Once the ductus arteriosus is reopened, the dose of PGE-1 may be titrated to the lowest effective dose. PGE-1 induces several side effects, including apnea, hyperthermia, hypotension, and thrombocytopenia. These side effects are dose dependent and are usually encountered with higher doses of PGE-1.

Stabilization of an infant presenting in circulatory collapse should follow the usual principles of resuscitation: **A**irway, **B**reathing, and **C**irculation. Effective stabilization often requires mechanical ventilator support and use of PGE-1 to reopen the ductus arteriosus. Other measures may include volume resuscitation, addition of inotropes to augment ventricular systolic function, correction of electrolyte and acid–base abnormalities, and maintaining glucose homeostasis. Laboratory tests to identify the extent of renal or hepatic injury should be undertaken along with serial arterial blood gas and lactate measurements.

Effectiveness of resuscitative efforts in this patient may be gauged by improvement in lower extremity pulses and blood pressure and normalization of blood gases.

CONCLUSION

Congenital heart disease is the most common birth malformation. Despite the numerous forms, neonates with CHD present in limited ways: cyanosis, shock, and tachypnea. A careful history and physical examination guided by a systematic approach will help formulate a clinical diagnosis without much difficulty.

SUGGESTED READINGS

Abu-Harb M, Hey E, Wren C: Death in infancy from unrecognized congenital heart disease, *Arch Dis Child Fetal Neonatal Ed* 71:3–7, 1994.

Ainsworth SB, Wyllie JP, Wren C: Prevalence and clinical significance of cardiac murmurs in neonates, *Arch Dis Child Fetal Neonatal Ed* 80:F43–F45, 1999.

Allan LD, Crawford DC, Chita SK: Familial recurrence of congenital heart disease in a prospective series of mothers referred for fetal echocardiography, *Am J Cardiol* 58: 334–337, 1986.

Ardrain GM, Dawes GS, Prichard MML, et al.: The effect of ventilation of the foetal lungs upon the pulmonary circulation, *J Physiol* 118:12–22, 1952.

Arlettaz R, Archer N, Wilkinson AR: Natural history of innocent heart murmurs in newborn babies: controlled echocardiographic study, *Arch Dis Child Fetal Neonatal Ed* 78:F166–F170, 1998.

Artman A, Mahony L, Teitel DF: *Neonatal cardiology*, 2nd ed, New York, NY, 2011, McGraw-Hill.

Benjamin JT, Romp RL, Carlo WA, et al.: Identification of serious congenital heart disease in neonates after initial hospital discharge, *Cong Heart Dis* 2(5):327–331, 2007.

Burd L, Deal E, Rios R, et al.: Congenital heart defects and fetal alcohol spectrum disorders, *Cong Heart Dis* 2(4): 250–255, 2007.

Burn J, Brennan P, Little J, et al.: Recurrence risks in offspring of adults with major heart defects: results from first cohort of British collaborative study, *Lancet* 351(9099):311–316, 1998.

cdcinfo@cdc.gov (homepage on the Internet). Centers for Disease Control and Prevention; Atlanta, GA. Available from http://www.cdc.gov/ncbddd/heartdefects/.

Cohen LS, Friedman JM, Jefferson JW: A reevaluation of risk of in utero exposure to lithium, *JAMA* 271(2): 146–150, 1994.

Edelstone DI, Rudolph AM: Preferential streaming of ductus venosus blood to the brain and heart in fetal lambs, *Am J Physiol* 237:H724–H729, 1979.

Friedberg MK, Silverman NH, Moon-Grady AJ, et al.: Prenatal detection of congenital heart disease, *J Peds* 155(1):26–31, 2009.

Hoffman JIE, Kaplan S: The incidence of congenital heart disease, *JACC* 39(12):1890–1900, 2002.

Jacobs JP, Jacobs ML, Mavroudis C, et al. Executive summary: The Society of Thoracic Surgeons Congenital Heart Surgery Database—Fourteenth Harvest—January 1, 2007-December 31, 2010. The Society of Thoracic Surgeons (STS) and Duke Clinical Research Institute (DCRI), Duke University Medical Center, Durham, NC, Spring 2011 Harvest.

Kaltman JR, Andropoulos DB, Checchia PA: Report of the Pediatric Heart Network and National Heart, Lung, and Blood Institute Working Group on the Perioperative Management of Congenital Heart Disease, *Circulation* 121:2766–2772, 2010.

Kemper AR, Mahle WT, Martin GR, et al.: Strategies for implementing screening for critical congenital heart disease, *Pediatrics* 128(5):1259–1267, 2011.

Lisowski LA, Verheijen PM, Copel JA: Congenital heart disease in pregnancies complicated by maternal diabetes mellitus, *Herz* 35:19–26, 2010.

Mackie AS, Jutras LC, Dancea AB, et al.: Can cardiologists distinguish innocent from pathologic murmurs in neonates? *J Pediatr* 154:50–54, 2009.

Mahle WT, Martin GR, Beekman III RH, et al.: Endorsement of Health and Human Services recommendation for pulse oximetry screening for critical congenital heart disease, *Pediatrics* 129(1):190–192, 2012.

Mahle WT, Newburger JW, Matherne P, et al.: Role of pulse oximetry in examining newborns for congenital heart disease: a scientific statement from the AHA and AAP, *Pediatrics* 124(2):823–836, 2009.

McCrindle BW, Shaffer KM, Kan JS, et al.: *Arch Pediatr Adolesc Med* 150:169–174, 1996.

Mielke G, Benda N: Cardiac output and central distribution of blood flow in the human fetus, *Circulation* 103: 1662–1668, 2001.

Øyen N, Poulsen G, Boyd HA, et al.: Recurrence of congenital heart defects in families, *Circulation* 120(4):295–301, 2009.

Rudolph AM: *Congenital diseases of the heart: clinical physiological considerations*, 3rd ed, Chichester, West Sussex, UK, 2009, Wiley-Blackwell.

Tararbit K, Houyel L, Bonnet D, et al.: Risk of congenital heart defects associated with assisted reproductive technologies: a population-based evaluation, *Eur Heart J* 32(4):500–508, 2011.

van der Linde D, Konings EEM, Slager MA, et al.: Birth prevalence of congenital heart disease worldwide. A systematic review and meta-analysis, *J Am Coll Cardiol* 58:2241–2247, 2011.

Wren C, Reinhardt Z, Khawaja K: Twenty-year trends in diagnosis of life-threatening neonatal cardiovascular malformations, *Arch Dis Child Fetal Neonatal Ed* 93(1): F33–F35, 2008.

Wren C, Richmond S, Donaldson L: Presentation of congenital heart disease in infancy: implications for routine examination, *Arch Dis Child Fetal Neonatal Ed* 80:F49–F53, 1999.

PERSISTENT PULMONARY HYPERTENSION OF THE NEWBORN AND HYPOXEMIC RESPIRATORY FAILURE

Bobby Mathew, MBBS • Satyan Lakshminrusimha, MD

The fetus is in a state of "physiologic pulmonary hypertension." The PaO_2 in the descending aorta of the fetus is approximately 20 to 25 mmHg with an oxygen saturation (SaO_2) of 55% to 58% (Figure 17-1). In spite of being "hypoxemic" (low PaO_2 levels relative to postnatal standards), the fetus can deliver adequate oxygen to its tissues and is not hypoxic. Oxygen delivery (DO_2) is dependent on cardiac output (CO) and oxygen content of the blood (CaO_2). The fetus maintains adequate oxygen delivery to its tissues by the following physiologic adaptations: (1) presence of fetal hemoglobin (HbF) with high affinity for oxygen; (2) higher hemoglobin levels in a term fetus compared to children and adults resulting in a higher CaO_2 at any given oxygen saturation level; and (3) high cardiac output. During fetal life, the placenta is the organ of gas exchange. The difference in oxygen saturation (a measure of oxygen uptake from the organ of gas exchange) between the umbilical vein (80%) and umbilical artery (58%) during fetal life (Figure 17-1) is similar to the difference between the pulmonary vein/aorta (95%) and pulmonary artery (70%) in an adult.

Similar to the adult lung, the placenta receives approximately 40% to 45% of combined ventricular output. The lungs receive 8% to 10% of combined ventricular output in fetal lambs and approximately 25% in near-term human fetuses (Rasanen, Wood, Weiner, Ludomirski, & Huhta, 1996). After birth and following initiation of air breathing, pulmonary blood flow markedly increases (Lakshminrusimha & Steinhorn, 1999) resolving the fetal "physiologic pulmonary hypertension" (Lakshminrusimha, 2012). In infants with an adverse event *in utero* or with abnormalities of pulmonary transition at birth, pulmonary hypertension persists into the newborn period resulting in persistent pulmonary hypertension of the newborn (PPHN) leading to hypoxemic respiratory failure (HRF).

The following case studies discuss the presentation, clinical features, and management of PPHN and HRF.

CASE STUDY 1

A 32-year-old woman with gestational diabetes is admitted to a community hospital at 37½ weeks' gestation following rupture of membranes. She weighs 225 pounds and has a healthy 2-year-old boy born by cesarean section. A repeat cesarean section is performed for late decelerations. The baby weighs 8 pounds and 8 ounces (3855 grams) and is brought to the nursery at 2 hours of age for hypoglycemia. He is noted to be tachypneic with a respiratory rate of 82/minute. His oxygen saturation (SpO_2) is 83% in room air and he is placed in a hood with 30% oxygen. His SpO_2 continues to be low at 85% and the inspired oxygen concentration is gradually increased in steps to 45% to achieve saturations in the 90s. A chest x-ray is obtained (Figure 17-2) and the regional perinatal center is called for transport.

EXERCISE 1

QUESTION

1. What is the most likely cause for hypoxemia and tachypnea in this infant?
   a. Surfactant deficiency and respiratory distress syndrome (RDS)
   b. Retained fetal lung liquid and transient tachypnea of the newborn (TTN)
   c. Infection with pneumonia
   d. Atelectasis
   e. Cardiac failure

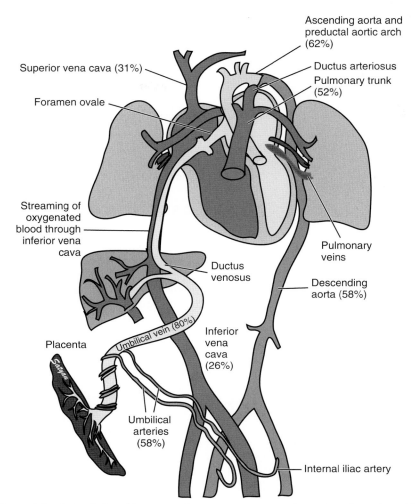

FIGURE 17-1 ■ **Normal fetal circulation.** The approximate oxygen saturation values in various blood vessels are shown in parentheses. Darker shade indicates lower oxygen saturation. There are three major vascular shunts that maintain the fetal circulatory pattern. (i) Ductus venosus shunts oxygenated blood from the umbilical venous circulation directly to the inferior vena cava. This oxygenated blood is preferentially streamed through the inferior vena cava and the right atrium towards the foramen ovale. (ii) Foramen ovale shunts oxygenated blood from the right atrium to the left atrium. Subsequently, this blood enters the left ventricle and ascending aorta and supplies the coronaries and the brain. (iii) Deoxygenated blood in the pulmonary artery bypasses the lungs through the ductus arteriosus and enters the descending aorta. (Copyright © 2015 Bobby Mathew, Satyan Lakshminrusimha. Published by Elsevier Inc. All rights reserved.)

ANSWER

1. **b.** This infant has several risk factors for respiratory distress at birth.
   - Early-term delivery (37⁶/₇ and 38⁶/₇ weeks postmenstrual age [PMA]) is associated with a higher risk of respiratory distress and admission to the neonatal intensive care unit (NICU) (Engle, 2011). The American College of Obstetrics and Gynecology (ACOG) strongly recommends against induction and elective cesarean section prior to 39 completed weeks of gestation (Spong et al., 2011) and has recently updated the guidelines for medically indicated late-preterm and early term

deliveries ("Committee opinion no. 560: medically indicated late-preterm and early-term deliveries," 2013).
   - Maternal diabetes increases the risk of surfactant deficiency and RDS.
   - Delivery by cesarean section also increases the risk of respiratory distress. The additive effect of cesarean section on respiratory morbidity is higher at 37 weeks compared to 39 or 40 weeks' gestation. Vaginal delivery is associated with a rapid reduction in fetal PVR at birth. Delivery by elective cesarean section (Ramachandrappa & Jain, 2008; Sulyok & Csaba, 1986) delays the decrease

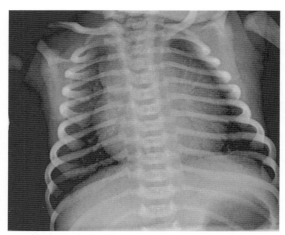

FIGURE 17-2 ■ **Chest x-ray from Case Study 1 obtained at 2.5 hours of age showing 10-rib expansion and some bilateral streakiness.** (Copyright © 2015 Bobby Mathew, Satyan Lakshminrusimha. Published by Elsevier Inc. All rights reserved.)

in pulmonary arterial pressure (Figure 17-3) and increases the risk for PPHN (Wilson et al., 2011). Compared to matched controls, infants with PPHN are more likely to have been delivered by cesarean section (Hernandez-Diaz, Van Marter, Werler, Louik, & Mitchell, 2007). The early term gestational age and the initial chest x-ray appearance in this patient are suggestive of retained lung liquid and TTN (Guglani, Lakshminrusimha, & Ryan, 2008). The chest x-ray shows expansion to 10 ribs, and diffuse interstitial markings (streaky appearance). Although most cases of TTN are mild (requiring less than 40% oxygen with a short course lasting 2 to 3 days), some cases may be associated with more profound hypoxemia (Ramachandrappa & Jain, 2008) and is sometimes referred to as "malignant TTN." Abnormal shunting secondary to pulmonary hypertension or congenital heart disease should be "ruled out" in such cases by echocardiography.

PULMONARY VASCULAR TRANSITION AT BIRTH

The entry of air into the alveoli with crying and breathing improves oxygenation of the pulmonary vascular bed, thereby decreasing pulmonary vascular resistance (PVR) and increasing pulmonary blood flow (Teitel, Iwamoto, & Rudolph, 1990). The increase in pulmonary blood flow raises left atrial pressures above right atrial pressures, closing the foramen ovale. Removal of the low resistance placental bed from the systemic circulation at birth increases systemic vascular resistance (SVR).

PVR falls to approximately half of SVR within a few minutes after birth. As PVR becomes less than SVR, flow reverses across the ductus arteriosus and oxygenated blood flows from the aorta to the pulmonary artery. Over the first few hours the ductus arteriosus closes, largely in response to an increase in oxygen tension, and with this, the normal postnatal circulatory pattern is established. Vasodilator mediators such as nitric oxide (NO) and prostacyclin (PGI_2) are important mediators of pulmonary vascular transition at birth (Abman, Chatfield, Hall, & McMurtry, 1990).

CASE STUDY 1 (continued)

The transport team arrives 3 hours later. The baby's oxygen requirement has steadily increased to 95% oxygen by hood with saturations in the high 90s. Clinical examination reveals tachypnea (72/minute), grunting, and intercostal retractions. The arterial blood gas is as follows: pH 7.21, PCO_2 66 mmHg, and PO_2 52 mmHg. His chest x-ray is repeated and is shown in Figure 17-4, A. A decision is made to intubate the patient prior to transport.

EXERCISE 2

QUESTION

1. What is the most likely cause of hypoxemia and respiratory distress in this infant?
   a. PPHN
   b. Pneumonia
   c. Absorption atelectasis
   d. RDS/surfactant deficiency

ANSWER

1. **c.** The infant is now grunting, which suggests that he is trying to maintain a normal functional residual capacity. Respiratory deterioration in this infant can be secondary to any of the choices mentioned above. However, the administration of high ambient concentrations of oxygen without positive pressure can result in "absorption atelectasis" (Figure 17-5). Unlike nitrogen (the predominant gas in room air), oxygen is easily absorbed from the alveoli into the bloodstream, leading to alveolar collapse. Because of nitrogen's low solubility, very little diffuses across the alveolar capillary interface, and most of the inspired nitrogen stays in the alveolus helping to keep it open. When a high fractional inspired oxygen is used, the concentration of nitrogen in the inspired gas and in the alveolus is decreased. Oxygen absorption atelectasis leads to ventilation-perfusion (V/Q) mismatch, shunting, and hypoxemia. Therefore, it is important to avoid administration of high concentrations

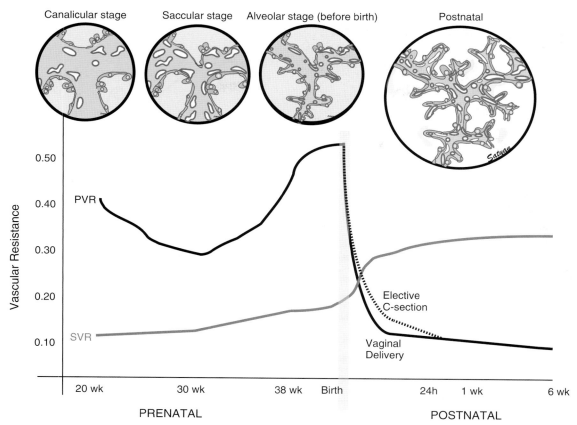

FIGURE 17-3 ■ **Changes in pulmonary vascular resistance (PVR) and systemic vascular resistance (SVR) during the last half of gestation and postnatal period.** During the canalicular phase of lung development, high PVR is caused by low density of vasculature. In the saccular stage, broad intersaccular septae contain the "double capillary network" and with increasing vascular density, PVR decreases. In the alveolar phase, despite the rapid increase in the number of small pulmonary arteries, high PVR is maintained by active vasoconstriction. After birth, lung liquid is absorbed and an air–liquid interphase is established with juxtaposition of capillaries and alveolar epithelium to promote effective gas exchange. Dashed line represents the delay in decrease of PVR observed following elective cesarean section. SVR markedly increases after clamping the umbilical cord and removal of the low-resistance placental circuit from the systemic circulation. (Copyright © 2015 Bobby Mathew, Satyan Lakshminrusimha. Published by Elsevier Inc. All rights reserved.)

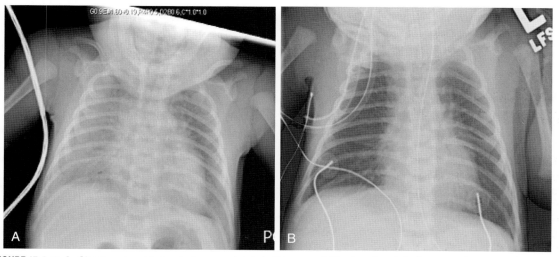

FIGURE 17-4 ■ **A,** Chest x-ray obtained at approximately 5 hours of life showing 8-9-rib expansion with increasing parenchymal densities. **B,** Chest x-ray obtained 1 hour after intubation and a dose of surfactant.

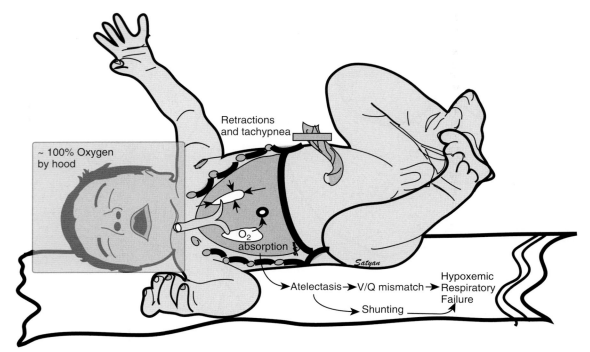

FIGURE 17-5 ■ **Absorption atelectasis—administration of a high concentration of inspired oxygen without positive pressure in an infant with respiratory distress—can lead to nitrogen washout and alveolar collapse.** Atelectasis can result in V/Q mismatch, shunting, and HRF with PPHN. (Copyright © 2015 Bobby Mathew, Satyan Lakshminrusimha. Published by Elsevier Inc. All rights reserved.)

of inspired oxygen (above 50% to 60%) without positive pressure (such as continuous positive airway pressure [CPAP]) in neonates with respiratory distress.

The x-ray appearance in Figure 17-4, *A* is consistent with the diagnosis of absorption atelectasis. It is also possible that this baby developed surfactant inactivation resulting in poor lung recruitment. The baby responded to initiation of mechanical ventilation and surfactant administration (see below) with improvement in oxygenation, and the relative contribution of these individual interventions cannot be determined.

CASE STUDY 1 (continued)

The baby is intubated by the transport respiratory therapist and placed on a conventional ventilator with positive end expiratory pressure (PEEP) of 6 cm H_2O, peak inspiratory pressure (PIP) of 18 cm H_2O at a rate of 35/minute. A dose of surfactant is administered. A subsequent x-ray prior to transfer shows improved aeration (Figure 17-4, B). The oxygen requirement is reduced to 35% with a right upper extremity (preductal) SpO_2 of 94%. On arrival to the Children's Hospital, the echocardiogram shows normal cardiac anatomy with left-to-right shunting at the patent ductus arteriosus

(PDA) and patent foramen ovale (PFO). An arterial blood gas drawn from the umbilical arterial line is as follows: pH of 7.49, $PaCO_2$ of 31 mmHg, PaO_2 of 60 mmHg. The ventilator rate is weaned to 30/minute and PIP is lowered to 16 cm H_2O after checking tidal volumes. The neonatologist discusses with the transport team and the residents the importance of avoiding hypocapnia and the effect of blood gases and ventilator settings on pulmonary blood flow.

EXERCISE 3

QUESTION

1. All of the following statements regarding the effect of pH, PO_2, and PCO_2 on pulmonary and cerebral circulation are correct EXCEPT:
   a. Hypoxia causes pulmonary vasoconstriction and cerebral vasodilation.
   b. Acute metabolic acidosis increases PVR and dilates the cerebral circulation.
   c. Acute respiratory acidosis increases PVR and dilates the cerebral circulation.
   d. Decreasing mean airway pressure (Paw) and reducing lung volume below functional residual capacity (FRC) increases PVR.
   e. Marked increase in Paw reduces cardiac output and cerebral blood flow.

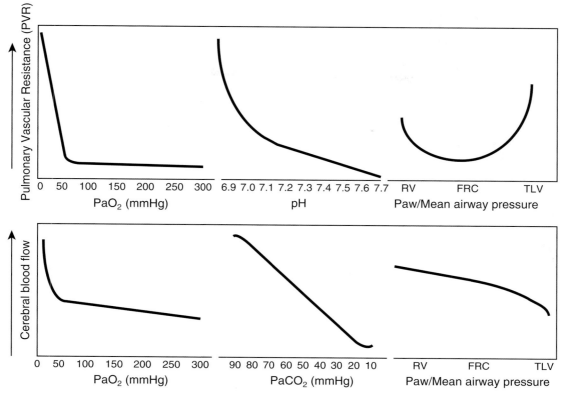

FIGURE 17-6 ■ **The effect of Pao$_2$, pH (or Paco$_2$), and mean airway pressure (Paw) on pulmonary vascular resistance (PVR, top panel) and cerebral blood flow (bottom panel).** Decrease in Pao$_2$ below 50 mmHg increases PVR by hypoxic pulmonary constriction and increases cerebral blood flow. Metabolic and respiratory acidosis cause pulmonary vasoconstriction and alkalosis causes pulmonary vasodilation. Increase in Paco$_2$ increases cerebral blood flow but acute metabolic changes in pH do not influence cerebral blood flow, as hydrogen ions do not easily diffuse across the blood brain barrier. Extremes of Paw increase PVR. PVR is minimal at functional residual capacity (FRC). Progressive increase in Paw toward total lung volume (TLV) reduces cardiac output by impeding venous return. Very low Paw reduces lung inflation to residual volume (RV), kinks extra-alveolar pulmonary vessels, and increases PVR. (Copyright © 2015 Bobby Mathew, Satyan Lakshminrusimha. Published by Elsevier Inc. All rights reserved.)

ANSWER

1. **b.** The systemic (cerebral) circulation responds to changes in blood gas parameters in a different manner compared to the pulmonary circulation (Figure 17-6). Hypoxia constricts pulmonary vessels and increases PVR. Normoxia dilates pulmonary vessels and decreases PVR but hyperoxia does not result in additional vasodilation (Lakshminrusimha et al., 2007; Lakshminrusimha et al., 2009; Rudolph & Yuan, 1966). The change point below which PVR increases is the alveolar PAO$_2$ that corresponds to the Pao$_2$ of 50 mmHg in neonatal animals without pulmonary hypertension and 60 mmHg in neonatal animal models of PPHN. Conversely, cerebral vasodilation occurs in response to decreased arterial oxygen content. Acidosis (both respiratory and metabolic) leads to pulmonary vasoconstriction and alkalosis (both respiratory and metabolic) causes pulmonary vasodilation. The

combination of acidosis and hypoxia results in exaggerated pulmonary vasoconstriction. Maintaining an arterial pH >7.30 will reduce pulmonary vasoconstriction in response to hypoxia (Rudolph & Yuan, 1966). Cerebral blood flow, on the other hand, decreases with respiratory alkalosis (approximately 4% reduction per mmHg decrease in Paco$_2$ in adults and a slightly lower degree in neonates). Changes in Paco$_2$ mediate alteration in cerebral blood flow by changing perivascular fluid pH in the brain (Figure 17-6 and Figure 17-7). Acute metabolic acid–base disturbances do not result in changes in cerebral blood flow, as H$^+$ ions do not cross the blood–brain barrier. However, in neonates with severe birth asphyxia, a rapid infusion of sodium bicarbonate causes cerebral perivascular alkalosis (owing to a leaky blood–brain barrier) and reduces cerebral blood flow (Lou, Lassen, & Fris-Hansen, 1978). Increasing Paw reduces

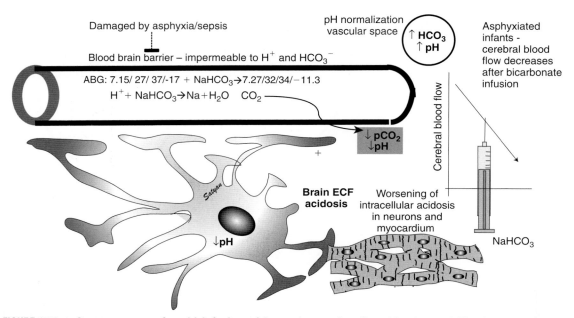

FIGURE 17-7 ■ **Consequences of rapid infusion of large doses of sodium bicarbonate.** The blood–brain barrier is normally impermeable to hydrogen ions and bicarbonate ions. However, CO_2 diffuses easily across the blood–brain barrier into the perivascular space. Acidosis in the perivascular extracellular fluid space in the brain causes cerebral vasodilation, and alkalosis in this space causes cerebral vasoconstriction. In conditions associated with acute metabolic acidosis with compensatory hypocapnia as seen in Case Study 6, low $PaCO_2$ results in cerebral vasoconstriction. Rapid correction of intravascular acidosis with rapid, large infusions of sodium bicarbonate results in increase in plasma pH, increase in $PaCO_2$, and reduction in base deficit. However, increased CO_2 diffuses across the blood–brain barrier causing perivascular acidosis in the brain. Diffusion of CO_2 also leads to intracellular acidosis in the neuronal cells, glial cells, and cardiac myocytes. In conditions associated with damage to the blood–brain barrier (as in asphyxia, hypoxia, and sepsis/meningitis), sodium bicarbonate may pass through the blood–brain barrier causing acute perivascular alkalosis and reduction in cerebral blood flow (Lou et al., 1978). Hence, caution must be exercised during alkali therapy. If sodium bicarbonate is absolutely needed, only small doses (such as 1 to 2 mEq/kg) should be infused, slowly and with careful monitoring of acid–base status. (Copyright © 2015 Bobby Mathew, Satyan Lakshminrusimha. Published by Elsevier Inc. All rights reserved.)

venous return and reduces cardiac output and cerebral blood flow. The effect of Paw on PVR is dependent on lung volume. At FRC, PVR is at its lowest and increases with atelectasis and hyperinflation (Figure 17-6).

The infant in this vignette has HRF with clinical signs of PPHN that responded to appropriate mechanical ventilation and surfactant. The differential diagnosis in such cases includes pulmonary parenchymal disease, congenital heart disease (CHD), and PPHN. Table 17-1 summarizes the distinguishing features of these conditions. Disorders of perinatal transition—such as retained fetal lung fluid, surfactant deficiency and/or inactivation, and PPHN—often coexist and contribute to HRF, especially in late-preterm (34⁶⁄₇ to 36⁶⁄₇ weeks PMA) and early term infants.

Chest x-rays are often helpful in the diagnosis in infants with HRF and some of the characteristic x-ray appearances for common neonatal respiratory disorders (Box 17-1) are described below. These descriptive terms are often used in the NICU and may provide a clue to the diagnosis.

Grainy: This is a classic description of RDS caused by surfactant deficiency. Grainy, translucent appearance of the lung fields is caused by the presence of microatelectasis interspersed with areas of hyperexpansion. Small alveoli have a tendency to collapse owing to increased surface tension in the absence of surfactant and inspired air empties into larger alveoli. Large alveoli have lower surface tension and continue to get larger (Laplace law) leading to a translucent, ground glass, or grainy appearance. The lungs are low volume (in nonintubated infants) and have air bronchograms (air in large airways superimposed on a background of granularity).

Streaky: A streaky appearance is characteristic of TTN with retained fetal lung liquid. Streaky interstitial shadowing associated with fluid in the horizontal fissure is the classic appearance of TTN. The lungs are usually well expanded or have an increased volume. This is caused by peribronchial cuffing and air trapping in expiration

TABLE 17-1   Differential Diagnosis of Hypoxemic Respiratory Failure in a Newborn Infant

	Lung Disease	PPHN	Cyanotic CHD
Respiratory distress	Present	Often present	Usually absent
Oxygen saturation (pulse oximetry) SpO$_2$	Improves with supplemental O$_2$	Labile, postductal SpO$_2$ may be lower than preductal SpO$_2$	Low fixed SpO$_2$ with minimal increase with supplemental O$_2$
PaCO$_2$	Elevated	Often elevated (except in "black lung" PPHN)	Usually normal/low
Hyperoxia test	PaO$_2$ often >150 mmHg	PaO$_2$ often >100 mmHg	PaO$_2$ often <100 mmHg
Hyperoxia–hyperventilation	PaO$_2$ often >150 mmHg	PaO$_2$ improves with hyperventilation	PaO$_2$ often <100 mmHg
Echocardiography	Normal	Structurally normal heart; RV hypertrophy, tricuspid regurgitation, bowing of interventricular septum to left, R→L or bidirectional shunt at PFO and/or PDA	Abnormalities in cardiac anatomy
Chest x-ray	Often associated with parenchymal densities	Depends on primary respiratory disease; reduced pulmonary vascularity in "black-lung" or idiopathic PPHN	Usually normal at birth; may be associated with abnormal cardiac silhouette and altered pulmonary vascularity

---

BOX 17-1   **The Differential Diagnosis of HRF and PPHN (Mnemonic: TACHyPneA)**

Transient tachypnea of the newborn/retained fetal lung fluid

Aspiration syndromes (meconium, blood or amniotic fluid, and **a**sphyxia)

Congenital anomalies (congenital diaphragmatic hernia)

Hyaline membrane disease/RDS

Pneumonia or sepsis

Air leaks

---

leading to hyperexpansion of the lungs (Guglani et al., 2008).

Black lung: In "black-lung" or idiopathic PPHN without parenchymal lung disease, lung fields are dark owing to decreased pulmonary vascularity. The lung fields may also appear black in infants with a pneumothorax secondary to anterior layering of lucent air in the pleural space.

Fluffy: In meconium aspiration syndrome (MAS), lung fields are overinflated with fluffy infiltrates in both lung fields. Aspirated meconium may exert a ball-valve effect leading to expiratory obstruction and air trapping.

Bubbly: Lung fields appear bubbly in pulmonary interstitial emphysema where air extravasates into the wall of the bronchi. A bubbly appearance may also be seen on the side of herniation in

congenital diaphragmatic hernia (CDH) owing to the presence of air in the intestines.

Hazy: The lung fields can appear hazy in infants with pneumonia and pulmonary hemorrhage.

Patchy: A patchy (nonhomogenous opacities) chest x-ray is suggestive of pneumonia. It is important to recognize that pneumonia caused by early-onset sepsis from group B streptococcal infection and gram-negative infections such as *Escherichia coli* can mimic other neonatal respiratory disorders such as RDS or MAS.

White-out appearance: A white-out appearance may be seen in diffuse extensive atelectasis of the lung. A similar appearance may be seen in obstructed total anomalous pulmonary venous return (TAPVR). The typical "snowman in a snowstorm" appearance is caused by pulmonary edema from obstruction of the pulmonary venous return associated with a supracardiac form of TAPVR. This condition may occasionally be confused with PPHN prior to obtaining an echocardiogram.

SYSTEMIC OXYGEN DELIVERY

An understanding of the basic principles of gas exchange and transport is crucial to assessing severity of PPHN and HRF. Figure 17-8 reviews the changes in oxygen levels through the process of oxygen transport from inspired gas to the mitochondria. This figure also illustrates the concept of systemic oxygen delivery (calculated by multiplying cardiac output with the

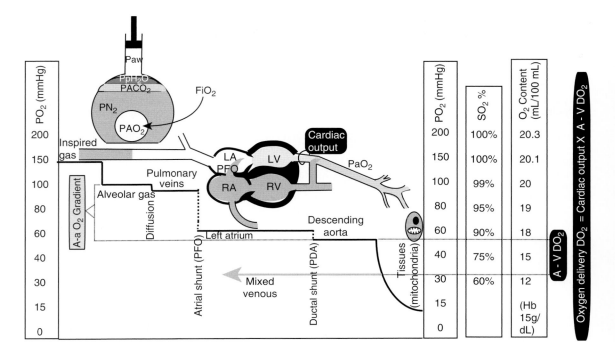

FIGURE 17-8 ■ Basics of gas exchange and transport. In this graph, the Y-axis represents PO_2 levels through the process of oxygen transport from inspired gas to the tissues and mitochondria. Approximate equivalent values for saturation (SO_2 in %) and oxygen content (in mL/dL assuming a hemoglobin level of 15 g/dL) are shown. The solid horizontal line shows approximate PO_2 values as oxygen moves from inspired gas to the alveolus. In the alveolus, oxygen is diluted by the presence of water vapor (ppH_2O), nitrogen, and carbon dioxide. There is a slight decrease in PO_2 as oxygen diffuses from the alveolus to the pulmonary capillary. In the left atrium, right-to-left shunt across the patent foramen ovale (PFO) decreases PO_2 in neonates with PPHN. A similar right-to-left shunt from pulmonary artery to aorta through the patent ductus arteriosus (PDA) further decreases the PO_2 in the postductal aorta. As the blood traverses the capillary, PO_2 decreases as oxygen diffuses into the tissues. The PO_2 values are low within the cell and mitochondria. The difference between arterial and venous oxygen content is called A-V DO_2 and is expressed in mL/dL. Multiplying A-V DO_2 with cardiac output provides systemic oxygen delivery (DO_2). (Copyright © 2015 Bobby Mathew, Satyan Lakshminrusimha. Published by Elsevier Inc. All rights reserved.)

difference between arterial and venous oxygen content A–V DO_2).

Systemic oxygen delivery = cardiac output ×
[(arterial oxygen content) − (venous oxygen content)]

Oxygen content = (oxygen bound to hemoglobin) + (oxygen dissolved in the plasma) in mL/dL

Oxygen content = (hemoglobin concentration g/dL × 1.34 × oxygen saturation) + (PO₂ in mmHg × 0.003) mL/dL

QUESTION

1. List the factors that determine oxygen delivery to the tissues in the order of importance.
   a. Dissolved oxygen
   b. Hemoglobin concentration
   c. Hemoglobin saturation
   d. Cardiac output

ANSWER

1. **d, b, c, a.** The cardiac output and hemoglobin concentration are the most important factors determining systemic oxygen delivery. The essential goal of management of PPHN is to maintain adequate delivery of oxygen to the tissues.

Assessment of Severity of PPHN/HRF

The severity of PPHN and HRF and response to treatment are objectively assessed by using four indices (Figures 17-8 and 17-9).

1. **Oxygenation index (OI):** This index includes factors that determine oxygenation (Paw) and concentration of inspired oxygen in the numerator and arterial oxygen tension in the denominator. This is one of the few indices that includes ventilator

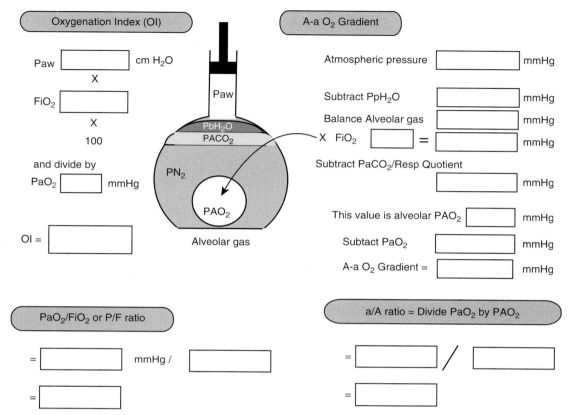

FIGURE 17-9 ■ **Worksheet for calculating severity of illness in PPHN/ HRF.** A full-term baby with meconium aspiration syndrome on a mean airway pressure (Paw) of 15 cm H_2O, FiO_2 of 1.0, $PaCO_2$ of 50 mmHg, and PaO_2 of 50 mmHg is cared for at the Women and Children's Hospital of Buffalo (atmospheric pressure – 747 mmHg).

(i) **Oxygenation index** is calculated by multiplying Paw × FiO_2 × 100 in the numerator. In the current patient, this value is 1500. Oxygenation index (OI) is calculated by dividing this number by PaO_2 of 50 mmHg. The OI is calculated to be 30 in this patient. This is the only index that takes Paw into consideration while determining the severity of HRF/PPHN.

(ii) **A-a gradient**: Subtracting PpH_2O (47 mmHg) from atmospheric pressure (747 mmHg) provides a value of 700 mmHg. Multiplying this value with FiO_2 of 1.0 will result in an alveolar pressure of 700 mmHg. Arterial $PaCO_2$ divided by the respiratory quotient (assumed to be 1.0 for neonates on glucose infusion) is subtracted (50 mmHg/1 = 50 mmHg) from 700 mmHg to provide the partial pressure of alveolar oxygen (PAO_2 – 650 mmHg in the current patient). Subtracting arterial PaO_2 (50 mmHg) from PAO_2 results in the A-a gradient of 600 mmHg.

(iii) An arterial to alveolar oxygen tension ratio (**a/A ratio**) is obtained by dividing PaO_2 by alveolar PAO_2. In the current patient, this ratio is 0.078.

(iv) **P/F ratio** (PaO_2/FiO_2 ratio) is often used to determine the severity of acute lung injury (ALI) and acute respiratory distress syndrome (ARDS) in children and adults. In the current patient, P/F ratio is 50 mmHg.

pressure and is commonly used in clinical trials to evaluate therapy in PPHN/HRF. The formula for calculating OI is given below and is illustrated in Figure 17-9 with an example.

$$OI = FiO_2 \times MAP \times 100/PaO_2$$

Some units assess the severity of PPHN/ HRF based on OI (Golombek & Young, 2010)
Mild – OI ≤15
Moderate – OI 15 to ≤25

Severe – OI 25 to ≤40
Very severe – OI >40 (with possible need for extracorporeal membrane oxygenation [ECMO])

2. **Alveolar-arterial oxygen gradient (A-a gradient or A-aDO_2):** This number estimates the gradient in the partial pressure of oxygen from the alveolus (PAO_2 – with an upper case "A" to denote alveolus) to the aorta (PaO_2 with a lower case "a" denote arterial) and is calculated as follows (also see Figure 17-9):

$A - aDO_2 = [(FiO_2) $ (barometric pressure $[\sim 760 \text{ mmHg}]$ − water vapor pressure $[47 \text{ mmHg}]) - PaCO_2/R] - PaO_2$ where R − respiratory quotient = 1 for neonates receiving glucose infusion).

Please refer to Figure 17-9 for a detailed explanation.

3. **a/A ratio:** This is a ratio of arterial to alveolar PO_2 and is commonly used in translational studies.

4. **P/F ratio:** This is commonly used in pediatric and adult critical care units to assess severity of acute lung injury (ALI) and/or acute respiratory distress syndrome (ARDS) and is obtained by dividing PaO_2 by FiO_2. The patients are categorized based on the severity of hypoxemia: Mild (>200 mmHg to ≤300 mmHg), moderate (>100 mmHg to ≤200 mmHg), and severe (PaO_2/FiO_2 ≤100 mmHg).

CASE STUDY 2

A 38-year-old woman at 34⅗ weeks' gestation with poorly controlled diabetes mellitus and previous history of stillbirth at 36 weeks is being evaluated at the high-risk antenatal clinic. An episode of prolonged fetal bradycardia is noted and emergency cesarean section performed. The baby needs CPAP in the delivery room for mild grunting and is transferred to newborn nursery in room air. The infant is tachypneic and has preductal saturations in the mid-80s. He is given 50% oxygen by hood with improvement in saturations to the mid-90s. The initial chest x-ray shows expansion to seven ribs, bilateral haziness with mild granularity, and fluid in the horizontal fissure. The baby is transferred to the NICU for further evaluation.

EXERCISE 5

QUESTION

1. What is/are the most likely diagnoses?
   a. RDS
   b. Retained fetal lung fluid and TTN
   c. Early-onset sepsis with pneumonia
   d. Pulmonary hypoplasia

ANSWER

1. **a** and **b.** This is a common scenario that presents to clinicians in the NICU and well-baby nursery. This baby has clinical symptomatology that straddles both RDS and TTN. However, late-preterm gestation and maternal diabetes put this

infant at greater risk of RDS. The presence of low lung volumes with granularity on chest x-ray suggests that RDS is the predominant cause of hypoxemia in this infant. This infant is born prematurely without labor and some degree of retained lung liquid should be expected.

CASE STUDY 2 (continued)

Following admission to the NICU the baby is placed on nasal CPAP 4 to 6 cm H_2O in 40% oxygen. The initial capillary blood gas is as follows: pH 7.28, PCO_2 55 mmHg, PO_2 62 mmHg. The baby continues to be tachypneic with moderate retractions and the CPAP is increased to 6 to 8 cm H_2O. The oxygen requirement gradually increases to 65% to maintain SpO_2 in the mid-90s. The arterial blood gas at 4 hours of age is as follows: pH 7.22, $PaCO_2$ 60 mmHg, PaO_2 48 mmHg, and base deficit of 4 mEq/L. The chest x-ray is repeated and shows decreased lung volumes and increased granularity. A complete blood count (CBC) with differential count and blood culture are obtained. The baby is started on ampicillin and gentamicin. The white blood cell count is 18,000/mm³ with an immature to total neutrophil ratio of 0.11, hematocrit 55%, and platelets 246,000/mm³. The oxygen saturation value in the right upper limb is 92% and in the right lower limb is 82%.

EXERCISE 6

QUESTION

1. What is the next step in the management of this infant?
   a. Request an echocardiogram to rule out cyanotic CHD or PPHN.
   b. Start inhaled NO via CPAP because this infant has clinical symptomatology consistent with PPHN.
   c. Endotracheal intubation and surfactant replacement.
   d. Maintain the current level of CPAP (6 to 8 cm of water) and repeat an arterial blood gas in 1 hour.
   e. Noninvasive positive pressure ventilation (NIPPV) via nasal cannula.

ANSWER

1. **c.** This infant has untreated RDS as evidenced by the clinical picture of respiratory distress with elevated $PaCO_2$ and increasing oxygen requirement. This infant has predisposing risk factors for RDS such as late-preterm gestation and maternal diabetes. The chest x-ray appearance confirms the diagnosis. The SpO_2 in the right upper limb is higher than that in the lower

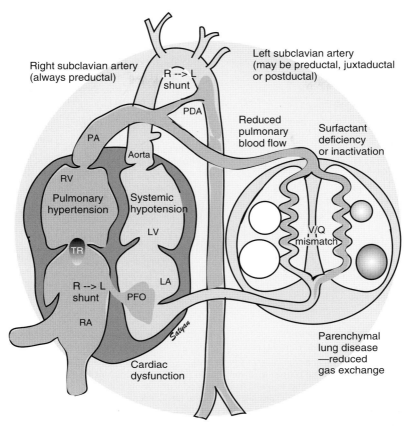

FIGURE 17-10 ■ **Hemodynamic changes in PPHN/HRF.** Surfactant deficiency (RDS) or inactivation (meconium aspiration or pneumonia) result in parenchymal lung disease and ventilation–perfusion (V/Q) mismatch. Increased pulmonary vascular resistance results in reduced pulmonary blood flow and right-to-left shunt through PDA and/or PFO. Pulmonary hypertension is often associated with systemic hypotension with septal deviation to the left. Cardiac dysfunction secondary to asphyxia, sepsis, or CDH may complicate HRF. The right subclavian artery (and blood flowing to the right upper extremity) is always preductal. The left subclavian artery may be preductal, juxtaductal, or postductal. Hence, preductal oxygen saturations should be obtained from the right upper extremity. *PA*, Pulmonary artery; *RV*, right ventricle; *LV*, left ventricle; *TR*, tricuspid regurgitation; *RA*, right atrium; *LA*, left atrium; *PDA*, patent ductus arteriosus; *PFO*, patent foramen ovale. (Copyright © 2015 Bobby Mathew, Satyan Lakshminrusimha. Published by Elsevier Inc. All rights reserved.)

limb. This suggests shunting across the ductus arteriosus from right (pulmonary artery) to left (aorta). Preductal oxygen saturations are often obtained from the right upper extremity. (The right subclavian artery always arises proximal to the ductus arteriosus; whereas the left subclavian occasionally can arise at or after the insertion of the ductus arteriosus; see Figure 17-10). The presence of a lower SpO₂ in the lower limb compared to the right upper limb is indicative of a right-to-left ductal shunt. An echocardiogram will be helpful if the infant does not respond to intubation, surfactant replacement, and alveolar recruitment.

CASE STUDY (continued)

The baby is intubated and receives a dose of surfactant. The initial ventilator settings are PIP of 20 cm H₂O, PEEP of 4 cm H₂O, pressure support of 12 cm H₂O, Paw of 10 cm H₂O, rate 40/minute, and inspiratory time of 0.35 seconds. There is minimal improvement in oxygen requirement following administration of surfactant. Umbilical arterial and venous lines are placed and the blood gas at 8 hours of age has a PaO₂ of 45 mmHg in 70% oxygen [oxygenation index = Paw (10) × FiO₂ (0.7) × 100/PaO₂ (45) = 15.6]

An echocardiogram is performed, which shows structurally normal heart with right ventricular systolic pressure of 55 mmHg. Right-to-left shunting is noted both at the foramen ovale and PDA (Figure 17-11, A). Inhaled NO is started at 20 ppm. The baby is reevaluated 15 minutes following initiation of inhaled NO and noted to have persistent oxygen requirement at 70%. Arterial blood gases repeated at 10 hours of age are as follow: pH of 7.22, PaCO₂ of 58 mmHg, PaO₂ of 64 mmHg, and a base deficit

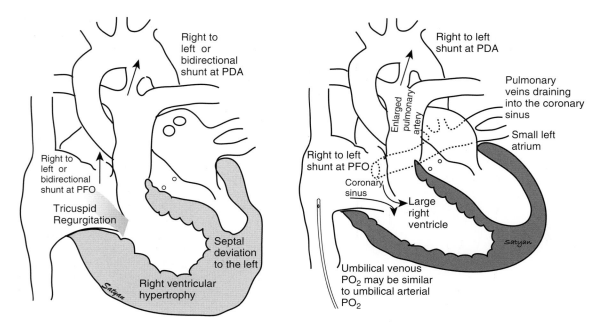

A. Echocardiographic features in PPHN

B. Total anomalous pulmonary venous return to coronary sinus

FIGURE 17-11 ■ **A,** Echocardiographic features of PPHN. Infants with significant PPHN often have a right-to-left or bidirectional shunt at the level of the patent foramen ovale (PFO) and/or patent ductus arteriosus (PDA). Tricuspid regurgitation (TR) jet is often noted and is used to estimated right ventricular systolic pressure. Right ventricular hypertrophy with deviation of interventricular septum to the left is commonly present. **B,** Cardiac findings in total anomalous pulmonary venous return (TAPVR) to the coronary sinus. Left atrium is small and pulmonary venous flow is diverted to the right atrium. The left atrium is filled by a right-to-left shunt across the PFO. The right ventricule and pulmonary artery are enlarged because of increased blood flow. Pulmonary arterial blood flows right-to-left across the PDA to the aorta. If the tip of the umbilical venous catheter is in the right atrium, PO_2 levels might be relatively high—similar to umbilical arterial sample—as oxygenated blood enters the right atrium. (Copyright © 2015 Bobby Mathew, Satyan Lakshminrusimha. Published by Elsevier Inc. All rights reserved.)

of 5 mEq/L. The chest x-ray shows poorly inflated lungs with bilateral ground-glass opacities.

EXERCISE 7

QUESTION

1. What is the most likely reason for poor response to inhaled NO in this infant?
   a. Missed diagnosis of cyanotic CHD
   b. Inadequate alveolar recruitment
   c. Surfactant protein B deficiency
   d. Pulmonary venous hypertension

ANSWER

1. **b.** The most likely reason for not responding to inhaled NO is inadequate alveolar recruitment. The persistent underinflation on chest x-ray is evidence of inadequate respiratory support. Increasing the PEEP, PIP, or inspiratory time are common strategies to increase Paw and oxygenation during conventional ventilation. The use of high-frequency ventilation with adequate

Paw can also achieve lung recruitment. It is unusual for cyanotic CHD to present with elevated $PaCO_2$. Surfactant protein B deficiency is a very rare condition and presents with intractable RDS in term infants. Pulmonary venous hypertension is usually secondary to obstruction to pulmonary venous drainage, mitral stenosis, or left ventricular dysfunction.

CASE STUDY 2 (continued)

The baby is placed on a high-frequency oscillator with the following settings: Paw of 12 cm H_2O, amplitude 30, frequency 12 Hz, and 50% O_2. Inhaled NO is continued at 20 ppm. A chest x-ray is repeated and shows inflation to eight ribs, symmetrical bilateral opacification, and normal heart size.

For inhaled NO to be effective, it has to be delivered to the site of action (i.e., to the vascular smooth muscle cell in the pulmonary arteriole through the respiratory tree). Failure to achieve lung recruitment prior to initiation of inhaled NO is a common cause for failure to sustain an oxygenation response.

CASE STUDY 2 (continued)

The baby is given another dose of surfactant, and lung is recruited by increasing the Paw to 16 cm H_2O with prompt improvement in oxygenation. The inspired oxygen concentration is weaned to 30%. The Paw is decreased to 14 cm H_2O. A repeat blood gas is as follows: pH of 7.33, $PaCO_2$ of 40 mmHg, PaO_2 of 98 mmHg.

Subsequently, the oxygen requirement is weaned to 21% and inhaled NO is weaned off over the next 20 hours. The baby is switched over to the conventional ventilator the following day and extubated 24 hours later to 30% oxygen by nasal cannula.

CASE STUDY 3

A 32-year-old gravida 2, para 0 mother is admitted in labor at 40 weeks' gestation with rupture of membranes. Meconium stained amniotic fluid (MSAF) is noted and induction of labor with oxytocin is commenced. Fetal tachycardia and loss of variability are observed and an emergency cesarean section is performed.

EXERCISE 8

QUESTION

1. What are the factors that determine the need for tracheal suctioning in infants born through MSAF?
   a. Consistency of meconium
   b. Duration of rupture of membranes
   c. Gestational age
   d. Nonvigorous state
   e. Cyanosis

ANSWER

1. **d.** Based on current neonatal resuscitation guidelines, infants who are depressed and nonvigorous (defined as having poor respiratory effort, poor tone, and heart rate less than 100/minute) should undergo tracheal suctioning. However, the evidence supporting suctioning of the trachea in depressed newborn infants is weak. In a large multicenter randomized trial, Wiswell and colleagues demonstrated that tracheal suctioning in the vigorous infant born through MSAF is not associated with reduction in the incidence or severity of MAS (Wiswell et al., 2000). Attempts at intubation in a vigorous infant may also cause laryngeal and/or oral trauma and precipitate vagal bradycardia.

CASE STUDY 3 (continued)

At birth this baby is apneic and limp with heart rate of 50/minute. Meconium is suctioned below the cords and positive pressure ventilation (PPV) is provided. The heart rate improves with PPV. Apgar scores are 1, 4, 5, and 7 at 1, 5, 10, and 15 minutes respectively. The cord pH is 7.02 with base deficit of 15 mEq/L. The baby is noted to have irregular gasping respirations and is placed on mechanical ventilation. Arterial blood gas at 1 hour of age is as follows: pH of 6.83, $PaCO_2$ of 76 mmHg, PaO_2 of 52 mmHg, and base deficit of 22.8 mEq/L. The infant requires 100% oxygen to maintain preductal saturations above 92%. Postductal saturations in the lower limb are 83%. The baby is placed on high-frequency oscillator with the following settings: MAP of 18 cm H_2O, amplitude 40 cm H_2O, frequency 9 Hz, and FiO_2 of 1.0. On neurologic examination, she is noted to have poor tone, absent reflexes, dilated nonreactive pupils, and absent Moro reflex. Whole-body hypothermia is initiated for features of severe hypoxic ischemic encephalopathy (HIE) and a target esophageal temperature of 33.5° C is achieved at 2.5 hours of age.

Her chest x-ray shows fluffy infiltrates with 9-10-rib expansion on both sides. A dose of surfactant is administered with minimal improvement in respiratory status. Systemic blood pressure is 52/36 (mean 44 mmHg). Arterial blood gas from an umbilical arterial catheter 2 hours after achieving hypothermia at 33.5° C is as follows: pH of 7.21, $PaCO_2$ of 54 mmHg, PaO_2 of 40 mmHg, and base deficit at 6.1 mEq/L.

EXERCISE 9

QUESTION

1. What is the most appropriate next step in the management of this infant?
   a. Increase pH by an infusion of sodium bicarbonate.
   b. Induce a respiratory alkalosis by increasing the ventilator frequency.
   c. Increase Paw to achieve 10-11-rib expansion.
   d. Inhaled NO
   e. Dopamine infusion

ANSWER

1. **d.** This baby has MAS (with HRF) and HIE. Both of these conditions predispose the infant to develop PPHN. The infant has clinical signs of PPHN with right-to-left shunting at the ductus arteriosus as evidenced by the difference in pre- and postductal saturation values. The concurrent multiple pathophysiologic processes in this infant present challenging issues in management. Metabolic acidosis is associated with pulmonary vasoconstriction and worsening of pulmonary hypertension (Figure 17-6). In the past, induction of respiratory and/or metabolic alkalosis was the mainstay of therapy for pulmonary hypertension. Although short-term pulmonary vasodilation is achieved with hyperventilation, infants managed with respiratory alkalosis have worse neurodevelopmental outcomes with a high incidence of

sensorineural deafness (Hendricks-Munoz & Walton, 1988). Sodium bicarbonate infusion improves intravascular pH but may cause paradoxical intracellular acidosis in tissues and is associated with decreased cerebral blood flow in infants with HIE (see Figure 17-7). In contrast to the conventional ventilator, increasing the frequency on the high frequency oscillator reduces tidal volume and increases $PaCO_2$. Adjusting the Paw on high-frequency oscillator to optimize lung inflation is critically important for oxygenation and ventilation. However, hyperexpansion is associated with decreased venous return and increased PVR (Figure 17-6) leading to deterioration in systemic oxygen delivery. There is no clinical indication for the use of dopamine in this infant. The mean blood pressure in this infant is within the normal limits for a newborn full-term infant. In addition, dopamine has vasoconstrictor effects both on systemic *and* pulmonary vasculature. In this case, initiation of inhaled NO to selectively dilate pulmonary vasculature may be the most effective therapy with least side effects. Inhaled NO is inactivated by hemoglobin and has no systemic vasodilator effect. Inhaled NO also reduces intrapulmonary right-to-left shunting by preferentially dilating blood vessels that supply well-ventilated alveolar units. This is referred to as the "microselective effect of inhaled NO" (Figure 17-12).

CASE STUDY 3 (continued)

Following initiation of inhaled NO, there is a transient improvement in oxygen saturations to 97%. However, within 30 minutes, preductal oxygen saturations decrease to 85%. Arterial blood gas values 2 hours after initiation of inhaled NO are as follows: pH of 7.17, $PaCO_2$ of 58 mmHg, PaO_2 of 59 mmHg, and base deficit of 7.3 mEq/L. The chest x-ray shows increased haziness with mild cardiomegaly. An echocardiogram shows a right-to-left shunt at the level of the PDA but a left-to-right shunt at the PFO level associated with myocardial dysfunction and poor contractility.

EXERCISE 10

QUESTION

1. Which of the following factors contributes to poor response to inhaled NO in this patient with MAS and HIE?
    a. Whole-body hypothermia results in pulmonary vasoconstriction
    b. Liver dysfunction from asphyxia impairs response to inhaled NO
    c. Left ventricular dysfunction with pulmonary venous hypertension
    d. Coexisting acute tubular necrosis and renal dysfunction

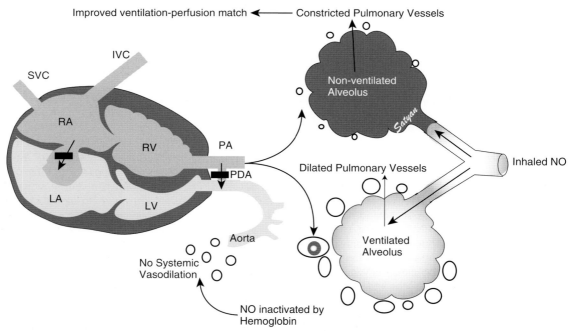

FIGURE 17-12 ■ **Selective and microselective action of inhaled nitric oxide (NO).** Inhaled NO is a selective dilator of the pulmonary circulation without any significant systemic vasodilation, as it combines with hemoglobin to form methemoglobin. As it is an inhaled vasodilator, it selectively enters the well ventilated alveoli, improves blood flow to these alveoli, and reduces V/Q mismatch (microselective effect). (Copyright © 2015 Bobby Mathew, Satyan Lakshminrusimha. Published by Elsevier Inc. All rights reserved.)

TABLE 17-2	Differential Diagnosis of Hypoxemia in a Neonate Based on the Direction of Shunt at Atrial and Ductal Level on Echocardiography		
Diagnosis	**Ductal Shunt**	**Atrial Shunt**	**Management**
Parenchymal lung disease and V/Q mismatch and intrapulmonary shunt	L → R	L → R	Lung recruitment, specific therapy (antibiotics for pneumonia, surfactant for RDS) Inhaled NO may be beneficial by correcting V/Q mismatch
PPHN	R → L	R → L	Oxygenation, correction of acidosis, and inhaled NO
Left ventricular dysfunction (common in diaphragmatic hernia, asphyxia, and sepsis) (Kinsella, 2008; Sehgal, Athikarisamy, & Adamopoulos, 2011)	R → L	L → R	Inotropes and vasodilators (Milrinone)
Tricuspid atresia/stenosis or pulmonic atresia/stenosis	L → R	R → L	PGE1 + Surgery
TAPVR (total anomalous pulmonary venous return) (Lakshminrusimha et al., 2009)	R → L (Large PA)	R → L (small LA and *no tricuspid regurgitation*)	Surgery

Modified from Lakshminrusimha S, Kumar VH: Diseases of pulmonary circulation. In Fuhrman BP, Zimmerman JJ, editors: Pediatric critical care, 4th ed, Philadelphia, PA, 2011, Elsevier/Saunders, pp 632-656.

ANSWER

1. **c.** Hypothermia induces both pulmonary and systemic vasoconstriction. However, currently there are no data to suggest that therapeutic hypothermia increases the incidence of PPHN or failure to respond to inhaled NO in patients with asphyxia. The patient in this vignette has ventricular dysfunction. Patients with HRF and PPHN typically have a right-to-left shunt at the level of PDA and PFO (see Figure 17-10). In the presence of left ventricular dysfunction, left atrial pressures are elevated resulting in a left-to-right shunt at the foramen ovale (Table 17-2). An elevated left atrial pressure results in pulmonary venous hypertension. Administration of inhaled NO to a patient with pulmonary venous hypertension can result in flooding of the pulmonary capillary bed and worsening of pulmonary edema resulting in clinical deterioration (Kinsella, 2008). It has been suggested that an "inodilator" such as milrinone may be more effective than inhaled NO in improving left ventricular function and reducing pulmonary venous hypertension (Lakshminrusimha & Steinhorn, 2013) (Figure 17-13).

Three case series report the effectiveness of milrinone in improving oxygenation in NO-resistant PPHN (Bassler, Choong, McNamara, & Kirpalani, 2006; McNamara, Laique, Muang-In, & Whyte, 2006; McNamara, Shivananda, Sahni, Freeman, & Taddio, 2012). Unlike inhaled NO, which acts through cGMP, milrinone inhibits phosphodiesterase 3A (PDE3A, Figure 17-14) in pulmonary arterial smooth muscle cells and cardiac myocytes and increases the level of a different second messenger, cAMP, resulting in pulmonary vasodilation and improved ventricular function.

CASE STUDY 3 (continued)

With respiratory deterioration, inhaled NO is discontinued and patient is started on milrinone infusion at 0.33 mcg/kg/min following a loading dose of 50 mcg/kg over 30 minutes. After 2 hours, the dose of milrinone is escalated to 0.66 mcg/kg/min. A repeat echocardiogram obtained 24 hours after initiation of milrinone shows improved cardiac function. Following 3 days of therapy with milrinone, the patient is weaned from the oscillator to conventional ventilator.

Meconium staining of amniotic fluid occurs in 5% to 25% of normal pregnancies. Risk factors for in utero meconium passage include postmaturity, placental insufficiency, fetal distress, and intrauterine growth restriction. Gasping occurs with asphyxia and causes particulate meconium to be aspirated into the airways. MAS occurs in about 5% of infants born through MSAF. The incidence of MAS has decreased in recent years due to the reduction in number of postterm deliveries. The pathophysiology of MAS includes a combination of mechanical effects from airway obstruction, chemical pneumonitis, inflammation, surfactant inactivation, and increased PVR. The practice of suctioning of the oropharynx upon delivery of the head does not reduce the incidence or severity of MAS and is no longer recommended (Fraser et al., 2005; Vain et al., 2004). Intratracheal suctioning for

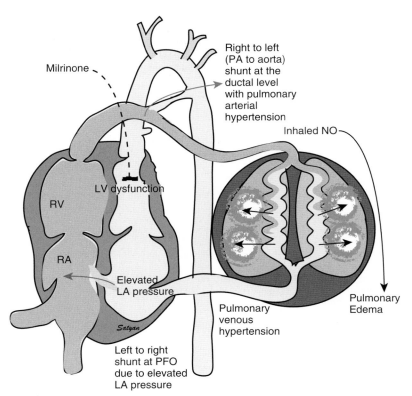

FIGURE 17-13 ■ **Pulmonary hemodynamic changes in the presence of left ventricular dysfunction.** Left ventricular (LV) dysfunction is occasionally associated with asphyxia, sepsis, or diaphragmatic hernia. In the presence of LV dysfunction, left atrial (LA) pressure is elevated resulting in a left-to-right shunt at the patent foramen ovale (PFO). Pulmonary venous hypertension leads to pulmonary edema. Administration of inhaled NO dilates pulmonary arteries and increases blood flow to the lungs without improving LV dysfunction or LA pressure. This results in worsening pulmonary edema and deterioration of respiratory status. Administration of milrinone improves diastolic and systolic function of the LV and improves pulmonary venous hypertension. (Copyright © 2015 Bobby Mathew, Satyan Lakshminrusimha. Published by Elsevier Inc. All rights reserved.)

meconium below the cords is reserved for nonvigorous infants born through MSAF. Infants with MAS are at high risk for PPHN, HRF, and air leaks.

The basic principles of management include assisted ventilation with avoidance of respiratory and metabolic acidosis, preventing hypoxia-induced pulmonary vasoconstriction and maintaining normal blood pressure and perfusion. As surfactant inactivation occurs with meconium aspiration, surfactant replacement should be considered in severe cases. Surfactant has been shown to decrease the need for ECMO in patients with MAS (Lotze et al., 1998). With the use of surfactant, inhaled NO and high-frequency oscillatory ventilation, there has been a marked reduction in patients needing ECMO for MAS. Infants who undergo ECMO for MAS have a much higher survival compared to infants with other indications for ECMO (Table 17-3).

CASE STUDY 3 (continued)

This neonate with asphyxia, MAS, and PPHN is undergoing whole-body cooling to a core temperature of 33.5° C. An arterial blood gas is drawn from the umbilical arterial line. The lab reports a pH of 7.41, $PaCO_2$ of 35 mmHg, and PaO_2 of 55 mmHg at 37° C. You call the lab supervisor and inform her that the baby's core temperature is 33.5° C.

EXERCISE 11

QUESTION

1. The lab supervisor corrects the blood gas results to the baby's temperature of 33.5° C. What changes do you expect with $PaCO_2$ at the baby's body temperature?
   a. The $PaCO_2$ decreases with hypothermia and correction to a temperature of 37° C results in an elevated value (40.5 mmHg).
   b. Temperature has no effect on $PaCO_2$ and no correction is necessary.
   c. The $PaCO_2$ increases with hypothermia and correction to a temperature of 37° C results in a depressed value (31.5 mmHg).

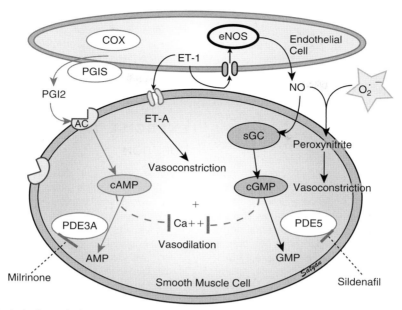

FIGURE 17-14 ■ Endothelium-derived vasodilators: prostacyclin (PGI₂), nitric oxide (NO), and vasoconstrictor (endothelin, ET-1). The enzymes, cyclooxygenase (COX) and prostacyclin synthase (PGIS) are involved in the production of prostacyclin. Prostacyclin acts on its receptor in the smooth muscle cell and stimulates adenylate cyclase (AC) to produce cyclic adenosine monophosphate (cAMP). Cyclic AMP is broken down by phosphodiesterase 3A (PDE 3A) in the smooth muscle cell. Milrinone inhibits PDE 3A and increases cAMP levels in pulmonary arterial smooth muscle cells and cardiac myocytes resulting in pulmonary (and systemic) vasodilation and inotropy. Endothelin is a powerful vasoconstrictor and acts on ET-A receptors in the smooth muscle cell and increases ionic calcium concentration. A second endothelin receptor (ET-B) on the endothelial cell stimulates NO release and vasodilation. Endothelial nitric oxide synthase (eNOS) produces NO, which diffuses from the endothelium to the smooth muscle cell and stimulates soluble guanylate cyclase (sGC) enzyme to produce cyclic guanosine monophosphate (cGMP). Cyclic GMP is broken down by PDE 5 enzyme in the smooth muscle cell. Sildenafil inhibits PDE5 and increases cGMP levels in pulmonary arterial smooth muscle cells. Cyclic AMP and cGMP reduce cytosolic ionic calcium concentrations and induce smooth muscle cell relaxation and pulmonary vasodilation. NO is a free radical and can avidly combine with superoxide anions to form a toxic vasoconstrictor, peroxynitrite. The bioavailability of NO in a tissue is determined by the local concentration of superoxide anions. Hyperoxic ventilation with 100% oxygen can increase the risk of formation of superoxide anions in the pulmonary arterial smooth muscle cells and limit the bioavailability of NO. (Copyright © 2015 Bobby Mathew, Satyan Lakshminrusimha. Published by Elsevier Inc. All rights reserved.)

TABLE 17-3 **Recent Data on Neonatal Respiratory ECMO Runs by Diagnosis (July 2008-December 2012)**

Diagnosis	Total Runs	Survived	% Survived
Congenital diaphragmatic hernia (CDH)	981	467	47.6%
Meconium aspiration syndrome (MAS)	516	490	95%
Persistent pulmonary hypertension of the newborn (PPHN)/persistent fetal circulation (PFC)	733	554	75.6%
Respiratory distress syndrome (RDS)	66	55	83.3%
Sepsis	106	69	65.1%
Pneumonia	48	24	50%
Air-leak syndrome	10	6	60%
Others	1391	951	68.4%
Total	3776	2598	68.8%

Data from ELSO Registry. Accessed January 08, 2013.

ANSWER

1. **a.** The clinician should pay particular attention to the changes in $PaCO_2$ with hypothermia for HIE. $PaCO_2$ decreases with hypothermia and correction to a temperature of 37° C results in an elevated $PaCO_2$ level. This can compromise cerebral blood flow and hence a higher corrected $PaCO_2$ should be accepted in these patients. In a retrospective study of patients enrolled in the whole-body cooling trial, Pappas and colleagues demonstrated an association between hypocarbia and poor neurodevelopmental outcome at 18 to 22 months (Pappas et al., 2011). A delicate balance exists between improving pulmonary blood flow and gas exchange and providing adequate cerebral perfusion to optimize neurodevelopmental outcome in infants with MAS, PPHN, and HIE (Figure 17-6).

CASE STUDY 4

A 19-year-old mother with poor prenatal care is admitted in labor a week prior to her expected date of delivery. A quick sonogram reveals that the fetus has a left sided diaphragmatic hernia. A 3245-gram male infant is born by spontaneous vaginal delivery. On examination, he has mild respiratory distress and a heart rate of 140 beats/minute. Auscultation reveals absence of breath sounds on the left with heart sounds shifted to the right. A Replogle suction tube is placed in the stomach. He is intubated with a 3.5-mm tracheal tube. An umbilical arterial line is placed and an arterial blood gas is drawn with the infant on conventional ventilation with the following settings: PIP of 23 cm H_2O, PEEP of 5 cm H_2O, Paw of 13 cm H_2O, rate of 40/minute, and inspired oxygen concentration of 70%. The arterial blood gas is as follows: pH 7.27, PCO_2 57 mmHg, and PO_2 29 mmHg. To assess the severity of his illness, calculate his oxygenation index using the formula given in Figure 17-9.

EXERCISE 12

QUESTION

1. What is the oxygenation index in this patient?
   a. 13
   b. 26
   c. 31
   d. 36
   e. 45

ANSWER

1. **c.**

CASE STUDY 4 (continued)

The chest x-ray shows herniated abdominal contents in the left hemithorax. There is mediastinal shift to the right. The right lung is expanded to nine ribs. Because of low oxygen saturations, the inspired oxygen concentration is steadily increased to 100%. His preductal and postductal saturations are 86% and 68% respectively. Therapy with inhaled NO at 20 ppm is initiated with no significant improvement in oxygenation.

EXERCISE 13

QUESTION

1. What is (are) the causes of poor response to inhaled NO in this patient?
   a. Decreased cross-sectional area of pulmonary vasculature
   b. Muscularization of arteries and "fixed" pulmonary hypertension
   c. Left ventricular dysfunction
   d. Target enzyme abnormalities
   e. Elevated levels of vasoconstrictors such as endothelin

ANSWER

1. **All of the above.** Infants with CDH have pulmonary hypoplasia and PPHN secondary to impaired pulmonary vascular development and increased muscularization of the pulmonary arterioles. Abnormalities of enzymes in the NO pathway (de Buys Roessingh et al., 2011) have been observed in animal models of CDH (Karamanoukian et al., 1996). Many infants with CDH also have abnormalities in left ventricular structure and function that can lead to pulmonary venous hypertension and may contribute to poor response to inhaled NO. Elevated endothelin (a powerful vasoconstrictor, Figure 17-14) levels have been observed in patients with CDH (Keller et al., 2010). The only randomized control trial evaluating the use of inhaled NO in CDH showed a higher need for ECMO in patients that received NO ("Inhaled nitric oxide and hypoxic respiratory failure in infants with congenital diaphragmatic hernia. The Neonatal Inhaled Nitric Oxide Study Group [NINOS]," 1997). Infants with CDH need frequent echocardiographic assessment of ventricular pressure and function during therapy. Corrective surgery is usually performed following adequate control of pulmonary hypertension.

ROLE OF ECHOCARDIOGRAPHY IN INFANTS WITH HRF

Hemodynamic profile assessed by functional echocardiography is extremely useful to diagnose, manage, and follow the changes with therapy in infants with HRF (El-Khuffash & McNamara,

2011). Pulmonary arterial pressure is estimated from the tricuspid regurgitation jet velocity. Using the modified Bernoulli equation, systolic right ventricular pressure (mmHg) is estimated as $4v^2$ + right atrial pressure, where "v" is the maximal velocity of tricuspid regurgitation jet in meters/second on continuous-wave Doppler echocardiogram (Yock & Popp, 1984). Right ventricular dysfunction caused by excessive afterload appears to be a major risk factor for poor outcome in HRF (Lapointe & Barrington, 2011) and may influence the velocity of the tricuspid regurgitation jet. Echocardiographic assessment of atrial and ductal level shunts assists in diagnosis and optimal management of a newborn presenting with hypoxemia (Table 17-2).

EXERCISE 14

QUESTION

1. Which of the following disorders associated with PPHN has the highest mortality following ECMO?
   a. Air-leak syndromes
   b. CDH
   c. MAS
   d. Surfactant deficiency leading to respiratory distress syndrome (RDS)
   e. Idiopathic "black-lung" PPHN

ANSWER

1. **b.** Of the various causes of PPHN listed in Box 17-1, CDH is associated with a high requirement for ECMO. Recent data from the Extracorporeal Life Support Organization (ELSO) registry shows that survival following ECMO is only 48% with CDH (compared to 95% with MAS).

   Diaphragmatic hernia occurs in about one in 3000 live births. Left sided diaphragmatic hernia is more common (85%) and is associated with better prognosis than right sided hernias (Gaxiola, Varon, & Valladolid, 2009). The overall rate of survival for CDH is approximately 68% and has not significantly improved over the last decade. The presence of a low observed to expected lung-to-head ratio (LHR) and presence of liver herniation into the chest on prenatal ultrasound carry poor prognosis in infants with CDH (Jani et al., 2007). Various fetal interventions are being investigated currently, including *in utero* tracheal occlusion to improve lung size.

   A systematic review of best practice has identified key elements of respiratory care in infants with CDH that are associated with improved outcomes (Logan, Rice, Goldberg, & Cotten, 2007). Gentle ventilation and permissive hypercapnia is being advocated to avoid high PIP and to reduce

volutrauma to the hypoplastic lungs. The goal is to achieve preductal saturations ≥85%, $PaCO_2$ ≤65 mmHg, pH ≥7.25, and adequate tissue perfusion by monitoring pH and lactate levels. Institution of high-frequency ventilation early or as a rescue mode once the preset limit of ventilator parameters fail to achieve adequate saturation values or $PaCO_2$ levels is important to decrease ventilator-induced lung injury. Studies of infants with PPHN maintaining high normal $PaCO_2$ (40 to 60 mmHg) indicate similar or better outcomes with less chronic lung disease in CDH (Dworetz, Moya, Sabo, Gladstone, & Gross, 1989; Wung, James, Kilchevsky, & James, 1985).

CASE STUDY 4 (continued)

In spite of maximal support with conventional ventilation and inhaled NO, this baby continues to exhibit hypoxemia. The arterial blood gas from the umbilical arterial line is as follows: pH of 7.15, $PaCO_2$ of 80 mmHg, PaO_2 of 27 mmHg. The baby is switched to the high-frequency oscillator. The parents are approached regarding the risks and benefits of ECMO. A head ultrasound, echocardiogram, PT, PTT, fibrinogen, and blood products are ordered.

EXERCISE 15

QUESTION

1. Which of the following findings would be considered a contraindication to ECMO?
   a. Echocardiogram showing evidence of biventricular dysfunction
   b. The presence of liver in the thorax on x-ray
   c. PT of 17.5 seconds and PTT of 100 seconds with a fibrinogen of 250 mg/dL from a heparinized umbilical arterial line
   d. A grade III intraventricular bleed on head ultrasound
   e. Single umbilical artery observed during umbilical catheterization

ANSWER

1. **d**. ECMO is prolonged cardiopulmonary bypass for neonates with reversible respiratory or cardiac failure who are unlikely to survive in spite of maximal medical management. Ventricular function assessment on echocardiogram is important in deciding the appropriate mode of ECMO (venovenous vs. venoarterial, see later and Table 17-4). Biventricular dysfunction is not a contraindication for ECMO. Prolonged PTT is likely related to contamination from heparin and this sample needs to be repeated with adequate "waste" draw. A grade III intraventricular

TABLE 17-4 Differences Between Venovenous (VV) and Venoarterial (VA) Extracorporeal Membrane Oxygenation (ECMO)

Criteria	VV ECMO	VA ECMO
Relationship between "artificial" lung and native lung	In series and replaces part or all of native lung function	In parallel with the native lungs and replaces part or all of both heart and lung function
Carotid artery ligation	Not necessary—results in better cerebral hemodynamics	Required—alters cerebral hemodynamics (reduced cerebral blood flow velocities and decreased cerebral oxygenation during right carotid cannulation and impaired autoregulation)
Embolic strokes	Minimal risk of embolic strokes (the risk is nonexistent if there is no interatrial communication)	Risk of embolic strokes
Indication	Preferred mode for neonatal respiratory failure	Primary cardiac dysfunction for providing partial or complete circulatory support, secondary cardiac failure from profound respiratory failure (some centers prefer VV ECMO for this indication), inability to place a 12 Fr double lumen cannula (because of size or mediastinal shift), shock/severe hypotension
Pressure in cerebral circulation	Normal	High, increasing the risk of reperfusion injury
Risk of reperfusion injury	Low	High risk of hyperoxic and hypocarbic reperfusion injury
Pulmonary blood flow	Maintained with well oxygenated blood	Decreased pulmonary blood flow
Systemic flow	Preservation of pulsatile arterial flow	Potential loss of pulsatile arterial flow (pulsatile flow can be maintained with partial bypass and good cardiac function)
PaO_2	45-80 mmHg	60-150 mmHg
Cardiac effects	Negligible (no change in RV preload or LV afterload)	Decreased LV preload and increased LV afterload
Coronary blood flow	Derived from LV/ascending aorta blood (oxygenated)	Derived from LV poorly oxygenated blood (prior to arterial catheter) and retrograde flow from the arterial cannula
Recirculation	Occurs secondary to single cannula flow dynamics and cannula position	Chance of recirculation is eliminated
Rate of stabilization	Slow stabilization	Instant stabilization

hemorrhage is likely to expand and deteriorate with anticoagulation and ECMO is contraindicated in this context.

During ECMO, oxygen delivery and gas exchange is maintained in the presence of pulmonary and/or cardiac dysfunction. Infants who survive show improvement in parenchymal lung disease, pulmonary vascular remodeling, and cardiac dysfunction during the ECMO course.

Two modalities of ECMO are used for neonatal respiratory failure: venovenous (VV) and venoarterial (VA). The differences between these two modalities are shown in Table 17-4 and Figure 17-15. In VV ECMO, an extracorporeal circuit is connected to the neonate's circulation by a double-lumen internal jugular venous cannula. VV ECMO augments oxygen delivery and Po_2 in the right atrium, right ventricle, and pulmonary circulation, thereby effecting a reduction in PVR. The reduction in PVR increases blood flow through the lung and returns oxygenated blood to the left atrium (Figure 17-15), left ventricle, and aortic root. In the aortic root, well-oxygenated blood flows into the coronary circulation and augments cardiac function and output. Therefore, VV ECMO provides some support for cardiac function and may be considered in neonates who require vasopressor

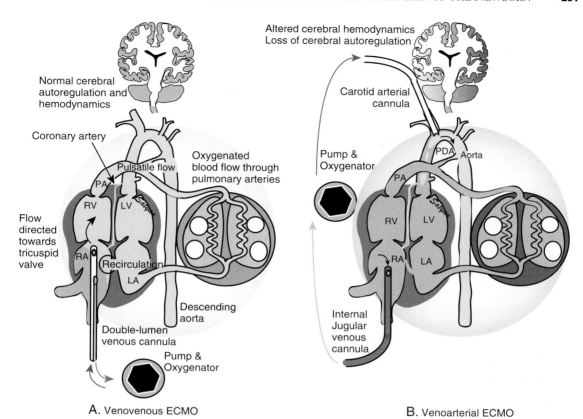

FIGURE 17-15 ■ Diagram of circulatory pattern and oxygenation of blood during venovenous VV (left panel) and venoarterial VA (right panel) ECMO. In VV ECMO, a double-lumen venous cannula is placed. Blood is drawn from the right atrium and pumped back into the right atrium with the flow directed toward the tricuspid valve. Because both input and output are through the same cannula, there is a risk of recirculation. Oxygenated blood perfuses the lung and returns to the left heart and the systemic circulation. Cerebral hemodynamics are preserved in VV ECMO. In VA ECMO, blood drains from the right atrium and is oxygenated and pumped back into the arch of aorta. The presence of a carotid arterial cannula results in disruption of cerebral autoregulation. The lung is perfused with deoxygenated blood. (Copyright © 2015 Bobby Mathew, Satyan Lakshminrusimha. Published by Elsevier Inc. All rights reserved.)

agents to support blood pressure (whose cardiac dysfunction might be related to hypoxemia). Rarely, conversion to VA ECMO is required in the event that cardiac output does not improve on VV ECMO.

ECMO in a critically ill, hypoxemic, and acidotic neonate with systemic heparinization is associated with a moderate risk of intracranial hemorrhage and bleeding. Preterm infants (<34 weeks' PMA) are generally excluded from receiving ECMO because of the high inherent risk of severe intracranial hemorrhage.

CASE STUDY 4 (continued)

In the patient with CDH, echocardiogram shows evidence of severe PPHN with right-to-left shunting through a patent foramen ovale and ductus arteriosus with slightly decreased ejection fraction. The infant requires 5 mcg/kg/min of dopamine. The head ultrasound is normal. An arterial blood gas on

a Paw of 15 cm H_2O, rate = 8 Hz and 100% oxygen is as follows: pH of 7.13, $Paco_2$ of 55 mmHg, Pao_2 of 30 mmHg. The atmospheric pressure in this NICU is 747 mmHg.

EXERCISE 16

QUESTION

1. Based on these findings, which of the following statements is TRUE?
   a. OI is >40 and $AaDO_2$ is >600 and the patient is a candidate only for VA ECMO.
   b. OI is >40 and $AaDO_2$ is >600 and the patient is a candidate for VV ECMO.
   c. OI is <40 and $AaDO_2$ is <600 and the patient is not a candidate for VA or VV ECMO.
   d. OI is >40 and $AaDO_2$ is <600 and the patient is a candidate for VA ECMO.
   e. This patient has CDH and has high mortality in spite of ECMO and hence ECMO is contraindicated.

ANSWER

1. **b**. To be eligible for ECMO, neonates should be greater than 34 weeks PMA (birth weight >2000 grams), ventilated for less than 10 days (i.e., less likely to have irreversible chronic lung disease), have a reversible pulmonary or cardiac disease, and be at high risk for dying. To predict which infants with respiratory disorders are at high risk of dying, OI and A-aDO$_2$ (Figure 17-9) are used to quantitate the degree of respiratory failure. An OI >40 (for >2 hours in 3 of 5 serial arterial blood gases) is predictive of a 60% to 80% risk of dying (Engle et al., 1993; "UK collaborative randomised trial of neonatal extracorporeal membrane oxygenation," 1996). Similarly, A-aDO$_2$ ≥630 for longer than 4 hours is predictive of about an 80% risk of dying. Many neonatal units prefer to cannulate patients for ECMO before the onset of severe cardiopulmonary decompensation in an attempt to improve outcome.

   Most ECMO centers exclude infants with PPHN if they have significant intracranial hemorrhage, medically unresponsive bleeding diathesis, irreversible major organ failure, a chromosomal abnormality, or syndrome associated with a high mortality rate or an extremely poor neurologic prognosis. While counseling families, it is important to understand that survival outcomes differ depending on the underlying diagnosis. Recent data from the ELSO registry (Table 17-3) show that mortality associated with ECMO is >50% with CDH.

   The most frequently observed complications in neonates receiving ECMO are intracranial hemorrhage/infarction, cannula site bleeding, surgical site bleeding, seizures, renal insufficiency, hypertension, and hyperbilirubinemia. Mechanical problems such as clots within the circuit are occasionally encountered.

   Long-term neurodevelopmental outcome at school age is generally encouraging for neonates with PPHN critical enough to receive inhaled NO or ECMO. Rosenberg and colleagues recently reported that among 109 school age survivors of PPHN (77 had received inhaled NO and 12 required ECMO), medical, neurodevelopmental, and social/emotional/behavioral outcome did not differ between children treated with inhaled NO, with or without ECMO, and those managed with no exposure to inhaled NO. Overall, 24% had respiratory problems, 60% had abnormal chest x-rays, and 6.4% had some sensorineural hearing loss. Overall, 9.2% of the cohort had a full-scale IQ less than 70 and 7.4% had an IQ ranging from 70 to 84 (Rosenberg et al., 2010). The U.K. collaborative trial randomized critically ill neonates either to transfer to a regional center for ECMO or continued conventional care at the local NICU. At 7-year follow up, mortality was significantly lower in the ECMO group with no increase in disability (McNally, Bennett, Elbourne, Field, & Group, 2006). The presence of neurodevelopmental and medical disabilities likely reflects the severity of the underlying illnesses experienced by these infants rather than complications of interventions received.

CASE STUDY 5

An ex 23-week small-for-gestational age infant at 38 weeks' PMA has severe bronchopulmonary dysplasia (BPD) and requires respiratory support with CPAP 6 to 8 cm and FiO$_2$ of 0.45. She was born to a 22-year-old mother following prolonged rupture of membranes for 3 weeks with oligohydramnios. The postnatal course was complicated with left sided grade 3 IVH, PDA that was surgically closed on Day 28, necrotizing enterocolitis with perforation, and an episode of ventilator-associated pneumonia. The baby has received multiple courses of antibiotics for presumed sepsis and experienced one episode of coagulase negative staphylococcal bacteremia.

EXERCISE 17

QUESTION

1. What are the underlying pathophysiologic mechanisms for persisting CPAP and oxygen requirements in this infant?
   a. Pulmonary hypoplasia secondary to oligohydramnios
   b. Impaired alveolarization
   c. Tracheo/bronchomalacia
   d. Increased airway reactivity
   e. Pulmonary hypertension

ANSWER

1. **All of the above.** With improved survival of extremely preterm infants, morbidities such as pulmonary hypertension are increasingly seen in this group of infants. Pulmonary hypertension is observed in 15% to 20% of extremely preterm infants (and approximately 25% to 37% of infants with BPD) (An et al., 2010; Slaughter, Pakrashi, Jones, South, & Shah, 2011). Prolonged duration of ventilation, intrauterine growth restriction, and oligohydramnios are risk factors associated with development of pulmonary hypertension. The pathophysiology of pulmonary hypertension in these infants is a combination of pulmonary hypoplasia and impaired vascular development. BPD is associated with reduced cross-sectional perfusion area with decreased arterial density

and abnormal muscularization of peripheral pulmonary arteries.

The onset of pulmonary hypertension in BPD is variable and can occur as late as 3 to 4 months of age (Bhat, Salas, Foster, Carlo, & Ambalavanan, 2012). A delay in diagnosis is associated with progressive pulmonary vascular disease, cor pulmonale, and high mortality. Echocardiographic screening for pulmonary hypertension should be considered for infants who are ventilated or require >30% oxygen or have radiologic evidence of BPD. The echocardiogram is usually performed at 1 month of age and every 4 weeks until discharge. Screening for pulmonary hypertension by echocardiography using the velocity of the tricuspid regurgitation jet for estimation of pulmonary pressures may be misleading (Mourani, Sontag, Younoszai, Ivy, & Abman, 2008). The presence of interventricular septal flattening and right ventricular hypertrophy are other echocardiographic markers for pulmonary hypertension. Cardiac catheterization is the gold standard for the diagnosis of pulmonary hypertension in these patients and should be considered prior to initiation of long-term therapy for pulmonary hypertension and to evaluate the response to different vasodilators.

The optimal intervention strategies for reversing early pulmonary hypertension or treating established pulmonary hypertension in BPD are not clear. Optimizing ventilator management to prevent periods of hypoxemia is very important to prevent further progression of pulmonary hypertension. This may involve setting higher oxygen saturation targets and providing long-term mechanical ventilator support in the most severely affected infants. Multiple therapies such as maintaining higher oxygen saturation targets, inhaled NO, sildenafil, prostacyclin and endothelin receptor antagonists have been tried with mixed results. A stepwise algorithm with the initiation of 20 ppm of inhaled NO, with addition of sildenafil and gradual increase in the dose to a maximum of 2 mg per kg q 6 hours to desired response followed by an attempt to wean off inhaled NO has been proposed (Abman & Nelin, 2012). When there is an inability to wean inhaled NO, the addition of endothelin receptor antagonist (bosentan) or prostacyclin analogue has been suggested. Mourani and colleagues demonstrated improvement in echocardiographic parameters in 88% of the patients with sildenafil therapy (Mourani & Abman, 2013; Mourani, Sontag, Ivy, & Abman, 2009). The recent U.S. Food and Drug Administration (FDA) "black box" warning about increased mortality among children treated with sildenafil for pulmonary hypertension has limited the use of phosphodiesterase inhibitors in this population (Abman et al., 2012). The importance of multidisciplinary care and nutritional interventions to foster lung development and healing in these patients cannot be overemphasized. At this time prevention remains the best strategy, and lung protective strategies employed very early in the neonatal course may decrease the incidence of this condition.

CASE STUDY 6

A 3-hour-old term male infant (birth weight of 3925 grams) born to a 32-year-old gravida 2, para 1 with adequate prenatal care develops respiratory distress with tachypnea and desaturations needing supplemental oxygen. The mother's antenatal culture for group B Streptococcus (GBS) was positive, and rupture of membranes occurred 8 hours prior to delivery; there was no maternal pyrexia in labor. He is transferred to the NICU and is placed in a hood with 60% oxygen; saturation values are in the mid-90s. He is started on antibiotics following blood cultures. A chest x-ray shows bilateral haziness with increased pulmonary vascularity and enlarged cardiothymic silhouette. Vital signs: temperature of 37.3° C, heart rate of 162/minute, respiratory rate of 80/minute, and BP of 59/40 mean 47 mmHg. An arterial blood gas is obtained and the results are as follows: pH of 7.27, PaCO$_2$ of 42 mmHg, PaO$_2$ of 45 mmHg in 60% oxygen. No murmur is audible on auscultation of the precordium. He appears comfortable but is tachypneic with mild intercostal retractions.

EXERCISE 18

QUESTION

1. What is the most appropriate next step in the management of this infant?
   a. Intubation and administration of surfactant
   b. Nasal CPAP
   c. Increase inspired oxygen concentration to 100%
   d. Echocardiogram

ANSWER

1. **b, c** (for hyperoxia test), and **d.** The differential diagnosis for the infant includes: (1) parenchymal lung disease such as pneumonia and early-onset sepsis; (2) idiopathic PPHN; and (3) cyanotic CHD, and is outlined in Table 17-1. Appropriate antibiotic therapy should be started for suspected sepsis. In spite of mild respiratory distress and tachypnea, the infant has a normal PaCO$_2$ and severe hypoxemia. This picture is more suggestive of PPHN or cyanotic CHD. A normal antenatal sonogram does not rule out

the possibility of cyanotic CHD. Although abnormalities such as hypoplastic left heart, septal defects, and single ventricle are commonly diagnosed antenatally, abnormalities of the vessels such as transposition of the great vessels, coarctation of the aorta, and anomalous pulmonary venous return may be missed.

CASE STUDY 6 (continued)

The infant is placed on nasal CPAP with 100% inspired oxygen to minimize respiratory distress and to perform a hyperoxia test. His blood pressure and perfusion are normal. An arterial blood gas is obtained from the right radial artery 30 minutes after placing on CPAP. The results are as follows: pH of 7.25, PaCO$_2$ of 46 mmHg. PaO$_2$ of 62 mmHg, with a base deficit of 7.3 mEq/L.

EXERCISE 19

QUESTION

1. How would you interpret the results of the hyperoxia test and what is the appropriate next step in management of this hypoxemic infant?
   a. The results are suggestive of severe parenchymal lung disease and the baby should be intubated and placed on mechanical ventilation.
   b. Hyperoxia test results confirm the presence of PPHN; intubation and inhaled NO should be administered.
   c. Hyperoxia test results are suggestive of PPHN or cyanotic CHD. Intravenous prostaglandin E1 (PGE1) therapy should be initiated. An echocardiogram should be ordered.
   d. Current management with nasal CPAP and 100% oxygen is appropriate as the PaO$_2$ is >60 mmHg.

ANSWER

1. **c.** A right radial arterial PaO$_2$ of <150 mmHg in 100% oxygen by CPAP is highly suggestive of cyanotic CHD or severe PPHN. It is important to immediately confirm these possibilities by an echocardiogram. Intravenous PGE1 therapy should be initiated to maintain ductal patency because ductal dependent CHD is a possibility. This agent also has pulmonary vasodilator effect and may be beneficial in PPHN. Common side effects of PGE1 include pyrexia and apnea.

CASE STUDY 6 (continued)

The baby is placed on intravenous PGE1 at 0.05 mcg/kg/min. Apneic spells are observed and he is intubated and placed on conventional ventilation.

The echocardiogram shows a large right ventricle, large main pulmonary artery, right-to-left shunt at the PFO and PDA, and a small left atrium. An estimate of pulmonary arterial pressure cannot be determined, as a tricuspid regurgitation jet is not observed. Based on these findings, severe PPHN is suspected. Intravenous PGE1 infusion is stopped and inhaled NO is administered at 20 ppm. An hour later, a repeat arterial blood gas from the umbilical arterial line is as follows: pH of 7.15, PaCO$_2$ of 27 mmHg, PaO$_2$ of 37 mmHg, and base deficit of 17 mEq/L. the metabolic acidosis is "corrected" with sodium bicarbonate (0.3 × base deficit × weight in kg = 0.3 × 3.9 × 17 = 20 mEq diluted 1:1) infused over 30 minutes.

EXERCISE 20

QUESTION

1. Treatment to induce rapid alkalinization of the blood may be complicated by which of the following?
   a. Intracellular acidosis
   b. Rapid fluctuation in cerebral blood flow
   c. Decrease in intravascular pH
   d. None of the above

ANSWER

1. **a** and **b.** Many infants with PPHN and HRF have a metabolic acidosis. Acidosis causes pulmonary vasoconstriction. In the past, it was a common practice to induce metabolic alkalosis but this strategy was associated with an increased need for ECMO (Walsh-Sukys et al., 2000). Rapid infusion of sodium bicarbonate is associated with fluctuations in cerebral blood flow and serum sodium levels. In addition, the CO$_2$ produced as a result of interaction between NaHCO$_3$ and acid diffuses across the blood–brain barrier and cell membranes resulting in perivascular acidosis in the brain and intracellular acidosis in neuronal cells and cardiac myocytes (Figure 17-7). Caution should be exercised during bicarbonate therapy (Aschner & Poland, 2008).

CASE STUDY 6 (continued)

The patient continues to remain hypoxemic despite correction of pH and inhaled NO. A repeat echocardiogram is obtained in preparation for ECMO. The cardiologist confirms earlier findings but cannot clearly track pulmonary veins to the left atrium. A computed tomography (CT) angiogram is performed and the diagnosis of anomalous drainage of pulmonary veins into the coronary sinus is confirmed (Figure 17-11, B). After surgical correction, he is discharged home at 20 days of age.

Infants with TAPVR mimic parenchymal lung disease (especially if obstructed) and PPHN. There are many clinical and echocardiographic features common to both conditions. Patients with TAPVR or PPHN can present with hypoxemia and respiratory distress. The chest x-ray may show coarse opacities. An echocardiogram shows a dilated pulmonary artery and right ventricle with right-to-left shunting at the foramen ovale and ductus arteriosus in both conditions. The presence of fixed hypoxemia (as opposed to labile hypoxemia in PPHN), presence of a small left atrium without draining pulmonary veins, and *absence* of tricuspid regurgitation should alert the physician to the possibility of TAPVR. Patients with TAPVR do not generally respond to an infusion of PGE1; however, some cases of infradiaphragmatic TAPVR associated with a closed ductus venosus respond with improved oxygenation.

This case illustrates the importance of continuous assessment and multidisciplinary evaluation of patients with PPHN and HRF.

OVERVIEW OF MANAGEMENT OF PPHN/ HRF AND PULMONARY VASODILATOR THERAPY

The pathophysiology of PPHN involves abnormalities in the lung, pulmonary vasculature, and cardiac function. Hence, therapy should address general supportive measures, optimal lung recruitment, cardiac support, and pulmonary vasodilation.

- PPHN and/or HRF with underlying parenchymal lung disease is a common problem in neonatal units. Appropriate diagnostic workup and specific therapy targeting the underlying lung disease such as pneumonia is important.
- Minimal stimulation, sedation, and analgesia are crucial to avoid episodes of hypoxemia. Labile hypoxemia is a characteristic feature of PPHN and excessive stimulation can precipitate hypoxic pulmonary vasoconstriction.
- Surfactant therapy is beneficial in patients with RDS and in conditions associated with surfactant inactivation, such as MAS (Lotze et al., 1998).
- Maintaining optimal oxygen levels and avoiding hypoxemia and hyperoxemia is vital during management of PPHN/HRF. Maintaining the PaO_2 in the 60 to 80 mmHg range and preductal oxygen saturation in the 90% to 97% range is recommended.

- Gentle ventilation to maintain $PaCO_2$ in the 40s to low 50s and avoiding acidosis (pH <7.30) has been associated with better outcomes.
- If it is not possible to maintain adequate ventilation and oxygenation with conventional ventilation, and if a high PIP (>25 cm H_2O) is required to keep $PaCO_2$ in the 40s to low 50s, many centers recommend switching to a high frequency oscillator or jet ventilator. Some centers prefer to use high-frequency ventilation as the primary mode of ventilation in the management of PPHN/HRF.
- Infants with clinical or echocardiographic evidence of PPHN (Figure 17-10 and 17-11, *A*) and infants with moderate to severe HRF benefit from pulmonary vasodilator therapy. Inhaled NO is currently the only FDA-approved specific pulmonary vasodilator for infants. The typical starting dose is 20 ppm. Optimal lung recruitment with the use of adequate PEEP, Paw, and/or surfactant is crucial for adequate and sustained response to inhaled NO. If inhaled NO results in improvement in systemic oxygenation, the FiO_2 should be gradually weaned, maintaining the SpO_2 in the 90% to 97% range. Inhaled NO is weaned in steps when the FiO_2 is ≤0.6 and PaO_2 is ≥60 mmHg or the SpO_2 is ≥90% as shown in Figure 17-16.
- Cardiac support with adequate volume infusion to avoid hypovolemia and inotropic support is essential. Deteriorating right ventricular and left ventricular function is a common cause for failure of medical management and need for ECMO in PPHN. It is important to remember that inotropes such as dopamine are not selective to systemic circulation and can result in pulmonary vasoconstriction.
- Intravenous sildenafil and/or intravenous milrinone (Figure 17-14) are not currently approved by the FDA. These promising therapeutic strategies are used by clinicians and centers with expertise in pulmonary vasodilator therapy.
- If PPHN/HRF does not respond to conventional medical management, early referral to an ECMO center is important.

CONCLUSION

Advances in respiratory management and pulmonary vasodilator therapy have reduced the need for ECMO for neonatal respiratory disorders. However, 20% to 40% of patients with PPHN/HRF fail to respond to conventional therapy and this failure rate is based on the primary underlying

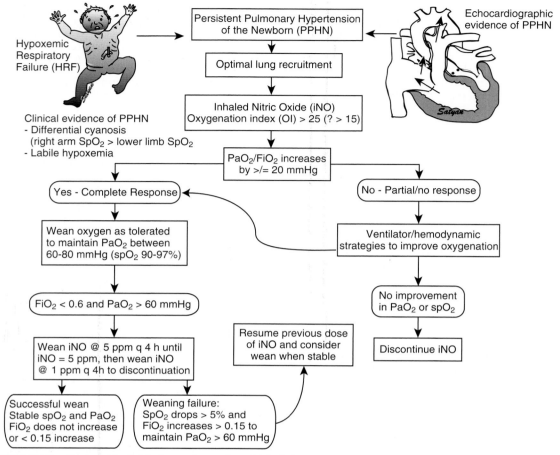

FIGURE 17-16 ■ **Protocol for initiation and weaning of inhaled nitric oxide in use at Women and Children's Hospital of Buffalo** (see text for details). (Adapted from Lakshminrusimha S, Kumar VH: Diseases of pulmonary circulation. In Fuhrman BP, Zimmerman JJ, editors: *Pediatric critical care,* 4th ed, Philadelphia, PA, 2011, Elsevier/Saunders, pp 632-656. Copyright © 2015 Bobby Mathew, Satyan Lakshminrusimha. Published by Elsevier Inc. All rights reserved.)

disease. Pulmonary hypertension associated with conditions such as CDH and BPD responds poorly to treatment and further studies are required to improve outcome in these conditions.

ACKNOWLEDGEMENT

The authors thank Drs. Veena Manja, Jayasree Nair, and Omar Al-Ibrahim for their critical review of the chapter.

SUGGESTED READING

Abman SH, Chatfield BA, Hall SL, McMurtry IF: Role of endothelium-derived relaxing factor during transition of pulmonary circulation at birth, *Am J Physiol* 259(6, Pt 2):H1921–1927, 1990.

Abman SH, Kinsella JP, Rosenzweig EB, Krishnan U, Kulik T, Mullen M, et al.: Implications of the U.S. Food and Drug Administration warning against the use of sildenafil for the treatment of pediatric pulmonary hypertension, *Am J Respir Crit Care Med* 187(6):572–575, 2012.

Abman SH, Nelin LD: Management of the infant with severe bronchopulmonary dysplasia. In Bancalari E, editor: *The newborn lung,*, Philadelphia, PA, 2012, Saunders Elsevier, pp 407–425.

An HS, Bae EJ, Kim GB, Kwon BS, Beak JS, Kim EK, et al.: Pulmonary hypertension in preterm infants with bronchopulmonary dysplasia, *Korean Circ J* 40(3):131–136, 2010.

Aschner JL, Poland RL: Sodium bicarbonate: basically useless therapy, *Pediatrics.* 122(4):831–835, 2008.

Bassler D, Choong K, McNamara P, Kirpalani H: Neonatal persistent pulmonary hypertension treated with milrinone: four case reports, *Biol Neonate* 89(1):1–5, 2006.

Bhat R, Salas AA, Foster C, Carlo WA, Ambalavanan N: Prospective analysis of pulmonary hypertension in extremely low birth weight infants, *Pediatrics* 129(3):e682–689, 2012.

Committee opinion no. 560: medically indicated late-preterm and early-term deliveries, *Obstet Gynecol* 121(4):908–910, 2013.

de Buys Roessingh A, Fouquet V, Aigrain Y, Mercier JC, de Lagausie P, Dinh-Xuan AT: Nitric oxide activity through guanylate cyclase and phosphodiesterase modulation is impaired in fetal lambs with congenital diaphragmatic hernia, *J Pediatr Surg* 46(8):1516–1522, 2011.

Dworetz AR, Moya FR, Sabo B, Gladstone I, Gross I: Survival of infants with persistent pulmonary hypertension without extracorporeal membrane oxygenation [comment], *Pediatrics* 84(1):1–6, 1989.

El-Khuffash AF, McNamara PJ: Neonatologist-performed functional echocardiography in the neonatal intensive care unit [review], *Semin Fetal Neonatal Med* 16(1):50–60, 2011.

Engle WA: Morbidity and mortality in late preterm and early term newborns: a continuum, *Clin Perinatol* 38(3):493–516, 2011.

Engle WA, Peters EA, Gunn SK, West KW, Langefeld C, Hui SL: Mortality prediction and interval until death in near-term and term neonates with respiratory failure, *J Perinatol* 13(5):368–375, 1993.

Fraser WD, Hofmeyr J, Lede R, Faron G, Alexander S, Goffinet F, et al.: Amnioinfusion for the prevention of the meconium aspiration syndrome, *N Engl J Med* 353(9):909–917, 2005.

Gaxiola A, Varon J, Valladolid G: Congenital diaphragmatic hernia: an overview of the etiology and current management, *Acta Paediatr* 98(4):621–627, 2009.

Golombek SG, Young JN: Efficacy of inhaled nitric oxide for hypoxic respiratory failure in term and late preterm infants by baseline severity of illness: a pooled analysis of three clinical trials, *Clin Ther* 32(5):939–948, 2010.

Guglani L, Lakshminrusimha S, Ryan RM: Transient tachypnea of the newborn, *Pediatr Rev* 29(11):e59–65, 2008.

Hendricks-Munoz KD, Walton JP: Hearing loss in infants with persistent fetal circulation, *Pediatrics* 81(5):650–656, 1988.

Hernandez-Diaz S, Van Marter LJ, Werler MM, Louik C, Mitchell AA: Risk factors for persistent pulmonary hypertension of the newborn, *Pediatrics* 120(2):e272–282, 2007.

Inhaled nitric oxide and hypoxic respiratory failure in infants with congenital diaphragmatic hernia: The Neonatal Inhaled Nitric Oxide Study Group (NINOS), *Pediatrics* 99(6):838–845, 1997.

Jani J, Nicolaides KH, Keller RL, et al.: Observed to expected lung area to head circumference ratio in the prediction of survival in fetuses with isolated diaphragmatic hernia, *Ultrasound Obstet Gynecol* 30(1):67–71, 2007.

Karamanoukian HL, Peay T, Love JE, Abdel-Rahman E, Dandonna P, Azizkhan RG, et al.: Decreased pulmonary nitric oxide synthase activity in the rat model of congenital diaphragmatic hernia, *J Pediatr Surg* 31(8):1016–1019, 1996.

Keller RL, Tacy TA, Hendricks-Munoz K, Xu J, Moon-Grady AJ, Neuhaus J, et al.: Congenital diaphragmatic hernia: endothelin-1, pulmonary hypertension, and disease severity, *Am J Respir Crit Care Med* 182(4):555–561, 2010.

Kinsella JP: Inhaled nitric oxide in the term newborn. [Review], *Early Hum Dev* 84(11):709–716, 2008.

Lakshminrusimha S: The pulmonary circulation in neonatal respiratory failure, *Clin Perinatol* 39(3):655–683, 2012.

Lakshminrusimha S, Russell JA, Steinhorn RH, Swartz DD, Ryan RM, Gugino SF, et al.: Pulmonary hemodynamics in neonatal lambs resuscitated with 21%, 50%, and 100% oxygen, *Pediatr Res* 62(3):313–318, 2007.

Lakshminrusimha S, Steinhorn RH: "Inodilators" in nitric oxide resistant PPHN [editorial], *Pediatr Crit Care Med* In press.

Lakshminrusimha S, Steinhorn RH: Pulmonary vascular biology during neonatal transition, *Clin Perinatol* 26(3):601–619, 1999.

Lakshminrusimha S, Swartz DD, Gugino SF, Ma CX, Wynn KA, Ryan RM, et al.: Oxygen concentration and pulmonary hemodynamics in newborn lambs with pulmonary hypertension, *Pediatr Res* 66(5):539–544, 2009.

Lakshminrusimha S, Wynn RJ, Youssfi M, Pabalan MJ, Bommaraju M, Kirmani K, et al.: Use of CT angiography in the diagnosis of total anomalous venous return, *J Perinatol* 29(6):458–461, 2009.

Lapointe A, Barrington KJ: Pulmonary hypertension and the asphyxiated newborn, *J Pediatr* 158(suppl 2):e19–24, 2011.

Logan JW, Rice HE, Goldberg RN, Cotten CM: Congenital diaphragmatic hernia: a systematic review and summary of best-evidence practice strategies, *J Perinatol* 27(9):535–549, 2007.

Lotze A, Mitchell BR, Bulas DI, Zola EM, Shalwitz RA, Gunkel JH: Multicenter study of surfactant (beractant) use in the treatment of term infants with severe respiratory failure. Survanta in Term Infants Study Group, *J Pediatr* 132(1):40–47, 1998.

Lou HC, Lassen NA, Fris-Hansen B: Decreased cerebral blood flow after administration of sodium bicarbonate in the distressed newborn infant, *Acta Neurol Scand* 57(3):239–247, 1978.

McNally H, Bennett CC, Elbourne D, Field DJ: Group, U. K. C. E. T. United Kingdom collaborative randomized trial of neonatal extracorporeal membrane oxygenation: follow-up to age 7 years, *Pediatrics* 117(5):e845–854, 2006.

McNamara PJ, Laique F, Muang-In S, Whyte HE: Milrinone improves oxygenation in neonates with severe persistent pulmonary hypertension of the newborn, *J Crit Care* 21(2):217–222, 2006.

McNamara PJ, Shivananda SP, Sahni M, Freeman D, Taddio A: Pharmacology of milrinone in neonates with persistent pulmonary hypertension of the newborn and suboptimal response to inhaled nitric oxide, *Pediatr Crit Care Med* 14(1): 74–84, 2013.

Mourani PM, Abman SH: Pulmonary vascular disease in bronchopulmonary dysplasia: pulmonary hypertension and beyond, *Curr Opin Pediatr* 25(3):329–337, 2013.

Mourani PM, Sontag MK, Ivy DD, Abman SH: Effects of long-term sildenafil treatment for pulmonary hypertension in infants with chronic lung disease, *J Pediatr* 154(3):379–384, 2009. 384 e371–372.

Mourani PM, Sontag MK, Younoszai A, Ivy DD, Abman SH: Clinical utility of echocardiography for the diagnosis and management of pulmonary vascular disease in young children with chronic lung disease, *Pediatrics* 121(2):317–325, 2008.

Pappas A, Shankaran S, Laptook AR, Langer JC, Bara R, Ehrenkranz RA, et al.: Hypocarbia and adverse outcome in neonatal hypoxic-ischemic encephalopathy, *J Pediatr* 158(5):752–758, 2011. e751.

Ramachandrappa A, Jain L: Elective cesarean section: its impact on neonatal respiratory outcome, *Clin Perinatol* 35(2):373–393, 2008.

Rasanen J, Wood DC, Weiner S, Ludomirski A, Huhta JC: Role of the pulmonary circulation in the distribution of human fetal cardiac output during the second half of pregnancy, *Circulation* 94(5):1068–1073, 1996.

Rosenberg AA, Lee NR, Vaver KN, Werner D, Fashaw L, Hale K, et al.: School-age outcomes of newborns treated for persistent pulmonary hypertension, *J Perinatol* 30(2):127–134, 2010.

Rudolph AM, Yuan S: Response of the pulmonary vasculature to hypoxia and H+ ion concentration changes, *J Clin Invest* 45(3):399–411, 1966.

Sehgal A, Athikarisamy SE, Adamopoulos M: Global myocardial function is compromised in infants with pulmonary hypertension, *Acta Paediatr* 101(4):410–413, 2012.

Slaughter JL, Pakrashi T, Jones DE, South AP, Shah TA: Echocardiographic detection of pulmonary hypertension in extremely low birth weight infants with bronchopulmonary dysplasia requiring prolonged positive pressure ventilation, *J Perinatol* 31(10):635–640, 2011.

Spong CY, Mercer BM, D'Alton M, Kilpatrick S, Blackwell S, Saade G: Timing of indicated late-preterm and early-term birth, *Obstet Gynecol* 118(2, Pt 1):323–333, 2011.

Sulyok E, Csaba IF: Elective repeat cesarean delivery and persistent pulmonary hypertension of the newborn, *Am J Obstet Gynecol* 155(3):687–688, 1986.

Teitel DF, Iwamoto HS, Rudolph AM: Changes in the pulmonary circulation during birth-related events, *Pediatr Res* 27(4, Pt 1):372–378, 1990.

UK collaborative randomised trial of neonatal extracorporeal membrane oxygenation: UK Collaborative ECMO Trail Group, *Lancet* 348(9020):75–82, 1996.

Vain NE, Szyld EG, Prudent LM, Wiswell TE, Aguilar AM, Vivas NI: Oropharyngeal and nasopharyngeal suctioning of meconium-stained neonates before delivery of their shoulders: multicentre, randomised controlled trial, *Lancet* 364(9434):597–602, 2004. http://dx.doi .org/10.1016/S0140-6736(04)16852-9.

Walsh-Sukys MC, Tyson JE, Wright LL, Bauer CR, Korones SB, Stevenson DK, et al.: Persistent pulmonary hypertension of the newborn in the era before nitric oxide: practice variation and outcomes, *Pediatrics* 105(1, Pt 1):14–20, 2000.

Wilson KL, Zelig CM, Harvey JP, Cunningham BS, Dolinsky BM, Napolitano PG: Persistent pulmonary hypertension of the newborn is associated with mode of delivery and not with maternal use of selective serotonin reuptake inhibitors, *Am J Perinatol* 28(1):19–24, 2011. http://dx.doi.org/ 10.1055/s-0030-1262507.

Wiswell TE, Gannon CM, Jacob J, Goldsmith L, Szyld E, Weiss K, et al.: Delivery room management of the apparently vigorous meconium-stained neonate: results of the multicenter, international collaborative trial, *Pediatrics* 105(1, Pt 1):1–7, 2000.

Wung JT, James LS, Kilchevsky E, James E: Management of infants with severe respiratory failure and persistence of the fetal circulation, without hyperventilation, *Pediatrics* 76(4):488–494, 1985.

Yock PG, Popp RL: Noninvasive estimation of right ventricular systolic pressure by Doppler ultrasound in patients with tricuspid regurgitation, *Circulation* 70(4):657–662, 1984.

CHAPTER 18

RENAL FAILURE IN NEONATES

Kimberly J. Reidy, MD • Fangming Lin, MD, PhD

The etiology of neonatal renal failure encompasses both chronic conditions such as congenital defects of the kidney and urinary tract, and acute insults such as hypoxia, ischemia, or drug toxicity leading to acute kidney injury (AKI) (Moghal et al., 2006). AKI in the neonate has been difficult to define, especially in the setting of prematurity, as standard definitions for both adult and pediatric patients rely on changes in serum creatinine and urine output (Fortenberry et al., 2013). During fetal development, the placenta provides renal-like clearance of plasma waste products. For the first day after birth, the newborn's creatinine predominantly reflects maternal renal function. Glomerular filtration rate is relatively low in newborn infants and changes rapidly over the first few weeks of life. Nephrogenesis continues in the normal fetus until 34 to 35 weeks' gestation and, thus, a "normal" serum creatinine is difficult to define for infants born prior to 34 weeks' gestation. In addition, neonatal AKI can present with severe oliguric or anuric renal failure that requires renal replacement therapy (RRT) but can also present with nonoliguric AKI, especially in the setting of injury from nephrotoxic medications. Thus, given that there is no standard definition for neonatal AKI and because nonoliguric AKI may be unrecognized by clinicians, it is challenging to determine the true incidence of neonatal AKI. Studies of neonatal AKI typically use a serum creatinine of 1.5 mg/dL or BUN >20 mg/dL as a cutoff indicating AKI for infants greater than 34 weeks' gestation, or urine output <1 mL/kg/hr (Fortenberry et al., 2013). By these definitions, AKI is reported to affect between 8% and 24% of infants cared for in neonatal intensive care units (NICUs) (Askenazi et al., 2009).

It has been increasingly recognized that neonatal AKI can lead to adverse long-term consequences. Neonatal AKI is associated with mortality rates as high as 25% and is even associated with increased mortality following NICU discharge (Koralkar et al., 2011). In addition, studies suggest that low birth weight,

prematurity, and neonatal AKI may lead to increased risk for microalbuminuria, hypertension, and chronic end-stage kidney disease later in life (Carmody & Charlton, 2013; Hoy et al., 2005).

CASE STUDY 1

A baby boy is born to a 19-year-old gravida 1, para 0 mother at 39 weeks' gestation. Mother sought late prenatal care, with her first visit at 20 weeks' gestation. Maternal testing: Rapid Plasma Reagin (RPR) negative, hepatitis B surface antigen negative, group B Streptococcus (GBS) colonization negative, and human immunodeficiency virus (HIV) negative. Pregnancy was complicated by intrauterine growth retardation (IUGR), anhydramnios at 29 weeks' gestation, and small kidneys with right hydronephrosis. Amniocentesis demonstrated a normal male karyotype. He was born via normal spontaneous vaginal delivery (NSVD), initially cried, then became apneic and bradycardic and required cardiopulmonary resuscitation and intubation. His Apgar scores were 6/7/8, and birth weight was 2875 grams. His blood urea nitrogen (BUN) and creatinine were 7 mg/dL and 1.6 mg/dL, respectively, on admission to the NICU.

EXERCISE 1

QUESTION

1. In addition to obtaining a kidney and bladder ultrasound, initial management for this patient should include:
   a. Restricting fluid to insensible water losses
   b. Initiating dialysis
   c. Consulting pediatric urology

ANSWER

1. **c.** There are three types of acute renal failure: prerenal, intrinsic renal, and postrenal failure. In a male infant with hydronephrosis and a history of anhydramnios, the most likely cause of renal failure is posterior urethral valves, which results from an obstruction at the level of the prostatic urethra. Once the obstruction is relieved by

TABLE 18-1 **Causes of Neonatal AKI**

Prerenal	Intravascular volume depletion
	Reduced renal perfusion, such as with heart failure
Intrinsic Renal	Nephrotoxic medications
	Acute tubular necrosis secondary to
	Hypoxia/ischemia/asphyxia
	Sepsis
	Hypotension
	Renal a/hypo/dysplasia
	Cystic kidney disease
	Vascular: renal arterial or vein thrombosis
Postrenal	Posterior urethral valves

placement of a Foley catheter, many neonates with posterior urethral valves will become poly-uric, not anuric. Thus, while it may be necessary to restrict fluid in caring for the anuric neonate, at this point it is unclear how much urine output this neonate is capable of producing (Table 18-1).

While dialysis may be necessary in caring for neonatal AKI, it is not correct for initial management of this infant. There are no clear indications for dialysis in this infant at this time.

Indications for dialysis:
- Fluid overload (congestive heart failure [CHF], pulmonary edema, severe hypertension)
- Intractable acidosis
- Hyperkalemia
- Uremic complications (hemorrhage, encephalopathy, etc.)
- Fluid removal to optimize nutrition and medication administration

The placenta provides renal-like clearance during fetal life. Thus, at birth, even a completely anephric neonate will have normal electrolytes and will not likely need dialysis immediately. Second, the creatinine at birth represents the maternal creatinine value and cannot be used to determine the neonate's renal function. In a healthy full-term newborn, the creatinine will typically decrease rapidly in the first few days after birth but may not reach its nadir until 10 days to 2 weeks of life. However, some neonates with posterior urethral valves will require dialysis in infancy. Thus, consulting a pediatric nephrologist to guide early management is beneficial. If the kidney and bladder ultrasound demonstrates a thickened and trabeculated bladder, a pediatric urologist will likely recommend placement of a Foley catheter to relieve the outflow tract obstruction until a definitive diagnosis is made by voiding cystourethrogram (VCUG). Surgical procedures, such as valve ablation, will be determined by the urologist.

CASE STUDY 1 (continued)

The patient was admitted to the NICU and was initially hypotensive, with a blood pressure of 50/20, and was started on dopamine for inotropic support. An echocardiogram on day of life 1 (DOL 1) showed a moderately dilated right atrium and left ventricle, small atrial septum defect with bidirectional flow, moderate right ventricular hypertrophy (RVH), and moderate patent ductus arteriosus (PDA) with right to left flow. A renal ultrasound showed bilateral small dysplastic kidneys and right hydronephrosis (Figure 18-1). Pediatric urology was consulted and a urinary catheter was placed. The nurse alerts you that the infant is hypoxic with retractions and on auscultation air entry into the lungs is decreased bilaterally.

EXERCISE 2

QUESTION

1. The most likely cause of respiratory distress in this infant is:
   a. Pulmonary edema
   b. Congestive heart failure
   c. Pneumothorax

ANSWER

1. **c.** Based on the history given, the infant is unlikely to have received enough fluids to develop pulmonary edema from fluid overload on the first day of life. The echocardiogram report gives no indication of decreased heart function that would suggest a cause for congestive heart failure. The amniotic fluid is required for lung development. Thus, renal dysplasia and urinary outflow tract obstruction leading to oligohydramnios or anhydramnios can result in pulmonary hypoplasia. These infants often require respiratory support postbirth. Pulmonary hypoplasia may increase the risk for respiratory complications, such as pneumothorax.

CASE STUDY 1 (continued)

The respiratory course was complicated by bilateral pneumothoraces (R>L) and required right chest tube placement, which was later removed. The patient was extubated on DOL 4 to nasal cannula with O_2 supplementation. A VCUG on DOL 5 showed posterior urethral valves, and bilateral severe reflux (Figure 18-2). The patient received 7 days of ampicillin and cefotaxime for possible sepsis and then was kept on ampicillin for urinary tract infection (UTI) prophylaxis. The patient was initially NPO on intravenous total parenteral nutrition (TPN).

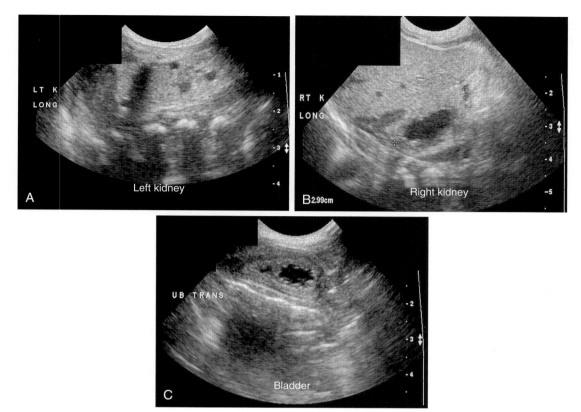

FIGURE 18-1 ■ Renal (**A** and **B**) and bladder (**C**) ultrasounds demonstrating bilateral small dysplastic kidneys and R hydronephrosis and thick-walled bladder.

FIGURE 18-2 ■ **A**, VCUG image for patient described in Case Study 1, which shows the dilated prostatic urethra (*arrow*), location of the urethral valve (*arrowhead*) and a small thick-walled bladder. The findings are consistent with posterior urethral valves. **B**, VCUG also reveals bilateral reflux into ureters and the renal collecting system.

EXERCISE 3

QUESTION

1. Which of the following kinds of feedings are optimal for this infant?
   a. Similac PM 60/40
   b. 22 calorie/ounce transitional formula
   c. Expressed breast milk
   d. Expressed breast milk supplemented with breast milk fortifier

ANSWER

1. **a** or **c.** The correct answer is either expressed breast milk or Similac PM 60/40. The kidneys are the major mechanism by which phosphorus is excreted. In the setting of renal insufficiency, phosphorus excretion decreases and the elevations in serum phosphorus stimulate secretion of parathyroid hormone. Secondary hyperparathyroidism and reduced formation of the active

form of vitamin D (1,25-(OH)$_2$-vitamin D) due to decreased 1-hydroxylation that occurs in the kidney can lead to complications such as defective bone mineralization (renal rickets) and long-term cardiovascular complications due to deposition of calcium and phosphorus in the vasculature. Both breast milk and Similac PM 60/40 have lower potassium, calcium, and phosphorus content, making these better choices for neonates with renal insufficiency. High-calorie–containing formulas and breast milk fortifiers contain higher levels of potassium, calcium, and phosphorus, and can lead to hyperkalemia and hyperphosphatemia in neonates with renal failure. In addition, following ablation of posterior urethral valves, many neonates will never recover function of the collecting ducts, which are the segments responsible for water reabsorption, and will become polyuric. These infants require additional free water intake to compensate for water loss in their diluted urine; thus, concentrated formulas (e.g., 22 to 24 kcal/oz versions) should be avoided in infants with persistently high urinary volumes and low urine specific gravity.

CASE STUDY 1 (continued)

The clinical course over the next two days was remarkable for hemodynamic instability and a low urine output. A head ultrasound study revealed two hyperechogenic foci in the midline, and flattening of the left ventricle. Table 18-2 lists other pertinent laboratory data and clinical information.

Physical Examination

Length 52 cm, Weight 3.75 kg, HC 33.5 cm
T 37.1° C, HR 149/minute, RR 60/minute, BP 81/58, O$_2$ sat 97%
General: Alert
HEENT: periorbital edema
Chest: bilateral decreased air entry, no retractions
Cardiovascular: normal S1, S2, and no murmur

Abdomen: soft, slightly distended, nontender, liver 1 cm palpable at RCM
Genitourinary: Tanner 1 male, Foley in place, scrotal edema, and right testicle not descended
Extremities: well perfused, edema bilaterally
Neurologic: normal

EXERCISE 4

QUESTION

1. The most appropriate next step in care for this infant is:
   a. Normal saline bolus to increase urine output
   b. Placement of a peritoneal dialysis catheter
   c. Palliative care

ANSWER

1. **b.** This infant has normal blood pressure and perfusion and does not appear to be volume depleted; instead, the infant is edematous and likely volume overloaded. A normal saline bolus should be avoided.

   This infant now has several indications for dialysis: volume overload and electrolyte abnormalities, including hyperkalemia. The infant has progressively worsening creatinine, indicative of poor renal function. In addition, the degree of dysplasia on renal ultrasound is marked, likely giving this infant a poor renal prognosis. Approximately one third of patients with posterior urethral valves will require dialysis in infancy. Renal transplant is not feasible until infants are large enough for their abdomens to accommodate the size of an adult kidney (usually when the infant weighs approximately 10 kg). Peritoneal dialysis (PD) is the preferred mode of dialysis for infants for several reasons (Zaritsky & Warady, 2011). First, providing adequate nutrition in infancy requires a significant daily fluid intake; PD allows

TABLE 18-2 **Major Laboratory and Clinical Findings**

Day	Na (mEq/L)	K (mEq/L)	Cl (mEq/L)	HCO$_3$ (mEq/L)	BUN (mg/dL)	Creatinine (mg/dL)	Calcium (mg/dL)	PO$_4$ (mg/dL)	Fluid intake (mL)	Fluid output (mL)	Other treatments
0	132	4.4	106	21	8	1.6	7.7		186	12	Hypotensive required fluid boluses and pressors
1	133	3.6	104	20	17	2	8.2		378	22	
2	129	3.4	91	25	37	3.3	9.1	3.4	297	98	
3	130	3.6	94	24	45	3.7	9.2	3.7	250	135	Furosemide started for fluid overload
4	132	3.3	94	29	50	3.8	10	3.2	281	177	
5	138	5.7	96	32	55	4.2	10.3	2.8	251	156	
6	150	6.5	98	34	64	4.9	10.3	4.1	240	80	

for this fluid and waste products to be removed daily. Second, infants often do not tolerate rapid fluid shifts during the 2 to 4 hours treatment of each hemodialysis session that is required once a day or every other day. In addition, hemodialysis often requires that a significant proportion (>10%) of the infant's blood volume (estimated 80 mL/kg) remain in the extracorporeal hemodialysis circuit. This can result in both hemodynamic instability and a requirement for transfusion of blood products, which will increase the risk for sensitization to donor antigens in future kidney transplants. Fluid removal by PD occurs daily over a longer period of time (usually 10 to 12 hours for infants on chronic PD). Of note, in the United States, chronic PD is typically performed by the parents at home using an automated cycler. This requires a significant time commitment from the parents to train (usually performed over a few weeks) and perform the dialysis procedures 7 nights a week, 365 days a year. A typical infant will remain on dialysis for over a year, as growth to reach a size amenable for transplantation is often slow in children with end-stage kidney disease.

The ethics of providing dialysis to neonates should always be a consideration, because this could indicate the potential need for lifelong RRT and ultimately renal transplantation. This infant was able to be extubated, suggesting that the degree of pulmonary hypoplasia was not life limiting and the infant appears to be neurologically intact without significant comorbidities. Thus, the infant would be a good candidate for dialysis. Neonatal survival at 1 year for those started on dialysis in infancy reaches approximately 85%, although there is a slightly worse prognosis for anuric infants. The most common causes of death are from cardiopulmonary causes and infection in this age group (North American Pediatric Renal Trials and Collaborative Studies, 2011).

EXERCISE 5

QUESTION

1. The mother asks you why her infant developed this condition. She is worried that it was because she traveled by airplane when she was pregnant, which she was advised not to do.

ANSWER

1. You reply that unless she had exposed to known teratogens during travel, it is more likely that genetic abnormalities may have caused the kidney and urinary tract malformations. Genetic

tests are recommended, especially if she considers having more children.

EMBRYONIC KIDNEY DEVELOPMENT

The kidneys are derived from the intermediate mesoderm. There are three sets of embryonic kidneys during embryogenesis: the pronephros (at 3 weeks' gestation), mesonephros (at 4 weeks' gestation), and metanephros (at 5 weeks' gestation; Figure 18-3). The pronephros and most of the mesonephros degenerate. The mesonephric duct (Wolffian duct) forms the epididymis, vas deferens, seminal vesicles, and ejaculatory ducts in males. The mature human kidneys develop from the metanephros. The ureteric bud, which is an outgrowth of the mesonephric duct, invades the metanephric mesenchyme and undergoes serial branching to form the collecting ducts. The tips of the ureteric bud induce nephron formation in the mesenchyme. Thus, the number of ureteric bud branches will influence nephron number. Defects in ureteric bud migration and branching can lead to congenital abnormalities of the kidneys (e.g., renal aplasia, hypoplasia, dysplasia) as well as urinary tract deformities such as ureteral pelvic junction (UPJ) or ureteral

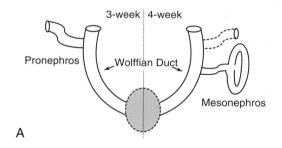

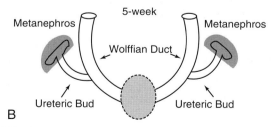

FIGURE 18-3 ■ **Embryonic kidney development. A,** The pronephros develops at 3 weeks' gestation and degenerates at about 4 weeks when the mesonephros forms. The mesonephros has transient secretory function, but the majority of its structures also degenerate. **B,** The metanephros that forms at 5 weeks' gestation subsequently develops into the mature kidney when the ureteric bud invades and induces nephrogenesis.

vesical junction (UVJ) obstruction and vesico-ureteral reflux.

The inductive signals originating from the ureteric bud stimulate mesenchymal to epithelial transition, and spheres of epithelial cells known as renal vesicles are the earliest form of the developing nephron. The developing nephrons go through a series of morphologic changes, forming a comma- and then S-shaped bodies. Segments of the S-shaped body will differentiate into the distal tubule, proximal tubule, and podocytes. Endothelial cells migrate into the cleft of the S-shaped body to form the glomerular endothelial cells. The molecular signals that drive nephrogenesis require reciprocal interactions between the ureteric bud and surrounding metanephric mesenchyme. Genetic defects in these signaling pathways can lead to abnormal development in the nephron and the collecting systems.

The first glomeruli form by 9 weeks, and nephrogenesis continues until 34 to 35 weeks' gestation. The ureters and bladder form around the same time as the metanephric kidney. Glomerular filtration begins at the gestational age of 9 to 10 weeks. Fetal urine is the major source of amniotic fluid from approximately 16 weeks' gestation onward. Thus, obstruction of urinary outflow (as may occur in posterior urethral valves) or renal aplasia/severe dysplasia leads to low urine production and will present with oligohydramnios during the pregnancy, which affects fetal lung development (lack of sufficient amniotic fluid diminishes fetal breathing and thoracic movement that is required for proper lung maturation).

Congenital abnormalities of the kidney and urinary tract (CAKUT) are the leading causes of end-stage renal disease (ESRD) in children in the United States (NAPRTCS reports). Obstructive uropathy from posterior urethral valves represents a major proportion of those children requiring dialysis in infancy. Posterior urethral valves are membranes at the junction of the prostatic and bulbar urethra. Although the pathophysiology of this condition is not fully understood, these membranes are thought to form during normal development. However, failure to recanalize during urethral development leads to bladder outlet obstruction. In the face of high-pressure obstruction, bladder differentiation is impaired, and a thick-walled bladder develops. The dilation of the prostatic urethra can lead to the classic keyhole sign on a fetal ultrasound. The bladder obstruction can result in vesicoureteral reflux, and the exposure of the developing kidneys to obstruction results in varying degrees of renal dysplasia. Although

some familial cases have been identified, the majority of cases of posterior urethral valves appear to be sporadic, and contributing genetic and environmental factors have not been clearly identified to date. New technologies, such as whole genome exome sequencing could help discover genetic mutations that underlie these malformations.

CASE STUDY 2

This is a 1-day old girl born at 26 weeks' gestation via a spontaneous vaginal delivery 2 days following premature rupture of membranes. Her birth weight was 750 grams and her Apgar scores were 6 and 5 at 1 and 5 minutes of life. She was intubated and given surfactant. After a blood specimen was drawn for culture, she was started on ampicillin and gentamicin and given intravenous (IV) fluid. She fails to pass urine in the first 24 hours after birth, and her blood pressures are persistently low at 30/20 mmHg.

EXERCISE 6

QUESTIONS

1. When should newborns pass the first urine after birth?

2. What should you do first to evaluate and treat this infant?

3. Is she at risk for gentamicin toxicity?

ANSWERS

1. Studies have shown that almost 100% of newborns have the first void within 24 hours after birth and nearly half of them void 8 hours after birth (Clark, 1977). Although very few infants of less than 32 weeks' gestation were documented in these studies and the time of the first void varies considerably, failing to pass urine beyond 24 hours should prompt the physician to evaluate and intervene for newborns of any gestational age.

2. She required resuscitation at birth and has a persistently low blood pressure that may be limiting perfusion of vital organs, including the heart and kidneys. Prolonged hypotension could serve as a prerenal etiology for acute ischemic and hypoxic injury to the kidney and should be corrected immediately. A normal saline infusion at 10 cc/kg (over 30 minutes) can be given at this time, and a repeated dose with the same volume could be considered if there is no significant improvement in the blood pressure. A renal

ultrasound is also recommended. She needs frequent monitoring of respiratory, cardiac, and fluid status. Placement of a Foley catheter is also recommended to drain the urine from the bladder and for subsequent monitoring of urine output.

3. Aminoglycosides are frequently used to treat infants with the possibility of sepsis due to their fast bactericidal effect, synergy with β-lactam antibiotics, and low cost. However, they can accumulate in tissues such as the kidney and the ear, causing nephrotoxicity and ototoxicity. Gentamicin is one of the most nephrotoxic and best studied aminoglycosides (Lopez-Novoa et al., 2011). The kidney excretes gentamicin, and its nephrotoxicity affects all compartments of the kidney. The incidence of gentamicin nephrotoxicity ranges from 10% to 25%. Risk factors contributing to its toxicity include reduced renal mass, intravascular volume depletion, long duration and high dose of treatment, and concomitant use of other nephrotoxic medications. Gentamicin causes apoptosis and necrosis of renal tubular cells, especially epithelial cells of the proximal tubules, by complex mechanisms including phospholipidosis, reduced ATP production in the mitochondria, and increased oxidative stress. Death of tubular cells results in tubular obstruction and increased hydrostatic pressure in the tubular lumen and the Bowman capsule, leading to a reduced filtration pressure gradient and low glomerular filtration rate (GFR). Cell death is accompanied by interstitial inflammation. Injury to epithelial cells interferes with ion transport, and may result in nonoliguric or polyuric renal failure. Excessive delivery of water and solutes to the distal nephron triggers tubuloglomerular feedback (tubuloglomerular feedback is one of several mechanisms the kidney uses to regulate glomerular filtration rate) further reducing GFR. In addition, gentamicin can cause direct functional alterations in the glomerulus and increase resistance of renal vasculature to reduce renal blood flow. Because its toxicity is usually related to blood concentration and duration of treatment, close monitoring of drug levels is required before subsequent administration, especially when renal compromise is suspected. In this case, our patient has an increased risk for gentamicin toxicity resulting from low nephron numbers attributed to prematurity, possible higher drug levels from decreased blood flow to the kidneys, and renal ischemic and hypoxic insult from the low blood pressure. Improving her systemic circulation with fluid and inotropic agents, if indicated, may help reduce renal injury.

MEASUREMENTS OF RENAL FUNCTION IN PREMATURE INFANTS

Serum creatinine is the sum of its generation from muscle metabolism and its excretion by the kidney. Clinicians use it to estimate renal function under steady state conditions. At birth, an infant's serum creatinine level reflects the maternal creatinine level (Quigley, 2012). Serum creatinine declines after birth to a new steady state level in about 2 weeks in full-term infants. However, premature infants can have an initial increase in serum creatinine and have a slower decline in creatinine level, which may take 5 to 6 weeks before reaching a steady state level (Thayyil et al., 2008). The initial increase in creatinine is largely due to its reabsorption of creatinine by renal tubules as a result of immature tubular function and does not always indicate AKI. For these reasons, serum creatinine in premature newborns cannot truly reflect GFR. The estimated GFR for a full term infant is about 26 mL/min/1.73M^2 and doubles by 2 weeks of age. The postnatal increase in GFR is mainly due to postnatal hemodynamic changes resulting in: (1) increased renal blood flow by the mechanisms of reduction of renal vascular resistance and elevation of systemic blood pressure; and (2) redistribution of renal blood flow from the medulla to the cortex. Because GFR is determined by the filtration rate at each nephron and premature infants (<35 weeks' gestation) have decreased numbers of filtering nephrons, premature infants have a lower GFR value. A prospective study of infants born at 27 to 31 weeks' gestation showed that the GFR slowly increased over the first month of life, and that the increase of GFR was inversely correlated to the gestational age (Vieux et al., 2010). At 7 days and 28 days postnatally, infants born at 27 weeks' gestation have a median GFR of 13.4 and 21.0 mL/min/1.73M^2, respectively. Risk factors for decreasing GFR in premature infants include the use of nephrotoxic medications, systemic hypotension, hypovolemia, perinatal asphyxia, sepsis, and intrauterine growth restriction.

Other important physiologic abnormalities in premature infants are a high fractional excretion of urinary sodium (FeNa) and relatively higher serum potassium value. FeNa can be as high as 5%, thus making it less useful in differentiating prerenal vs. intrinsic renal disease. The principal cells of the collecting duct are the final regulators for urinary sodium reabsorption and potassium excretion. The epithelial sodium channels (ENaC) of the principal cells are less responsive to aldosterone and have low sodium transport activity. The cause of the higher serum potassium levels is unclear, but is likely owing either to diminished excretion of potassium by the kidney or decreased levels of Na+/K+ ATPase allowing potassium to leak out of the intracellular compartment.

Urine concentrating ability is limited in newborns due to: (1) low response to antidiuretic hormone (ADH) in the collecting ducts; (2) lower medullary concentration gradient; and (3) shorter loops of Henle. Premature infants have a significantly lower GFR and less mature tubular transport function than full-term neonates. Although neonates can excrete urine with an osmolality of 50 mOsm/kg water, which is comparable to adults, they are only able to concentrate the urine to 600 mOsm/kg water, which is about half of the concentrating ability in adults (Calcagno et al., 1954). Urine concentrating ability reaches adult level by 2 years of age. In addition, neonates have increased amounts of insensible water loss through the skin, especially when they are placed under the warmer. The daily fluid requirement in neonates is greater when calculated based on body weight.

It is important to note that in neonates, the low GFR can also limit the ability to excrete free water. Human milk is low in sodium, but neonates are able to excrete a sufficient amount of free water absorbed from the milk. Hyponatremia can result when formula is diluted because neonates will drink larger volumes to meet their caloric needs. The proximal tubules in neonatal kidneys have lower rates of bicarbonate reabsorption, and therefore the serum bicarbonate will be lower in a neonate as compared to an adult. Similarly, glucose reabsorption in the proximal tubules is low. It is common to have renal glycosuria in infants born before 30 weeks' gestation. In contrast, neonates have more active phosphate reabsorption than adults, leading to a higher serum phosphorus concentration and a positive phosphorus balance needed for growth.

In summary, neonatal kidneys undergo functional maturation after birth. Full-term infants have more complete kidney structures, but premature infants born before 34 weeks have incomplete nephrogenesis (Hughson et al., 2003). One should bear in mind premature infants' unique renal physiology when administering medications and managing fluids, electrolytes, and nutrition.

CASE STUDY 2 (continued)

Her blood culture was negative at 48 hours and antibiotics were discontinued. By 72 hours of life, *her urine output was 1 cc/kg/hr and the serum creatinine value was 1.5 mg/L. She remained on a ventilator and had bounding pulse, an active precordium, and a loud continuous murmur. An echocardiogram shows a 3-mm PDA with left-to-right shunt and retrograde diastolic aortic flow.*

EXERCISE 7

QUESTIONS

1. Can a large PDA affect renal perfusion?

2. How does ibuprofen affect the kidney when it is used for PDA closure?

ANSWERS

1. PDA is a common complication in premature infants and is associated with increased risk for intraventricular hemorrhage, bronchopulmonary dysplasia, necrotizing enterocolitis, and death (Hamrick & Hansmann, 2010). A significant left-to-right shunt increases pulmonary blood flow and can contribute to a continued need for respiratory support. A reversal of diastolic blood flow from the descending aorta can result in compromised blood flow to organs distal to the descending aorta such as the kidney and the intestinal tract. In renal arteries, the velocity of diastolic blood flow can be diminished and, in some cases, retro-diastolic blood flow can be observed (Bomelburg et al., 1989). Low renal perfusion limits the excretion of metabolic products generated in underperfused organs, which contributes to profound metabolic acidosis.

2. All prostanoids (PGD2, PGE2, PGF2, PGI2, and thromboxane A2) are synthesized in the kidney by the action of cyclooxygenases (COX1 and COX2). Prostaglandin E2 is the main renal prostanoid and plays an important role in regulating renal vascular tone (hemodynamic effect) and salt and water excretion (tubular effect). Under stress conditions, such as dehydration, hypotension and cardiac failure, vasoconstrictors (angiotensin II, endothelin and catecholamines) are highly activated. It is essential that the vasodilatory PGE2 and PGI2 oppose the action of vasoconstrictors to maintain glomerular filtration rate by dilating afferent arterioles. Newborn kidneys have high pre- and postglomerular vascular resistance. They are more dependent on vasodilatory prostaglandins for normal renal function and therefore are more sensitive to adverse effects of nonsteroidal antiinflammatory drugs (NSAIDs) on the kidney (Antonucci & Fanos, 2009).

Ibuprofen inhibits PGE2 synthesis and is used to constrict an open PDA, leading to functional closure. Although studies on low birth weight infants have shown that ibuprofen is as effective as indomethacin in closing a PDA and may have a better safety profile relating to impaired renal, gastrointestinal and cerebral blood flow, it is important to remember that all NSAIDs can precipitate acute renal failure especially when other risk factors are present. In general, adverse renal effects induced by NSAIDs are usually reversible.

CASE STUDY 2 (continued)

As a result of her hemodynamically significant PDA, she received two doses of ibuprofen. Her urine output decreased to 0.3 cc/kg/hr. Her serum creatinine increased to 1.8 mg/dL in the next 24 hours and continued to increase to 2.2 mg/dL 72 hours after ibuprofen was given. She appears puffy but does not require higher ventilator support. An echocardiogram shows closure of the PDA.

EXERCISE 8

QUESTIONS

1. Which of the following statements about this infant's renal function is correct?
   a. She in acute renal failure and requires fluid restriction.
   b. This infant is not in renal failure. A rise in serum creatinine values is expected with ibuprofen and no intervention is needed at this time.
   c. Renal failure is present and diuretics should be used to increase urine output.

ANSWERS

1. **None of the above**. At this time, there is no universally accepted definition for AKI in premature infants mainly due to the lack of early biomarkers that can be standardized for clinical application (Askenazi et al., 2011). Serum creatinine does not increase until renal function is reduced by 25% to 50%. Its level can increase in the first few days after birth before its decline to a steady state over the next 5 to 6 weeks. Most neonatal AKI results in polyuric renal failure (urine output >1 mL/kg/hr), making urine output an unreliable measurement for renal function. Risk factors for AKI in this case include low perfusion pressure for the kidney from her PDA, use of NSAIDs, and prematurity. The fact that her urine output has decreased

from 1 cc/kg/hr to 0.3 cc/kg/hr while creatinine has progressively increased to 2.2 mg/dL makes the diagnosis of AKI (and renal failure) undisputable.

Loop diuretics inhibit the Na-K-2Cl co-transporter in epithelial cells of the thick ascending limb (TAL) to increase urine flow. Use of diuretics might facilitate fluid excretion to improve cardiopulmonary status and allow infants to receive fluid for medications and nutrition. However, diuretics do not improve GFR. There is no evidence to show that diuretics accelerate recovery from AKI. To exert its effect, furosemide needs to be filtered through the glomerular filtration barrier to reach to the lumen of the TAL. Renal failure limits the filtration of furosemide and reduces its effect. Although higher doses of furosemide can be given to overcome the low glomerular filtration, it increases the risks of furosemide accumulation in the circulation and ototoxicity. Diuretics can add to prerenal insult if the circulating volume is reduced. Current KDIGO (Kidney Disease Improving Global Outcomes) clinical practice guidelines for AKI recommend not using diuretics to prevent AKI or to treat AKI, except when they are required for managing fluid overload.

Fluid restriction should not be used unless the infant is felt to be fluid overloaded or there is persistent anuria.

CASE STUDY 2 (continued)

Her urine output improved to 1 cc/kg/hr and serum creatinine gradually improved to 0.8 mg/L at 3 weeks and 0.4 mg/dL at 5 weeks. She was weaned off mechanical ventilation. She is tolerating feeds and gaining weight appropriately. Her mother is expecting her to go home soon.

EXERCISE 9

QUESTION

1. What will you tell the family about her kidney condition?

ANSWER

1. She had an AKI and her kidney function is recovering to the level that allows her to excrete fluid and metabolic wastes. However, she has an increased risk for chronic kidney disease (CKD) and can develop hypertension. She should have long-term follow up with a pediatric nephrologist after being discharged from the NICU.

LONG-TERM RENAL CONSEQUENCE IN CHILDREN WITH PREMATURE BIRTH

With the advancement of neonatal intensive care, more premature infants can now live and be discharged safely from the NICU. However, it is clear that these survivors have unique requirements in their healthcare. Long-term kidney care is no exception. Clinical research and observational data indicate that premature birth and low birth weight are associated with an increased risk for CKD. As kidney formation does not complete until 34 weeks of gestation and the most robust nephrogenesis occurs in the third trimester, premature birth results in low nephron numbers and immature kidneys in both structure and function. Human autopsies from cases that include infants, children, and adults have shown that there is a more than 8-fold difference in glomerular numbers ranging from 220,000 to 1,825,000. A linear relationship exists between low birth weight and glomerular number (Figure 18-4) (Hughson et al., 2003). Each kilogram increase in birth weight is predicted to increase the glomerular number by 257,000. Extrauterine insults including nephrotoxic medications, infection, and hypotension can impair kidney development. Autopsy studies in infants with birth weights of less than 1000 grams show no evidence of new nephron formation 40 days after birth. Infants who experienced AKI have even lower numbers of glomerular counts. The volume of glomeruli is larger (oligomeganephronia) in children with premature birth. Hyperfiltration occurs in the small number of nephrons that have larger glomeruli, which leads to secondary focal glomerular sclerosis (FSGS). Proteinuria and hypertension can develop rapidly, which accelerates the progression of CKD and contributes to further declines in renal function. A systemic review indicates that adults born with low birth weight have a 70% increase in developing CKD and highlights the necessities of long-term renal care for children with premature birth (Carmody & Charlton, 2013).

It is worth noting that most infants discharged from the NICU have normal serum creatinine values, but the serum creatinine does not measure GFR accurately. Because of functional compensation, a loss of half of the nephron number leads to only a 20% to 30% decrease in GFR. At this time, there is neither a sensitive method to screen for renal impairment nor a general guideline for long-term renal care for NICU graduates. Collaborations among neonatologists, pediatricians, and nephrologists are crucial in identifying children at risk and implementing long-term care plans. Prematurity and a history of AKI warrant a nephrology clinic follow up. A simple urine test for albuminuria may detect glomerular lesions. Hypertension could be a sign of salt and water retention from low numbers of functional nephrons. Impaired linear growth could also reflect CKD. Although there are no specific treatments to regenerate damaged nephrons or prevent the development of CKD, early identification of children with CKD may help to reduce CKD-associated complications such as anemia, growth failure, renal osteodystrophy, impaired neurocognitive function, and poor quality of life. Parents can be educated to avoid nephrotoxic medications such as NSAIDs and obesity, both of which could adversely affect kidney function. As the children grow into adolescence, when stressful conditions exist, close monitoring and preparation for transition to adult nephrology services become an integral part of the long-term care.

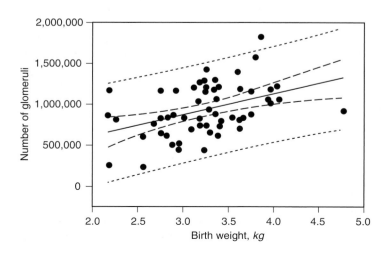

FIGURE 18-4 ■ The relationship between birth weight and total glomerular number. Symbols are (•) Nglom vs. birth weight; (——) Nglom vs. birth weight regression; (– – –) 95% regression CI; (- - -) regression prediction interval. The regression coefficient predicts a gain of 257,426 glomeruli per kg increase in birth weight, r = 0.423, P = 0.0012, N = 56. (From Hughson M, Farris AB III, Douglas-Denton R, Hoy WE, Bertram JF. Glomerular number and size in autopsy kidneys: the relationship to birth weight. *Kidney Int* 63:2113-2122, 2003.)

CASE STUDY 3

A 7-day old Twin A female born at 35 weeks' gestation was delivered via cesarean section for decreased fetal movements and abnormal fetal heart tracings. She was transferred from an outside hospital for management of AKI. At birth, she was limp and apneic with Apgar scores of 2 and 5 at 1 and 5 minutes of life. The birth weight was 2300 grams. She was intubated and placed on a ventilator. Immediately after birth, she was noted to be hypotensive and required IV vasopressor support. She received treatment with IV meropenem and acyclovir. Her serum creatinine values rose from 1.4 mg/dL at birth to 5.4 mg/dL at day 7. At that time she was oliguric with a urine output of only 22 cc in 24 hours despite receiving high doses of furosemide. She has gained 540 grams since birth and has severe anasarca and ascites. On admission to your hospital, her heart rate is 120 beats per minute and blood pressure is 58/28. Her serum chemistry values are as follows: Na 122 mEq/L, K 5.9 mEq/L, Cl 83 mEq/L, HCO$_3$ 15 mEq/L, BUN 52 mg/dL, and creatinine 5.4 mg/dL. Her liver transaminases and both direct and indirect bilirubin are elevated. Renal ultrasound shows enlarged echogenic kidneys (R kidney 5 cm, L kidney 5.6 cm). A head ultrasound study demonstrates no acute hemorrhage.

EXERCISE 10

QUESTION

1. What is the next best step for management of this infant's elevated serum potassium concentration and metabolic acidosis?
   a. Calcium chloride
   b. Sodium bicarbonate
   c. Sodium polystyrene sulfonate (Kayexalate) by mouth

ANSWER

1. **b.** A serum potassium concentration of 5.9 mEq/L is unlikely to induce electrocardiogram (ECG) changes and by itself is not an indication for calcium chloride. IV calcium is indicated in the setting of hyperkalemia and ECG changes. Treatment of acidosis with sodium bicarbonate will likely drive the potassium into cells and decrease the serum potassium concentration. Oral administration of sodium polystyrene sulfonate is generally avoided in neonates because of potential intestinal complications, and would not be a first-line choice for management of this infant's serum potassium.

NEONATAL HYPERKALEMIA AND MANAGEMENT

Hyperkalemia (K >6.0 mEq/L) can be a life-threatening complication of neonatal AKI. Premature neonates have decreased GFR and relative resistance to aldosterone, limiting their ability to excrete potassium. Therefore, reducing potassium intake by elimination of potassium from TPN or intravenous fluid (IVF) and/or use of low potassium formula (Similac PM 60/40 or breast milk) is an important precaution in the management of neonatal AKI. Administration of sodium polystyrene resins can be used to achieve the exchange of potassium for sodium, but direct oral or rectal administration should be avoided in neonates as it has been reported to cause intestinal ischemia, obstruction, and perforation. Potassium intake can be further decreased by mixing sodium polystyrene with Similac PM 60/40 or breast milk allowing the potassium to precipitate out. After allowing the precipitate to settle, the supernatant is decanted for oral/gastric administration (so that there is no direct administration of the resin).

For acute management of hyperkalemia, an ECG should be performed to evaluate the effects of hyperkalemia on the heart's electrical activity. Calcium gluconate should be administered in the presence of ECG changes. As concomitant acidosis will drive potassium out of cells and elevate the serum potassium, sodium bicarbonate should be administered to treat acidosis, but is not used when metabolic acidosis is not present. Administration of IV glucose and insulin can be used in the acute setting to stimulate potassium entry into cells and temporarily lower serum potassium. However, insulin and glucose will not enhance excretion of potassium. In the nonanuric patient, IV furosemide can be administered to increase potassium excretion. More recently, inhaled albuterol (salbutamol) has been used to treat infants with elevated serum potassium values. Small randomized clinical trials indicate the drug is effective, but is has not been evaluated in a large randomized trial. If medical management fails, dialysis will be indicated for potassium removal.

EXERCISE 11

QUESTION

1. When would you consider RRT?

ANSWER

1. This case illustrates that the etiology of neonatal AKI is most often multifactorial, as hypoxia,

hypotension, sepsis, and nephrotoxic medications likely all contributed to the development of AKI. As in many cases of neonatal AKI secondary to perinatal asphyxia and sepsis, this infant has multiorgan dysfunction, with respiratory failure and hepatic insufficiency. Despite initial resuscitation, this infant likely has developed severe acute tubular necrosis, and unfortunately her oliguric renal failure has not improved. Medical management with high-dose furosemide and fluid restriction was unsuccessful and she remains severely oliguric (0.3 mL/kg/hr) with fluid overload. Therefore, this renal insufficiency and fluid overload will likely not respond to further medical management, indicating the need for RRT.

Continuous renal replacement therapy (CRRT) is designed to provide continuous support (i.e., 24 hours/day) of renal function, analogous to the continuous respiratory support provided by a ventilator (Bunchman et al., 2008; Goldstein, 2011). Although CRRT is often thought of as continuous venovenous hemofiltration (CVVH) or continuous venovenous hemodiafiltration (CVVHDF), it can also include continuous PD. Acute PD often requires immediate use of a peritoneal catheter, which has a high risk of leaks and infection. Thus, initial exchange volumes will need to be small, and this limits the effectiveness of acute PD for clearance and fluid removal. Although extending PD continuously for 24 hours may overcome its inadequacies, there are some cases where this still will not provide sufficient therapy. In addition, small exchange volumes often require manual PD exchanges by NICU nurses, which further increases the risks of infection.

CVVH and CVVHDF can be provided to neonates. However, the mortality rates in NICU patients needing CVVH are higher (up to 75%) compared to older patients in the pediatric ICU (about 40%). At the present time, commercially available hemofiltration systems are not designed for neonates. The circuits require that >10% of the infant's blood volume is extracorporeal. Thus, infants on CVVH/CVVHDF will generally require priming of the circuit with blood products to reduce the risk of developing hypotension.

EXERCISE 12

QUESTION

1. Which of the following vascular accesses is the preferred route for initiating CVVHDF in the neonate?
   a. Two 5F umbilical artery and venous catheters (UAC/UVC)
   b. Femoral double lumen 7F catheter
   c. Internal jugular double lumen 7F catheter
   d. Subclavian double lumen 7F catheter

ANSWER

1. **b or c.** Vascular access is often the major limiting factor when performing CVVH or CVVHDF in neonates, especially in the setting of anasarca (Bunchman et al., 2008; Goldstein, 2011). Vascular resistance is inversely proportional to the fourth power of the radius of the catheter; thus, the smallest catheters will have the highest resistance to blood flow. The shortest, widest catheter that can be placed is desirable. Smaller catheters and the small size of neonates may limit blood flow rates, increasing the risk of clotting the circuit. While using 5F catheters for CVVH in the umbilical artery and vein has been reported, it is often unsuccessful, and many clinicians advocate for double lumen 7F catheters as the better alternative.

Whenever placing a central line in a neonate with renal failure, one should always consider the future possibility of chronic renal failure requiring arteriovenous fistulas (AVF) for hemodialysis or kidney transplant. Thus, an internal jugular catheter is preferred, as subclavian catheters may result in venous stenosis that will preclude AVF placement on the arm. Femoral catheters are not ideal because of higher risk of catheter malfunction from kinking or increased resistance secondary to increased intraabdominal pressure. Femoral catheters may also lead to vascular stenosis that may limit the ability to attach a future transplanted kidney to those vessels. However, in neonates, internal jugular access may not be feasible and it is not uncommon to use femoral access. In small neonates, two single lumen femoral catheters have been used if the placement of a double lumen 7F catheter is not possible.

CASE STUDY 3 (continued)

The severe anasarca precluded placement of a vascular access catheter. A PD catheter was placed and acute PD was initiated with 35 cc exchange volumes and 40-minute dwell time. Ultrafiltration was successful and the infant became less edematous and was more alert. She was weaned off ventilator support. She remained oliguric and a permanent PD catheter was placed. She was started on Similac PM 60/40 for feeds. However, after a few days, the PD became less effective (less ultrafiltrate was observed) and the infant developed worsening edema.

EXERCISE 13

QUESTION

1. The next intervention is to:
   a. Increase the dextrose concentration in the PD fluid
   b. Decrease the dextrose concentration in the PD fluid
   c. Give a dose of furosemide

ANSWER

1. **a.** The dextrose concentration in the dialysate drives the osmotic gradient to enable ultrafiltration and fluid removal, so the recommended step would be to increase the dextrose concentration. Decreasing the dextrose concentration will decrease the osmotic gradient, leading to less ultrafiltration. However, dextrose concentrations higher than 1.5% in the dialysate should only be used for a short period of time, as a high concentration (e.g., 4.25% dextrose-containing PD solutions) can lead to peritoneal membrane damage, resulting in dialysis failure. In oliguric and anuric infants with severe ATN, additional furosemide is unlikely to result in sufficient fluid removal.

CASE STUDY 3 (continued)

After raising the dextrose concentration to 4.25% in the dialysate, fluid removal was increased and the patient became less edematous over the next few days.

EXERCISE 14

QUESTION

1. What is the best study of the options below to assess the likelihood of this infant recovering renal function?
   a. Serum creatinine
   b. Renal ultrasound
   c. Doppler ultrasound of renal arteries

ANSWER

1. **c.** Recovery from acute tubular necrosis can take weeks to months. Severe ischemic injury can also result in cortical necrosis and poor renal perfusion, which may be identified by examination of renal arterial blood flow by Doppler ultrasound. Increased echogenicity on renal ultrasound may be present in both reversible and irreversible renal failure and cannot alone be used to determine renal prognosis. As creatinine is cleared by PD, changes in creatinine while on PD may not reflect intrinsic renal function. In addition to renal blood flow studies, increased urine output can be a useful indicator of returning renal function for a neonate on dialysis.

CASE STUDY 3 (continued)

A repeat renal ultrasound demonstrated good arterial blood flow to both kidneys. Over the course of the following week, urine output increased to 2 cc/kg/hr and dialysis was discontinued. Serum creatinine gradually decreased to 0.2 mg/dL. After discharge, the patient received follow up in the outpatient nephrology clinic.

SUGGESTED READINGS

Antonucci R, Fanos V: NSAIDs, prostaglandins and the neonatal kidney, *J Matern Fetal Neonatal Med* 22(Suppl 3): 23–26, 2009.

Askenazi DJ, Ambalavanan N, Goldstein SL: Acute kidney injury in critically ill newborns: what do we know? What do we need to learn? *Pediatr Nephrol* 24(2):265–274, 2009.

Askenazi DJ, Koralkar R, Levitan EB, et al.: Baseline values of candidate urine acute kidney injury biomarkers vary by gestational age in premature infants, *Pediatr Res* 70: 302–306, 2011.

Bomelburg T, Jorch G: Abnormal blood flow patterns in renal arteries of small preterm infants with patent ductus arteriosus detected by Doppler ultrasonography, *Eur J Pediatr* 148:660–664, 1989.

Bunchman TE, Brophy PD, Goldstein SL: Technical considerations for renal replacement therapy in children, *Semin Nephrol* 28(5):488–492, 2008.

Calcagno PL, Rubin MI, Weintraub DH: Studies on the renal concentrating and diluting mechanisms in the premature infant, *J Clin Invest* 33:91–96, 1954.

Carmody JB, Charlton JR: Short-term gestation, long-term risk: prematurity and chronic kidney disease, *Pediatrics* 131:1168–1179, 2013.

Clark DA: Times of first void and first stool in 500 newborns, *Pediatrics* 60:457–459, 1977.

Fortenberry JD, Paden ML, Goldstein SL: Acute kidney injury in children: an update on diagnosis and treatment, *Pediatr Clin North Am* 60(3):669–688, 2013.

Goldstein SL: Advances in pediatric renal replacement therapy for acute kidney injury, *Semin Dial* 24(2):187–191, 2011.

Hamrick SE, Hansmann G: Patent ductus arteriosus of the preterm infant, *Pediatrics* 125:1020–1030, 2010.

Hoy WE, Hughson MD, Bertram JF, Douglas-Denton R, Amann K: Nephron number, hypertension, renal disease, and renal failure, *J Am Soc Nephrol* 16:2557–2564, 2005.

Hughson M, Farris III AB, Douglas-Denton R, Hoy WE, Bertram JF: Glomerular number and size in autopsy kidneys: the relationship to birth weight, *Kidney Int* 63: 2113–2122, 2003.

Koralkar R, Ambalavanan N, Levitan EB, McGwin G, Goldstein S, Askenazi D: Acute kidney injury reduces survival in very low birth weight infants, *Pediatr Res* 69:354–358, 2011.

Lopez-Novoa JM, Quiros Y, Vicente L, Morales AI, Lopez-Hernandez FJ: New insights into the mechanism of aminoglycoside nephrotoxicity: an integrative point of view, *Kidney Int* 79:33–45, 2011.

Moghal NE, Embleton ND: Management of acute renal failure in the newborn, *Semin Fetal Neonatal Med* 11(3):207–213, 2006.

North American Pediatric Renal Trials and Collaborative Studies (NAPRTCS): *2011 annual report*. https://web.emmes.com/study/ped/annlrept/annlrept.html.

Ohlsson A, Walia R, Shah S: Ibuprofen for the treatment of patent ductus arteriosus in preterm and/or low birth weight infants, *Cochrane Database Syst Rev* (1):CD003481, 2008.

Quigley R: Developmental changes in renal function, *Curr Opin Pediatr* 24:184–190, 2012.

Thayyil S, Sheik S, Kempley ST, Sinha A: A gestation- and postnatal age-based reference chart for assessing renal function in extremely premature infants, *J Perinatol* 28:226–229, 2008.

Vieux R, Hascoet JM, Merdariu D, Fresson J, Guillemin F: Glomerular filtration rate reference values in very preterm infants, *Pediatrics* 125:e1186–e1192, 2010.

Zaritsky J, Warady BA: Peritoneal dialysis in infants and young children, *Semin Nephrol* 31(2):213–224, 2011.

CHAPTER 19

NEONATAL SEIZURES

Renée A. Shellhaas, MD, MS

Neonatal seizures affect 1.5 to 3.5 per 1000 live term infants and are distinct from seizures in older children and adults. Most often, neonates have acute symptomatic seizures—the seizures reflect underlying acute or subacute cerebral dysfunction, rather than an epilepsy syndrome. Also, unlike seizures in older patients, neonatal seizures are usually subclinical. In this chapter, we will review the differential diagnosis of abnormal paroxysmal events in neonates (many of which are not seizures), causes of neonatal seizures, typical seizure semiologies, diagnostic testing, and treatment for electrographically confirmed seizures.

ESSENTIAL FEATURES OF THE HISTORY AND PHYSICAL EXAMINATION FOR NEONATES WITH SUSPECTED SEIZURES

History

It is important with any critically ill neonate that the history encompass the antepartum period, labor, and delivery. The mother's health history (hypertension, diabetes, need for medications of any kind, substance use and abuse, trauma, infections), mother's gravity and parity, as well as history of fetal demise or stillbirths must all be ascertained. Prenatal care and antepartum fetal testing are important to ascertain, because they can provide clues regarding timing of a potential injury to the fetus/neonate. Pertinent issues in the peripartum period include risk factors for neonatal sepsis (e.g., maternal fever, prolonged rupture of membranes, group B *Streptococcus* [GBS] colonization), abnormal progression of labor, use of medications that could influence neonatal behavior (e.g., magnesium or narcotics), meconium staining of amniotic fluid, and mode of delivery (precipitous delivery, requirement for operative vaginal delivery or cesarean section). Postnatal considerations include initial assessments of the infant (e.g., Apgar scores, need for and duration of resuscitation) and the subsequent clinical course.

Timing of Seizure Onset

It can be helpful to organize and prioritize the diagnostic considerations according to the timing of seizure onset (Table 19-1), although this method is not perfect because many conditions can overlap specified time periods. Physical examination for an infant with suspected neurologic disease must include both a detailed general examination and a thorough neurologic examination. Pertinent elements of the general examination include:

- Vital signs
- Growth parameters (especially noting head size in relation to body size)
- Assessment of the anterior fontanel (a bulging fontanel or splayed sutures suggest increased intracranial pressure)
- Dysmorphic features
- Heart murmurs (congenital heart disease is a major risk factor for perinatal stroke)
- Skin lesions (e.g., rashes to suggest infection, or features of neurocutaneous diseases like tuberous sclerosis or hypomelanosis of Ito)
- Genitourinary examination (certain genetic epilepsy syndromes have associated genital anomalies)
- Joint contractures (suggesting long-standing restriction of movements *in utero*)

The neurologic examination must include assessments of each of the following:

- Mental status (awake, alert, lethargic, irritable, stupor, coma)
- Cranial nerve functioning (pupils, corneal reflexes, extraocular movements, facial expressions, response to loud sounds, tongue movements, palate elevation, suck, swallow, phonation)
- Motor function (muscle bulk, tone, and strength, including power and symmetry of movements)
- Sensation (e.g., facial sensation is intact to light touch if touching the cheek precipitates a rooting reflex)
- Primitive reflexes (Moro, suck, grasp, root, etc.)
- Deep tendon reflexes

TABLE 19-1 **Neonatal Seizure Etiologies, Classified According to Typical Time of Seizure Onset***

Peak Time of Seizure Onset	Common Neonatal Seizure Etiologies
Within 24 hours of birth	Hypoxic ischemic encephalopathy Bacterial meningitis Sepsis TORCH** infections Direct effects of maternal drugs (e.g., cocaine) Transient metabolic disturbances (e.g., hypoglycemia, hypocalcemia) Intracranial hemorrhage Cerebral dysgenesis Pyridoxine dependent epilepsy
24 to 72 hours	Meningoencephalitis Drug withdrawal (neonatal abstinence syndrome) Intraventricular hemorrhage (mainly preterm infants) Nonketotic hyperglycinemia Sepsis Urea cycle disorders Perinatal arterial ischemic stroke Cerebral venous sinus thrombosis
72+ hours	Inborn errors of metabolism Sepsis Herpes simplex virus encephalitis Kernicterus

*Note that many of these etiologies may present across several of these arbitrary time cut-offs.
**"TORCH" infections include toxoplasmosis, rubella, cytomegalovirus, and herpes simplex virus.

TABLE 19-2 **Clinical Appearances of Neonatal Seizures and Other Episodic Neonatal Behaviors**

Seizures	Subtle Seizures*	Non-Seizure Events
Focal clonic jerking**	Apnea (most often with associated eye deviation or other signs)	Benign neonatal myoclonus (events occurring only during sleep)
Multifocal clonic jerking	Sucking, chewing	Jitteriness
Focal tonic events	Swimming, bicycling	Non-seizure apnea
Myoclonus	Isolated tonic eye deviation	Clonus
Rarely infantile spasms	Isolated episodic elevated heart rate or blood pressure (unusual)	Opisthotonos or other types of posturing

*The signs listed under this heading are sometimes manifestations of seizures, but are often nonictal paroxysmal events.
**Focal clonic jerking is the most reliable clinical manifestation of neonatal seizures. Note that *neonates virtually never have generalized convulsions.*

DIFFERENTIAL DIAGNOSIS OF ABNORMAL PAROXYSMAL EVENTS IN NEONATES

Seizures in newborn infants can be the first sign of serious neurologic disease or systemic illness. It is of critical importance to understand the semiologies that are most—and least—likely to represent neonatal seizures (Table 19-2). Abnormal paroxysmal events in a neonate should prompt an emergent evaluation with immediate treatment of the underlying cause (if possible). However, many paroxysmal events are not, in fact, seizures. Since the diagnostic evaluation of neonatal seizures is often invasive, and anticonvulsant medications can have significant side effects, awareness of common non-seizure semiologies and etiologies of paroxysmal movements is critical.

CASE STUDY 1

A 3500-gram male infant was delivered at 39 weeks estimated gestational age to a 28-year-old primigravida mother, after a pregnancy complicated only by maternal group B streptococcal colonization. His mother received adequate antibiotic prophylaxis during labor. The infant was delivered vaginally and appeared healthy, with a normal physical examination and Apgar scores of 9 at both 1 and 5 minutes of life. He was cared for in the well-baby nursery and discharged to home with his mother after 36 hours.

One week later, he developed unusual episodes characterized by brief, sudden, jerking movements of his arms and legs. These occurred in clusters lasting between 1 and 5 minutes while he was sleeping. Between events, he seemed healthy. He was breastfeeding every 3 hours and appeared well hydrated.

At his pediatrician's office, the baby was well-appearing and weighed 3600 grams. His head circumference was 35.5 cm and his vital signs were normal. While he was sleeping in his mother's arms, he suddenly developed a series of arrhythmic jerking movements of his left arm, followed by the left leg and then the right arm. The pediatrician lifted him to the examination table and undressed him. The infant cried and the movements stopped.

CASE STUDY 2

A 3500-gram male infant was delivered at 39 weeks' estimated gestational age to a 28-year-old gravida 4, para 1 (three spontaneous first trimester abortions) mother, after an uncomplicated pregnancy. He was delivered vaginally and appeared well, with a normal physical examination and Apgar scores of 9 at both 1 and 5 minutes of life. He was discharged home at 48 hours of life, after receiving routine prenatal care.

At his routine follow up with his pediatrician on Day 6, the infant weighed 3400 grams and appeared sleepy and dehydrated. He was afebrile but tachycardic. His mother expressed feelings of depression and stated that breastfeeding was not going as well as she had hoped. While he was sleeping in his mother's arms, he suddenly developed rhythmic jerking of the left arm, followed by the left leg and then the right arm. The pediatrician lifted him to the examination table and undressed him. The infant did not arouse, but the movements ceased.

DIAGNOSTIC POSSIBILITIES FOR UNUSUAL PAROXYSMAL EVENTS IN NEONATES

EXERCISE 1

QUESTION

1. Consider the two infants in Case Studies 1 and 2. For each newborn, decide whether you think the infant has seizures and make a differential

diagnosis list and select the most likely diagnosis and the most important diagnosis (i.e., the one you can't afford to miss).

ANSWER

1. The histories for cases 1 and 2 are quite similar, yet the etiologies of the two infants' paroxysmal events are entirely different. Case 1 is that of a healthy-appearing neonate whose only risk factor is his mother's group B *Streptococcus* colonization (which was adequately treated). The key piece of history is that the events occurred during sleep and ceased once the infant was awoken. In the context of a completely healthy infant, the history of myoclonic jerks that only occur during sleep is sufficient for a diagnosis of benign neonatal sleep myoclonus.

Classic teaching is that movements caused by seizures are not suppressed by gentle restraint of the affected limb, whereas non-seizure movements are easily extinguished. For example, a newborn that is simply jittery, such as an infant with neonatal abstinence syndrome, will have prominent low-amplitude and high-frequency limb movements and an exaggerated Moro reflex. The jittery movements are magnified by internal and external stimuli, but are calmed by gentle restraint. Contrary to this classic teaching, the movements of benign neonatal sleep myoclonus frequently continue despite restraint of the limb. Waking the infant, and observing the cessation of myoclonic movements is the key feature of both the history and examination.

If the diagnosis is in question then a full evaluation is warranted. Scenarios in which a diagnosis of benign neonatal sleep myoclonus ought to be questioned include an ill-appearing infant, abnormal vital signs, abnormal mental status or focal neurologic abnormalities on physical examination, risk factors for infection (such as maternal group B streptococcal infection), etc. Seizures can occur during both wakefulness and sleep, another key diagnostic distinction.

The neonate in Case Study 2 was ill-appearing, lethargic, and dehydrated. His mother also reported poor feeding. In this case, the pediatrician should have high suspicion that the episode of multifocal clonic jerking was a neonatal seizure. As in most neonates with seizures, the seizures are symptomatic of underlying cerebral dysfunction. Appropriate treatment will rely on rapid identification of the etiology and correction of any reversible process. The infant in Case Study 2 was dehydrated and lethargic, which raises numerous diagnostic possibilities,

TABLE 19-3 Etiologies of Neonatal Seizures*

Infectious	Metabolic	Cerebrovascular	Congenital Brain Malformations	Genetic/Syndromic Epilepsies
Meningitis (bacterial) Encephalitis (viral) Central nervous system "TORCH" infections**	Hypoglycemia Hypocalcemia Hypernatremia or hyponatremia Inborn errors of metabolism Hypoxic-ischemic encephalopathy	Intraventricular hemorrhage Intraparenchymal hemorrhage Subdural hematoma Subarachnoid hemorrhage Arterial ischemic stroke Cerebral sinovenous thrombosis	Multiple types, including: • Malformations of cortical development (e.g., lissencephaly, focal cortical dysplasia) • Disorders of prosencephalic development (e.g., holoprosencephaly)	Benign familial neonatal convulsions Pyridoxine dependent epilepsy Early myoclonic epilepsy of infancy Ohtahara syndrome

*There are many other etiologies of neonatal seizures. This list is not meant to be exhaustive. Rather, it is intended to provide an overview of the scope of diagnoses that underlie neonatal seizures.
**"TORCH" infections include toxoplasmosis, rubella, cytomegalovirus, and herpes simplex virus.

including electrolyte abnormalities, hypoglycemia, infection, inborn errors of metabolism, cerebrovascular abnormalities, etc. A list of diagnostic considerations is presented in Table 19-3. For this infant, neuroimaging revealed a venous sinus thrombosis—perhaps related to an inherited thrombophilia given his mother's history of multiple miscarriages—and the events were confirmed to be multifocal seizures.

DIAGNOSTIC TESTING FOR SUSPECTED NEONATAL SEIZURES

A critical distinction between neonatal seizures and seizures among older children is that *most neonatal seizures are subclinical*—they have no externally apparent manifestations. This phenomenon is well described by many research teams; most report that 50% to 80% of electrographically confirmed neonatal seizures are subclinical. It should not be surprising that most neonatal seizures have no clinically apparent sign. After all, a preverbal infant cannot describe an unusual visual phenomenon arising from an occipital seizure or a sense of déjà vu caused by a temporal lobe seizure.

Although most neonatal seizures are subclinical and can only be diagnosed accurately by electroencephalography (EEG), *most abnormal neonatal movements are not seizures*. Even the most experienced clinicians often misdiagnose unusual paroxysmal events as seizures.

Both healthy and sick neonates have many and varied unusual movements, which most often have no EEG correlate and thus are not seizures. This does not mean these events are normal. Indeed, opisthotonic posturing is an ominous sign. However, because they are not seizures, such events should not be treated with anticonvulsant medication. Accurate diagnosis of neonatal seizures and non-seizure events is critical, both to ensure adequate treatment for infants with seizures and to avoid administering anticonvulsants to those whose events are not seizures.

The diagnosis of neonatal seizures is made based on clinical findings and EEG. When seizures are suspected, multiple facets of evaluation and treatment must occur simultaneously: (1) accurate diagnosis of the events of concern (e.g., seizure versus nonepileptic paroxysmal event), which is most accurately characterized by EEG; (2) determination of the etiology of the events of concern (e.g., sepsis, electrolyte abnormalities, acquired or congenital brain abnormalities); and (3) empiric treatment of the most likely etiologies (e.g., antibiotics, adequate hydration). Here, we discuss characterization of the events of concern first, but in clinical practice additional diagnostic evaluation and treatment occur in tandem.

CASE STUDY 3

A 35-week gestational age infant was delivered via caesarian section to a 25-year-old primigravida mother whose labor was complicated by fever and severe abdominal pain. The infant was lethargic, with frequent apneic episodes, and a single epi-sode of focal tonic stiffening of the left arm. Placen-tal pathology confirmed chorioamnionitis.

CASE STUDY 4

A 40-week gestational age infant was transferred from a referring hospital for evaluation of intraven-tricular hemorrhage. He has depressed mental sta-tus and is intubated and sedated. A brain magnetic resonance imaging (MRI) is scheduled in 2 hours.

CASE STUDY 5

A 39-week gestational age infant was delivered to a 30-year-old multiparous mother who admits to polysubstance abuse during the pregnancy. The infant is now 2 days old and she is jittery and has frequent episodes of full body stiffening and crying. Blood and cerebrospinal fluid cultures are negative.

EXERCISE 2

QUESTIONS

Options for diagnosis of neonatal seizures include bedside (clinical) observation, routine-length electroencephalography (EEG), conventional video-EEG monitoring, and amplitude-integrated EEG. For each of the following cases, decide which electrodiagnostic test is indicated.
1. Case Study 3
2. Case Study 4
3. Case Study 5

ANSWERS

1. The infant in Case Study 3 is at very high risk for sepsis and meningitis, which raises concern for acute symptomatic seizures. The episodes of apnea could be ictal, or could be unrelated to seizures. The episode of tonic stiffening of the left arm is likely a focal seizure. The depressed mental status may be accentuated by subtle or subclinical seizures. The best, most appropriate testing for this neonate is conventional video-EEG monitoring. If no seizures are recorded, and the EEG background remains stable, then monitoring can be discontinued after 24 hours. If seizures are identified on the EEG, then moni-toring should continue until the infant remains seizure-free for 24 hours.

2. The neonate in Case Study 4 is at high risk for seizures, due to the intracranial hemorrhage. He has depressed mental status, which raises con-cern for subclinical status epilepticus. However, he will need to be transported to MRI in 2 hours

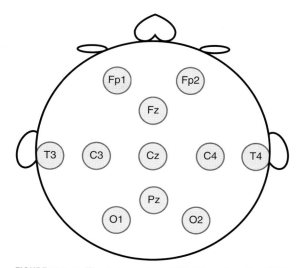

FIGURE 19-1 ■ **The international 10-20 system for EEG electrode placement, modified for neonates.** EEG electrodes are placed in the positions indicated. By convention, odd numbers indicate the left side of the head, even numbers the right, and "z" indicates the midline. In addition, a respiratory channel and single-channel electrocardiogram are required for accurate interpretation of the study. Time-locked video is usu-ally recorded, and extraoculogram and electromyog-raphy channels are often useful.

and cannot have EEG leads in place during the MRI scan, because the leads contain metal. In this case, using amplitude-integrated EEG to screen for status epilepticus before he is transported to MRI is a reasonable option. Conventional EEG monitoring can begin after the MRI.

3. The infant in Case Study 5 likely has neonatal abstinence syndrome. Although this raises the risk for neonatal seizures, the events of con-cern are not focal, which lessens the chances that they represent seizures. The episodes are occurring very frequently, so they are likely to be captured during a routine-length neonatal EEG. If several (three or four) typical events are recorded and are not seizures, and the EEG background is normal or nearly normal, then a routine EEG may be adequate for this infant.

Conventional EEG monitoring is the gold standard for the diagnosis and quantification of neonatal seizures. Electrodes are placed accord-ing to the International 10-20 system, modified for neonates (Figure 19-1), with extracerebral leads including a respiratory channel and elec-trocardiogram. These extracerebral channels are crucial for assessment of behavioral state and identification of extracerebral artifacts. Extra-oculogram and surface electromyography leads are often helpful, but are not always required.

BOX 19-1   **Indications for Neonatal EEG Monitoring**

1. Evaluation of abnormal paroxysmal events
   - Focal clonic, focal tonic, or multifocal clonic events*
   - Intermittent, isolated, forced eye deviation
   - Myoclonus
   - Unexplained paroxysmal autonomic abnormalities (e.g., paroxysmal tachycardia or hypertension)
   - Brainstem-release phenomena (e.g., oral automatisms or bicycling movements)
   - Other stereotyped abnormal movements
2. Surveillance for subclinical seizures
   - Initial diagnosis
   - Assessment of treatment response to anticonvulsant medications**
   - Evaluation for seizure recurrence during or after weaning of anticonvulsant medications
3. Assessment of EEG background abnormalities
   - Provide supporting evidence for estimation of prognosis
   - Amplitude-integrated EEG is well-suited for this purpose
   - Serial routine-length conventional EEGs may also be adequate for this purpose

*These are the most reliable seizure semiologies in neonates.
**More than 50% of neonates with clinically apparent seizures will have electroclinical dissociation (clinical signs vanish while electrographic seizures continue) after phenobarbital or phenytoin are administered.

BOX 19-2   **Sample High-Risk Clinical Circumstances That Should Prompt Consideration of Neonatal EEG Monitoring**

- Acute neonatal encephalopathy
  - Encephalopathy following suspected perinatal asphyxia
  - Encephalopathy after cardiopulmonary resuscitation
- Risk for acute brain injury *combined with* clinical encephalopathy
  - Severe pulmonary disease, such as severe persistent pulmonary hypertension
  - Extracorporeal membrane oxygenation (ECMO)
  - Complex congenital heart defects requiring early surgery
- Central nervous system infection
  - Meningoencephalitis
  - Infants at high risk for central nervous system infection (for example, encephalopathy in the context of chorioamnionitis, or maternal herpes simplex virus colonization)
- Intracranial hemorrhage *combined with* clinical encephalopathy
  - Subarachnoid, subdural, or intraventricular hemorrhage
  - Clinical suspicion for acquired brain injury
- Inborn errors of metabolism (suspected or confirmed)
- Perinatal stroke (suspected or confirmed)
- Sinovenous thrombosis (suspected or confirmed)
- Genetic or syndromic disorders involving the brain
  - Cerebral dysgenesis
  - Dysmorphic features with associated microcephaly

Time-locked video recording is strongly recommended, both for the differential diagnosis of paroxysmal clinical events and to assist in distinguishing artifacts (e.g., chest physical therapy can create rhythmic EEG artifacts that can be mistaken for a seizure if no video is available). A bedside observer is also key. This individual should alert the EEG reviewer to clinically important events (e.g., paroxysmal episodes or administration of neuroactive medications) by pressing a patient event marker and/or documenting on a bedside flow sheet.

Indications for neonatal EEG monitoring are outlined in Box 19-1. EEG monitoring is resource-intensive and requires specialized equipment and available staff for implementation and interpretation. Not every sick neonate can or should be monitored. Instead, this technology should be reserved for those at highest risk for seizures. Examples of scenarios in which EEG monitoring ought to be considered are presented in Box 19-2. Note that one theme among these scenarios is that of an infant with risk factors for central nervous system dysfunction who *also has encephalopathy* (e.g., an infant who is well-appearing and whose mother had group B streptococcal colonization likely does not need EEG monitoring, but if the infant develops abnormal mental status, then EEG monitoring to evaluate for subtle or subclinical seizures would be reasonable).

The most appropriate duration of EEG recording depends on the indication for testing.

TABLE 19-4 Guidelines for EEG Monitoring Duration

Indication for EEG Monitoring	Suggested Duration of EEG Monitoring
Evaluate for electrographic seizures	24 hours*
Monitoring after confirmation of electrographic seizures	Until the neonate has been seizure-free for 24 hours**
Differential diagnosis of paroxysmal events	Until 3 to 4 typical events have been recorded and determined not to be seizures
Characterization of the EEG background	Serial routine-length (60-minute) EEGs are typically appropriate for this indication

*After 24 hours, if there have been no seizures and the EEG background is stable, then monitoring can usually be discontinued.
**Unless, in consultation with a neurologist, a decision is made to stop EEG monitoring sooner (for example, in an infant with cerebral dysgenesis who is not expected to become completely seizure-free).

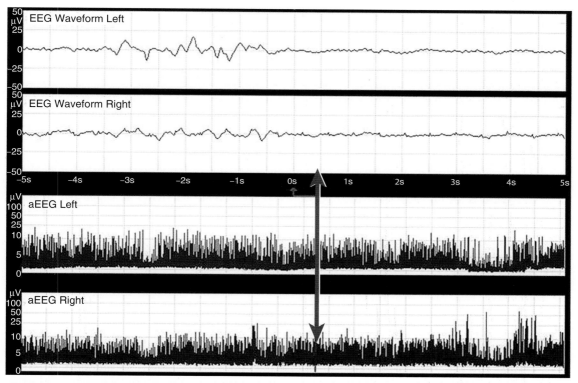

FIGURE 19-2 ■ **Dual channel amplitude-integrated EEG (aEEG) recorded from a full-term infant.** The top two panels display 10 seconds of "raw" EEG, whereas the bottom two panels display 3 hours of aEEG. The *arrow* indicates the point on the aEEG that corresponds to the raw EEG panels.

In general, a *routine-length neonatal EEG is insufficient to screen for seizures*. A normal—or nearly normal—EEG background does not preclude a diagnosis of seizures and so should not dissuade a clinician from ordering EEG monitoring for an infant in whom there is significant concern for seizures. Suggested guidelines for EEG duration are presented in Table 19-4.

Because access to conventional EEG monitoring can be limited, particularly on weekends and in the evenings, many neonatologists employ amplitude-integrated EEG (aEEG) for evaluation of the electrographic background and to screen for seizures. aEEG utilizes filters to reduce high (>15 Hz) and low (<2 Hz) frequencies, and also rectifies and smooths the EEG signal and displays the tracing on a semi-logarithmic display at 6 cm/hour (Figure 19-2). aEEG can be recorded independently from—or in parallel with—conventional EEG. If a single channel aEEG is to be recorded in isolation, biparietal electrode positions are recommended because these overly the cerebrovascular watershed zones. Most modern aEEG equipment displays dual channel tracings, recorded from left and right central and parietal electrodes.

In some neonatal intensive care units (NICUs), aEEG and conventional EEG are recorded simultaneously. Most often, this is accomplished by displaying the digital aEEG trend on the bedside monitor for review by the primary clinical team, while the full conventional EEG is recorded and interpreted off-line by a clinical neurophysiologist. This approach allows NICU staff to identify concerning patterns in the aEEG background and contact the clinical neurophysiologist for confirmation of the findings.

aEEG can provide prognostically significant data regarding the electrographic background. Because the tracing is displayed on a markedly compressed time scale, the reviewer can assess multiple hours of recording on a single screen. aEEG has been studied in numerous clinical scenarios, including hypoxic ischemic encephalopathy (HIE), prematurity, and sepsis. Major advantages of aEEG, compared with conventional EEG monitoring, include its relatively simple implementation at the bedside and the lack of requirement for an immediately available, experienced clinical neurophysiologist. However, there is an important learning curve and a rigorous program for continuous quality improvement is strongly recommended. Ideally, aEEG should be considered a tool that complements, but does not replace, conventional EEG monitoring (Glass, 2013).

aEEG background is interpreted according to one of two classification systems: a simple system based on the amplitude of the upper and lower margins of the aEEG band (al Naqeeb, 1999); or a complex system of pattern recognition that adapts terminology from conventional EEG interpretation (Hellström-Westas, 2006). Although there is better interindividual reliability using the simple system, the complex system offers richer texture in aEEG interpretation.

Although aEEG is certainly useful for electrographic background interpretation and assessment of the evolution of background patterns over extended time periods, its use for seizure detection is controversial. Neonatal seizures are, by nature, brief and spatially restricted. More than half of neonatal seizures last less than 90 seconds, which translates to approximately 1.4 mm on a typical aEEG screen display. Although using dual (vs. single) aEEG channels and concurrent display of the corresponding "raw" EEG improves seizure detection, novices are less likely than experts to detect seizures on aEEG. A dual

channel aEEG recording that captured several prolonged seizures is displayed in Figure 19-3.

Most studies report relatively good specificity, but the sensitivity of aEEG for seizure detection is quite low. Some studies discuss the sensitivity of aEEG for detecting *seizure positive records* (i.e., at least one seizure is detected in an aEEG tracing known to contain seizures), whereas others report the sensitivity and specificity for detection of *individual seizures*. Single-channel aEEG, without the corresponding raw EEG, has about 25% to 50% sensitivity for detecting *seizure positive aEEG records* and about 25% to 40% sensitivity for *individual seizure* detection. Adding a second aEEG channel, along with the raw EEG traces, improves sensitivity to about 75% for expert aEEG reviewers. Because of the limited sensitivity for seizure detection, aEEG is not a substitute for conventional EEG monitoring for the purpose of seizure detection, although it is likely better than no electroencephalographic monitoring at all. The high specificity is reassuring, because this implies that few infants are likely to be treated with anticonvulsant medications based on aEEG monitoring when they do not, in fact, have seizures.

aEEG is best used when conventional EEG is not available or is not practical or feasible. When seizures are suspected on aEEG, corroboration with conventional EEG is suggested in order to confirm the diagnosis and guide treatment decisions.

ADDITIONAL DIAGNOSTIC EVALUATION

For any infant in whom a diagnosis of neonatal seizures is being considered, a full sepsis evaluation is strongly recommended (to include cultures of blood, urine, and cerebrospinal fluid) and antibiotics should be administered until the cultures are proved to be negative. Electrolyte and glucose levels should also be measured emergently, and corrected if abnormal. However, anticonvulsant medications are not always immediately mandatory. If the episodes in question are not clinically felt to be definite seizures, then antiseizure treatment can sometimes be deferred until a definitive diagnosis is made (sepsis evaluation should not be postponed, however).

Diagnostic testing for neonates with confirmed or suspected seizures must be tailored to the individual clinical scenario. Most often, the seizures are a symptom of an underlying problem rather than a sign of a neonatal epilepsy syndrome. The most appropriate laboratory testing and neuroimaging, as well as the treatment and

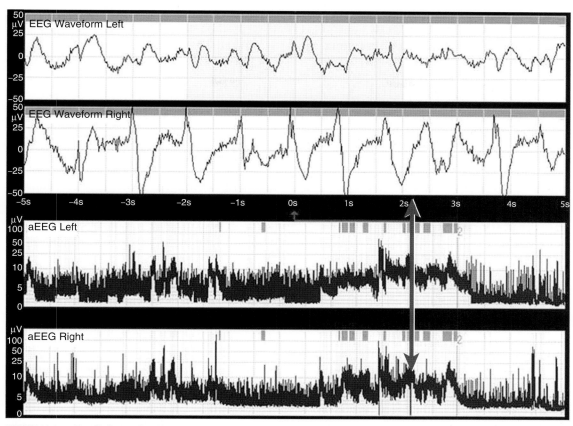

FIGURE 19-3 ■ **Dual channel amplitude-integrated EEG (aEEG) recorded from a 39-week gestational age infant with hypoxic-ischemic encephalopathy.** The top two panels are 10 seconds of "raw" EEG, whereas the bottom two panels are 3 hours of the left and right aEEG. The *arrow* indicates the portion of the aEEG traces corresponding to the raw EEG display. There is a seizure in the right hemisphere.

prognosis of neonates with seizures, depend on the clinical scenario.

Virtually always, infection should be suspected as the underlying etiology of neonatal seizures. Therefore, blood cultures and a complete blood count and differential are required. Unless the infant is too medically unstable, a lumbar puncture is also necessary to assess the cerebrospinal fluid for bacterial culture, cells, protein, and glucose. If a lumbar puncture is not feasible, then the infant should be treated presumptively for bacterial meningitis. In the proper clinical circumstances, the infant should also be treated for presumed herpes simplex virus (HSV) encephalitis, and an HSV PCR should be sent from the cerebrospinal fluid. Serum electrolytes and glucose levels should be evaluated, in order to identify easily reversible causes of seizures, such as hypoglycemia. Serum liver and kidney function tests should be assessed, because they can provide hints at the underlying diagnosis and may influence treatment decisions (e.g., one might choose to avoid high-dose phenobarbital if the infant has significant hepatic dysfunction).

If the etiology of the seizures is not immediately obvious, after the above basic laboratory evaluation is complete, then testing for metabolic disorders is warranted (e.g., lactate, pyruvate, ammonia, plasma amino acids, urine organic acids, and sometimes cerebrospinal fluid for neurotransmitters, lactate, and amino acids). Genetic testing should be considered in some circumstances (e.g., chromosomal microarray in the case of dysmorphic features and comorbid seizures, or specific gene testing in the case of particular malformations of cortical development or constellations of congenital anomalies).

In most emergency departments and NICUs, it is fairly easy and quick to obtain a cranial ultrasound at the infant's bedside. Although ultrasound cannot provide detailed brain imaging, it can be used to assess for obvious hemorrhage or hydrocephalus. Generally, computed tomography (CT) of the head is not undertaken in newborns because of concerns about radiation. Instead, MRI is the preferred neuroimaging test for neonates with seizures. Diffusion-weighted imaging can be particularly informative during the first days after an acquired brain injury, but if the MRI must be deferred one must avoid imaging during the phase of pseudonormalization (the timing of which will vary, depending on the injury and the use of therapeutic hypothermia, but is typically 6 to 8 days for normothermic and 11 to 12 days for cooled infants). MRI is also essential to delineate the extent of congenital brain malformations. MR venography can be employed to assess for cerebral venous sinus thrombosis, whereas MR angiography can be helpful in cases of arterial ischemic stroke.

TREATMENT OF NEONATAL SEIZURES

CASE STUDY 6

A 38-week gestational age female, weighing 3000 grams, has confirmed bacterial meningitis. Your clinical team monitors her with conventional video EEG, because of her high-risk clinical scenario and concurrent depressed mental status. The EEG confirms the presence of subclinical focal seizures arising from multiple locations.

EXERCISE 3

QUESTION

1. Consider the following case. Outline your treatment algorithm for the neonate with confirmed electrographic seizures. What is your first-line agent? What will you prescribe if your first treatment does not control the seizures?

ANSWER

1. Phenobarbital is generally the first-line anticonvulsant medication. If this is not effective, then follow the algorithm outlined in Figure 19-4.

By definition, a neonatal seizure is a discrete electrographic event that is distinct from the EEG background, evolves in location, morphology, and/or frequency, and *lasts at least 10 seconds* (Figures 19-5 and 19-6). An electroclinical seizure is an electrographic seizure that has corresponding clinical signs (but clinical signs are not required for an electrographic event to be classified as a seizure). Episodes that have no associated correlate on EEG should not be considered seizures. Rather, these are paroxysmal non-seizure events.

Individual neonatal seizures are rarely prolonged. Most neonatal seizures last less than 90 seconds. Therefore, neonatal status epilepticus

is defined as the presence of electrographic seizures during at least 50% of a 1-hour EEG epoch. Historically, there has been some debate regarding the clinical importance of neonatal seizures. In animal models, there is evidence that neonatal seizures accentuate underlying brain injury, with long-term adverse consequences. Seizures are a risk factor for unfavorable outcomes in human neonates with HIE, and higher seizure burden is associated with worse outcomes in several clinical scenarios. Neonatal seizures are also a risk factor for pharmacoresistance among older children who develop epilepsy. Therefore, contemporary clinical practice generally dictates that neonatal seizures be treated with anticonvulsant medications. In the past, many clinicians treated only clinically apparent seizures, however current recommendations are that seizure diagnosis and treatment be made on the basis of EEG findings (i.e., electrographic seizures should be treated).

There is little scientific evidence to guide the treatment of neonatal seizures. A single randomized controlled trial demonstrated that phenobarbital and phenytoin have equally incomplete efficacy, providing complete seizure control in only about 45% of neonates with electrographic seizures (Painter et al., 1999). Despite this disappointing result, phenobarbital remains the first-line treatment for neonatal seizures. Typically, the infant is given a bolus loading dose of 20 to 30 mg/kg. The treatment response is assessed and additional loading doses may be administered, depending on side effects and efficacy, before a maintenance dose of 4 to 6 mg/kg/day is initiated.

There is considerable variability in clinical practice for second- and third-line treatment options. A suggested algorithm is outlined in Figure 19-4. Traditionally, fosphenytoin is the most widely accepted second-line agent. Advantages include known efficacy and side-effect profile. Disadvantages include somewhat limited efficacy (about 45% response rate), propensity to induce arrhythmias, and extremely variable intestinal absorption (thus requiring intravenous administration). It is crucial to follow free and total phenytoin levels, because critically ill neonates often have low protein binding and so will have higher than expected free phenytoin levels even when the total level appears modest.

There has been an increasing trend toward treating neonatal seizures with levetiracetam. The potential advantages of levetiracetam include the lack of drug-drug interactions, presumed safety in infants with hepatic dysfunction, and easy oral or intravenous administration.

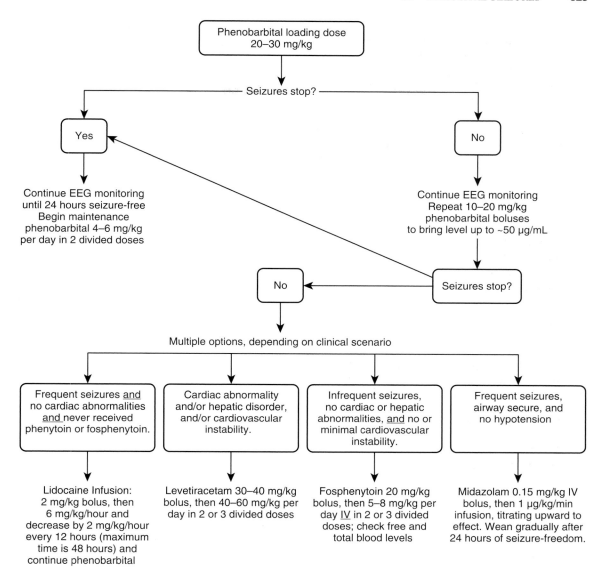

FIGURE 19-4 ■ **Suggested treatment algorithm for neonatal seizures.** For almost all cases, phenobarbital is the first-line treatment. If there is an anticipated delay in obtaining phenobarbital or any of the second- or third-line medications, and the infant is having frequent seizures, a dose of lorazepam (0.05 to 0.1 mg/kg) may be administered in the interim.

To date, however, the appropriate loading and maintenance doses for neonates have not been clarified. Also, importantly, the efficacy of levetiracetam for neonatal seizure treatment is unknown. The doses suggested in Figure 19-4 are derived from the available literature (case series and retrospective reviews) and personal experiences, and should not be considered class 1 (or 2 or 3) evidence. Ongoing clinical trials should provide evidence to guide dosing and delineate efficacy, but those results are not presently available (as of February 2014).

For infants whose seizures have not responded to high doses of phenobarbital, intravenous infusions of midazolam or lidocaine can be considered. Treatment algorithms for both of these medications have been published (outlined in Figure 19-4) and a limited body of evidence supports their use in neonates. Note, however, that because of the risk of arrhythmia, *lidocaine should never be used to treat seizures in a neonate who has received fosphenytoin/phenytoin or who has congenital heart disease.*

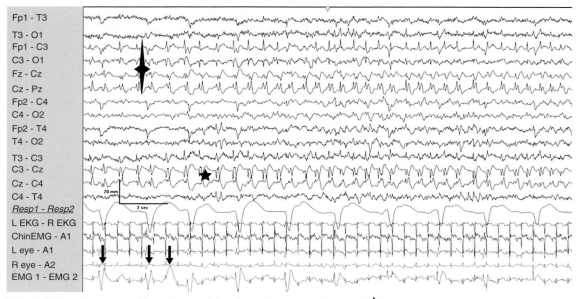

FIGURE 19-5 ■ **Electrographic seizure arising from the central vertex (★), with a field to the left central and occipital regions (↓).** The *arrows* highlight the movement detected on the electromyography channel, and the nurse indicated that the infant had jerking of the head during this seizure.

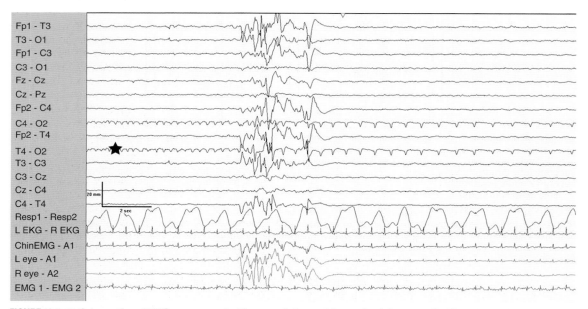

FIGURE 19-6 ■ **Conventional EEG was recorded from an infant with cerebral dysgenesis.** There is a subclinical right occipital seizure, indicated by the *star*.

TREATING NEONATAL SEIZURES IN THE CONTEXT OF THERAPEUTIC HYPOTHERMIA

CASE STUDY 7

A 37-week infant is born via emergency caesarian section resulting from placental abruption. The infant's Apgar scores are 1, 2, and 5 at 1, 5, and 10 minutes, respectively. She has lip-smacking

movements, concerning for seizures, and is moderately encephalopathic upon arrival in your NICU. You determine that she meets clinical criteria for whole body hypothermia as a neuroprotective strategy.

EXERCISE 4

QUESTION

1. Are there special considerations required for dosing of anticonvulsant medications during

therapeutic hypothermia? Consider the following case. How would you manage the seizures?

ANSWER

1. Phenobarbital dosing does not require adjustment for infants undergoing therapeutic hypothermia. However, other medication dosing might need to be customized.

    Therapeutic hypothermia has become the standard of care for infants with acute HIE. Many of these infants (~40% in the initial cooling trials) have seizures, which are typically subclinical. These seizures are a marker of increased risk for poor neurodevelopmental outcomes. Many centers routinely monitor these patients with conventional EEG throughout cooling and rewarming. Because hypothermia is associated with physiologic changes in liver and kidney function, and can alter cytochrome P450 enzyme function, it is important to consider whether medication dosing must be adjusted during cooling.

    Evidence from population pharmacokinetic modeling showed that the hypothermia does not alter pharmacokinetic parameters for phenobarbital. Therefore, traditional phenobarbital dosing (i.e., beginning with a 20 to 30 mg/kg loading dose, with repeated boluses as necessary, followed by standard maintenance doses) is appropriate initial therapy for infants with seizures who are being treated with therapeutic hypothermia.

    However, a study of lidocaine pharmacokinetics suggested that the dose should be modified somewhat if the infant is cooled. For infants weighing 2.0 to 2.5 kg, begin with a 2 mg/kg bolus, followed by consecutive continuous infusions of 6 mg/kg/hour (for 3.5 hours), 3 mg/kg/hour (for 12 hours), 1.5 mg/kg/hour (for 12 hours). For neonates weighing 2.5 to 4.5 kg, begin with the same 2 mg/kg bolus, followed by 7 mg/kg/hour (for 3.5 hours), 3.5 mg/kg/hour (for 12 hours), 1.75 mg/kg/hour (for 12 hour), before stopping the infusion (van den Broek, 2013).

WHEN CONVENTIONAL TREATMENT DOESN'T WORK

CASE STUDY 8

A 36-week gestational age infant presented on the first day of life with frequent focal seizures, manifest as ictal apnea with occasional focal clonic limb jerking. The interictal EEG is markedly abnormal, with high-amplitude multifocal spikes and no normal patterns. The brain MRI and initial tests of infection and electrolyte disturbances are all normal. Treatment with phenobarbital, fosphenytoin, levetiracetam, and midazolam has not controlled the seizures.

EXERCISE 5

QUESTION

1. What is your approach when the usual anticonvulsant medications fail to control the seizures? How would you proceed with the infant in Case Study 8?

ANSWER

1. In this case, refocusing on identifying the underlying seizure etiology is essential. Once the etiology is known, it will direct your management.

    When initial approaches to treatment of neonatal seizures are not effective, the first step is to return to the basics: what is the etiology? Most often, the answer is unknown. Once the most common etiologies are ruled out (e.g., the infant is known not to be septic or to have meningitis, there is no obvious lesion on appropriate neuroimaging testing, there are no dysmorphic features, etc.), then a search for other rare etiologies must be undertaken.

    One essential diagnostic consideration is pyridoxine-dependent seizures. This is a treatable autosomal recessive epilepsy syndrome, associated with mutations of ALDH7A1. Affected neonates present in the first days of life with pharmacoresistant seizures. They usually also have profoundly abnormal interictal (between-seizure) EEG patterns. The diagnosis can be made by administering 100 mg of intravenous pyridoxine during EEG monitoring. In neonates with pyridoxine dependency, the seizures cease and the EEG patterns improve after just a few minutes. If there is no response after the first dose of pyridoxine, then repeated doses should be administered every few minutes (maximum 500 mg total). Oxygen saturation and vital signs must be monitored, as cardiovascular collapse has been described with high-dose intravenous pyridoxine administration. If the seizures resolve, then a diagnosis of pyridoxine-dependent seizures is presumed and the infant should be maintained on pyridoxine indefinitely (approximately 15 mg/kg/day in two divided doses). Standard anticonvulsant medications can be weaned off, and the diagnosis should be confirmed with genetic testing.

DURATION OF ANTICONVULSANT THERAPY

EXERCISE 6

QUESTION

1. Once an infant's seizures are well-controlled, how long should antiseizure medications be continued? What factors should play roles in your decision-making process?

ANSWER

1. The duration of treatment depends on several factors: etiology, ease of attaining seizure control and number of anticonvulsant medications required, and overall goals of care.

   Most neonatal seizures are acute symptomatic seizures. As such, they often flare for several days and then resolve. Whether the seizures would have stopped spontaneously or were controlled because of medications is often uncertain. Equally uncertain, in many cases, is the appropriate duration of anticonvulsant therapy. Several factors are important in the decision-making process:
   - What is the etiology of the seizures?

   An infant whose seizures are attributable to transient hypoglycemia (e.g., infant of a diabetic mother whose initial glucose was very low, but now has normal glucose levels and a normal neurologic examination) might not need any treatment with anticonvulsant medication. A newborn with HIE, whose seizures occurred on the first day of life and resolved rapidly with low-dose phenobarbital, might safely come off of this medication before NICU discharge. On the other hand, a neonate with lissencephaly and associated treatment-resistant epilepsy is likely to require lifelong anticonvulsant treatment.
   - How difficult were the seizures to control?

   If the seizures were easily controlled, the infant has a normal examination, a follow up EEG is normal or nearly normal, and neuroimaging does not reveal a major abnormality, then discontinuing the anticonvulsant medication quickly is quite reasonable. Conversely, if the seizures were difficult to control, and/or multiple medications were required, and/or the infant has an abnormal neurologic examination, EEG, and/or neuroimaging, then discontinuing all anticonvulsants is not prudent. In this case, simplification of the medication regimen by reducing to a minimum number of medications may be the best short-term goal.
   - What are the anticipated risks and benefits for continued treatment?

   A history of neonatal seizures is a significant risk factor for the later development of epilepsy.

However, chronic epilepsy may not develop for many years and there is no current evidence that prolonged treatment with an anticonvulsant is protective. Additionally, the medications of choice for children with epilepsy are usually quite different from the drugs used for acute symptomatic neonatal seizures (e.g., oxcarbazepine for childhood focal epilepsy syndromes, or adrenocorticotropic hormone (ACTH) for infantile spasms). Finally, there is concern that some of the anticonvulsant drugs, especially phenobarbital, may have deleterious effects on the developing brain by inducing abnormal neuronal apoptosis. All of the anticonvulsants can also cause sedation, which can in theory interfere with daily activities and potentially contribute to long-term developmental delays.

Conversely, there are risks to having ongoing, uncontrolled seizures. Concerns about anticonvulsant medications' potential adverse effects on neurodevelopment must be tempered by the fact that uncontrolled epilepsy is also associated with unfavorable development. If elements of the history, neuroimaging, EEG, and/or examination findings suggest a high risk for ongoing seizures, then most clinicians recommend continuing the medication. Such infants should be reassessed regularly by a pediatric neurologist to determine whether the continued treatment is adequate and/or warranted.

NEURODEVELOPMENTAL PROGNOSIS AFTER NEONATAL SEIZURES

EXERCISE 7

QUESTION

1. You are about to have a family meeting with the parents of a newborn infant with acute symptomatic seizures. They want to know their baby's prognosis. What are you going to tell them?

ANSWER

1. The risk of death or significant neurodevelopmental disability can be difficult to estimate, but it is the parents' most important concern. Although one can never be absolutely sure about the prognosis of any particular neonate, there are some data that can inform the discussion. Discussions of predicted outcome must be informed by the infant's gestational and postmenstrual ages, the etiology of the seizures, how easily the seizures are controlled with medications, as well as EEG

and neuroimaging data. The risk for adverse outcomes is quite high, particularly for neonates with meningitis, severe HIE, congenital anomalies, or neonatal epilepsy syndromes.

If all etiologies are considered, acute mortality for neonates with seizures ranges from 25% to 40%, with higher risk among preterm infants. Developmental delays and cerebral palsy are diagnosed in about two thirds of affected children by ages 2 to 3 years. Postneonatal epilepsy, in which the acute symptomatic seizures subside but recurrent unprovoked seizures develop, has been reported in 17% to 56% of children who had neonatal seizures (compared with 1% of the general population). In general, the harder the acute symptomatic seizures are to control, and the higher the seizure burden, the worse the prognosis. Similarly, the more foci of seizure onset, the more diffuse the cerebral injury, and the more likely the child will have significant neurodevelopmental disability.

CONCLUSION

Neonatal seizures are quite common, but they are difficult to diagnose by clinical observation alone. EEG monitoring is the gold standard for neonatal seizure diagnosis, but can be complemented by amplitude-integrated EEG in certain circumstances. A concerted effort to search for, and treat, the underlying cause of the seizures is mandatory. The first-line treatment for neonatal seizures is usually phenobarbital, with second- and third-line treatments selected based on the clinical scenario. The underlying etiology and response to treatment are crucial predictors of long-term neurodevelopmental outcome.

SUGGESTED READINGS

al Naqeeb N, et al.: Assessment of neonatal encephalopathy by amplitude-integrated electroencephalography, *Pediatrics* 103(6):1263–1271, 1999.

Bittigau P, et al.: Antiepileptic drugs and apoptotic neurodegeneration in the developing brain, *Proc Natl Acad Sci USA* 99(23):15089–15094, 2002.

Blume HK, Garrison MM, Christakis DA: Neonatal seizures: treatment and treatment variability in 31 United States pediatric hospitals, *J Child Neurol* 24(2):148–154, 2009.

Castro Conde JR, et al.: Midazolam in neonatal seizures with no response to phenobarbital, *Neurology* 64:876–879, 2005.

Chapman KE, Raol YH, Brooks-Kayal AR: Neonatal seizures: controversies and challenges in translating new therapies from the lab to the isolette, *Eur J Neurosci* 35:1857–1865, 2012.

Fenichel GM, editor: *Neonatal Neurology*, 4th ed, Philadelphia, PA, 2007, Churchill Livingstone Elsevier.

Glass HC, et al.: Neonatal seizures: treatment practices among term and preterm infants, *Pediatr Neurol* 26(2):111–115, 2012.

Glass HC, Wusthoff CJ, Shellhaas RA. Amplitude integrated EEG: the child neurologist's perspective. *J Child Neurol*. In press.

Hellström-Westas L, de Vries LS, Rosen I: *Atlas of Amplitude-Integrated EEGs in the Newborn*, 2nd ed., London, UK, 2008, Informa Healthcare.

Hellström-Westas L, et al.: Amplitude-integrated EEG classification and interpretation in preterm and term infants, *NeoReviews* 7(2):e76–e87, 2006.

Holmes GL: The long-term effects of neonatal seizures, *Clin Perinatol* 36(4):901–914, 2009.

McBride MC, Laroia N, Guillet R: Electrographic seizures in neonates correlate with poor neurodevelopmental outcome, *Neurology* 55:506–514, 2000.

Painter MJ, et al.: Phenobarbital compared with phenytoin for the treatment of neonatal seizures, *N Engl J Med* 341:485–489, 1999.

Painter MJ, et al.: Neonates with seizures: what predicts development? *J Child Neurol* 27(8):1022–1026, 2012.

Shellhaas RA, et al.: The American Clinical Neurophysiology Society's Guideline on Continuous Electroencephalography Monitoring in Neonates, *J Clin Neurophysiol* 28(6):611–617, 2011.

Shellhaas RA, et al.: Population pharmacokinetics of phenobarbital in infants with neonatal encephalopathy treated with therapeutic hypothermia, *Pediatr Crit Care Med* 14(2):194–202, 2013.

Shellhaas RA, Clancy RR: Characterization of neonatal seizures by conventional and single channel EEG, *Clin Neurophysiol* 118:2156–2161, 2007.

Shellhaas RA, Saoita AI, Clancy RR: The sensitivity of amplitude-integrated EEG for neonatal seizure detection, *Pediatrics* 120(4):770–777, 2007.

Silverstein FS, Ferriero DM: Off-label use of antiepileptic drugs for the treatment of neonatal seizures, *Pediatr Neurol* 39:77–79, 2008.

van den Broek MPH, et al.: Anticonvulsant treatment of asphyxiated newborns under hypothermia with lidocaine: efficacy, safety, and dosing, *Arch Dis Child Fetal Neonatal Ed* 98(4):F341–F345, 2013.

van den Broek MPH, et al.: Pharmacokinetics and clinical efficacy of phenobarbital in asphyxiated newborns treated with hypothermia, *Clin Pharmacokinet* 51:671–679, 2012.

CHAPTER 20

INTRAVENTRICULAR HEMORRHAGE

Andrew Whitelaw, MD, FRCPCH

Bleeding from the germinal matrix in and around the ventricles of the brain is one of the common serious complications of very preterm birth. Although some authors prefer to use "periventricular hemorrhage" to include hemorrhages that do not enter the ventricles, the term "intraventricular hemorrhage" (IVH) is usually applied to all germinal matrix hemorrhages, even the minority that do not rupture into the lumen of the ventricles. Research-based improvements in perinatal care have substantially reduced the percentage of preterm infants with IVH, but the increased survival of extremely immature infants <28 weeks means that there are more infants at risk of IVH. Although the reduction in IVH can be considered one of the success stories of perinatal medicine, it remains an important cause of morbidity and mortality. Intraventricular hemorrhage is rare in term infants. Furthermore, it has a completely different pathogenesis and clinical course from those in small preterm infants and will be discussed separately.

INTRAVENTRICULAR HEMORRHAGE IN THE PRETERM INFANT

IVH in preterm infants increases in risk <33 weeks' gestational age. In some instances, the amount of blood lost may be large enough to result in hypovolemia, hypotension, and death. Large hemorrhages are often followed by progressive ventricular enlargement (dilatation) and/or parenchymal hemorrhagic infarction in the adjacent periventricular white matter and these serious complications carry a high risk of subsequent neurodevelopmental impairment.

Hemorrhage may be restricted to the subependymal germinal matrix (Figure 20-1, *A*), may enter the lateral ventricles (intraventricular hemorrhage) (Figure 20-1, *B*), or may give rise to periventricular hemorrhagic infarction through the mechanism of obstruction to the terminal vein.

IVH was first described as a postmortem diagnosis and assumed to be a fatal event in preterm infants. Diagnosis during life was first made possible by computed tomography (CT) scan and then by ultrasound. Papile grading of IVH (Table 20-1, Figure 20-2) using CT scan has been applied to ultrasound and has been widely accepted.

CASE STUDY 1

A 32-year-old woman in her second pregnancy was admitted to your hospital's high-risk obstetrical service at 25 weeks' gestation. The fetus was in a breech presentation. The mother asked to talk to a neonatologist because she wanted to find out what could happen to her baby after delivery. She had heard that very premature babies were often disabled and asked what was the most common type of brain damage suffered by babies born at 25 weeks. You replied that bleeding into the ventricles of the brain was one of the most common problems. She then asked if anything could be done before or during the birth to minimize the risk.

EXERCISE 1

QUESTIONS

1. Why is the risk of IVH increased in very preterm infants and not in term infants or older children who are ill?

2. What is the overall risk of IVH at 25 weeks' gestation with modern perinatal care?

3. Which interventions before or during preterm delivery have been shown in randomized trials to reduce the risk of IVH?

Pathology of IVH in Preterm Infants

ANSWERS

1. The germinal matrix produces neuronal precursors during gestational weeks 10 to 20 and then produces glial precursor cells. Whereas the

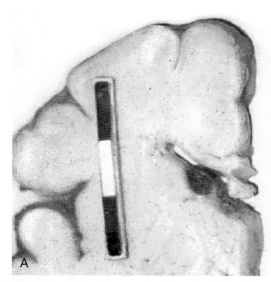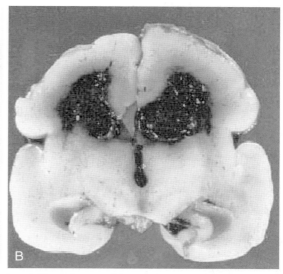

FIGURE 20-1 ■ **A,** Postmortem preterm brain (right hemisphere). There is a small hemorrhage in the subependymal germinal matrix. **B,** Postmortem preterm brain. There is massive hemorrhage with distention of the lateral and third ventricles.

TABLE 20-1	**Papile Grading of IVH**
Grade	**Description**
Grade I	Hemorrhage confined to the subependymal germinal matrix in the caudothalamic groove (Figure 20-2, *A*)
Grade II	Hemorrhage in germinal matrix and a small amount within the ventricular lumen, with the clot occupying less than 50% of the ventricular lumen and not distending the ventricular system (Figure 20-2, *B*)
Grade III	Germinal matrix hemorrhage with a large amount of clot (>50% of ventricular lumen) distending the ventricular system (Figure 20-2, *C*)
Grade IV	Germinal matrix and intraventricular hemorrhage in apparent continuity with hemorrhage into the periventricular white matter (Figure 20-2, *D*)

germinal matrix is producing new brain cells, it requires a rich blood supply; however, the blood vessels are structurally immature and not designed to last a lifetime. The intraventricular hemorrhage does not arise from an arterial aneurysm but from capillaries or small venules in which endothelial cells are poorly supported by pericytes. The endothelial cells have gaps between them and lack connective tissue and muscle support. The basal lamina is immature and there is a deficiency of glial fibrillary acidic protein in the astrocyte-end-feet. By the time the infant has reached term gestation, the germinal matrix has done its job of producing brain cells and almost disappears.

Diminished autoregulation of blood flow in the cerebral circulation is another variable that increases the risk of rupturing the germinal matrix vessels. Healthy individuals can (auto) regulate cerebral blood flow so that it remains constant despite variations in blood pressure. However, very preterm infants with respiratory distress syndrome (RDS) are usually unable to autoregulate cerebral blood flow. Struggling to breathe (with or without mechanical ventilation) generates wide swings in intrathoracic pressure, which are transmitted directly to the fragile vessels in the germinal matrix. As a result, the arterial pressure and cerebral blood flow velocity fluctuate. In addition, hypercapnia in infants with RDS produces cerebral vasodilatation, and acute swings in PcO_2 further destabilize cerebral blood flow. Once bleeding has started, it may continue unchecked as the premature skull can expand without increasing pressure enough to tamponade the hemorrhage. Formation of intraventricular clot may consume coagulation factors and platelets, which cannot be rapidly replaced, resulting in secondary coagulopathy.

In addition, IVH may give rise to periventricular hemorrhagic infarction through the mechanism of obstruction to the terminal vein (Figure 20-3). The venous drainage from the periventricular white matter occurs via the terminal vein through the germinal matrix. A large hematoma at that location will obstruct the terminal vein, thus raising venous pressure in the periventricular white matter. If there is a concurrent episode of hypotension, perfusion in the periventricular white matter will be reduced because of the raised venous pressure leading to

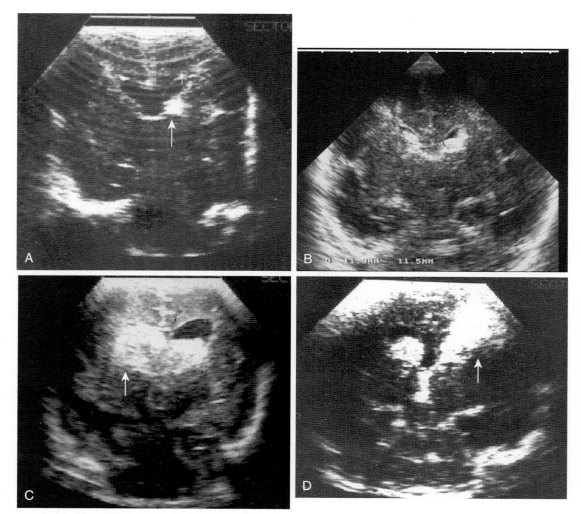

FIGURE 20-2 ■ **A,** Coronal ultrasound scan showing a small hemorrhage (arrowed) in the subependymal germinal matrix. Grade 1 IVH. **B,** Coronal ultrasound scan showing small amounts of blood clot in both lateral ventricles without ventricular distention. Grade II IVH. **C,** Coronal ultrasound scan showing large amounts of blood clot (arrowed) in both lateral ventricles with distention. Grade III IVH. **D,** Coronal cranial ultrasound scan showing a large amount of blood in the third and both lateral ventricles with some distention. In addition there is a large periventricular echodensity (arrowed) in apparent continuity with the lateral ventricle. Grade IV IVH.

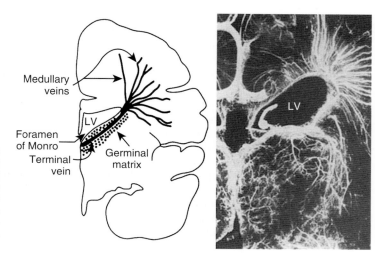

FIGURE 20-3 ■ Schematic diagram showing that the medullary arranged in a fan-shaped distribution, draining blood from the periventricular white matter into the terminal vein that courses through the germinal matrix. (From Volpe JJ: *Neurology of the newborn,* 5th ed, Philadelphia, PA, 2008, Saunders, p 521.)

a hemorrhagic infarction. Furthermore, because of the raised venous pressure, secondary bleeding can occur into the infarcted area.

2. In the early 1980s, a number of studies found that nearly 50% of all infants with birth weight <1500 grams had IVH. Since then, the incidence of IVH has decreased markedly in infants with birth weights 1000 to 1500 grams but, during the same period, survival of extremely low birth weight infants has increased. This means that there are more infants at highest risk. About 26% of infants in the U.S. Neonatal Network with birth weights 500 to 749 grams had IVH in the 1990s with 13% being severe. There does not appear to have been a further decrease in IVH during the past decade. In the Vermont-Oxford Network, 6.2% of infants with birth weights 500 to 1500 grams had a serious (grade III or IV) intraventricular hemorrhage in 2000 to 2001 and in 2008 to 2009. Allowing for infants >1500 grams who also have IVH would mean there are approximately 6000 new cases of grade III and IV IVH annually in the United States. The EXPRESS study from Sweden documented the course of infants below 27 weeks' gestation across the whole of Sweden between 2004 and 2007. At 25 weeks' gestation, despite universal availability of high-quality perinatal care, 12% had severe IVH.

3. Antenatal corticosteroids before preterm delivery have shown a very consistent reduction in IVH, including severe IVH in many randomized trials (Roberts, 2006). The effect applies across a wide range of gestational ages (<37 weeks) and with different corticosteroid regimens. However, the most commonly used treatment was a total dose of 24 mg betamethasone administered over a 24-hour period. For optimal effect the first dose had to have been given at least 24 hours before delivery. Delayed clamping of the umbilical cord, allowing transfusion of blood from the placenta, has been shown to reduce the incidence of IVH (Rabe, 2012). Antenatal vitamin K has been investigated in seven randomized clinical trials, but a metaanalysis did not show a significant benefit (Crowther, 2010).

CASE STUDY 1 (continued)

M was given two doses of betamethasone 12 hours apart. After 36 hours, contractions started and her temperature rose to 38° C. A female infant was delivered by emergency cesarean section, weighing 740 grams with a head circumference of 23 cm. Umbilical cord clamping was not delayed and an umbilical vein blood sample showed pH 7.25 with a base deficit of 4 mmol/L. She had a heart rate of 60 beats per minute with no spontaneous respiration,

or muscle tone. Following bag and mask ventilation with 21% oxygen, the heart rate increased to 100 beats per minute but she remained cyanotic. After placement of a pulse oximeter, her limbs and trunk were wrapped in a plastic bag to reduce heat loss. The pulse oximeter showed a saturation value of 60%. Raising the inspired oxygen to 70% increased the saturation (SaO_2) to 92%. Apgar scores were 3 at 1 minute and 6 at 5 minutes. She was intubated and given prophylactic surfactant via the endotracheal tube. By age 20 minutes, her inspired oxygen fraction was reduced to 35%. She maintained a SaO_2 of 92% and heart rate of 120 beats per minute.

She was mechanically ventilated at 40 breaths per minute and transferred to the neonatal intensive care unit (NICU). On arrival, her rectal temperature was 35.8° C, heart rate 126 beats per minute, blood pressure 24 mmHg, and SaO_2 of 91%; the inspired oxygen was 35%. An umbilical artery blood gas showed a pH of 7.24, PaO_2 of 49 mmHg, and PCO_2 of 43 mmHg. A cranial ultrasound scan was performed at 3 hours of age (Figure 20-4).

EXERCISE 2

QUESTIONS

1. Are there any evidence-based postnatal interventions to prevent IVH?

2. Would you order a cranial ultrasound scan on admission to the NICU?

3. What additional risk factors for IVH have become apparent at this stage?

4. Identify the numbered structures in the cranial ultrasound Figure 20-4.

5. Which findings on the scan point to the infant being very preterm? Does the scan show any significant abnormality?

ANSWERS

1. Evidence-based postnatal interventions to prevent IVH include:
   a. For ventilated preterm infants with evidence of asynchronous respiratory efforts, neuromuscular paralysis with pancuronium has been shown to reduce the incidence of IVH. Uncertainty remains, however, regarding the long-term pulmonary and neurologic effects, and regarding the safety of prolonged use of pancuronium in ventilated newborn infants.
   b. Volume-targeted ventilation may reduce IVH when compared with the more traditional pressure-limited ventilation; however, larger randomized trials are needed.

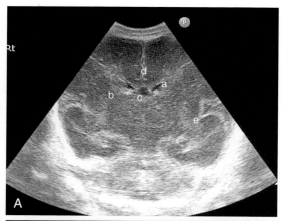

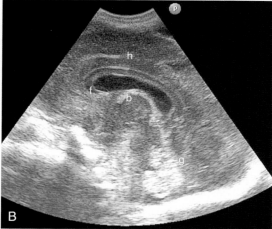

FIGURE 20-4 ■ **A**, Case 1. Coronal ultrasound scan at 3 hours. **B**, Sagittal scan at 3 hours.

c. Indomethacin promotes maturation of blood vessels in the germinal matrix and blunts swings in blood pressure and cerebral blood flow. Randomized clinical trials have shown a reduction in IVH but a metaanalysis and the largest trial showed no reduction in neurologic disability (Fowlie, 2010).

d. Phenobarbital modulates blood pressure fluctuations and may have some free radical scavenging function. It has been tested in 11 postnatal trials with inconsistent results. However, the metaanalysis and the largest trial did not find any reduction in IVH.

e. Ethamsylate improves platelet function and enhances capillary basement membrane stability but clinical trials showed no reductions in mortality or neurodevelopmental impairment despite the reduction in intraventricular hemorrhage in infants <35 weeks' gestation.

f. Vitamin E has free radical scavenging action. Supplementation in preterm infants reduced the risk of intracranial hemorrhage, but increased the risk of sepsis. Evidence does not support the routine use of vitamin E supplementation by intravenous route at high doses.

2. Routine cranial ultrasound scanning of very preterm infants on admission to the NICU is not regarded as essential because it is argued that the scan does not affect treatment and most IVH occurs after the time of admission. However, we have found that scanning a high-risk infant on admission to the NICU is useful because: (a) diagnosis (or absence) of IVH immediately after birth helps discussions with parents later when they ask when and how injury occurred; (b) diagnosis of a substantial IVH immediately after birth increases the focus on prevention of any further injury including attention to coagulation and platelets; and (c) significant antenatal injury (cyst or dilated ventricles) or a congenital or antenatally acquired abnormality may be shown. A normal cranial ultrasound scan on admission does not, of course, mean that injury will not occur later in the neonatal period.

3. The infant has increased risk of IVH because:
   a. Umbilical cord clamping was not delayed
   b. Apgar score was low
   c. Temperature <36° C
   d. Arterial blood pressure was initially low

4. a. Lateral ventricle
   b. Choroid plexus
   c. Cavum septi pellucidi
   d. Interhemispheric fissure
   e. Sylvian fissure
   f. Corpus callosum
   g. Cerebellum
   h. Cingulate sulcus

5. The wide-open sylvian fissure and the almost straight cingulate sulcus indicate very early gestation.

CASE STUDY 1 (continued)

10 mL/kg of normal saline was given to increase the blood pressure, but the mean arterial blood pressure remained low (24 mmHg). Intravenous dopamine was started at 5 mcg/kg/minute with no effect. The rate of infusion was then increased to 10 mcg/kg/min and the mean arterial blood pressure rose to 30 mmHg. By 12 hours of age, the oxygen requirement increased to 50% and a second dose of surfactant was administered. The oxygen requirement fell to 30% and remained at that level. A cranial ultrasound scan was ordered on Day 3 (Figure 20-5).

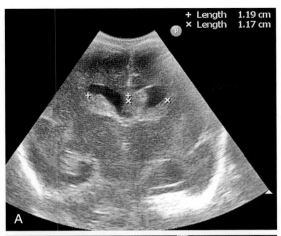

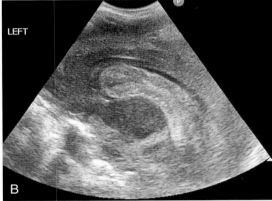

FIGURE 20-5 ■ A, Coronal ultrasound scan on Day 3. **B,** Parasagittal scan on Day 3. The crosses show the points for measuring ventricular width.

EXERCISE 3

QUESTIONS

1. Does surfactant replacement therapy change the risk of IVH?

2. Describe the abnormal findings shown in Figure 20-5.

3. What measurements are used to document the size of the cerebral ventricles in newborns and what are the normal limits? Are this infant's ventricular sizes within normal limits?

ANSWERS

1. Surfactant therapy reduces mortality but does not reduce the incidence of IVH.

2. There is a large amount of intraventricular blood clot, particularly on the parasagittal view, where the clot occupies >50% of the ventricular lumen and is distending the ventricle. This is a grade III IVH. There is no apparent parenchymal change.

The third ventricle is not dilated and there is no midline shift.

3. Ventricular width (also known as ventricular index) is the most widely used measurement of ventricular size in newborns. It measures the distance from the midline to the lateral border of the ventricle (Figure 20-5, *A*). Figure 20-6 demonstrates the 97th percentile according to gestational (or postmenstrual) age. This infant's ventricular widths measure 11.9 and 11.7 mm, both of which exceed the 97th percentile.

CASE STUDY 1 (continued)

It was possible to reduce the dopamine progressively and then discontinue it.

The infant remained ventilator dependent but without further major deterioration in gas exchange or circulation over the next 14 days. On Day 9 a course of indomethacin was given to close a symptomatic patent ductus arteriosus. The head circumference was measured daily. A cranial ultrasound scan (Figure 20-7) was carried out at 14 days of age. The head circumference was 23 cm.

EXERCISE 4

QUESTIONS

1. What has happened to ventricular size and shape between Figures 20-5 and 20-7?

2. How can one tell if ventricular enlargement is driven by expanding cerebrospinal fluid (CSF) or is a result of atrophy?

3. What are the mechanisms that cause ventricular dilatation and the associated white matter injury?

4. When should one intervene to decrease the ventriculomegaly?

5. Which treatment interventions to decrease ventriculomegaly are evidence-based?

6. Which other treatments are used but without evidence from randomized trials of efficacy?

ANSWERS

1. The lateral ventricles now have a rounded (ballooned) shape and the temporal horns are clearly enlarged. Intraventricular blood clots are still visible. The ventricular width has increased to 15.2 and 15.4 mm, clearly >4 mm over the 97th percentile. The third ventricle has now widened to 6.79 mm. Normally the third

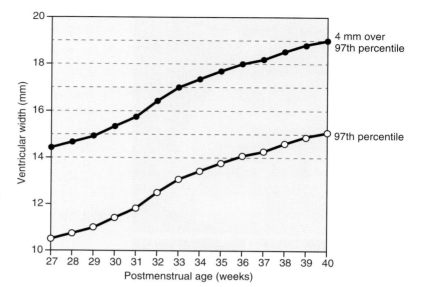

FIGURE 20-6 ■ **Ventricular width (ventricular index) plotted against gestational age.** The bottom line is the 97th percentile, and the top line is 4 mm over the 97th percentile. (From Whitelaw A, Aquilina K. Management of post-haemorrhagic ventricular dilatation. *Arch Dis Child* 2012;97:230.)

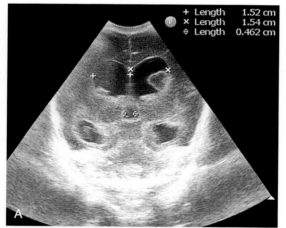

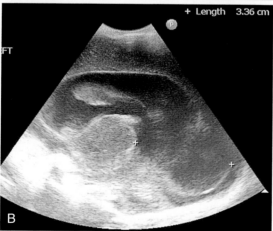

FIGURE 20-7 ■ **A**, Coronal ultrasound scan on Day 14. Crosses indicate ventricular width. **B**, Parasagittal scan on Day 14. Crosses indicate the thalamo-occipital distance.

ventricle is hardly visible on coronal view and width is no more than 2 mm. Figure 20-7, *B* shows the huge enlargement of the ventricle posteriorly. This finding is illustrated by the thalamo-occipital dimension, which should not exceed 24 mm.

2. On a single scan it can be difficult to know immediately if large ventricles are caused by too much CSF or a shrinking brain. However CSF-driven ventricular dilatation may be rapid, resulting in ballooned ventricles. Head growth eventually accelerates (although it may not in the first 1 to 2 weeks) and if pressure is measured, it exceeds 8 cm water. Ventricular dilatation due to atrophy is never rapid, often gives irregular ventricular shape, does not cause head accelerated head growth, and CSF pressure is not >8 cm water.

3. Posthemorrhagic ventricular dilatation is initially due to multiple small blood clots clogging up the channels of CSF reabsorption. The initial phase is followed by a repair reaction mediated, at least in part, by transforming growth factor beta (TGF-β), a cytokine that upregulates the genes for extracellular matrix proteins such as laminin, fibronectin, and vitronectin. TGF-β is stored in platelets (in the intraventricular blood clot) and is slowly released over weeks into the CSF. In addition, TGF-β is synthesized in periventricular cells as a response to injury. The deposition of extracellular matrix proteins in the subarachnoid space and CSF reabsorption channels has been likened to pouring cement or glue down a drain. At least four processes can be identified as potentially injuring

periventricular white matter in posthemorrhagic ventricular dilatation (PHVD).

   a. Premature infants have soft compliant skulls and ventriculomegaly can progress with minimal increases in intracranial pressure (ICP). However, when ICP rises above 12 mmHg, cerebral perfusion is often impaired.

   b. Enlarging ventricles produce physical distortion and edema in the periventricular white matter and this may impair myelination.

   c. The breakdown of hemoglobin results in release of free (non–protein-bound) iron into the CSF where it can injure brain cells by promoting free radical injury. The larger the hemorrhage, the more iron is released.

   d. Following IVH, high concentrations of pro-inflammatory cytokines are found in the CSF for many weeks and inflammation is a well-recognized mechanism of white matter injury.

4. If there is evidence of raised ICP, which is symptomatic (persistent and marked irritability, reduced responsiveness, or clinical seizures), then an intervention is required to lower pressure. If there is no indication of raised ICP, the indications for intervention are not universally agreed upon. However, ventricular width 4 mm over the 97th percentile (on each side) has been widely used as a criterion for treatment in clinical trials.

5. Repeated lumbar puncture/ventricular puncture; diuretic therapy with acetazolamide and furosemide; intraventricular injection of streptokinase; and drainage, irrigation, and fibrinolytic therapy (DRIFT) have been tested in randomized trials. None have shown any short-term benefit, e.g., reduction in shunt surgery, but irrigation and fibrinolytic therapy significantly reduced severe cognitive disability at 2 years.

6. Tapping a ventricular reservoir, subgaleal shunt insertion, external ventricular drainage, third ventriculostomy, and choroid plexus coagulation have all been used to treat PHVD but without evidence of efficacy in randomized clinical trials.

CASE STUDY 1 (continued)

A lumbar puncture was carried out on Day 15. The opening pressure with the infant quiet and very gently restrained was 11 cm water (8 mmHg) and 8 mL of cola-colored CSF was obtained with a closing pressure of 3 cm water (2 mmHg). The CSF protein was 600 mg/dL and the CSF glucose was 20 mg/dL (blood glucose 60 mg/dL). On Day 16 the head circumference increased to 23.5 cm. Another lumbar puncture was carried out.

EXERCISE 5

QUESTIONS

1. What is average daily increase in head circumference at this gestation?

2. What are the normal limits for CSF pressure in newborn infants? Is there a serious risk of coning (brain herniation) during a lumbar puncture in a newborn infant with raised ICP?

3. What is the significance of a CSF glucose of 20 mg/dL?

ANSWERS

1. The average increase in head circumference is about 1 mm/day at this gestation. The rate slows to about 0.5 mm/day at 40 weeks' gestation.

2. If an infant is not crying and is not being restrained on the abdomen or neck, CSF pressure at lumbar or ventricular puncture should not exceed 6 mmHg (about 8 cm water). Coning is extremely rare in newborn infants because:

   a. ICP rarely rises very high (by standards of childhood and adulthood) because of the compliant skull

   b. Sick infants are commonly intubated before undergoing a lumbar puncture

   c. The infant is horizontal when tapped

   Thus fear of coning should not deter a clinically indicated LP.

3. CSF glucose is normally well over 50% of blood glucose. 20 mg/dL is a low CSF glucose value (assuming the infant is not hypoglycemic). After an IVH has occurred, it is normal to have a low CSF glucose for many weeks.

CASE STUDY 1 (continued)

On Day 18, the head circumference increased to 23.9 cm. A cranial ultrasound showed a small increase in ventricular measurements. A lumbar puncture was carried out. The opening pressure was 10 cm water (8 mmHg). Only 2 mL of cola-colored CSF could be obtained.

On the same day, the decision was made to place a ventricular access device, an Ommaya reservoir. 8 mL of CSF were removed at the time of placement. From Day 19 to 23, 10 mL/kg were removed from the reservoir each day. Subsequently 10 mL/kg CSF were removed only on days the head circumference increased significantly. On Day 24, the CSF contained 100 white cells/mL (mainly polymorphonuclear leukocytes) and a culture grew

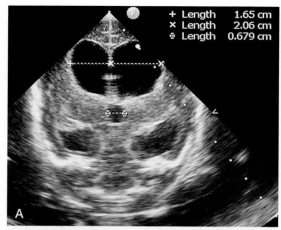

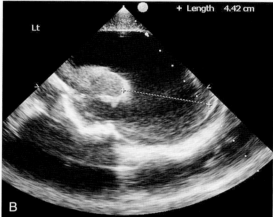

FIGURE 20-8 ■ **A,** Coronal ultrasound scan on Day 35. **B,** Parasagittal scan on Day 35. Crosses indicate the thalamo-occipital distance.

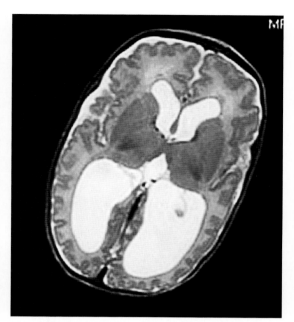

FIGURE 20-9 ■ Case 1. MRI T2 axial view at term.

coagulase-negative staphylococci. Vancomycin and gentamicin were injected into the ventricles using the reservoir, which was then removed. Intravenous vancomycin and gentamicin were given for 10 days. Intermittent ventricular taps were carried out when head circumference increased; the CSF was consistently negative on culture. On Day 35 head circumference was 31 cm. A cranial ultrasound scan was carried out (Figure 20-8). A second ventricular reservoir was then inserted and 10 mL/kg/day of CSF were removed. At 40 weeks' gestation, the head circumference was 36 cm. The reservoir was not entered for 3 days; however, the head circumference increased by 6 mm. A magnetic resonance imaging (MRI) brain scan was obtained (Figure 20-9) after which a ventriculoperitoneal shunt was inserted. At age 2 years her Psychomotor Development Index was 55 and her Mental Development Index was below 50. She could walk but had no speech and had significant problems with vision.

EXERCISE 6

QUESTIONS

1. In an infant with a ventricular reservoir, what are the indications for CSF removal? How much CSF should be taken?

2. Describe the significant findings in the MRI scan.

3. Why was the eventual neurodevelopmental outcome worse than suggested by the scan on Day 3?

ANSWERS

1. The purpose for inserting a ventricular reservoir is to enable the removal of sufficient CSF to normalize ICP and to prevent any further enlargement of the ventricles and excessive head enlargement. The standard procedure is to remove 10 mL/kg CSF over 10 (or more) minutes. Rapid removal of CSF can cause midline shift and precipitate secondary bleeding. Taking more than 20 mL/kg CSF at one tap may result in clinical deterioration. The frequency of taps should be adjusted in order to prevent any further ventricular enlargement and to achieve normal head growth over 7 days. When the ventricles are very large, the goal is to reduce ventricular size to 4 mm over the 97th percentile.

2. The ventricles are bilaterally enlarged, particularly in the occipital region, the left slightly more than

the right. Periventricular white matter is correspondingly reduced. There is still a small amount of germinal matrix hemorrhage. Signal from the posterior limb of the internal capsule is present.

3. The scan on Day 3 showed grade III IVH but without any apparent parenchymal changes. There are three additional factors that increase the risk of brain injury and disability: prolonged ruptured membranes with maternal pyrexia, progressive posthemorrhagic ventricular dilatation eventually requiring shunt surgery, and CSF infection associated with the ventricular reservoir. The infant did not exhibit severe motor delay and this is consistent with the internal capsule being present. The marked loss of periventricular white matter in the occipital region is associated with later visual processing problems.

CASE STUDY 2

A pregnant woman, N, had an uneventful pregnancy until placental abruption at 27 weeks' gestation. An emergency caesarean section was carried out, but there was no time to give antenatal corticosteroids. The infant was male, birth weight 1100 grams, and had Apgar scores of 1 at 1 minute, 3 at 5 minutes, and 3 at 10 minutes. He was intubated, ventilated, and given cardiac compressions in the first 2 minutes of life. Surfactant was given into the trachea. The cord blood pH was 7.01 with base deficit 15 mmol/L. Despite the early surfactant administration, he developed respiratory distress syndrome with inspired oxygen requirements of 50% to 60%. He was administered pancuronium and ventilated with a time cycled, pressure-limited ventilator. At 20 hours his oxygen saturations fell despite 95% oxygen, breath sounds were diminished over the right lung, and a right-sided pneumothorax was confirmed by transillumination. The mean arterial blood pressure fell to 23 mmHg. A chest drain was inserted on the right side with an improvement in oxygenation. A dopamine infusion was started at 10 mcg/kg/min and then increased to 15 mcg/kg/min. After 4 hours, the mean arterial pressure was restored to 30 mmHg. At 24 hours, a blood sample showed: hemoglobin 10 g/dL, white blood cells 30,000/mcL, platelets 56,000/mcL, prothrombin time 27 seconds, and activated partial thromboplastin time (APTT) 60 seconds. Packed red cells, platelets, and fresh frozen plasma were given intravenously. A cranial ultrasound was carried out at 24 hours (Figure 20-10).

Intermittent cycling movements of the legs were observed and then flexion/extension movements of the left hand. You suspected seizure activity and this was confirmed by EEG. A dose of 20 mg/kg of phenobarbital was infused intravenously over 20

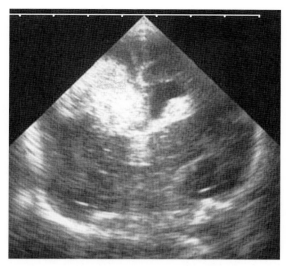

FIGURE 20-10 ■ Case 2. Coronal ultrasound scan on Day 2.

minutes and the seizure activity ceased clinically and electrically.

EXERCISE 7

QUESTIONS

1. What are the significant findings in the scan (Figure 20-10)?

2. The mother asks what the scan means for her son's later development. What can you tell her at this stage?

ANSWERS

1. There is a grade IV IVH on the right, with blood in the left and third ventricles. There is no parenchymal injury on the left and no midline shift.

2. The injury in the brain tissue on the right is large and its location means that control of movement in the left leg and left arm will be affected. There is a wide range of later development with this grade of injury. He may or may not be able to walk. The brain injury also means there is an increased risk of epilepsy. It is more difficult to predict mental development. If later scanning confirms no injury in the brain tissue on the left, mental function can be in the normal range. Repeated scanning will also be important because there is a high risk of hydrocephalus. If that happens, additional interventions will be needed and the risk of disability will be increased.

CASE STUDY 2 (continued)

He did not require a ventricular reservoir or a ventriculoperitoneal shunt and had no significant

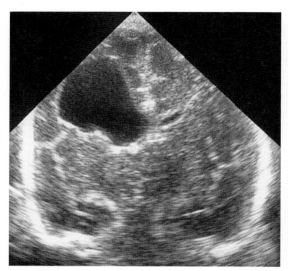

FIGURE 20-11 ■ Case 2. Coronal ultrasound scan at term.

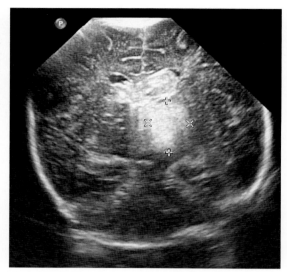

FIGURE 20-12 ■ Case 3. Coronal ultrasound scan at 3 days.

infection at any stage. Figure 20-11 shows a cranial ultrasound scan at term gestation. He developed a left hemiparesis but walked at age 2 years. He subsequently had two nonfebrile seizures and was treated with carbamazepine for 2 years with no recurrence. At 9 years of age, he was doing well academically and he could swim 200 meters. Functional MRI scanning showed that he had relocated motor cortical function from the right hemisphere to the left. Thus the left hemisphere was controlling the left hand, arm, and leg.

INTRAVENTRICULAR HEMORRHAGE IN THE TERM INFANT

CASE STUDY 3

A primigravida woman went into labor at 41 weeks' gestation. There were some late decelerations of the fetal heart rate but a fetal blood sample showed pH 7.26. There was meconium stained liquor in the second stage. A male infant weighing 3750 grams was delivered by vacuum extraction. Apgar scores were 6 at 1 minute, 8 at 5 minutes, and 9 at 10 minutes. Cord pH was 7.28. He was examined by a neonatologist. No congenital abnormalities were found and his tone, activity, and responsiveness were within normal limits. He was allowed to go with his mother to the postpartum ward. She worked hard on establishing breastfeeding, but found him rather irritable. At 24 hours of age he was observed to have clonic movements for 3 minutes and became transiently cyanotic. He was admitted to the NICU. Examination showed a weak

suck and some hypotonia. A cranial ultrasound scan was carried out on Day 2 (Figure 20-12).

EXERCISE 8

QUESTIONS

1. What abnormalities are visible on the ultrasound scan?

2. What underlying diagnoses should be considered and what further investigations are indicated?

3. Apart from anticonvulsant therapy, should any other treatment be considered?

ANSWERS

1. There is a large amount of intraventricular blood, which is distending the lateral ventricles. In addition, there is a large echodensity (hemorrhagic infarction) in the left thalamus and basal ganglia area.

2. One possibility is a bleeding disorder. Either thrombocytopenia (alloimmune) or an inherited coagulation-factor deficiency should be ruled out. Therefore a platelet count, prothrombin time, and APTT are needed. Another possibility is a cranial sinus thrombosis, which produces bleeding by raised venous pressure in the choroid plexus and central gray matter. MR imaging with MR venography will be needed.

3. If a bleeding tendency were shown, then appropriate replacement of platelets or coagulation factors is urgent. In cranial sinus thrombosis

there is a risk of the thrombosis extending, thus producing an increased secondary infarction. This has been the argument for anticoagulation with low–molecular weight heparin but most clinicians have not dared to do this because of fear of rebleeding. Serial scanning and head circumference measurements will be needed to detect progressive ventricular dilatation.

SUGGESTED READINGS

Crowther CA, Crosby DD, Henderson-Smart DJ: Vitamin K prior to preterm birth for preventing neonatal periventricular haemorrhage, *Cochrane Database Syst Rev* (1):CD000229, 2010 Jan 20.

Fowlie PW, Davis PG, McGuire W: Prophylactic intravenous indomethacin for preventing mortality and morbidity in preterm infants, *Cochrane Database Syst Rev* (7):CD000174, 2010 Jul 7.

Papile L, Burstein J, Burstein R, Koffler H: Incidence and evolution of subependymal and intraventricular hemorrhage: a study of infants with birth weights less than 1500 g, *J Pediatr* 92:529–534, 1978.

Rabe H, Diaz-Rossello JL, Duley L, Dowswell T: Effect of timing of umbilical cord clamping and other strategies to influence placental transfusion at preterm birth on maternal and infant outcomes, *Cochrane Database Syst Rev* (8):CD003248, 2012 Aug 15.

Roberts D, Dalziel S: Antenatal corticosteroids for accelerating fetal lung maturation for women at risk of preterm birth [review], *Cochrane Database Syst Rev* (3):CD004454, 2006 Jul 19.

Volpe JJ: *Neurology of the newborn*, 5th ed, Philadelphia, PA, 2008, Saunders, p 521.

Whitelaw A: Periventricular hemorrhage: a problem still today, *Early Hum Dev* 88:965–969, 2012.

Whitelaw A, Aquilina K: Management of posthaemorrhagic ventricular dilatation, *Arch Dis Child Fetal Neonatal Ed* 97(3):F229–F233, 2012.

CHAPTER 21

SURGICAL EMERGENCIES IN THE NEWBORN

Calvin J. Young, MD • Michael G. Caty, MD, MMM • Robert A. Cowles, MD

A variety of surgical emergencies occur in neonates. Rapid identification of surgically treatable conditions and subsequent surgical consultation can significantly affect patient outcomes. This chapter discusses many of the major newborn emergencies that require urgent surgical evaluation and intervention. Not all conditions necessarily require operative treatment; however, the surgeon often remains an important member of the multidisciplinary team. The text is divided into sections based upon common patient presentations. Each section begins with a descriptive case followed by a discussion of important issues, treatment options, and expectations. Necrotizing enterocolitis (NEC), the most common abdominal emergency in the premature newborn, is discussed in detail in a separate section of this book and therefore will not be covered here.

EMERGENCIES OF THE TRACHEA, ESOPHAGUS, AND THORAX

CASE STUDY 1

A newborn male in the well-baby nursery is noted to immediately vomit his initial feedings and appears to have excessive oral and pharyngeal secretions. An orogastric tube is placed but does not advance because of resistance. The infant is nearly full term but no other prenatal history is immediately available. An anteroposterior chest x-ray shows the orogastric tube is coiled in the proximal esophagus (Figure 21-1).

EXERCISE 1

QUESTIONS

1. Which of the following is/are appropriate next steps in the care of this newborn?
   a. Replacement of the orogastric tube until it clearly passes into the stomach
   b. Formal upper gastrointestinal (GI) barium contrast study to assess for patency of esophagus, stomach, and duodenum

   c. Endotracheal intubation
   d. Change in formula and reattempt oral feedings
   e. None of the above

2. Which of the following should have been evaluated during his prenatal ultrasound?
   a. Volume of amniotic fluid
   b. Size of fetal stomach
   c. Cardiac anatomy
   d. Renal anatomy
   e. All of the above

3. Based on the information available, what is the diagnosis?
   a. Isolated (pure) esophageal atresia without fistula
   b. Esophageal atresia with distal tracheoesophageal fistula
   c. Esophageal atresia with proximal tracheoesophageal fistula
   d. Pyloric stenosis
   e. Tracheal stenosis

4. Which of the following evaluations should be obtained immediately after the diagnosis is made and prior to any operative intervention?
   a. A spinal ultrasound
   b. Renal ultrasound
   c. Echocardiogram
   d. Barium enema
   e. **a**, **b**, and **c** only

5. What is the most important factor affecting outcome of a newborn with esophageal atresia and tracheoesophageal fistula?
   a. Presence of imperforate anus
   b. Severity of congenital heart disease
   c. Size of the patent ductus arteriosus
   d. Gestational age ≥37 weeks
   e. Evidence of a small stomach on prenatal ultrasound

ANSWERS

1. **e.**

2. **e.**

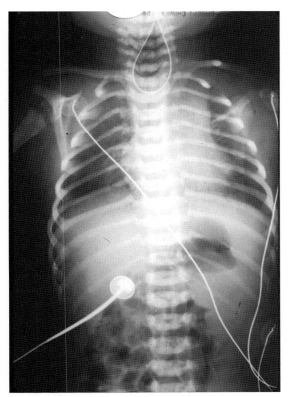

FIGURE 21-1 ■ **Newborn with intolerance of initial oral feeding.** The orogastric tube cannot be advanced. The x-ray shows the tube coiled in the proximal esophagus and the presence of distal bowel gas.

3. **b.**

4. **c.**

5. **b.**

Esophageal atresia with tracheoesophageal fistula (EA/TEF) occurs in about 1 in 2500 births and results from abnormal or incomplete separation of the trachea from the esophagus during development (Moore, 1988). Newborns with esophageal atresia with (or without) tracheoesophageal fistula usually present with excessive drooling and poor tolerance of initial oral feedings. The presence of polyhydramnios with a diminutive fetal stomach can suggest esophageal atresia, but definitive prenatal diagnosis is not routine. An attempt at placement of an orogastric tube that is met with unusual resistance and failure to advance is a classic finding. Radiographic evidence includes a chest x-ray showing the orogastric tube coiled in the proximal esophagus. Additionally, a dilated, air-filled proximal esophagus can also commonly be appreciated on chest x-ray (Figure 21-1) (Azizkhan, 1992; O'Neill, 2004). These findings are sufficient to make a diagnosis of esophageal atresia. Formal

upper GI contrast studies or further attempts to pass a nasogastric tube can be hazardous and are discouraged (Azizkhan, 1992).

Once a diagnosis of esophageal atresia is made, a survey for associated anomalies should be conducted. EA/TEF is part of the VAC-TERL (Vertebral, Anal, Cardiac, Tracheo-Esophageal, Renal, Limb) association and, therefore, a specific search for these abnormalities should be undertaken, with evaluation of the cardiac anatomy being most time sensitive. The search for associated anomalies can be completed with a careful physical examination, plain x-rays, ultrasound (spinal and renal), and an echocardiogram. The child's respiratory function should be supported as conservatively as possible. Intubation with positive pressure ventilation should be avoided unless absolutely necessary, as much of the tidal volume in this scenario would be lost via the fistula (if present) into the stomach. If intubation and mechanical ventilation are necessary, a surgeon should be contacted in the event that an urgent gastrostomy or ligation of the fistula becomes necessary.

EA/TEF can have five different anatomic varieties (Figure 21-2), with the most common being an esophageal atresia and distal tracheo-esophageal fistula. Any variation that includes a distal fistula should show air in the GI tract, often in a normal configuration. Conversely, those patients with a pure or isolated esophageal atresia have a gasless abdomen on an abdominal x-ray (Figure 21-3). Patients with EA/TEF and other GI anomalies such as duodenal atresia or anorectal malformation should be surgically evaluated with urgency since decompression of the GI tract is often impossible.

Operative repair of EA/TEF most often involves a right thoracotomy with esophageal anastomosis and closure of the tracheoesophageal fistula. In some cases, several operative procedures are required. In pure esophageal atresia without fistula the first operation is commonly a feeding gastrostomy, as there is often a large gap between the two esophageal ends. The gastrostomy can be used to initiate enteral feedings for nutritional optimization prior to further operative intervention. Newborns with concurrent EA/TEF, severe congenital heart disease, and very low birth weight are particularly challenging cases and have been shown to be poor candidates for full one-stage repair (Spitz, 1994). These frail newborns may benefit from a staged approach beginning with a decompressive gastrostomy, with or without division of the tracheoesophageal fistula, followed by complete repair at a later time.

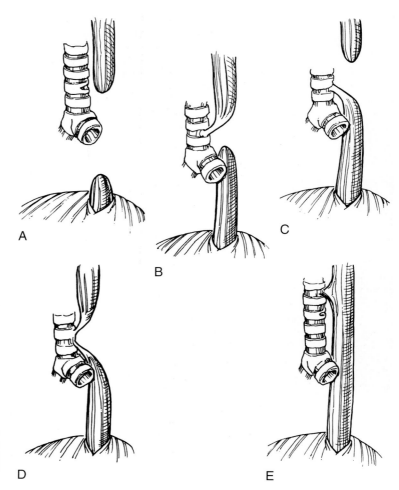

FIGURE 21-2 ■ Classification of different forms of esophageal atresia without tracheoesophageal fistula (**A**) and with tracheoesophageal fistula (**B-E**).

CASE STUDY 2

You are called to the neonatal intensive care unit (NICU) for a term baby in severe respiratory distress. The baby has a scaphoid abdomen, and an antenatal ultrasound suggests an abnormal stomach position.

EXERCISE 2

QUESTIONS

1. What is the most appropriate initial diagnostic test?
   a. Chest computed tomography (CT)
   b. Abdominal magnetic resonance imaging (MRI)
   c. Plain radiograph including abdomen and chest
   d. Umbilical vein venogram
   e. Umbilical artery angiogram

2. After the initial chest x-ray, the pre- and postductal oxygen saturation monitors read 90% and 65%, respectively, while the infant is on the ventilator with an FiO$_2$ of 1.0. The initial treatment plan should include which of the following?
   a. Emergency thoracotomy in the NICU
   b. Pharmacologic paralysis and high-pressure ventilation
   c. Extracorporeal membrane oxygenation (ECMO)
   d. Gentle mechanical ventilation without paralysis to minimize barotrauma
   e. Bilateral chest tubes

ANSWERS

1. **c.**

2. **d.**

The most common location for a congenital diaphragmatic hernia (CDH) is posterolateral. These occur in about 1 in every 4000 newborns and most (80%) are on the left side. Because abdominal contents have herniated into the chest cavity early in gestation, patients with CDH have respiratory insufficiency secondary

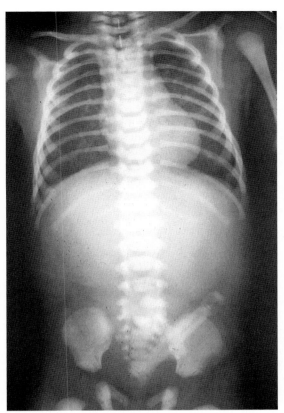

FIGURE 21-3 ■ X-ray findings in esophageal atresia without fistula. Note the orogastric tube in the proximal esophagus and the absence of gas in the abdomen.

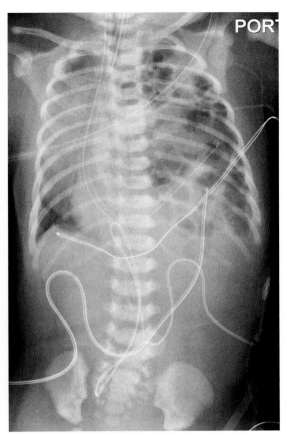

FIGURE 21-4 ■ Left posterolateral congenital diaphragmatic hernia (CDH). The heart is displaced to the right and the left chest is filled with loops of intestine. Note the course of the orogastric tube suggesting an intrathoracic position of the stomach.

to lung hypoplasia and pulmonary hypertension. Poorly oxygenated blood is "shunted" into the systemic circulation via the foramen ovale and the patent ductus arteriosus (PDA). Both lungs are compressed owing to mass effect exerted by the intrathoracic viscera and can be further damaged by the use of high ventilator pressures. Histologically these lungs exhibit immaturity as well. In selected cases, inhaled nitric oxide can help lower the high pulmonary vascular resistance, but is often not helpful.

Many CDH are discovered before birth on routine prenatal ultrasound, which allows for a planned delivery at a neonatal referral center (Adzick, 1985). Prenatal intervention (tracheal occlusion) has been studied, but is still investigational (Harrison, 2003). At birth, a scaphoid abdomen is often described and radiographs show intestine in the chest cavity (Figure 21-4). Cystic lung lesions may occasionally be mistaken for CDH. These conditions can be differentiated by passing a nasogastric tube or by an upper GI series demonstrating GI contents in the thoracic cavity.

All newborns with CDH require operative intervention. The timing of surgery has changed over time from being an immediate emergency procedure to a planned procedure, days after birth, once evidence of pulmonary hypertension has resolved (Boloker, 2002; Clark, 1998). Monitoring pre- and postductal oxygen saturations is useful in this regard. ECMO is reserved for those babies who fail all ventilator and pharmacologic strategies. Please see Chapter 17 for additional information on management.

EMERGENCIES OF THE ABDOMINAL WALL

CASE STUDY 3

You are contacted by a community hospital where a 34-week gestation, 1900-gram boy with an abdominal wall defect was just delivered. The child is vigorous and appears healthy with no other obvious

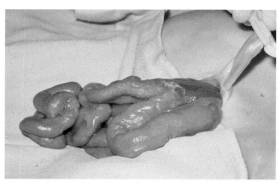

FIGURE 21-5 ■ **Appearance of the exposed bowel in gastroschisis.** The thickened and abnormal appearance of the bowel is classic as is the location of the defect just to the right of the umbilicus.

abnormalities. The pediatrician caring for this newborn tells you that there is a large amount of intestine outside the baby's abdomen and that the bowel appears thickened, stiff, and leathery (Figure 21-5). The actual defect is difficult to visualize under the loops of exposed intestine. The vital signs are appropriate and there is no respiratory distress.

EXERCISE 3

QUESTIONS

1. This case description most classically illustrates what kind of abdominal wall defect?
   a. Ruptured umbilical hernia
   b. Omphalocele
   c. Gastroschisis
   d. Pentalogy of Cantrell
   e. Epigastric hernia

2. Appropriate instructions for the outside institution prior to transfer include which of the following?
   a. Placement of nasogastric tube
   b. Placement of an umbilical arterial catheter
   c. Coverage of the exposed intestine with a plastic bowel bag
   d. **a** and **c** only
   e. **a**, **b**, and **c**

3. Upon arrival, the child is clinically stable and you identify the lesion as gastroschisis. The baby is prepared for the operating room for attempt at primary closure of the defect. Appropriate preparation of this baby for surgical closure of the defect includes which of the following?
   a. Endotracheal intubation
   b. Establishing secure access for intravenous fluids
   c. Positioning of the bowel to avoid kinking of the mesenteric blood supply
   d. Placing the newborn in a warmed environment
   e. All of the above

4. Which of the following abnormalities are described in association with gastroschisis?
   a. Hypoplastic left sided heart syndrome
   b. Small intestinal atresia
   c. Anomaly of intestinal rotation
   d. Biliary atresia
   e. **b** and **c** only

5. Which are signs that the baby is developing abdominal compartment syndrome?
   a. Decreasing urine output
   b. Increasing P_{CO_2}
   c. Firmness on abdominal examination
   d. Venous congestion of the lower extremities
   e. All of the above

ANSWERS

1. **c.**

2. **d.**

3. **e.**

4. **e.**

5. **e.**

The major abdominal wall defects seen in neonates include omphalocele and gastroschisis. Inguinal and umbilical hernias are considered milder abdominal wall defects but can become surgical emergencies in the NICU. Both types of major defects can be seen on prenatal ultrasound, giving the neonatologist and surgeon time to plan the perinatal and postnatal care (Langer, 2003; O'Neill, 2004; Wilson, 2004). Gastroschisis can be differentiated from omphalocele based on several aspects (O'Neill, 2004). First, the size and location of the defect is different. The defect in gastroschisis is often small and located to the right of the umbilical cord (see Figure 21-5). Additionally, in neonates with gastroschisis a membrane does not cover the herniated abdominal contents. In contrast, an omphalocele defect is central and often larger, with a covering membrane (Figure 21-6).

The postnatal care for children with abdominal wall defects is critical and should begin in the delivery room. Evaluation of the defect and its contents is often easy. Prior to transfer to a center where definitive care can be administered, the abdominal contents should be wrapped in a warm saline-soaked gauze and placed in a plastic bowel bag to prevent loss of heat and fluid. Also, placement of a nasogastric tube is recommended in order to prevent aspiration or gaseous distention of the stomach and bowel. Finally, secure intravenous access should be obtained and volume resuscitation should be carefully monitored

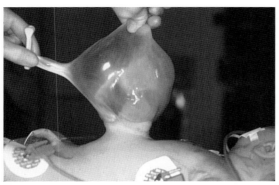

FIGURE 21-6 ■ Moderate sized omphalocele with a covering membrane. Both the stomach and bladder have been decompressed in preparation for closure of the defect.

because fluid loss can be significant, especially in infants with gastroschisis due to the exposed viscera. Because the surgical approach to abdominal wall defects involves manipulation of the umbilical cord stump, umbilical vessel catheters are discouraged.

The neonate should be kept in a warm environment to minimize fluid loss and coagulopathy. The herniated abdominal viscera often falls over one side of the child's body. Effort should be made to secure the bowel in a position that avoids kinking of the mesenteric vessels. This will minimize swelling of the viscera. A screen for concomitant anomalies should be performed, especially when an omphalocele is present. Omphalocele can be associated with congenital heart disease and hypoglycemia, and this information is important to the anesthesiologist and surgeon. Gastroschisis, on the other hand, is associated with intestinal atresia and an anomaly of intestinal rotation and fixation.

After successful surgical closure of an abdominal wall defect, the size of the abdominal cavity may not accept the previously herniated viscera without sequelae. When size mismatch is severe, a condition known as abdominal compartment syndrome (ACS) can occur (Wilson, 2004). ACS occurs when intraabdominal hypertension leads to end-organ insufficiency. ACS can hinder venous return, renal perfusion, and respiratory mechanics. Although no exact intraabdominal pressure measurement has been correlated with ACS, a decreasing urine output, increasing peak ventilator pressure, increasing PCO_2, and a firm abdomen are clues that ACS may be present. Often, the lower extremities become edematous and develop obvious signs of venous congestion when ACS is present. Reopening the abdomen may be necessary in cases in which ACS is present.

CASE STUDY 4

A 30-week gestation, newborn male has been stable in the NICU and preparations are being made for discharge home. You are alerted by the nurse who states that the child has vomited several times and appears very uncomfortable. When you examine the baby, you notice that the abdomen is nontender but quite distended. There is a reducible umbilical hernia; however, the right groin area appears noticeably larger and firmer than the left. The testes are descended bilaterally.

EXERCISE 4

QUESTIONS

1. What is the most likely diagnosis?
   a. Hydrocele
   b. Left inguinal hernia
   c. Right inguinal hernia
   d. Intussusception
   e. None of the above

2. What is the most likely cause of the baby's problem?
   a. Straining due to constipation
   b. Failed or incomplete closure of the processus vaginalis
   c. Viral infection
   d. All of the above
   e. None of the above

3. You make the diagnosis at 6 in the evening and attempt to reduce the hernia but without success. At this point, what would you do next?
   a. Request a surgeon see the infant later that day and continue to feed the infant.
   b. Place a nasogastric tube and ask for an immediate surgical consultation.
   c. Observe the infant over the next 4 to 6 hours.
   d. Administer a suppository.
   e. None of the above

4. What is/are the acceptable treatment options for an incarcerated inguinal hernia in an infant?
   a. Always emergent operation
   b. Simple reduction followed by planned operation
   c. Attempted reduction with emergent operation if unsuccessful
   d. **b** or **c**
   e. Reduction, discharge home, followed by elective operation

ANSWERS

1. **c.**

2. **b.**

3. **a.**

4. **d.**

Vomiting in the newborn can be the result of many conditions. In the case cited, the physical exam finding of a right groin mass that cannot be reduced suggests an incarcerated right inguinal hernia. Inguinal hernias are common and are the result of a persistently patent processus vaginalis. Crying or straining can often make an inguinal hernia more obvious but does not cause hernias themselves.

When concerned for the presence of an incarcerated inguinal hernia, a surgeon should be contacted as soon as possible. Because the incarcerated hernia can contain intestine, bladder, omentum, and ovary (in females), it is important to attempt reduction of the hernia as soon as possible. Prolonged incarceration can lead to venous congestion and edema of the incarcerated contents, making later attempts to reduce the hernia more difficult. Reduction of an incarcerated inguinal hernia is often possible before surgery. Gentle but constant pressure on the incarcerated contents in the direction of the inguinal ring is usually successful. The person reducing the hernia will feel a definite return of the entire contents of the hernia sac into the abdominal cavity and resolution of the groin bulge. If bedside reduction is not successful, administration of sedation with a repeat attempt at reduction may be considered in the appropriate setting. In cases where reduction of the hernia is possible either with or without sedation, the hernia should be repaired within 48 hours. Most surgeons would recommend against discharging a newborn with a previously incarcerated inguinal hernia prior to repair because of high incidence of recurrent incarceration (Gahukamble, 1996).

Only when a hernia is not reducible, despite sedation and attempts by the pediatric surgeon, is the child taken to the operating room for urgent operative repair. A standard inguinal incision is used. The incarcerated contents are inspected for signs of ischemia at operation and a decision is made regarding the need for intestinal resection. The operation is often more difficult than an elective inguinal hernia repair and the internal inguinal ring is sometimes opened. Incarcerated inguinal hernias are associated with higher rates of recurrence and testicular loss. For this reason, exploration of the contralateral groin should be avoided and only considered if a clear, obvious inguinal hernia is present.

GASTROINTESTINAL EMERGENCIES

CASE STUDY 5

A 1-week-old newborn is irritable and has several episodes of bilious emesis after the most recent

feeding. He is tachycardic but otherwise the vital signs are stable. The physical examination reveals a full abdomen but no marked abnormality.

EXERCISE 5

QUESTIONS

1. What is the appropriate next step in this case?
   a. Evaluate the infant for possible gastroesophageal reflux with a pH probe.
   b. Start treatment with a proton pump inhibitor.
   c. Perform ultrasound examination of the pylorus.
   d. Perform upper GI contrast study.
   e. Change oral feedings to a soy-based formula.

2. Which of the following is (are) true about intestinal malrotation and midgut volvulus?
   a. They always occur at the same time.
   b. Emergent operation is recommended if either is found to be present.
   c. Neither condition can be asymptomatic.
   d. Both conditions can cause bilious emesis.
   e. Plain abdominal x-rays are very helpful in the diagnosis.

ANSWERS

1. **d.**

2. **d.**

CASE STUDY 6

A 2.5-kg newborn had been in the nursery for 2 days for treatment of presumed sepsis. There was no record of prenatal care at your hospital. He initially fed well but on the third day of life had two episodes of green-colored emesis.

EXERCISE 6

QUESTIONS

1. Bilious emesis can be associated with which of the following?
   a. Intestinal stenosis
   b. Imperforate anus
   c. Hirschsprung disease
   d. Malrotation with volvulus
   e. All of the above

2. What should be the first initial radiographic study for this baby?
   a. Abdominal ultrasound
   b. Upper GI contrast study
   c. Contrast enema (CE)
   d. Chest x-ray
   e. Brain MRI

3. A nasogastric tube is placed and returns thick, bilious material. The initial radiographic study

excludes malrotation but shows significantly dilated loops of bowel. At this point, what is the most appropriate follow up study?
   a. Abdominal ultrasound
   b. Upper GI contrast study
   c. Contrast enema (CE)
   d. Chest x-ray
   e. Brain MRI

4. In this case, what does the presence of an unobstructed small caliber colon on CE suggest?
   a. Small bowel atresia
   b. Imperforate anus
   c. Duodenal atresia
   d. Meconium ileus
   e. **a** or **d**

ANSWERS

1. **e.**

2. **b.**

3. **c.**

4. **e.**

The causes of intestinal obstruction in the neonate are varied and can be related to either mechanical or functional abnormalities. When bilious emesis is witnessed or when a history of bilious emesis in a newborn is obtained, it is imperative that the physician first exclude malrotation, as this is a potentially life-threatening condition. Although malrotation with or without volvulus is classically associated with bilious emesis, all other forms of mechanical or functional intestinal obstruction distal to the ampulla of Vater can present with bilious emesis as well. The main causes of intestinal obstruction in the newborn include intestinal atresia (duodenal, small intestinal, colonic), malrotation with volvulus, meconium ileus, meconium plug, Hirschsprung disease, and imperforate anus. In general, the diagnosis of most types of anorectal malformations ("imperforate anus") is made after a focused clinical examination of the child's perineum. In the case described, the first step in management is insertion of a nasogastric tube for decompression and to decrease the risk of aspiration.

After a careful physical examination, the first radiographic study should be an upper gastrointestinal (UGI) contrast study to evaluate for anomalies of rotation. On the scout film, the general size of the bowel loops and distribution of enteric gas can suggest a diagnosis. A "double-bubble" sign is virtually pathognomonic for duodenal atresia or duodenal stenosis (Figure 21-7), and a "gasless" abdomen has been described in malrotation with volvulus.

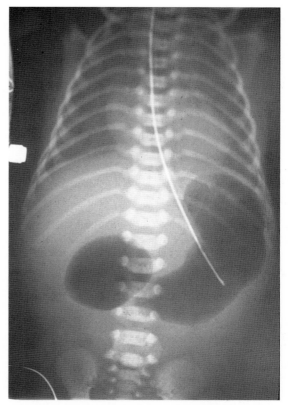

FIGURE 21-7 ■ Abdominal x-ray in suspected duodenal atresia confirms the "double bubble" sign.

Despite this, a plain abdominal x-ray can be deceiving and care must be taken when interpreting the plain x-ray. The UGI delineates the course of the esophagus, stomach, and duodenum. The fixation of the duodenum in its retroperitoneal location with the ligament of Treitz coursing to the left of the spinal column excludes malrotation. If the ligament of Treitz does not cross the midline, then the child has malrotation (Figure 21-8). If, in addition, there is a high-grade obstruction of the mid- or distal duodenum, then malrotation may be complicated by volvulus, although malrotation is not necessarily complicated by volvulus every time (Figure 21-9). The combination of malrotation and volvulus warrants immediate emergency surgical treatment (Rescorla, 1990). Ultrasound, CT scan, and MRI should be discouraged, as they are not as useful and are much more difficult to obtain than UGI study. On occasion, a UGI study is obtained for an unrelated reason, and a previously unrecognized malrotation is identified. In this scenario, if the malrotation is not causing symptoms, surgical treatment can be rendered on a nonemergent basis.

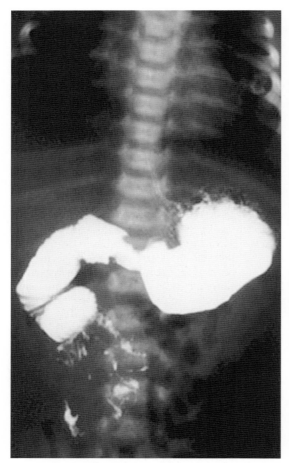

FIGURE 21-8 ■ **Upper GI contrast study reveals an abnormality of intestinal rotation with failure of the Ligament of Treitz to cross the midline.** Note the passage of contrast distally.

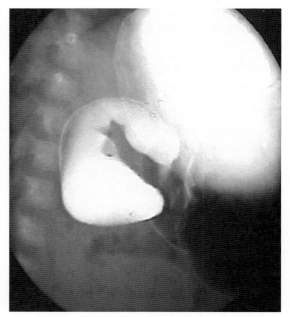

FIGURE 21-9 ■ **Upper GI contrast study showing an abnormality of rotation for complete duodenal obstruction concerning for malrotation and volvulus.**

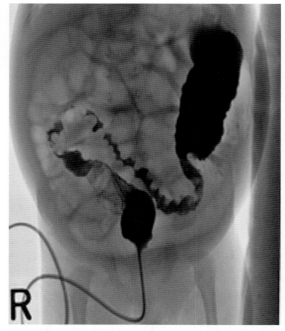

FIGURE 21-10 ■ **This contrast enema clearly shows the transition zone in an infant with Hirschsprung disease.**

If the initial UGI study shows normal bowel rotation or if there is low suspicion for malrotation at the outset, then a retrograde contrast enema (CE) is the next study of choice. As with the UGI study, the scout film can show dilated small bowel (atresia), calcifications (complicated meconium ileus), or a dilated colon (Hirschsprung disease). On the CE, the size of the colon is evaluated, as are the presence or absence of transition areas. A microcolon is most commonly associated with small bowel atresia and meconium ileus. In small bowel atresia, the contrast fills the microcolon but does not enter the dilated loops of intestine in a retrograde fashion. In meconium ileus, the CE may demonstrate meconium pellets in the colon, suggesting the diagnosis. In addition, contrast material may enter the dilated proximal bowel, excluding a mechanical atresia with the potential of having a therapeutic effect. In Hirschsprung disease,

the CE has been an important diagnostic tool for many years. A transition zone can be identified at the level where aganglionosis begins (Figure 21-10). If a transition zone is present or if the clinical suspicion is high, a rectal biopsy to confirm the diagnosis of Hirschsprung disease is indicated (Swenson, 2002).

CASE STUDY 7

A 2-day-old, 650-gram, 25-week gestation newborn has a newly distended abdomen despite the presence of a functioning orogastric tube. The vital signs are stable, oxygen saturation is 95% on nasal continuous positive airway pressure (CPAP), and urine output is adequate. Plain abdominal x-rays, including a cross-table lateral view, reveal a large amount of free intraperitoneal air (Figure 21-11).

EXERCISE 7

QUESTIONS

1. What are possible cause(s) of this baby's free intraperitoneal air?
   a. CPAP
   b. Gastric perforation
   c. Spontaneous intestinal perforation
   d. **b** and **c**
   e. None of the above

2. What is the next step in the management of this neonate?
   a. Repeat abdominal x-rays in 4 hours.
   b. Obtain a surgical consultation.
   c. Reposition the orogastric tube.
   d. Decrease CPAP support.
   e. Evacuate the intraperitoneal air with a small percutaneous drain.

ANSWERS

1. **d.**

2. **b.**

Pneumoperitoneum in the severely premature newborn (as in the case described) can be caused by a variety of conditions. One should assume that the extraluminal air is secondary to a perforated hollow viscous unless there is an obvious reason to believe otherwise (such as recent abdominal surgery or dissection of air from a pneumothorax). Spontaneous intestinal perforation (SIP), gastric perforation, and necrotizing enterocolitis (NEC) are responsible for a majority of cases (Grosfeld, 1996). Infrequently, intrathoracic air from a pneumothorax can track into the abdomen and cause pneumoperitoneum. Standard endotracheal ventilation and CPAP are not thought to be causes of pneumoperitoneum. NEC is the most common cause of intestinal perforation in premature newborns, but SIP is particularly associated with very low birth weight infants, especially those who receive perinatal steroids and indomethacin (Gordon, 2001; Pumberger, 2002; Stark, 2001). A definitive diagnosis of gastric perforation is difficult to make prior to surgery, but massive pneumoperitoneum is often noted on the preoperative abdominal x-rays of neonates with gastric perforation.

When pneumoperitoneum is identified, an urgent surgical consultation should be obtained. In most cases, surgical exploration will be performed, sometimes in the NICU. On selected occasions, when the neonate is unstable or unable to undergo laparotomy, the surgeon will elect to place a small drain in the abdominal cavity. The drain will allow evacuation of air and fluid and will provide a temporary treatment. Placement of the drain can be challenging and should only be performed by a surgeon. Once the neonate stabilizes, definitive operative intervention can be considered.

AIRWAY EMERGENCIES

CASE STUDY 8

A 28-week gestational age fetus is noted on a prenatal ultrasound to have a large, complex neck mass

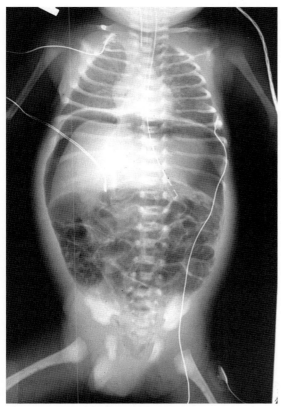

FIGURE 21-11 ■ **Premature infant with free intraperitoneal air.**

and evidence of polyhydramnios. You are consulted predelivery to be part of the multidisciplinary care team for this child.

EXERCISE 8

QUESTION

1. Which of the following treatment strategies are important to consider while planning for delivery of this child?
   a. Immediate endotracheal tube intubation at the time of delivery
   b. Preparation for immediate tracheostomy in the delivery room
   c. Planned ex utero intrapartum treatment (EXIT) procedure
   d. Consult surgeon after delivery for urgent mass resection on arrival to NICU
   e. **a**, **b**, and **c**

ANSWER

1. **e.**

Head and neck masses in children are common and usually benign in nature. However, as in the case described, even a benign mass can become a neonatal emergency when there is risk of airway compromise (Figure 21-12). Fetal head and neck (cervical) teratomas represent 3% to 5% of all teratomas and have an incidence of 1 in 35,000 to 200,000 live births (Tonni, 2010). Teratomas of the head and neck are frequently found in the anterior and midline as opposed to other types of head and neck masses like lymphatic malformations, hemangiomas, and bronchial cysts, which are found in the posterior and lateral regions. Other components of the differential diagnosis should include congenital goiter, foregut duplication cyst, and branchial cleft cyst.

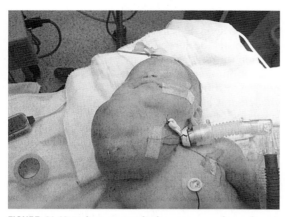

FIGURE 21-12 ■ **Large cervical mass causing airway compression.** This infant required tracheostomy placement for airway control perinatally.

Diagnosis of these masses is frequently accomplished in the prenatal period with ultrasound as early at 15 to 17 weeks' gestation, but more frequently in the late second or third trimester. Three-dimensional ultrasound can help with delivery planning by accurately describing the location and extension of the mass. Additionally, prenatal MRI has been advocated in complex cases where the lesion has intracranial involvement. Large teratomas have been associated with polyhydramnios secondary in esophageal compression and interference with fetal swallowing.

Management of these lesions requires a multidisciplinary team to be present at delivery. Caesarean section should be planned and upon delivery, endotracheal intubation or immediate tracheostomy should be performed before the umbilical cord is clamped. This sequence of events is called the ex utero intrapartum treatment (EXIT) procedure. Once the airway is secured in this manner, definitive resection of the mass can be performed once the infant is stabilized.

OTHER IMPORTANT FETAL MASSES

CASE STUDY 9

A 20-week gestation fetus is noted to have a sacral mass on a prenatal ultrasound. There are no signs of hydrops and the family is referred for prenatal counseling.

EXERCISE 9

QUESTION

1. Which of the following is/are characteristic of newborns presenting with sacrococcygeal teratomas?
   a. An incidence of 1 in 5000 births, similar to most other congenital anomalies
   b. Excellent function and cosmetic result following operative resection
   c. Potential for heart failure
   d. High incidence of malignancy
   e. None of the above

ANSWER

1. **c.**

Sacrococcygeal teratomas represent 35% to 60% of all teratomas and are the most common tumor in the neonate with an incidence of 1 in 35,000 to 40,000 live births. The differential diagnosis for masses in this region should include teratomas and meningoceles. Diagnosis is often made on prenatal ultrasound, frequently in the second

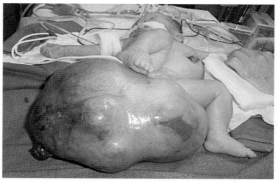

FIGURE 21-13 ■ **Sacrococcygeal teratoma (SCT) with a large external component.**

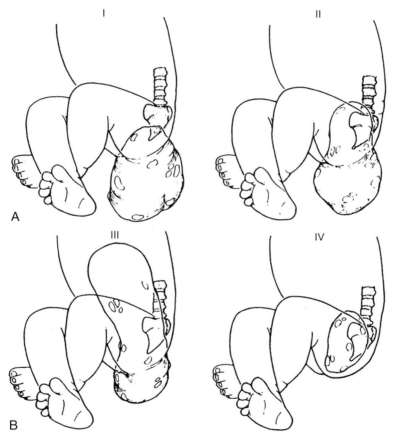

FIGURE 21-14 ■ **Altman classification of SCT.** Type I tumors are entirely external and type IV tumors are entirely internal.

trimester. Although small teratomas have little effect in utero, large vascular tumors (Figure 21-13) are associated with a higher mortality rate owing to premature delivery or tumor rupture. Overall, if diagnosed in utero, neonatal survival rates exceed 90%.

Although the majority of neonates with sacrococcygeal teratomas are asymptomatic, those with high-output heart failure, disseminated intravascular coagulopathy (DIC), or tumor rupture and bleeding will require urgent intervention by intensive care physicians and surgeons (Laberge, 2010).

As shown in Figure 21-14, sacrococcygeal teratomas are classified based on their extent of intra- and extrapelvic involvement. Frequently, children with strictly intrapelvic teratomas have a delay in diagnosis. These children can present with nonspecific symptoms such as urinary retention, constipation, or failure to thrive (Laberge, 2010). Children with obvious teratomas in this location should undergo resection of the mass as soon as they are medically fit for the procedure because the risk of malignancy at birth is low, around 10%. Those patients with delayed diagnoses have a greater risk of malignancy (Laberge, 2010).

SUGGESTED READINGS

Adzick NS, Harrison MR, Glick PH, et al.: Diaphragmatic hernia in the fetus: prenatal diagnosis and outcome in 94 cases, *J Pediatr Surg* 20:357, 1985.

Azizkhan RG: Esophageal atresia and distal tracheoesophageal fistula in a neonate, *Postgrad Gen Surg* 4:1–4, 1992.

Boloker J, Borteman D, Wung JT, Stolar CJH: Congenital diaphragmatic hernia in 120 infants treated consecutively with permissive hypercapnia, spontaneous respiration and elective repair, *J Pediatr Surg* 37:357, 2002.

Clark RH, Hardin WD, Hirschl RB, et al.: Current surgical management of congenital diaphragmatic hernia: a report for the Congenital Diaphragmatic Hernia Study Group, *J Pediatr Surg* 33:1004, 1998.

Gahukamble DB, Khamage AS: Early versus delayed repair of reduced incarcerated inguinal hernias in the pediatric population, *J Pediatr Surg* 31:1218–1220, 1996.

Gordon PV, Young ML, Marshall DD: Focal small bowel perforation: An adverse effect of early postnatal dexamethasone therapy in extremely low birth weight infants, *J Perinatol* 21:156–160, 2001.

Grosfeld JL, Molinari F, Chaet M, et al.: Gastrointestinal perforation and peritonitis in infants and children: experience with 179 cases over ten years, *Surgery* 120:650–655, 1996.

Harrison MR, Keller RL, Hawgood SB, et al.: A randomized trial of fetal endoscopic tracheal occlusion for severe fetal congenital diaphragmatic hernia, *N Engl J Med* 349:1916–1924, 2003.

Laberge J, Puligandla P, Shaw K: Teratomas, dermoids, and other soft tissue tumors. In Holcomb III GW, Murphy JP, Ostlie DJ (editors): *Ashcraft's pediatric surgery*, ed 5, Philadelphia, PA, 2010, Elsevier, pp 915–935.

Langer JC: Abdominal wall defects, *World J Surg* 27:117–124, 2003.

Moore KL: *The developing human; clinically oriented embryology*, Philadelphia, PA, 1988, Saunders, pp 207–216.

O'Neill JA, Grossfeld JL, Fonkalsrud EW, Coran AG: Abdominal wall defects. In *Principles of pediatric surgery*, St. Louis, MO, 2004, Mosby, pp 423–431.

O'Neill JA, Grossfeld JL, Fonkalsrud EW, Coran AG: Congenital abnormalities of the esophagus. In *Principles of pediatric surgery*, St. Louis, MO, 2004, Mosby, pp 385–394.

Pumberger W, Mayr M, Kohlhauser M, et al.: Spontaneous localized intestinal perforation in very-low-birth-weight infants: a distinct clinical entity different from necrotizing enterocolitis, *J Am Coll Surg* 195:796–803, 2002.

Rescorla FJ, Shedd FJ, Grosfeld JL, et al.: Anomalies of intestinal rotation in childhood: analysis of 447 cases, *Surgery* 108:710–715, 1990.

Spitz L, Kiely EM, Morecroft JA, Drake DP: Oesophageal atresia: at-risk groups for the 1990s, *J Pediatr Surg* 29:723–725, 1994.

Stark AR, Carlo WA, Tyson JE, et al.: Adverse effects of early dexamethasone treatment in extremely-low-birth-weight infants, *N Engl J Med* 344:95–101, 2001.

Swenson O: Hirschsprung's disease: a review, *Pediatrics* 109:914–918, 2002.

Tonni G, De Felice C, Centini G, Ginanneschi C: Cervical and oral teratoma in the fetus: a systematic review of etiology, pathology, diagnosis, treatment and prognosis, *Arch Gynecol Obstet* 282(4):355–361, 2010. http://dx.doi.org/10.1007/s0040-101-1500-7. Epub May 15, 2010.

Wilson RD, Johnson MP: Congenital abdominal wall defects: an update, *Fetal Diagn Ther* 19:385–398, 2004.

CHAPTER 22

NECROTIZING ENTEROCOLITIS

Eric B. Ortigoza, MD, MSCR • Josef Neu, MD

Necrotizing enterocolitis (NEC) is a devastating gastrointestinal disease that affects predominantly premature infants. It is one of the most enigmatic and feared diseases in the neonatal intensive care unit (NICU). The prevalence of this disease is about 7% among infants born at less than 32 weeks' gestation with birth weights between 500 and 1500 grams (Erasmus et al., 2002; Guillet et al., 2006; Holman et al., 2006; Horbar et al., 2002). Within hours after onset of initial symptoms, it can progress rapidly to septic shock, necrosis of the intestines, and death. The mortality of NEC is 20% to 30%, with the greatest mortality among infants who require surgery (Fitzgibbons et al., 2009). Because of the severity of this disease, many practitioners are concerned that enteral feeding is associated with the development of NEC. This concern has resulted in increased duration of intravenous nutrition, thus increasing the infection rate, cholestasis, and length of stay among infants who never develop NEC. It also is strongly associated with adverse neurodevelopmental outcomes (Stoll et al., 2002).

CASE STUDY 1

Baby girl BK (birth weight 1750 grams) was born via spontaneous vaginal delivery at 31 weeks to a mother whose prenatal course was complicated by preterm premature rupture of membranes 2 weeks before delivery and a positive vaginal culture for Chlamydia. The mother received a single dose of azithromycin and two doses of betamethasone before delivery. Apgar scaores were 8 and 9 at 1 and 5 minutes of life, respectively. Soon after delivery, the neonate became dusky and was admitted to the NICU with mild respiratory distress syndrome. She initially required continuous positive airway pressure (CPAP) and an FiO$_2$ of 0.6, but over the next 9 days, the baby was weaned from CPAP to room air. Ampicillin and gentamicin were administered for 2 days and both were stopped when cultures revealed no growth. Erythromycin was also administered because of inadequate treatment of maternal chlamydial infection. Feedings were started on

Day 2 of life with an initial volume of 20 mL/kg/day, divided every 3 hours, and were gradually advanced to full enteral feeds over the next 7 days. On Day 12 of life, she had a bilious gastric residual of 27 mL. Physical exam revealed an increased abdominal girth from 22 to 27 cm, a firm and distended abdomen, and a stool that tested positive for blood. Laboratory studies revealed a white blood count of 11,800/mm^3 with 45% mature neutrophils and 25% band forms. The hemoglobin concentration was 12 g/dL and the platelet count was 190 × 10^9/L. An arterial blood gas revealed pH 7.34, PaCO$_2$ 47, PaO$_2$ 147, and base excess -0.5. Serum electrolytes were normal. The abdominal x-ray revealed intestinal intramural and portal venous air, consistent with NEC (Figure 22-1). The baby was started on vancomycin and gentamicin, a nasogastric tube was placed to low intermittent suction, and a surgery consultation was obtained.

EXERCISE 1

QUESTION

1. Which of the following combination of signs and symptoms is most suggestive of surgical NEC?
   a. Baby with feeding intolerance, abdominal distension, bloody stools after 8 to 10 days of age, and a normal abdominal x-ray
   b. Baby has no clinical signs or symptoms but babygram includes an incidental finding of pneumatosis intestinalis
   c. Infant with bilious gastric residual and "free" intraperitoneal air on abdominal x-ray
   d. Infant with dilated loops of bowel on abdominal x-ray, abdominal distension, and nonbilious residuals

ANSWER

1. **c.** "Classic" NEC in a preterm infant includes feeding intolerance, abdominal distension, and bloody stools after 8 to 10 days of age, but these signs are not adequate to make the diagnosis of the disease. Pathognomonic findings on abdominal radiography are pneumatosis

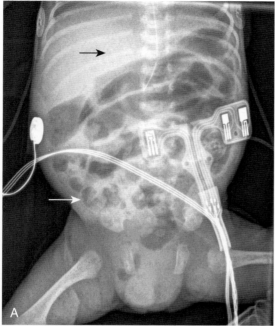

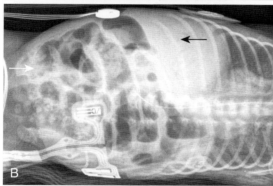

FIGURE 22-1 ■ **Neonate with NEC. A,** Supine radiograph obtained at presentation shows generalized bowel dilatation with gas, intramural gas (*white arrow*), and portal venous gas (*black arrow*). **B,** Left lateral decubitus radiograph obtained at presentation shows generalized bowel dilatation with gas, intramural gas (*white arrow*), and portal venous gas (*black arrow*).

intestinalis, portal venous gas, or both. Early imaging signs that raise suspicion for NEC include dilated loops of bowel, paucity of gas, and gas-filled loops of bowel that do not change with repeated radiographs. Establishing the diagnosis is difficult because of the lack of universally reliable diagnostic criteria. Two systems have been developed to assist in the diagnosis of NEC: Bell's Staging Criteria (modified) and the criteria published by the Vermont Oxford Network *Manual of Operations*. Both systems have strengths and weaknesses. We recommend the use of the terms "medical" and "surgical NEC" and that the term "Stage 1 NEC"

from Bell's Staging Criteria no longer be used because it does not indicate a definable pathologic entity. The baby in this case has medical NEC, but needs to undergo interventions (see treatment strategies section) and be followed closely because of the potential progression to surgical NEC.

CASE STUDY 1 (continued)

Over the next several days, despite broad-spectrum antibiotics, the baby's condition worsened, requiring intubation, mechanical ventilation, and packed red blood cells to correct hypovolemia and anemia. The baby eventually stabilized over several hours and was managed medically, without surgical intervention. A blood culture obtained at the time of the bilious residual grew Enterobacter cloacae. After a week of total parenteral nutrition, enteral feedings were restarted and advanced slowly. Once full feeding volume was achieved, the baby developed feeding intolerance manifested by increased gastric residuals and abdominal distension. She was otherwise asymptomatic.

EXERCISE 2

QUESTION

1. This recent feeding intolerance can represent what complication of NEC?
   a. Recurrent NEC
   b. Stricture formation
   c. Gastroesophageal reflux
   d. Lactose intolerance

ANSWER

1. **b.** The feeding intolerance is suggestive of stricture formation. Less common signs include the persistence of blood in the stool and recurrent episodes of bacteremia.

CLINICAL PRESENTATION OF NEC

The gestational age of an infant is inversely related to the prevalence rate of NEC. The smallest and most premature infants are at greatest risk (Lin & Stoll, 2006). Premature infants also tend to get NEC later compared to full-term infants. The more premature the infant, the later this condition occurs after birth (Neu, 2005b).

Several different entities are termed "NEC" and this includes term babies who may have ischemic bowel disease, infants with bovine protein intolerance, and infants with spontaneous intestinal perforations, all of which have different etiologies. The heterogeneity of these entities

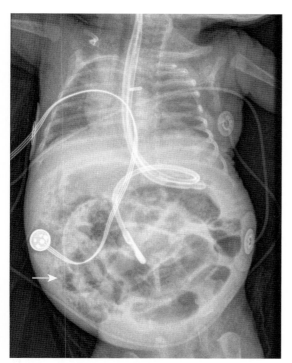

FIGURE 22-2 ■ Supine radiograph of the abdomen obtained in a neonate with NEC. The bowel is dilated with gas. The bubbly pattern of gas seen mainly in the right lower quadrant represents intramural gas (*white arrow*).

has led to confusion and has not been helpful in finding the cause and subsequent treatment of the most common form of this disease. "Classic" NEC in a preterm infant includes feeding intolerance, abdominal distension, and bloody stools usually after 8 to 10 days of age, but these signs are not adequate to make the diagnosis of the disease. Pathognomonic findings on abdominal radiography are pneumatosis intestinalis, portal venous gas, or both (Figures 22-1, *A*; 22-1, *B*; and 22-2). Early imaging signs that raise suspicion for NEC include dilated loops of bowel, paucity of gas, and gas-filled loops of bowel that do not change with repeated radiographs. However, "free air" outside the bowel signifies advanced NEC. Within hours, symptoms rapidly progress from subtle signs to abdominal discoloration, intestinal perforation, and peritonitis, leading to shock (Neu & Walker, 2011).

Establishing the diagnosis is difficult because of the lack of universally reliable diagnostic criteria. Bell and colleagues first described a staging system in 1978, a systematic description of NEC that was subsequently modified (Bell et al., 1978; Walsh & Kliegman, 1986). Bell's staging system includes three stages. Stage 1 criteria are nonspecific findings that include feeding intolerance, mild abdominal distension, or both. Stage 2 criteria include radiographic findings of pneumatosis intestinalis. Stage 3 criteria include a perforated viscus that may or may not be associated with intestinal necrosis, thus making the distinction with spontaneous intestinal perforation difficult, unless necrosis is directly visualized by the surgeon or evaluated histologically.

Another classification system that defines NEC more specifically is published in the Vermont Oxford Network *Manual of Operations* (Rees et al., 2010). This manual describes clinical and radiographic findings. To establish the diagnosis, it is required to have one or more findings from each type (clinical and radiographic). The clinical findings include bilious gastric aspirate or emesis, abdominal distension, and occult gross blood in the stool. The imaging findings include pneumatosis intestinalis, hepatobiliary gas, and pneumoperitoneum. However, severe NEC that requires surgery can develop without radiographic evidence of pneumatosis intestinalis or portal venous gas (Epelman et al., 2007). We recommend that use of the terms "medical" and "surgical NEC" are adequate and the term "Stage 1 NEC" no longer be used because it does not indicate a definable pathologic entity. Medical NEC is diagnosed with definitive findings radiographically or by ultrasound (pneumatosis intestinalis or portal venous gas) and surgical NEC is diagnosed at the time of surgery by direct visualization of necrotic bowel or histologic confirmation if the bowel is not obviously necrotic to the surgeon.

LABORATORY FEATURES

Laboratory tests are used to aid in the diagnosis, but are nonspecific to NEC. These laboratory features include leukopenia, thrombocytopenia, hyponatremia, hypokalemia, increased C-reactive protein levels, metabolic acidosis, disseminated intravascular coagulopathy (DIC), and glucose instability. They may be helpful in determining progression of severity of the disease.

Urinary markers such as intestinal fatty acid binding protein (I-FABP) and claudin-3 (indicating loss of integrity of intestinal barrier) and the fecal marker calprotectin (representing intestinal inflammation) are high in neonates suspected to have NEC who later develop the disease. Of the three markers, only I-FABP is related to disease severity. However, screening for NEC before clinical signs develop is not useful because I-FABP is not elevated before a clinical suspicion exists (Thuijls et al., 2010).

OTHER DETECTION TECHNOLOGIES

Plain abdominal radiographs are the current standard for confirming the diagnosis of NEC. However, it usually reflects a late finding of the disease. Because of the fulminant nature of NEC, any delay in the diagnosis prevents early intervention. There is a need for new, safe detection methods that are both sensitive and specific to early signs of NEC. Abdominal ultrasonography is showing promise in early detection of NEC by being able to depict intraabdominal fluid, bowel wall thickness, and bowel wall perfusion. However, state-of-the-art equipment and an experienced sonographer who masters the meticulous technique are essential (Bohnhorst et al., 2010; Dilli et al., 2010; Epelman et al., 2007).

CASE STUDY 2

Baby girl CJ (birth weight 1110 grams) is a twin born at 31 weeks' gestation to a 29-year-old mother whose pregnancy was complicated by severe discordance due to twin-to-twin transfusion. Baby girl CJ is the donor twin. A cesarean section was performed because of the growth discordance. Apgar scores were 5 and 9 at 1 and 5 minutes of life, respectively. The baby initially required nasal CPAP of 6 cm H_2O and an FiO_2 of 0.3. Overnight, she was weaned off CPAP to room air. Breast milk feedings were started on Day 2 of life at a volume of 10 mL/kg/day, divided every 3 hours. On Day 3 of life, the baby was noted to have a small bilious gastric residual with a slight increase in abdominal girth of 1 cm. She was also noted to have hyperglycemia. The abdominal radiograph showed intraperitoneal air.

EXERCISE 3

QUESTION

1. What is the most likely diagnosis?
   a. Spontaneous intestinal perforation
   b. NEC
   c. Meconium peritonitis
   d. Barotrauma

ANSWER

1. **a.** Spontaneous intestinal perforation usually occurs in the first few days of life. The majority of patients who develop this type of perforation have never been enterally fed or have received only minimal feedings. In addition, coadministration of indomethacin and glucocorticoids significantly increases the risk (Attridge et al., 2006a; Stark et al., 2001; Watterberg et al., 2004). The exact cause of spontaneous intestinal perforation is still

unclear, but the prognosis for affected neonates is usually good when they are diagnosed and treated early.

CASE STUDY 2 (continued)

Baby CJ was taken to the operating room where she was found to have an ileal perforation. An enterostomy was performed and CJ was reanastomosed 1 month later.

DIFFERENTIAL DIAGNOSIS

NEC is characterized by intestinal inflammation and its endpoint is ischemic necrosis, systemic inflammatory response syndrome (SIRS), and multiorgan system failure (Sharma et al., 2007). This excessive inflammatory process is initiated in the intestine, which is highly immunoreactive, and extends systemically, affecting distant organs like the brain, increasing the affected infant's risk of neurodevelopmental delays (Hintz et al., 2005; Salhab et al., 2004).

Spontaneous intestinal perforation represents a different disease entity with a different pathogenesis. It usually occurs in the first few days after birth and is not associated with enteral feedings (Attridge et al., 2006b; Stark et al., 2001). However, spontaneous intestinal perforation has been associated with the combined administration of indomethacin and glucocorticoids (Attridge et al., 2006a; Stark et al., 2001; Watterberg et al., 2004). Only minimal intestinal inflammation and necrosis are present with low levels of serum inflammatory cytokines. The exact cause of spontaneous intestinal perforation is still unclear, but it has been suggested that it is most likely due to a thromboembolic or ischemic phenomenon (Sharma et al., 2010).

CASE STUDY 3

Baby boy AR (birth weight 1800 grams) was born at 31 weeks by emergent cesarean section because of maternal vaginal bleeding and placental abruption. The mother had a positive cervical culture for group B Streptococcus and received perioperative antibiotics. Apgar scores were 6 and 8 at 1 and 5 minutes of life, respectively. He was placed on CPAP and his respiratory symptoms resolved after several hours. Enteral feedings were started on Day 2 of life using premature 24 kcal formula at 20 mL/kg/day divided every 3 hours. Feeds were advanced by 20 mL/kg/day daily as tolerated. On Day 5 of life, he had an episode of bradycardia and a 35 mL bilious gastric residual. His vital signs consisted of tachycardia and blood pressure of 29/14 with a capillary refill of 4 seconds. On physical exam, he was grayish appearing with cool extremities. His abdomen was distended, tender to palpation, with absent bowel sounds. The baby was grunting with labored respirations, becoming increasingly cyanotic despite an FiO_2 of 0.9.

EXERCISE 4

QUESTION

1. Which of the following next steps should receive the highest priority?
   a. Order a complete blood count, c-reactive protein, blood cultures, and arterial blood gas.
   b. Obtain an abdominal x-ray.
   c. Consult surgery.
   d. Perform endotracheal intubation and ventilation, administer a bolus of normal saline, and place a nasogastric tube to low-intermittent suction.

ANSWER

1. **d.** This infant is unstable and needs to be resuscitated. He is in shock and exhibiting signs of respiratory failure. A bolus of normal saline must be administered to support blood pressure and intubation should be performed for respiratory failure. A nasogastric tube should then be placed to low-intermittent suction to decompress the bowel and enhance perfusion of the bowel wall (by decreasing bowel wall tension) and to permit more effective ventilation (by decreasing intraabdominal pressure). The surgical team also needs to be notified as soon as possible after this initial stabilization.

CASE STUDY 3 (continued)

The abdominal x-ray demonstrated pneumatosis intestinalis (Figure 22-2).

EXERCISE 5

QUESTION

1. After blood cultures are obtained and NEC is suspected, what are the antibiotics of choice?
   a. Ampicillin and gentamicin
   b. Ampicillin, gentamicin, and metronidazole
   c. Vancomycin and gentamicin
   d. Vancomycin, gentamicin, and metronidazole

ANSWER

1. **a.** The authors recommend starting ampicillin and gentamicin although some clinicians replace ampicillin with vancomycin if *Staphylococcus epidermidis* is suspected. If the baby continues to worsen while on ampicillin and gentamicin or there are clear signs of peritonitis, clindamycin or metronidazole should be started to improve the coverage for anaerobic organisms.

CASE STUDY 3 (continued)

Two hours later, Baby boy AR is taken to the operating room because "free air" is seen on the abdominal x-ray (Figure 22-3). He now has a diagnosis of NEC with small bowel necrosis. A third of his small bowel is resected owing to necrosis.

EXERCISE 6

QUESTION

1. What is the major cause of significant long-term morbidity in babies who have intestinal resection for NEC?
   a. Spontaneous intestinal perforation
   b. Stricture formation
   c. Short bowel syndrome
   d. Intestinal adhesions

ANSWER

1. **c.** NEC that requires bowel resection may result in short bowel syndrome. This syndrome results in a decreased ability to absorb nutrients that are necessary for growth. For a neonate to survive on enteral nutrition, the remaining small bowel needs to undergo intestinal adaptation, a process by which the remaining intestine increases its ability to absorb nutrients (Matarese & Steiger, 2006). The presence of the ileocecal valve and the length of the remaining small bowel determine the potential of the small bowel to adapt. Adaptation can occur with a small bowel length as short as 11 cm if the ileocecal valve

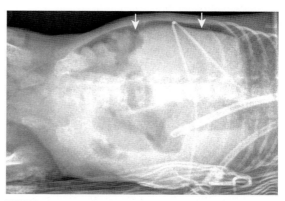

FIGURE 22-3 ■ **Left lateral decubitus radiograph of the abdomen obtained in a neonate with NEC.** Free intraperitoneal gas is present (*arrows*).

is intact. Without the ileocecal valve, adaptation can occur with a small bowel length of 15 cm (Quiros-Tejeira et al., 2004; Vargas et al., 1987). However, absence of the ileocecal valve is associated with longer duration of parenteral nutrition (Chaet et al., 1994; Goulet et al., 1991).

CURRENT TREATMENT STRATEGIES

Once NEC is diagnosed, medical or surgical management may be required based on the clinical presentation (Table 22-1). Medical intervention includes abdominal decompression, bowel rest, broad-spectrum intravenous antibiotics, and intravenous hyperalimentation. Surgical intervention is generally required in patients with intestinal perforation or deteriorating clinical or biochemical status. Of note, persistent acidosis, continued deterioration of platelet and white blood cell counts, and fixed bowel loops suggest intestinal necrosis and dead bowel (Neu, 2012). Surgical procedures involve either a drain

placement or exploratory laparotomy with resection of diseased bowel, and enterostomy with creation of a stoma. Great controversy exists whether exploratory laparotomy is preferable to peritoneal drain placement (Moss et al., 2006) but evidence suggests that laparotomy is preferred if clinical and imaging data suggest intestinal necrosis (Rees et al., 2010; Sharma et al., 2004).

CASE STUDY 4

Baby boy EG (birth weight 755 grams) was born at 25 weeks' gestation to a 25-year-old mother with preterm premature rupture of membranes for 10 days and a positive cervical culture for group B Streptococcus. Apgar scores were 1, 1, and 6 at 1, 5, and 10 minutes of life, respectively. He was intubated endotracheally during the resuscitation and received surfactant, broad-spectrum antibiotics, and indomethacin for prophylaxis against intraventricular hemorrhage. Over the next several days, his condition improved, and on Day 4 of life enteral feedings were started with a volume less than

---

TABLE 22-1 Diagnostic Criteria and Treatment of Necrotizing Enterocolitis

Diagnosis and Signs and Symptoms	Treatment Strategy
Suspected Necrotizing Enterocolitis	
Abdominal distention without radiographic evidence of pneumatosis intestinalis, portal venous gas, or free intraperitoneal air	Close clinical observation for increased abdominal distention and feeding intolerance
Unexpected onset of feeding intolerance	Consideration of bowel decompression and brief discontinuation of feeding (e.g., 24 hr); abdominal radiograph (anteroposterior and left lateral decubitus); monitoring of white-cell, differential, and platelet counts (sudden decreases suggest progression of disease); consideration of blood cultures and short course of intravenous antibiotics
Definitive Medical Necrotizing Enterocolitis	
Abdominal distention with pneumatosis intestinalis, portal venous gas, or both	Bowel decompression and discontinuation of enteral feedings for approximately 7-10 days
Other radiographic signs such as fixed, dilated loops of intestine and ileus patterns are not pathognomonic but should be treated as such	Close monitoring of white-cell, differential, and platelet counts (sudden decreases suggest progression of disease); blood culture and intravenous antibiotics for 7-10 days; close monitoring of abdominal radiographs (anteroposterior and left lateral decubitus); notification of surgical team
Surgical Necrotizing Enterocolitis	
Free intraperitoneal air on abdominal radiograph after initial medical signs and symptoms	Exploratory laparotomy with resection if necessary
Persistent ileus pattern, abdominal distention, and radiographs that show an absence of bowel gas, coupled with deteriorating clinical and laboratory values (e.g., decreasing neutrophil and platelet counts)	Placement of drain

From Neu J, Walker WA: Necrotizing enterocolitis, N Engl J Med 364(3):255-264, 2011; adapted from Bell MJ, Ternberg JL, Feigin RD, et al.: Neonatal necrotizing enterocolitis. therapeutic decisions based upon clinical staging, Ann Surg 187(1):1-7, 1978; and Walsh MC, Kliegman RM: Necrotizing enterocolitis: treatment based on staging criteria, Pediatr Clin North Am 33(1):179-201, 1986.

10 mL/kg/day, divided every 3 hours. He tolerated feeds well until Day 7 of life, when he was noted to have abdominal distension, and a bilious gastric residual. Physical examination revealed a heart rate of 150 beats per minute, a blood pressure of 52/38 mmHg, and marked abdominal distension. Ventilator settings included a rate of 10, PIP of 12, PEEP of 4, and FiO$_2$ of 0.3. Laboratory studies revealed an elevated white blood cell (WBC) count of 22,800 (70% mature neutrophils, 1% band forms), a platelet count of 265,000, and a hematocrit of 32%.

EXERCISE 7

QUESTION

1. Which of the following risk factors is associated with an increased risk of "classic NEC" in premature babies?
   a. Low Apgar scores
   b. Abnormal microbial intestinal colonization
   c. Enteral feeds during indomethacin administration
   d. Umbilical artery catheterization

ANSWER

1. **b.** The predisposing factors associated with "classic NEC" in premature babies include genetics, intestinal immaturity, imbalanced microvascular tone, abnormal microbial intestinal colonization, and a highly dysregulated immunoreactive intestinal mucosa. In premature babies, low Apgar scores, indomethacin administration, minimal enteral feedings, episodes of apnea or bradycardia, and umbilical artery catheterization do not increase the risk for NEC (Moss et al., 2008; Neu 2005a; C.M. Young et al., 2011).

CASE STUDY 4 (continued)

The abdominal x-ray shows dilated loops of bowel without intramural air or "free" air.

EXERCISE 8

QUESTION

1. What should be the management plan for this patient?
   a. Obtain a surgical consultation.
   b. Resume feedings and perform serial physical examinations.
   c. Perform serial physical examinations, serial abdominal radiographs, and serial laboratory studies.
   d. Perform serial physical examinations and serial abdominal radiographs and start empiric antibiotics

ANSWER

1. **c.** This patient needs to be monitored for progression of the disease, shock, and intestinal perforation. The best way to do this is by frequent serial physical examinations, serial abdominal radiographs (left lateral decubitus) every 6 to 8 hours, and laboratory studies to observe for signs of worsening thrombocytopenia, a decreased WBC count, or worsening metabolic acidosis.

CASE STUDY 4 (continued)

Baby boy EG did not have any evidence of pneumatosis intestinalis on the initial abdominal decubitus x-ray. In addition, two follow up films were read as normal. However, he eventually developed "free" air on a subsequent x-ray.

The lack of pneumatosis intestinalis on the initial and follow-up x-rays suggests the likelihood of a disease process other than NEC. In the operating room, the baby was found to have a malrotation with midgut volvulus and perforation of the dilated proximal bowel loop. Malrotation with midgut volvulus is a less common cause of intestinal perforation but it is a surgical emergency. In addition to signs of bowel obstruction, these babies can present with pneumatosis intestinalis and bloody stools secondary to vascular compromise of the bowel. This case illustrates how essential it is for the clinician to be vigilant of other pathologic states that initially can mimic NEC.

PATHOGENESIS

The pathogenesis of "classical" NEC is not entirely understood; however, epidemiologic observations suggest a multifactorial etiology (Lin & Stoll, 2006; Neu & Walker, 2011). Predisposing factors include genetics, intestinal immaturity, imbalanced microvascular tone, abnormal microbial intestinal colonization, and a highly dysregulated immunoreactive intestinal mucosa (Neu, 2012).

Intestinal Immaturity

The preterm infant is predisposed to intestinal injury because of dysmotility, immaturity of digestion, absorption, immune defenses, barrier function, and circulatory regulation (Martin & Walker, 2006; Nanthakumar et al., 2000; Neu, 2007). Gastric acid secretion is decreased in the preterm infant and has been associated with a greater occurrence of NEC, especially in babies whose gastric acid secretion is further limited by histamine-2 blocker administration (Guillet et al., 2006).

TABLE 22-2   Measures to Prevent Necrotizing Enterocolitis

Evidence of Efficacy and Safety	Evidence of Efficacy but Questionable Safety	Evidence of Efficacy in Animal Models but Not in Humans	Proposed Efficacy but Lacking Evidence
Breast milk feeding	Enteral aminoglycosides	Anticytokines	Prebiotics (derived from plants and breast milk)
Nonaggressive enteral feeding	Probiotics	Growth factors	Microbial components and toll-like-receptor agonists
	Glucocorticoids		Glutamine, n-3 fatty acids
	Arginine		

From Neu J, Walker WA: Necrotizing enterocolitis, N Engl J Med *364(3):255-264, 2011; adapted from Neu J: Neonatal necrotizing enterocolitis: an update,* Acta Paediatr Suppl *94(449):100-105, 2005; and Grave GD, Nelson SA, Walker WA, et al.: New therapies and preventive approaches for necrotizing enterocolitis: report of a research planning workshop,* Pediatr Res *62(4):510-514, 2007.*

Preterm infants have an exaggerated inflammatory response to luminal microbes. This excessive inflammatory response alters the protective barrier of the intestine. After initial postnatal microbial colonization, the human intestine may be able to adapt to the increased microbial stimulation by increasing the expression of toll-like receptor 4 (TLR-4) (Fusunyan et al., 2001). TLR-4 is a key receptor for gram-negative organisms. However, an important regulatory factor (IκB) for the transcription factor nuclear factor κB (NF-κB), which modulates inflammation, is underexpressed (Afrazi et al., 2010; Claud et al., 2004). This leads to an excessive and inappropriate inflammatory response that leads to intestinal injury and NEC (Martin & Walker, 2006). In addition, high serum levels of several cytokines and chemokines that recruit inflammatory cells have been reported in patients with NEC (Markel et al., 2006; Sharma et al., 2007). One of these cytokines, interleukin-8, is produced by epithelial cells and mediates the migration of neutrophils to the inflammatory site (Markel et al., 2006). The activation of these neutrophils can cause necrosis and increased production of acute-phase proteins in the gut (Mukaida, 2000).

Microbial Colonization

Inappropriate postnatal microbial colonization in preterm infants is thought to be an important risk factor for NEC (Claud & Walker, 2001; Morowitz et al., 2010). In support of this hypothesis is the observation that NEC does not occur until at least 8 to 10 days after birth, several days after anaerobic bacteria have colonized the intestinal tract. Furthermore, germ-free animals do not develop NEC (Morowitz et al., 2010; Schwiertz et al., 2003) and infants with NEC frequently have concomitant bacteremia and endotoxemia (Schwiertz et al., 2003). However, no specific organism has been implicated

consistently. Studies suggest an association between NEC, unusual intestinal microbial species, and less diverse microbiota, especially when a history of previous prolonged antibiotic therapy exists. New non–culture-based technologies being used in studies of NEC should help us determine the precise nature of this dysbiosis (Alexander et al., 2011; Cotten et al., 2009; Mai et al., 2011; Mshvildadze et al., 2010; Wang et al., 2009).

Hypoxia-Ischemia

Prospective and epidemiologic studies do not support that perinatal hypoxic-ischemic events—including low Apgar scores, episodes of apnea or bradycardia, umbilical artery catheterization, enteral feedings, and indomethacin—increase the risk of NEC (Moss et al., 2008; Neu 2005a; C.M. Young et al., 2011). In fact, premature infants generally do not develop NEC until their second week of life, making it very unlikely that perinatal hypoxic-ischemic events have any role in NEC 2 weeks after birth.

PREVENTATIVE APPROACHES

Many approaches have been proposed for the prevention of NEC, including the withholding of enteral feedings, using enteral antibiotics, feeding maternal breast milk (Sullivan et al., 2009), administering probiotic and/or prebiotic agents, and administering growth factors, anticytokine agents, and glucocorticoids (Table 22-2).

The concept of withholding enteral feedings comes from clinical experience and retrospective reviews that suggest an increased risk of NEC when feedings are rapidly increased (Anderson & Kliegman, 1991; Berseth et al., 2003). However, recent data suggest that withholding enteral feedings may be dangerous because it leads to intestinal atrophy, increased gut permeability and inflammation, prolonged use of intravenous hyperalimentation, and increased late-onset sepsis (Moss et al., 2008). A safer approach is to initiate low-volume feedings that are appropriate for gestational age and increase them gradually. This approach to feeding would not be contraindicated while the infant is on ventilator support, using umbilical catheters, or receiving indomethacin or dopamine (Neu & Zhang, 2005).

Infection control measures are essential for preventing the spread of NEC in the NICU. Some small studies have used oral aminoglycosides as prophylaxis against outbreaks; however, the concern for the emergence of resistant organisms prohibits prophylactic use of antibiotics (Egan et al., 1976; Grylack & Scanlon, 1978). In fact, recent studies suggest that prolonged use of empiric antibiotics results in an increase in the incidence of NEC (Cotten et al., 2009).

Probiotic Agents

Although several trials suggest that probiotics may decrease the incidence of NEC (Bin-Nun et al., 2005; Dani et al., 2002; Deshpande et al., 2010; Lin et al., 2005), probiotics have not been shown to decrease NEC-related mortality definitively and may increase the incidence of sepsis in infants with birth weights less than 750 grams (Lin et al., 2008). It would be wise to exert caution in the use of probiotics in preterm infants (Neu, 2011), especially because no evidence exists in support of such use from any large, adequately powered, prospective, single-protocol, randomized, double-blind trial.

Prebiotic Agents

Prebiotics are nutrients that enhance the growth of potentially beneficial intestinal microbes (Gibson, 1998). These nutrients include the oligosaccharides inulin, galactose, fructose, lactulose, and their combinations (Sherman et al., 2009). These compounds appear to alter the consistency and frequency of stools, but it is unclear how efficacious they are at preventing NEC. Prebiotics enhance the proliferation of gut flora like bifidobacteria, but these compounds require an appropriately colonized gut (lacking in very low birth weight premature infants) (Moro et al., 2002).

Microbial Components that Modulate Inflammation

Dead microbes may be as effective as live microbes in modulating excessive inflammatory stimuli (Li et al., 2009; Lopez et al., 2008; Zhang et al., 2005; Zhang et al., 2006). In fact, one study in preterm infants showed a decreased incidence of NEC when inactivated probiotics were administered (Awad et al., 2010).

FUTURE DIRECTIONS

Because of the fulminant nature of NEC, preventative approaches—rather than new treatment strategies—are more likely to provide a reduction of NEC-associated mortality and morbidity. Effective preventative strategies will depend on the use of clear diagnostic criteria that are used consistently to differentiate NEC from other entities like spontaneous intestinal perforation and intestinal injury in term infants. To help establish and apply these diagnostic criteria, it is necessary to develop highly sensitive and specific biomarkers (Young et al., 2009) and new monitoring technologies aimed at detecting factors that identify an infant at increased risk (Oh et al., 2010).

SUGGESTED READINGS

Afrazi A, Sodhi CP, Richardson W, et al.: New insights into the pathogenesis and treatment of necrotizing enterocolitis: toll-like receptors and beyond, *Pediatr Res* 69(3):183–188, 2010.

Alexander VN, Northrup V, Bizzarro MJ: Antibiotic exposure in the newborn intensive care unit and the risk of necrotizing enterocolitis, *J Pediatr* 159(3):392–397, 2011.

Anderson DM, Kliegman RM: The relationship of neonatal alimentation practices to the occurrence of endemic necrotizing enterocolitis, *Am J Perinatol* 8(1):62–67, 1991.

Attridge JT, Clark R, Walker MW, et al.: New insights into spontaneous intestinal perforation using a national data set: (1) SIP is associated with early indomethacin exposure, *J Perinatol* 26(2):93–99, 2006a.

Attridge JT, Clark R, Walker MW, et al.: New insights into spontaneous intestinal perforation using a national data set: (2) two populations of patients with perforations, *J Perinatol* 26(3):185–188, 2006b.

Awad H, Mokhtar H, Imam SS, et al.: Comparison between killed and living probiotic usage versus placebo for the prevention of necrotizing enterocolitis and sepsis in neonates, *Pak J Biol Sci* 13(6):253–262, 2010.

Bell MJ, Ternberg JL, Feigin RD, et al.: Neonatal necrotizing enterocolitis. Therapeutic decisions based upon clinical staging, *Ann Surg* 187(1):1–7, 1978.

Berseth CL, Bisquera JA, Paje VU: Prolonging small feeding volumes early in life decreases the incidence of necrotizing enterocolitis in very low birth weight infants, *Pediatrics* 111(3):529–534, 2003.

Bin-Nun A, Bromiker R, Wilschanski M, et al.: Oral probiotics prevent necrotizing enterocolitis in very low birth weight neonates, *J Pediatr* 147(2):192–196, 2005.

Bohnhorst B, Kuebler JF, Rau G, et al.: Portal venous gas detected by ultrasound differentiates surgical NEC from other acquired neonatal intestinal diseases, *Eur J Pediatr Surg* 21(1):12–17, 2010.

Chaet MS, Farrell MK, Ziegler MM, et al.: Intensive nutritional support and remedial surgical intervention for extreme short bowel syndrome, *J Pediatr Gastroenterol Nutr* 19(3):295–298, 1994.

Claud EC, Lu L, Anton PM, et al.: Developmentally regulated IkappaB expression in intestinal epithelium and susceptibility to flagellin-induced inflammation, *Proc Natl Acad Sci U S A* 101(19):7404–7408, 2004.

Claud EC, Walker WA: Hypothesis: inappropriate colonization of the premature intestine can cause neonatal necrotizing enterocolitis, *FASEB J* 15(8):1398–1403, 2001.

Cotten CM, Taylor S, Stoll B, et al.: Prolonged duration of initial empirical antibiotic treatment is associated with increased rates of necrotizing enterocolitis and death for extremely low birth weight infants, *Pediatrics* 123(1):58–66, 2009.

Dani C, Biadaioli R, Bertini G, et al.: Probiotics feeding in prevention of urinary tract infection, bacterial sepsis and necrotizing enterocolitis in preterm infants. A prospective double-blind study, *Biol Neonate* 82(2):103–108, 2002.

Deshpande G, Rao S, Patole S, et al.: Updated meta-analysis of probiotics for preventing necrotizing enterocolitis in preterm neonates, *Pediatrics* 125(5):921–930, 2010.

Dilli D, Suna Oguz S, Erol R, et al.: Does abdominal sonography provide additional information over abdominal plain radiography for diagnosis of necrotizing enterocolitis in neonates? *Pediatr Surg Int* 27(3):321–327, 2010.

Egan EA, Mantilla G, Nelson RM, et al.: A prospective controlled trial of oral kanamycin in the prevention of neonatal necrotizing enterocolitis, *J Pediatr* 89(3):467–470, 1976.

Epelman M, Daneman A, Navarro OM, et al.: Necrotizing enterocolitis: review of state-of-the-art imaging findings with pathologic correlation, *Radiographics* 27(2):285–305, 2007.

Erasmus HD, Ludwig-Auser HM, Paterson PG, et al.: Enhanced weight gain in preterm infants receiving lactase-treated feeds: a randomized, double-blind, controlled trial, *J Pediatr* 141(4):532–537, 2002.

Fitzgibbons SC, Ching Y, Yu D, et al.: Mortality of necrotizing enterocolitis expressed by birth weight categories, *J Pediatr Surg* 44(6):1072–1075, 2009. discussion 1075–1076.

Fusunyan RD, Nanthakumar NN, Baldeon ME, et al.: Evidence for an innate immune response in the immature human intestine: toll-like receptors on fetal enterocytes, *Pediatr Res* 49(4):589–593, 2001.

Gibson GR: Dietary modulation of the human gut microflora using prebiotics, *Br J Nutr* 80(4):S209–S212, 1998.

Goulet OJ, Revillon Y, Jan D, et al.: Neonatal short bowel syndrome, *J Pediatr* 119(1, pt 1):18–23, 1991.

Grave GD, Nelson SA, Walker WA, et al.: New therapies and preventive approaches for necrotizing enterocolitis: report of a research planning workshop, *Pediatr Res* 62(4):510–514, 2007.

Grylack LJ, Scanlon JW: Oral gentamicin therapy in the prevention of neonatal necrotizing enterocolitis. A controlled double-blind trial, *Am J Dis Child* 132(12):1192–1194, 1978.

Guillet R, Stoll BJ, Cotten CM, et al.: Association of H2-blocker therapy and higher incidence of necrotizing enterocolitis in very low birth weight infants, *Pediatrics* 117(2):e137–e142, 2006.

Hintz SR, Kendrick DE, Stoll BJ, et al.: Neurodevelopmental and growth outcomes of extremely low birth weight infants after necrotizing enterocolitis, *Pediatrics* 115(3):696–703, 2005.

Holman RC, Stoll BJ, Curns AT, et al.: Necrotising enterocolitis hospitalisations among neonates in the United States, *Paediatr Perinat Epidemiol* 20(6):498–506, 2006.

Horbar JD, Badger GJ, Carpenter JH, et al.: Trends in mortality and morbidity for very low birth weight infants, 1991-1999, *Pediatrics* 110(1, pt 1):143–151, 2002.

Li N, Russell WM, Douglas-Escobar M, et al.: Live and heat-killed Lactobacillus rhamnosus GG: effects on proinflammatory and anti-inflammatory cytokines/chemokines in gastrostomy-fed infant rats, *Pediatr Res* 66(2):203–207, 2009.

Lin HC, Hsu CH, Chen HL, et al.: Oral probiotics prevent necrotizing enterocolitis in very low birth weight preterm infants: a multicenter, randomized, controlled trial, *Pediatrics* 122(4):693–700, 2008.

Lin HC, Su BH, Chen AC, et al.: Oral probiotics reduce the incidence and severity of necrotizing enterocolitis in very low birth weight infants, *Pediatrics* 115(1):1–4, 2005.

Lin PW, Stoll BJ: Necrotising enterocolitis, *Lancet* 368(9543):1271–1283, 2006.

Lopez M, Li N, Kataria J, et al.: Live and ultraviolet-inactivated Lactobacillus rhamnosus GG decrease flagellin-induced interleukin-8 production in Caco-2 cells, *J Nutr* 138(11):2264–2268, 2008.

Mai V, Young CM, Ukhanova M, et al.: Fecal microbiota in premature infants prior to necrotizing enterocolitis, *PLoS One* 6(6):e20647, 2011.

Markel TA, Crisostomo PR, Wairiuko GM, et al.: Cytokines in necrotizing enterocolitis, *Shock* 25(4):329–337, 2006.

Martin CR, Walker WA: Intestinal immune defences and the inflammatory response in necrotising enterocolitis, *Semin Fetal Neonatal Med* 11(5):369–377, 2006.

Matarese LE, Steiger E: Dietary and medical management of short bowel syndrome in adult patients, *J Clin Gastroenterol* 40(Suppl 2):S85–S93, 2006.

Moro G, Minoli I, Mosca M, et al.: Dosage-related bifidogenic effects of galacto- and fructooligosaccharides in formula-fed term infants, *J Pediatr Gastroenterol Nutr* 34(3):291–295, 2002.

Morowitz MJ, Poroyko V, Caplan M, et al.: Redefining the role of intestinal microbes in the pathogenesis of necrotizing enterocolitis, *Pediatrics* 125(4):777–785, 2010.

Moss RL, Dimmitt RA, Barnhart DC, et al.: Laparotomy versus peritoneal drainage for necrotizing enterocolitis and perforation, *N Engl J Med* 354(21):2225–2234, 2006.

Moss RL, Kalish LA, Duggan C, et al.: Clinical parameters do not adequately predict outcome in necrotizing enterocolitis: a multi-institutional study, *J Perinatol* 28(10):665–674, 2008.

Mshvildadze M, Neu J, Shuster J, et al.: Intestinal microbial ecology in premature infants assessed with non-culture-based techniques, *J Pediatr* 156(1):20–25, 2010.

Mukaida N: Interleukin-8: an expanding universe beyond neutrophil chemotaxis and activation, *Int J Hematol* 72(4):391–398, 2000.

Nanthakumar NN, Fusunyan RD, Sanderson I, et al.: Inflammation in the developing human intestine: A possible pathophysiologic contribution to necrotizing enterocolitis, *Proc Natl Acad Sci U S A* 97(11):6043–6048, 2000.

Neu J: The 'myth' of asphyxia and hypoxia-ischemia as primary causes of necrotizing enterocolitis, *Biol Neonate* 87(2):97–98, 2005a.

Neu J: Neonatal necrotizing enterocolitis: an update, *Acta Paediatr Suppl* 94(449):100–105, 2005b.

Neu J: Gastrointestinal development and meeting the nutritional needs of premature infants, *Am J Clin Nutr* 85(2):629S–634S, 2007.

Neu J: Routine probiotics for premature infants: let's be careful!, *J Pediatr* 158(4):672–674, 2011.

Neu J, editor: *Gastroenterology and nutrition: neonatology questions and controversies*, ed 2, Philadelphia, PA, 2012, Elsevier.

Neu J, Walker WA: Necrotizing enterocolitis, *N Engl J Med* 364(3):255–264, 2011.

Neu J, Zhang L: Feeding intolerance in very-low-birth-weight infants: what is it and what can we do about it? *Acta Paediatr Suppl* 94(449):93–99, 2005.

Oh S, Young C, Gravenstein N, et al.: Monitoring technologies in the neonatal intensive care unit: implications for the detection of necrotizing enterocolitis, *J Perinatol* 30(11):701–708, 2010.

Quiros-Tejeira RE, Ament ME, Reyen L, et al.: Long-term parenteral nutritional support and intestinal adaptation in children with short bowel syndrome: a 25-year experience, *J Pediatr* 145(2):157–163, 2004.

Rees CM, Eaton S, Khoo AK, et al.: Peritoneal drainage does not stabilize extremely low birth weight infants with perforated bowel: data from the NET Trial, *J Pediatr Surg* 45(2):324–328, 2010, discussion 328–329.

Salhab WA, Perlman JM, Silver L, et al.: Necrotizing enterocolitis and neurodevelopmental outcome in extremely low birth weight infants <1000 g, *J Perinatol* 24(9):534–540, 2004.

Schwiertz A, Gruhl B, Lobnitz M, et al.: Development of the intestinal bacterial composition in hospitalized preterm infants in comparison with breast-fed, full-term infants, *Pediatr Res* 54(3):393–399, 2003.

Sharma R, Hudak ML, Tepas III JJ, et al.: Prenatal or postnatal indomethacin exposure and neonatal gut injury associated with isolated intestinal perforation and necrotizing enterocolitis, *J Perinatol* 30(12):786–793, 2010.

Sharma R, Tepas III JJ, Hudak ML, et al.: Neonatal gut barrier and multiple organ failure: role of endotoxin and proinflammatory cytokines in sepsis and necrotizing enterocolitis, *J Pediatr Surg* 42(3):454–461, 2007.

Sharma R, Tepas III JJ, Mollitt DL, et al.: Surgical management of bowel perforations and outcome in very low-birth-weight infants (< or =1,200 g), *J Pediatr Surg* 39(2):190–194, 2004.

Sherman PM, Cabana M, Gibson GR, et al.: Potential roles and clinical utility of prebiotics in newborns, infants, and children: proceedings from a global prebiotic summit meeting, New York City, June 27-28, 2008 *J Pediatr* 155(5):S61–S70, 2009.

Stark AR, Carlo WA, Tyson JE, et al.: Adverse effects of early dexamethasone in extremely-low-birth-weight infants. National Institute of Child Health and Human Development Neonatal Research Network, *N Engl J Med* 344(2):95–101, 2001.

Stoll BJ, Hansen N, Fanaroff AA, et al.: Late-onset sepsis in very low birth weight neonates: the experience of the NICHD Neonatal Research Network, *Pediatrics* 110(2, pt 1):285–291, 2002.

Sullivan S, Schanler RJ, Kim JH, et al.: An exclusively human milk-based diet is associated with a lower rate of necrotizing enterocolitis than a diet of human milk and bovine milk-based products, *J Pediatr* 156(4):562–567, 2009, e561.

Thuijls G, Derikx JP, van Wijck K, et al.: Non-invasive markers for early diagnosis and determination of the severity of necrotizing enterocolitis, *Ann Surg* 251(6):1174–1180, 2010.

Vargas JH, Ament ME, Berquist WE: Long-term home parenteral nutrition in pediatrics: ten years of experience in 102 patients, *J Pediatr Gastroenterol Nutr* 6(1):24–32, 1987.

Walsh MC, Kliegman RM: Necrotizing enterocolitis: treatment based on staging criteria, *Pediatr Clin North Am* 33(1):179–201, 1986.

Wang Y, Hoenig JD, Malin KJ, et al.: 16S rRNA gene-based analysis of fecal microbiota from preterm infants with and without necrotizing enterocolitis, *ISME J* 3(8):944–954, 2009.

Watterberg KL, Gerdes JS, Cole CH, et al.: Prophylaxis of early adrenal insufficiency to prevent bronchopulmonary dysplasia: a multicenter trial, *Pediatrics* 114(6):1649–1657, 2004.

Young C, Sharma R, Handfield M, et al.: Biomarkers for infants at risk for necrotizing enterocolitis: clues to prevention? *Pediatr Res* 65(5, pt 2):91R–97R, 2009.

Young CM, Kingma SD, Neu J: Ischemia-reperfusion and neonatal intestinal injury, *J Pediatr* 158(Suppl 2):e25–e28, 2011.

Zhang L, Li N, Caicedo R, et al.: Alive and dead Lactobacillus rhamnosus GG decrease tumor necrosis factor-alpha-induced interleukin-8 production in Caco-2 cells, *J Nutr* 135(7):1752–1756, 2005.

Zhang L, Li N, des Robert C, et al.: Lactobacillus rhamnosus GG decreases lipopolysaccharide-induced systemic inflammation in a gastrostomy-fed infant rat model, *J Pediatr Gastroenterol Nutr* 42(5):545–552, 2006.

INDEX

Page numbers followed by *f*, *t*, and *b* indicate figures, tables, and boxes, respectively.